Evidence-Based Neonatal Infections

Website: Evidence-Based Medicine Series

The Evidence-Based Medicine Series has a website at:

www.evidencebasedseries.com

Where you can find:

- Links to companion websites with additional resources and updates for books in the series
- Details of all new and forthcoming titltes
- Links to more Evidence-Based products: including the Cochrane Library, Essential Evidence Plus, and EBM Guidelines.

How to access the companion sites with additional resources and updates:

- Go to the Evidence-Based Series site: **www.evidencebasedseries.com**
- Select your book from the list of titles shown on the site
- If your book has a website with supplementary material, it will show an icon Companion Website next to the title
- Click on the icon to access the website

Evidence-Based Neonatal Infections

David Isaacs
Senior Staff Specialist
Department of Infectious Diseases and Microbiology
The Children's Hospital at Westmead
Sydney, NSW; and
Clinical Professor in Paediatric Infectious Diseases
University of Sydney
Australia

WILEY Blackwell

BMJ|Books

BMJ Books is an imprint of BMJ Publishing Group Limited, used under licence by John Wiley & Sons.

Registered office: John Wiley & Sons, Ltd, The Atrium, Southern Gate, Chichester, West Sussex, PO19 8SQ, UK

Editorial offices: 9600 Garsington Road, Oxford, OX4 2DQ, UK
The Atrium, Southern Gate, Chichester, West Sussex, PO19 8SQ, UK
111 River Street, Hoboken, NJ 07030-5774, USA

For details of our global editorial offices, for customer services and for information about how to apply for permission to reuse the copyright material in this book please see our website at www.wiley.com/wiley-blackwell

Library of Congress Cataloging-in-Publication Data

Isaacs, David, 1950– author.
Evidence-based neonatal infections / David Isaacs.
p. ; cm.
Includes bibliographical references and index.
ISBN 978-0-470-65460-6 (pbk.)
I. Title.
[DNLM: 1. Communicable Diseases–Handbooks. 2. Infant, Newborn, Diseases–therapy–Handbooks.
3. Evidence-Based Medicine–Handbooks. WS 39]
RJ254
618.92′01–dc23

2013026696

A catalogue record for this book is available from the British Library.

Wiley also publishes its books in a variety of electronic formats. Some content that appears in print may not be available in electronic books.

Cover design by Meaden Creative

Set in 9.5/12pt Minion by Aptara Inc., New Delhi, India
Printed and bound in Malaysia by Vivar Printing Sdn Bhd

1 2014

Contents

About the Author

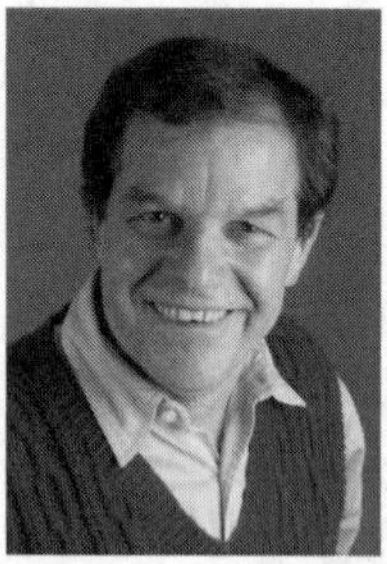

David Isaacs was born in London and has an identical twin brother, Stephen, who is a child psychiatrist. They went to different schools and once swapped schools for a day. His mother was also a child psychiatrist and his father, Alick Isaacs, discovered interferon in 1957. David trained as a general paediatrician in London and Sydney and in paediatric infectious diseases in Oxford. He moved to Sydney in 1989 to head the new Department of Immunology and Infectious Diseases at the Royal Alexandra Hospital for Children, but was the only member of the Department. He is a Clinical Professor in Paediatric Infectious Diseases at the Children's Hospital at Westmead and at the University of Sydney. His research is mainly in neonatal infections, respiratory viral infections, immunization and bioethics. He loves writing and has published extensively, over 300 original peer-reviewed papers and 10 books on paediatric infectious diseases, neonatal infections, immunizations and ethics. This is the third book he has written on neonatal infections, but the first to use a systematic evidence-based approach.

Preface

This book is aimed primarily at clinicians working with neonates, although I hope policymakers will also be interested. It is based on evidence from the literature but also on over 30 years attending neonatal unit ward rounds to learn, advise and teach about neonatal infections.

My special thanks to Dr Phil Britton and Dr David Andresen of the Children's Hospital at Westmead for their extraordinary but characteristic generosity in reading all the chapters and their invariably helpful and incisive advice. I would also like to thank Professor Craig Mellis of the University of Sydney and Professor Ruth Gilbert of the Institute of Child Health in London for help with the chapter on evidence and Associate Professor Ben Marais of the Children's Hospital at Westmead for his help with the section on tuberculosis. I would also like to thank John Yeats and Paul de Sensi from the Children's Hospital at Westmead for help with medical imaging.

I would like to thank my wife Carmel and my children for putting up with me spending long hours researching and writing this book.

Finally, I would like to acknowledge all my colleagues in neonatology who have shared their knowledge and discussed the management of neonatal infections. I dedicate this book to you, the neonatologists at the coal face making the difficult clinical decisions. I hope this book helps a bit.

David Isaacs
University of Sydney

CHAPTER 1
How to search for evidence

1.1 Obstacles to searching for evidence

Clinicians who do not search the literature for evidence quote lack of time[1–5] and lack of knowledge as the main constraints.[6, 7]

In this brief chapter, we will suggest a rapid and easy approach to searching for evidence. For more detail, one journal publication[8] and three books[9–11] can be consulted.

1.2 Sources of evidence

1.2.1 The Cochrane library

The Cochrane Collaboration was established in 1993 and named for the British epidemiologist Archie Cochrane. It is an international non-profit making organization which publishes online evidence about health care in the Cochrane Library including almost 5000 systematic Cochrane Reviews. Cochrane Reviews of treatment interventions are usually restricted to randomized controlled trials (RCTs) because this is the best study design to avoid bias. The Cochrane Library is free in developing countries, in the United Kingdom (where the NHS pays for it) and in Australia (paid for by the Federal Government). In the United States, access requires a subscription, but many libraries and hospitals subscribe so that it is readily available to many clinicians. The Cochrane Library website is http://www.thecochranelibrary.com/.

For the evidence for an intervention, search the Cochrane Library (Figure 1.1) first by typing your topic into the box marked SEARCH THE COCHRANE LIBRARY and clicking on Go. Try different search terms because they will give different information.

1.2.2 Medline and PubMed

PubMed is provided free by the US National Library of Medicine and the National Institutes of Health and gives access to the comprehensive database Medline to anyone with internet access. The website is http://www.pubmed.gov/.

The best approach to find evidence is to use the **Clinical Queries** option in PubMed. Click on Clinical Queries, under PubMed Tools, currently in the centre of the PubMed home page (Figure 1.2), which brings up a new screen (Figure 1.3). Enter your search terms into the Search box and click on SEARCH. PubMed automatically finds RCTs in the first column (set the Category to "therapy" and Scope to "narrow" to find RCTs) and systematic reviews including Cochrane reviews in the middle column (Figure 1.3). Ignore the third column (only used by geneticists). Experiment with search terms until you find the best ways of expanding or narrowing the search to find what you want.

1.3 Statistical terms and explanations

Cluster randomized trial: a trial in which a group of individuals is randomized. For example, whole villages could be randomized to have a study intervention or no intervention, rather than individuals. The village becomes the unit of randomization. Outcomes are compared between those who do and do not receive the intervention.

Confidence Intervals (CI): a way of quantifying measurement uncertainty. This is usually expressed as the 95% CI, which means that the true value will be within the range 95% of the time. If the Relative Risk of dying with treatment compared with placebo is 0.50 (95%

Evidence-Based Neonatal Infections, First Edition. David Isaacs.

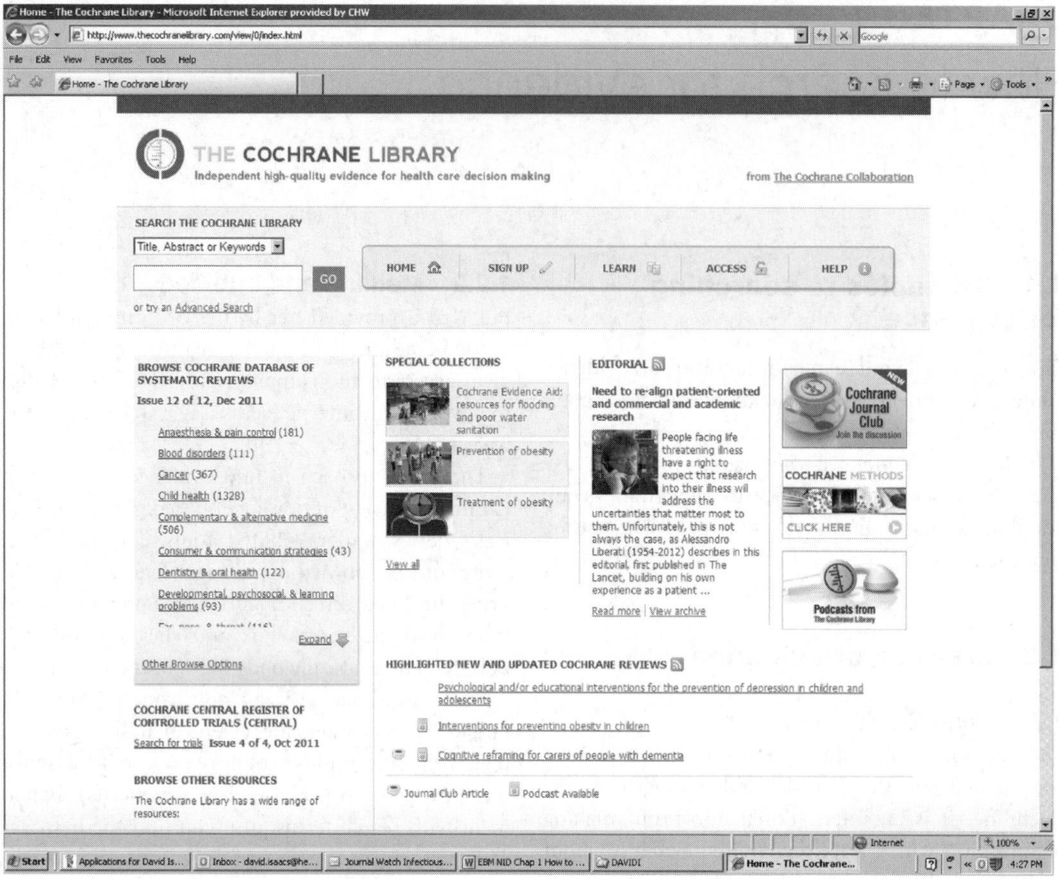

Figure 1.1 The Cochrane Library home page (2013).

CI 0.20–0.75), the treatment reduces the risk of dying by 50%, and 95% of the time it will reduce the risk by somewhere between 20% and 75%.

Negative predictive value (NPV): the proportion of subjects with a negative test result who are correctly diagnosed. The negative predictive value of a test for sepsis is a reflection of the test sensitivity and the incidence of sepsis in the population. The higher the negative predictive value of a test, the safer it is to use a negative test result as a basis to withhold treatment. If a test for sepsis has an NPV of 100%, then no child with sepsis will have a false negative result and all septic children will be identified by the test.

Number Needed to Treat (NNT): the number of patients you need to treat in order to achieve one extra favourable outcome. For example, if 19 of 20 patients treated with antibiotics for an infection get better compared with 14 of 20 treated with placebo, five extra patients get better for every 20 treated so the NNT is 20/5 or 4.

Odds Ratio (OR): the ratio of the odds of having the outcome in the treated group compared to the odds of having it in the control group. For example:

- If 100 of 1000 treated patients have persistent symptoms, the odds of persistent symptoms are 100/900 or 0.11 (11%).
- If 300 of 1000 untreated/placebo patients in the same study have persistent symptoms, the odds are 300/700 or 0.43 (43%).
- The odds ratio (OR) is 0.11/0.43 which is 0.26.

Positive predictive value (PPV): the proportion of subjects with a positive test result who are correctly

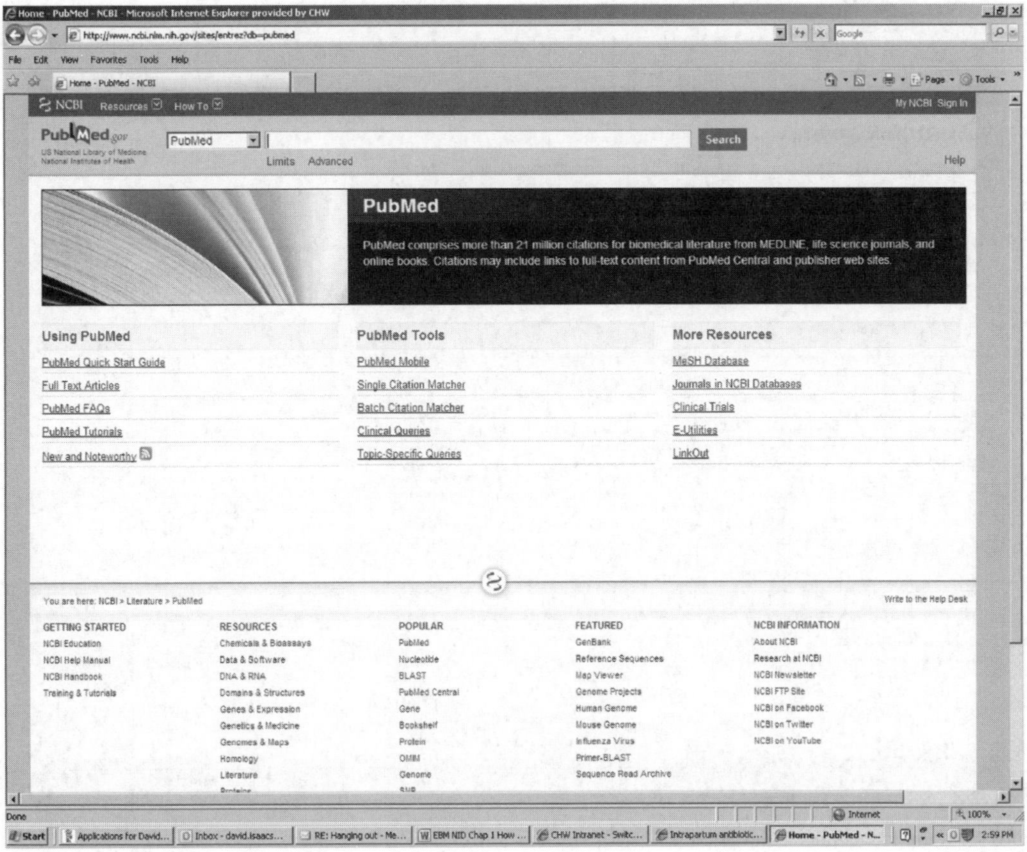

Figure 1.2 PubMed home page (2013).

diagnosed. The positive predictive value of a test for sepsis is a reflection of the test specificity and the incidence of sepsis in the population. If all infants with a positive test result receive antibiotics, for example, the higher the positive predictive value of a test for sepsis, the fewer children without sepsis will receive antibiotics.

Relative Risk or Risk Ratio (RR): the ratio of the risk in the treated group to the risk in the control group. For example:

- If 100 of 1000 treated patients have persistent symptoms, the risk of persistent symptoms is 100/1000 or 0.1 (10%).
- If 300 of 1000 untreated/placebo patients in the same study have persistent symptoms, the risk is 300/1000 or 0.3 (30%).
- The Relative Risk or Risk Ratio is 0.1/0.3 which is 0.33.

[When the event rate is 10% or lower, the OR and RR are similar. For more common events, the difference between OR and RR becomes wider, with the RR always closer to one. In general, it is preferable to use RR.[11]]

Sensitivity: the sensitivity of a test is the proportion of true positives correctly identified by the test (e.g. the percentage of infected infants who are correctly identified as having infection).

Specificity: the specificity of a test is the proportion of negatives correctly identified by the test (e.g. the percentage of healthy infants who are correctly identified by a sepsis test as not having infection).

1.4 Useful websites

The Cochrane Library: www.thecochranelibrary.com
Clinical Evidence: www.clinicalevidence.com
MEDLINE via PubMed: www.pubmed.gov

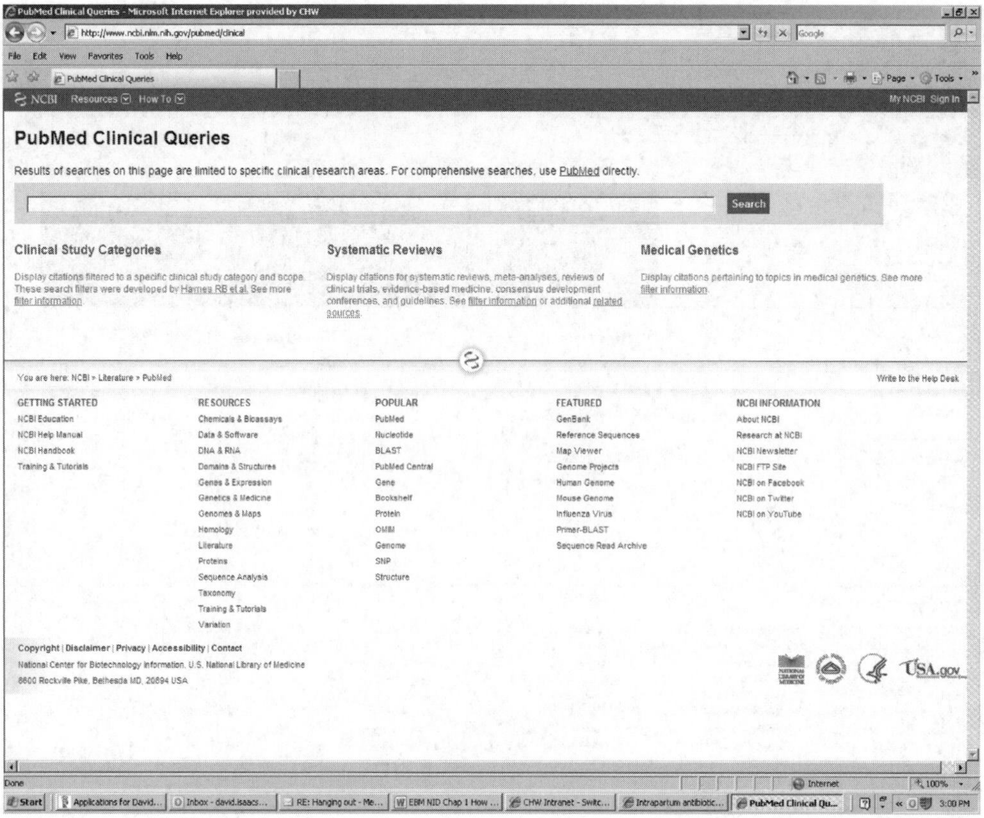

Figure 1.3 PubMed Clinical Queries page (2013).

GRADE working group:
www.gradeworkinggroup.org

[N.B. This chapter is adapted from Chapter 1 of reference 10 and we acknowledge some repetition.]

References

1. Dawes M, Sampson U. Knowledge management in clinical practice: a systematic review of information seeking behavior in physicians. *Int J Med Inf* 2003; 71:91–95.
2. Riordan FAI, Boyle EM, Phillips B. Best paediatric evidence; is it accessible and used on-call?. *Arch Dis Child* 2004; 89:469–471.
3. D'Alessandro DM, Kreiter CD, Peterson MW. An evaluation of information-seeking behaviors of general pediatricians. *Pediatrics* 2004; 113:64–69.
4. Ely JW, Osheroff JA, Ebell MH, Chambliss ML, Vinson DC. Obstacles to answering doctors' questions about patient care with evidence: qualitative study. *BMJ* 2002; 324:1–7.
5. Coumou HC, Meijman FJ. How do primary care physicians seek answers to clinical questions? A literature review. *J Med Libr Assoc* 2006; 94:55–60.
6. Caldwell PHY, Bennett T, Mellis C. Easy guide to searching for evidence for the busy clinician. *J Paed Child Health* 2012; 48:1095–1100.
7. Cotten CM, Taylor S, Stoll B, et al. Prolonged duration of initial empirical antibiotic treatment is associated with increased rates of necrotizing enterocolitis and death for extremely low birth weight infants. *Pediatrics* 2009; 123:58–66.
8. Isaacs D. How to do a quick literature search. *J Paed Child Health* 2013; 49: In press.
9. Moyer VA (ed). *Evidence-based pediatrics and child health*, 2nd edn. London: BMJ Books, 2004.
10. Isaacs D. *Evidence-based pediatric infectious diseases.* Oxford, Blackwell Publishing, 2007.
11. Strauss SE, Glasziou P, Richardson WS, Haynes RB. *Evidence-based medicine. How to practice and teach EBM*, 4th edn. Edinburgh: Elsevier Churchill Livingstone, 2011. ISBN 978-0-7020-3127-4.

CHAPTER 2
Epidemiology

2.1 Incidence and mortality

Neonatal infections are an important and sadly neglected cause of mortality and morbidity globally. In 2008, neonatal infections caused an estimated 29% of the 3.6 million neonatal deaths worldwide[1] (see Figure 2.1 and Table 2.1) or about one million deaths, almost all in developing countries.[1] Neonates comprised 41% of the estimated 8.8 million deaths in children under 5 years old worldwide in 2008.[1] Community-based studies in developing countries attribute up to 42% of neonatal deaths in the community to infection.[2]

The mortality from neonatal infections is considerably lower in resource-rich countries. Intrapartum antibiotic use to prevent group B streptococcus (GBS) infection has reduced mortality significantly in countries with a high incidence.[2–4]

Newborn babies have rates of infection as high as children and adults whose immunity is compromised for almost any other reason, including most oncology patients and the elderly. Although newborn babies, and particularly pre-term newborns, are immunocompromised, additional factors contribute to the high rates of neonatal infection and will be considered in Section 2.2.

Knowledge of the incidence of neonatal infections is important for planning preventive and intervention strategies and for comparisons within and between countries, which can help inform clinical practice and help assess the quality of care. However, such comparisons are not necessarily straightforward.

In developing countries, most deliveries occur in the home, so hospital-based studies of incidence and aetiology may give misleading or inaccurate results. Infections are usually diagnosed clinically without cultures, and deaths from infection are frequently underreported. Community studies report rates of clinical neonatal sepsis ranging from 49 per 1000 live births in babies >24 hours old in Guatemala to 170 per 1000 live births in rural India.[2] The reported rate of blood culture-confirmed cases is far lower: a minimum of 5.5 per 1000 live births in a rural hospital in Kenya,[5] a highly uncertain figure because of incomplete sampling. Infection-specific mortality rates reported in 32 studies varied from 2.7 per 1000 live births in South Africa to 38.6 per 1000 in Somalia.[2]

In industrialized Western countries where most de liveries occur in hospital, hospital-based studies of incidence are more representative.

The reported incidence of neonatal infection depends on how neonatal infection is defined and reported. Definitions may vary considerably. Examples include how contaminants in blood cultures and cerebrospinal fluid (CSF) are defined; whether or not contaminants are excluded; whether or not clinical sepsis with evidence of raised inflammatory markers is accepted as being infection; and whether infections are confined to positive cultures of blood and/or CSF or also include positive cultures from normally sterile sites, such as urine, bone, joint fluid or pulmonary fluid.

2.1.1 Early-onset infection

It is conventional to divide the reporting of neonatal infections into early- and late-onset infections. Early infections are presumed to be due to organisms acquired from the mother shortly before (e.g. Listeria) or at the time of birth (e.g. GBS) whereas

Evidence-Based Neonatal Infections, First Edition. David Isaacs.

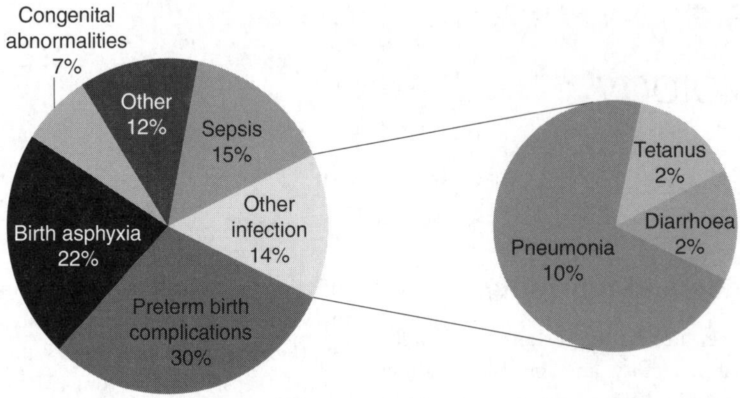

Figure 2.1 Global causes of neonatal deaths. Adapted from Reference 1 with permission from Elsevier. Copyright © 2010 Elsevier.

late infections are primarily caused by environmental organisms, acquired nosocomially (i.e. in hospital) or in the community. However, 'early onset' has been defined as anything from the first 2 days to the first 7 days after birth. Furthermore, environmental organisms may grow from blood cultures in the first 48 hours after birth, while the classic early-onset organisms like GBS and Listeria can cause late- as well as early-onset sepsis. Methicillin-resistant *Staphylococcus aureus* (MRSA), originally confined to hospitals or patients associated with hospitals, is a common community-acquired pathogen in many countries and can colonize pregnant women and cause both early- and late-onset neonatal infections.

There are two major considerations in defining early-onset infection, clinical and epidemiologic.

Table 2.1 Causes of death in neonates globally.

Cause of death	Number of deaths in millions (%)
Pre-term birth complications	1.033 (29%)
Birth asphyxia	0.814 (22%)
Sepsis	0.521 (15%)
Other	0.409 (11%)
Pneumonia	0.386 (11%)
Congenital abnormalities	0.272 (8%)
Diarrhoea	0.079 (2%)
Tetanus	0.059 (2%)
TOTAL	3.575

Source: Adapted from Reference 1 with permission from Elsevier. Copyright © 2010 Elsevier.

Question: Does it matter how we define early-onset infection clinically?

The clinical problem with defining early-onset infection as infections in the first 7 days after birth, as opposed to those in the first 48 hours say, comes if the empiric antibiotic regimen for early-onset sepsis does not cover organisms that may be acquired from 3 to 7 days. For example, say penicillin and gentamicin are recommended for early-onset sepsis, gentamicin has only modest anti-staphylococcal activity so this regimen provides little cover against *S. aureus* infections. Yet data from Western countries[6, 7] show that *S. aureus* bloodstream infections are not uncommon between days 3 and 7 (Figures 2.2 and 2.3).

Recommendation: It is critical for the clinician that empiric antibiotic regimens reflect the local epidemiology and cover the organisms likely to cause sepsis.

Question: Is there a correct way of reporting early-onset infection?

The incidence of early-onset infections is conventionally reported as the number of infections per 1000 live births in a defined period, for example, the number of infections in babies born in a maternity hospital (excluding babies transferred from other hospitals or home) divided by the number of live births over a

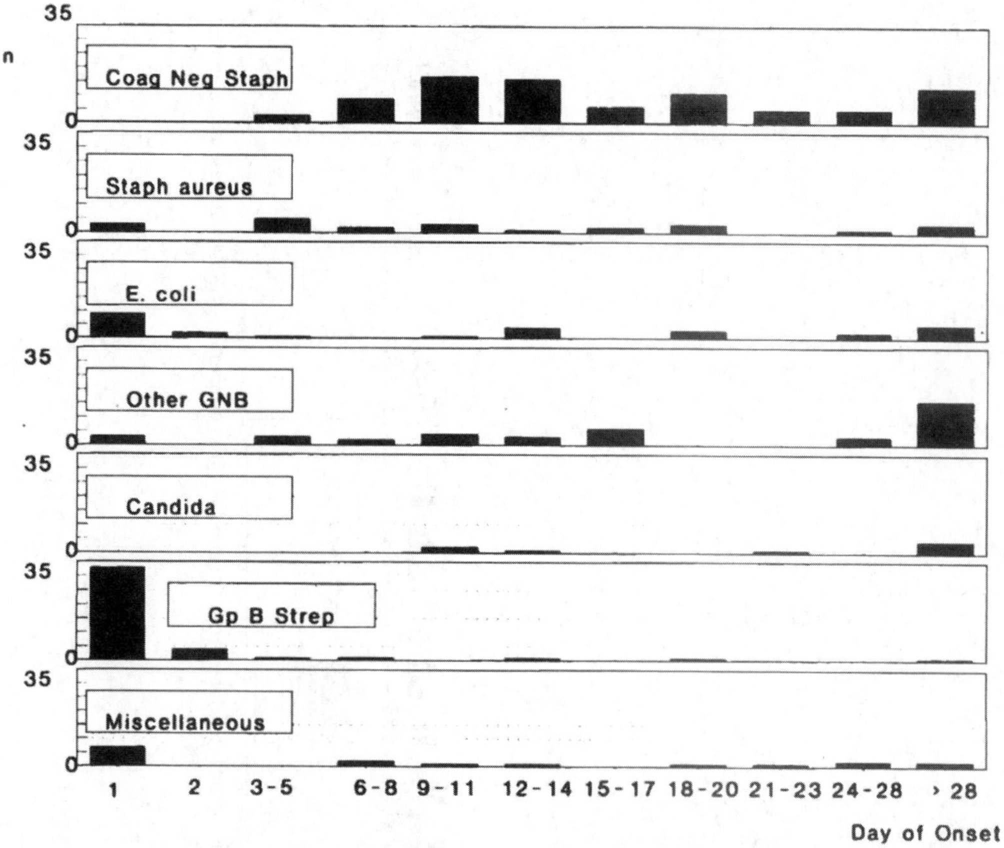

Figure 2.2 Timing of neonatal infection by organism. Adapted from Reference 6. CoNS, Coagulase-negative staphylococci; Other GNB, Other Gram-negative bacilli; Gp B Strep, Group B streptococci.

defined time period. Various countries have established neonatal infection surveillance networks, including Australia,[6] the United Kingdom,[7] Canada (http://www.canadianneonatalnetwork.org/portal/), the US National Institute of Child Health and Human Development (http://www.nichd.nih.gov),[3] Germany (http://www.nrz-hygiene.de/surveillance/kiss/neo-kiss/) and the Vermont Oxford Network (http://www.vtoxford.org/) has established a global network. The Australian, Canadian and US NICHD report all neonatal infections, whereas the other networks focus on low birth-weight babies in tertiary centres. Comparisons depend on definitions and completeness of reporting.[6–8]

Data on early infections inform public health interventions. For example, the rate of early-onset GBS infection determines whether or not prevention strategies are cost-effective.[9–12] Epidemiology should be a critical driver of public health.

The clinician wants data to inform empiric choice of antibiotics. Whether organisms are reported separately[6] (Figure 2.2) or all organisms combined on a single day[7] (Figure 2.3), clearly there is some overlap between organisms likely to have been maternally and those probably nosocomially acquired. An alternative approach is to separate infections into those in babies <48 hours old (early onset), in babies aged 3–7 days (intermediate sepsis) and in babies >7 days (late sepsis).[8]

Failure to exclude contaminants can give misleading results. For example, one single-centre study reported coagulase-negative staphylococci (CoNS) as their commonest cause of early-onset neonatal infection.[10] Excluding all likely contaminants (e.g. CoNS, diphtheroids, micrococci, α-haemolytic streptococci and anaerobes) is probably not valid, because these organisms occasionally cause serious infection, even

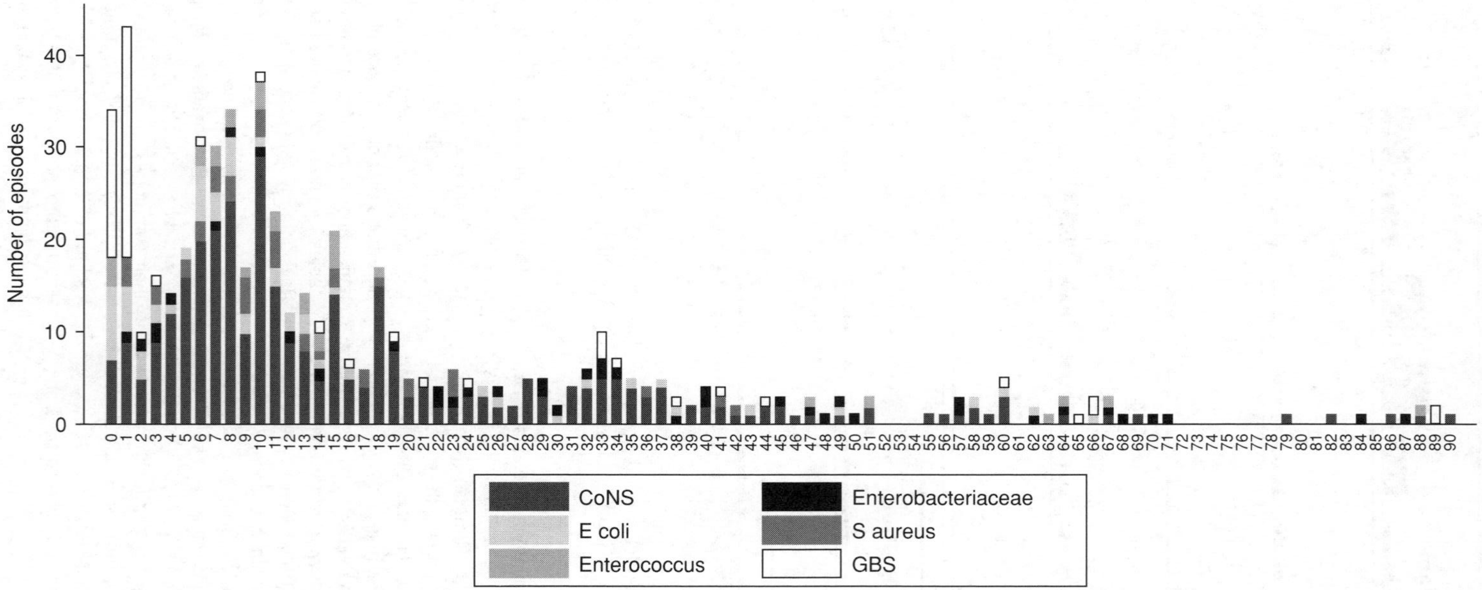

Figure 2.3 Pathogens according to the day of onset of infection, UK 2006–2008. Reprinted from Reference 7 with permission. CoNS, Coagulase-negative staphylococci; GBS, Group B streptococci.

meningitis. One option is to include all organisms cultured while acknowledging most are probably contaminants.[7] Another possibility is to use a combined clinical and laboratory definition of infection, and only report likely contaminants if the baby also has abnormal laboratory parameters, for example, elevated C-reactive protein (CRP), abnormal white cell or platelet count.[6]

In Western countries, early-onset infection is mainly due to GBS, although less frequently in countries using intrapartum antibiotic chemoprophylaxis, Gram-negative enteric bacilli (Enterobacteriaceae), notably *Escherichia coli*, and miscellaneous other organisms, including streptococci, which are mostly sensitive to penicillin or gentamicin.[4, 6, 7]

In stark contrast, most early-onset infections in developing countries are due to Klebsiella species, *E. coli*, other Gram-negative enteric bacilli and *S. aureus*.[13] Intriguingly, and for unknown reasons, this pattern of organisms, with little variation, is reported commonly from Africa, Asia, Latin America and the Middle East.[13] GBS is rare in resource-poor countries,[13] although an important cause of early-onset sepsis in some Asian countries.[9]

Self-evidently, it is vital to know the local organisms and their resistance patterns to develop rational empiric antibiotic policies for babies with suspected sepsis.

Recommendation: There is no single correct epidemiologic way of reporting early-onset infection, but reporting the date of onset would improve comparison of rates.

2.1.2 Late-onset infection

Late-onset neonatal infection can be caused by organisms associated with neonatal intensive care and acquired nosocomially (*nosocomos* means hospital in Greek), for example, CoNS and water-loving Gram-negative bacilli; by maternally acquired organisms that colonize the baby at birth and invade later, for example, GBS and Listeria; or by community organisms, including respiratory, gastrointestinal and Salmonella and skin organisms.[13]

In industrialized Western countries, the major burden of late-onset neonatal sepsis is in babies in neonatal intensive care units (NICU). The incidence of late sepsis is inversely related to gestational age and birth weight[14] (see Figure 2.4). Incidence can also be reported in terms of the proportion of babies admitted to NICU who develop sepsis, usually around 2–5%,

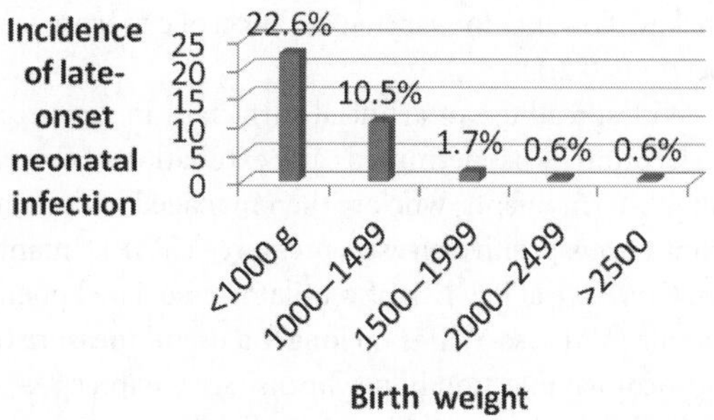

Figure 2.4 Incidence of late-onset neonatal infection by birth weight. Data from Reference 14.

depending on the NICU population.[7–14] In one study, annual rates of late sepsis ranged from 2.4% to 4.5% of NICU admissions in different NICUs, a difference which was statistically significant, but no longer significant after stratifying for birth weight.[14]

Rates of late-onset neonatal sepsis in industrialized countries may be reported as the proportion of babies admitted to neonatal units who develop sepsis or the proportion of all live born babies who develop sepsis, if these data are known. However, even after allowing for birth weight, the comparisons may be confounded by population variation. The risk of infection increases with the duration of neonatal unit stay, particularly if intensive care is needed. Stratification by birth weight allows for this, because low birth-weight infants stay longer. However, other more mature infants may require intensive care, for example, those needing gastrointestinal surgery.

In industrialized countries, the reported rate of late-onset neonatal infection in neonatal units is most useful when definitions of sepsis are standardized. Even then, comparisons between hospitals are only truly valid when variations in patient populations have been taken into account.[15, 16]

A refinement of crude comparisons of overall rates of late sepsis is to compare specific infections that are felt to reflect good hygiene in intensive care. An example is the use of rates of **central line-associated bacteraemia** (CLAB), also called **central line-associated blood stream infections (CLABSI)**.[15] A CLAB is defined as a bacteraemic infection caused by an organism like CoNS in a baby with a central line *in situ* and no other explanation for the infection. The rate can be reported as the number of CLAB's per 1000 line days, which makes allowance for varying duration of exposure (see Section 20.2.1).

Widespread use of artificial surfactant in resource-rich countries has permitted early extubation of almost all pre-term infants, who are then managed with nasal continuous positive airways pressure (CPAP). Infants on CPAP are at low risk of ventilator-associated pneumonia (VAP), so VAP is no longer a useful measure of nosocomial infection in newborns (see Chapter 8).

In developing countries, the reliability of reported infection rates depends on factors such as definitions, case ascertainment, population selection, whether or not babies are cultured and the reliability of the microbiology laboratory.[2] A review of 32 studies from developing countries found considerable study heterogeneity, making comparisons difficult.[2] Many studies did not distinguish early from late sepsis. Clearly, more accurate data based on standardized methods are needed.

2.1.2.1 Organisms causing late sepsis

In most Western countries, CoNS now cause just over 50% of all late-onset neonatal infections, even when likely contaminants are excluded. Most CoNS infections occur in low birth-weight infants and are central line-associated.[6, 7, 14, 15] The major pathogens causing the remainder of late-onset infections are Gram-negative enteric bacilli (Enterobacteriaceae) and *S. aureus* (methicillin-sensitive or MRSA). Other important but rarer causes of late-onset sepsis include enterococci (faecal streptococci), Listeria, Candida and miscellaneous rarer organisms.[6, 7, 14, 15]

In developing countries, there are limited data on home deliveries, but in a non-Cochrane review the four most common pathogens reported with almost equal frequency after 7 days of age were *S. aureus*, GBS, *Streptococcus pneumoniae* and non-typhoidal Salmonella species.[13]

2.2 Pathogenesis

2.2.1 Pregnancy

Pregnancy is an immunosuppressed state. The pregnant woman does not want to mount an immune response that would harm the foetus, so her cell-mediated immunity is reduced. Evidence of this impairment is the pregnant woman's increased susceptibility to infections which require cellular immunity for optimal recovery, such as viral infections (e.g. chickenpox, influenza, HIV) and intracellular bacterial infections (Listeria, tuberculosis). If the pregnant woman is infected with an intracellular pathogen during pregnancy, the baby may be infected transplacentally (e.g. *Listeria monocytogenes*; *Mycobacterium tuberculosis*; congenital infections caused by CMV, rubella, *Toxoplasma gondii*, *Treponema pallidum*, VZV) or perinatally (e.g. HIV, HSV, VZV, *M. tuberculosis*).

2.2.2 Chorioamnionitis

Chorioamnionitis is one of several terms used for intrauterine infection in the second half of pregnancy, others being intra-amniotic infection, amniotic fluid infection, placental infection and intrapartum infection. Clinical chorioamnionitis, with signs such as fever, tachycardia, uterine tenderness and foul-smelling amniotic fluid, occurs in anything from 1% to 10% or more of pregnancies, depending on the population studied.[17] Membrane rupture and/or labour frequently ensue.

Romero described four stages of ascending intrauterine infection, (a) cervical colonization/infection with pathologic bacteria, including bacterial vaginosis; (b), ascending infection from the cervix or vagina to the decidua (endometrium), (c) bacterial invasion of chorionic blood vessels and amniotic fluid and (d) foetal infection to cause pneumonia and often bacteraemia. Histopathologic chorioamnionitis can be diagnosed by histologic examination of the placenta and precedes defined clinical chorioamnionitis.

Only a relatively small proportion of babies born to mothers diagnosed with chorioamnionitis have proven early-onset bacteraemia.[17] Nevertheless, chorioamnionitis has a profound effect on neonatal outcome because it can induce pre-term labour, probably because the causative microorganisms produce prostaglandins and related substances. Pre-term birth predisposes the baby to early- and late-onset infections, and is associated with an increased risk of cerebral palsy[18] and bronchopulmonary dysplasia.[19]

A Cochrane systematic review provides strong evidence that giving maternal antibiotics for pre-term rupture of membranes significantly reduces chorioamnionitis (by 34%) and reduces the numbers of babies born within 2 days (29% reduction) and 7 days (21% reduction).[20] Neonatal infection is also reduced by a third (Relative Risk, RR = 0.67, 95% CI 0.52–0.85). Interestingly, β-lactam antibiotics, particularly amoxicillin–clavulanic acid, were associated with a more than fourfold increased risk of neonatal necrotizing enterocolitis (RR 4.72, 95% CI 1.57–14.23), whereas erythromycin was not,[20] an observation driven by the findings of the large ORACLE study.[21]

2.2.3 Early-onset sepsis

The intrauterine environment is usually sterile. However, if chorioamnionitis leads to ascending infection, although the foetus does not breathe *in utero*, the foetal lungs are fluid-filled and thus exposed to infected amniotic fluid. Early-onset sepsis caused by GBS, one of the major causes of early sepsis, almost always presents with early-onset pneumonia, even if the baby may sometimes also be bacteraemic and may even develop meningitis. This implies that the commonest route of infection in early-onset GBS infection is via the lung, either antenatally or by aspiration of maternal secretions during the birth process.

Other organisms associated with chorioamnionitis, such as *E. coli*, other Gram-negative bacilli, enterococci and anaerobes, generally cause early-onset sepsis without pneumonia. Indeed, apart from GBS pneumonia, most early-onset bacterial infections are nonfocal. This implies that the intra-amniotic organism is able to invade the baby's bloodstream. A baby with early-onset septicaemia is almost without exception colonized with the same organism, implying that colonization of the foetus' mucosal surfaces commonly precedes bacteraemia.

Transplacental infection is also possible. Babies born with *L. monocytogenes* infection are often bacteraemic and may present with rash and hepatosplenomegaly, suggesting transplacental infection. Their mothers are often febrile and sometimes shown to be bacteraemic, reinforcing the importance of transplacental Listeria infection. However, babies born with Listeria infection do sometimes have a significant respiratory illness with radiologic changes, suggesting that pulmonary aspiration may sometimes play a role in the pathogenesis of early-onset neonatal Listeria infection.

The maternal birth canal is colonized with a great variety of organisms that usually do not infect the mother but can potentially infect the baby. Babies not already exposed to intrauterine infection become colonized perinatally with bacteria and other organisms. While these usually remain commensals, they may occasionally cause late infection. If the mother's birth canal or perineum is colonized with potentially virulent organisms (e.g. MRSA, Salmonella, Pseudomonas) a baby colonized perinatally may develop sepsis rapidly.

Whenever considering why one person and not another develops an infection, it is necessary to consider three main factors: the host, the environment and the organism. The risk factors for early-onset sepsis reflect a combination of host factors (the more pre-term the baby, the higher the risk of sepsis), environmental risk factors (maternal risk factors) and virulence of the organism (maternal colonization with potent neonatal pathogens such as GBS, group A streptococci, HSV, etc.).

Risk factors for developing early-onset neonatal infection

A literature search of Medline via PubMed and Clinical Queries for systematic reviews and observational studies using the search term 'early-onset neonatal infections', category 'prognosis', scope 'broad' found 23 systematic reviews and 320 studies. Most of the studies were not relevant, but it was possible to identify risk factors from selected papers (Table 2.2). Although cohort studies are generally more valid for ascertaining risk factors, a case-control study is a more practical study design because early-onset sepsis is relatively uncommon.

Prior to intrapartum antibiotic prophylaxis, a systematic review of a number of studies of risk factors for early-onset neonatal GBS infection identified maternal colonization with GBS and prematurity as the major risk factors.[22] The risk increased with decreasing gestational age; the OR for infection was 4.8 for any baby <37 weeks of gestation and 21.7 for babies <28 weeks of gestation.[22] Other risk factors were prolonged rupture of membranes (PROM) >18 hours (OR 7.3), and intrapartum maternal fever >37.5°C (OR 4.0).[22]

A subsequent large nested case-control study of babies of 34 weeks of gestation or more concentrated on maternal risk factors.[23] There was no increased risk of early-onset neonatal infection when the highest maternal temperature was <38°C, but the risk increased rapidly above 38°C and was highest >39°C, although such fever was rare. The risk of sepsis

Table 2.2 Risk factors for early-onset neonatal infection.

Risk factors for early-onset neonatal infection
Prematurity: risk increases with decreasing gestation and birth weight
Spontaneous pre-term onset of labour
Spontaneous pre-term rupture of membranes
Prolonged rupture of membranes (increases with increasing duration >12 hours)
Maternal intrapartum fever >38°C
Maternal clinical chorioamnionitis
Vaginal examinations during labour
Maternal urinary tract infection
Maternal vaginal discharge
Maternal colonization with group B streptococcus (GBS)
Previous baby with early-onset GBS infection

Source: From References 22–25.

increased steadily with increasing duration of rupture of membranes greater than 12 hours.[23] The relationship between gestational age and sepsis showed a U-shaped curve, with the risk increasing with decreasing gestational age and increasing when gestation exceeded 42 weeks.[23] Any intrapartum antibiotic given >4 hours before delivery decreased the risk of early-onset neonatal infection compared with no antibiotic or antibiotic <4 hours before delivery.[23]

A case-control study from Pakistan found that maternal fever and vaginal examinations during labour were risk factors for early-onset sepsis, as in Western countries, but also found maternal urinary tract infection and vaginal discharge were risk factors in the developing country setting studied.[24]

2.2.4 Late-onset sepsis

The risk factors for late-onset sepsis reflect a combination of host factors (the more pre-term the baby, the higher the risk of sepsis), environmental risk factors (exposure to organisms and to factors like indoor pollution) and virulence of the organism (e.g. Pseudomonas in neonatal units, GBS acquired at birth or post-natally and causing invasive disease later in the first month,[25] and *M. tuberculosis* in developing countries).

The major risk factors for late-onset sepsis in industrialized countries relate to neonatal intensive care, because although only about 5–9% of babies in Europe and 12–13% of babies in the United States are born pre-term,[26] they are by far the most numerous babies to develop late-onset neonatal infection.

In resource-poor countries, most babies are born at home, and very different risk factors apply. However, although hospital-acquired neonatal infections in developing countries have the same risk factors as in Western countries, reported rates are 3–20 times higher than in Western countries.[27]

Host risk factors common to neonates in resource-poor and resource-rich countries are prematurity and anatomic abnormalities. Babies born with abnormal urinary tracts are at increased risk of urinary tract infection,[25] babies with abnormal gastrointestinal tracts are at increased risk of obstruction and of ischemic damage leading to infection and babies with obstructive pulmonary abnormalities such as sequestration are at increased risk of pneumonia (Table 2.3).

Risk factors for developing late-onset neonatal infection

A search of Medline via PubMed and Clinical Queries (see Chapter 1) for systematic reviews and case-control studies using the search term 'late-onset neonatal infections', category 'prognosis', scope 'broad' found 12 systematic reviews and 180 studies.

A non-Cochrane review article on risk factors for late-onset sepsis in premature infants[28] identified factors related to the causative organism, intensive care and preventative factors.

Late-onset bloodstream infections with Gram-negative bacilli and fungi are associated with increased mortality compared with matched, uninfected babies, whereas those with Gram-positive organisms, particularly CoNS, are not.[29] Pseudomonas is more virulent than other Gram-negative bacilli, with a mortality of 52–74% compared with 10–25% for other Gram-negative bacilli.[30–32]

The use and duration of central venous catheters is a clear risk factor for bloodstream infections with bacteria, notably CoNS, *S. aureus* and Gram-negative bacilli and with Candida. The review article noted that in a study of nosocomial infections in infants <1500 g,

Table 2.3 Risk factors for late-onset neonatal infection.

Risk factors for late-onset neonatal infection
All babies:
Prematurity: risk increases with decreasing gestation and birth weight
Anatomical, for example, urinary tract or gastrointestinal abnormalities
Exposure to organisms of high pathogenicity
Hospital-based:
Use and duration of parenteral nutrition
Use and duration of invasive mechanical ventilation
Use and duration of central venous catheters
Use of H2 blocker/proton pump inhibitors
Poor infection control
Colonization with virulent organisms, for example, Pseudomonas
Community-based:
HIV infection
Exposure to indoor air pollution (tobacco, chimney stoves)

Source: From References 28–31.

infection was significantly associated with lower birth weight, respiratory distress syndrome and duration of parenteral nutrition and was significantly lower if enteral feeds were started earlier.[33]

Risk factors for late-onset Gram-negative sepsis were considered in two case-control studies. A US study of low birth-weight infants (<1500 g) reported significant associations with the duration of central venous catheter >10 days, nasal CPAP, use of H2 blocker/proton pump inhibitors and gastrointestinal tract pathology.[34] A UK study found that mechanical ventilation, the use and duration of total parenteral nutrition, and the use and duration of a central venous catheter were significantly associated with Gram-negative infection by univariate analysis, but only the duration of total parenteral nutrition before infection remained significant by multivariate logistic regression analysis.[35]

An intriguing retrospective cohort analysis of twins born from 1994 to 2009 examined concordance rates for late-onset neonatal sepsis in monozygotic and dizygotic twins, and used logistic regression to look at genetic and non-genetic factors. They found that decreasing birth weight, occurrence of respiratory distress syndrome and the duration of total parenteral nutrition were significant non-genetic risk factors for infection.[36] Further analysis suggested that 49% of the variance in risk of sepsis was due to genetic factors and 51% due to environmental factors.[37]

There is intense research interest in how genetic factors influence the risk of neonatal sepsis. A study of T-cell cytokine production from 1 to 21 days of age in 996 extremely low birth-weight babies <1000 g found babies with bloodstream infection had significantly lower levels of the inflammatory cytokine IL-17 and higher levels of the regulatory cytokines IL-6 and IL-10. After adjusting for confounding variables, the ratio of regulatory to inflammatory cytokines was a significant risk factor for developing late-onset sepsis.[36] The genetic basis for the differing cytokine patterns awaits elucidation.

Some of the above-mentioned risk factors are effectively unavoidable once the baby is born: small, sick pre-term babies are at increased risk of infection. However, it may be possible to initiate early enteral feeds and thereby shorten the duration of parenteral nutrition and central venous catheters and it is also possible to avoid using H2 blocker/proton pump inhibitors.

In developing countries, the bulk of late-onset neonatal infections occur at home and are caused by bacterial infection, pneumonia, diarrheal illness and tetanus[1] (Figure 2.1). Factors that predispose to infection should be considered in terms of the host, the organism and the environment. Host factors include babies born prematurely and babies with underlying problems with immunity, particularly HIV infection. Exposure to organisms of high pathogenicity is an important issue which depends both on virulence of the organisms and environmental exposure. Newborns exposed to *M. tuberculosis* at or soon after birth are at high risk of developing tuberculosis. Other pathogenic organisms, including pyogenic organisms like *S. aureus* and group A streptococcus, intracellular bacteria like Salmonella, viruses and protozoa can cause late-onset neonatal infections. Environmental factors that increase the risk of the baby developing symptomatic infection include indoor air pollution from tobacco smoke and from open wood cooking fires.[38]

2.3 Outcome of neonatal infection

The long-term outcome of neonatal infections depends on many factors, of which the most important are the gestational age of the infant; early- versus late-onset infection; resource-rich versus resource-poor setting; presence of meningitis; and the timing and appropriateness of antibiotic therapy. Mortality was considered in Section 2.1 and many aspects of outcome will be considered under the relevant chapters regarding specific organs infected and specific organisms.

A large US multi-centre study conducted by the National Institute of Child Health Development Neonatal Research Network followed up 6093 infants born weighing 401–1000 g at 18–22 months of age. Infants were classified as uninfected ($n = 2161$), clinical infection alone ($n = 1538$), sepsis ($n = 1922$), sepsis and necrotizing enterocolitis ($n = 279$) or meningitis ($n = 193$). Compared with uninfected infants, all four infection groups were significantly more likely to have adverse neurodevelopmental outcomes, including cerebral palsy and visual impairment.[39] Neonatal infection was also associated with impaired head growth. The data were analysed by infecting organism group: CoNS, other Gram positive organisms, Gram negative bacilli and fungi. All adverse neurodevelopmental outcomes except hearing impairment but including microcephaly were higher among infected children in all pathogen groups. Hearing impairment was significantly higher in infants with Gram-negative and fungal infections.[39]

2.4 Prevention of neonatal infections

Prevention of neonatal infections will be considered in detail in Chapters 22 and 23.

References

1. Black R, Cousens S, Johnson HL, et al. Global, regional, and national causes of child mortality in 2008: a systematic analysis. *Lancet* 2010; 375:1969–1987.
2. Thaver D, Zaidi AK. Burden of neonatal infections in developing countries: a review of evidence from community-based studies. *Pediatr Infect Dis J* 2009; 28:S3–S9.
3. Lukacs S, Schoendorf KC, Schuchat A. Trends in sepsis-related mortality in the United States, 1985-1998. *Pediatr Infect Dis J* 2004; 23:599–603.
4. Stoll BJ, Hansen NI, Sanchez PJ, et al. Early onset neonatal sepsis: the burden of Group B streptococcal and *E. coli* disease continues. *Pediatrics* 2011; 127:817–826.
5. Berkley JA, Lowe BS, Mwangi I, et al. Bacteremia among children admitted to a rural hospital in Kenya. *N Engl J Med* 2005; 352:39–47.
6. Isaacs D, Barfield C, Grimwood K, McPhee AJ, Minutillo C, Tudehope DI. Systemic bacterial and fungal infections in infants in Australian neonatal units. Australian Study Group for Neonatal Infections.*Med J Aust* 1995; 162: 198–201.
7. Vergnano S, Menson E, Kennea N, et al. Neonatal infections in England: the NeonIN surveillance network. *Arch Dis Fetal Neonatal Ed* 2011; 96:F9–F14.
8. Viswanathan R, Singh AK, Basu S, Chatterjee S, Sardar S, Isaacs D. Multi-drug resistant Gram negative bacilli causing early neonatal sepsis in India. *Arch Dis Fetal Neonatal Ed* 2012; 97:F182–F187.
9. Tiskumara R, Fakharee SH, Liu CQ, et al. Neonatal infections in Africa. *Arch Dis Fetal Neonatal Ed* 2009; 94:F144–F148.
10. Mohle-Boetani JC, Schuchat A, Plikaytis BD, Smith JD, Broome CV. Comparison of prevention strategies for neonatal group B streptococcal infection. A population-based economic analysis. *J Am Med Assoc* 1993; 270:1442–1448.
11. Colbourn TE, Asseburg C, Bojke L, et al. Preventive strategies for group B streptococcal and other bacterial infections in early infancy: cost effectiveness and value of information analyses. *Br Med J* 2007; 335:655.
12. Edwards RK, Jamie WE, Sterner D, Gentry S, Counts K, Duff P. Intrapartum antibiotic prophylaxis and early-onset sepsis patterns. *Infect Dis Obstet Gynecol* 2003; 11:221–216.
13. Zaidi AKM, Thaver D, Ali AS, Khan TA. Pathogens associated with sepsis in newborns and young infants in developing countries. *Pediatr Infect Dis J* 2009; 28:S10–S18.
14. Isaacs D, Barfield C, Clothier T, et al. Late-onset infections of infants in neonatal units. *J Paediatr Child Health* 1996; 32:158–161.
15. Stover BH, Shulman ST, Bratcher DF, Brady MT, Levine GL, Jarvis WR; Pediatric Prevention Network. Nosocomial infection rates in US children's hospitals' neonatal and pediatric intensive care units. *Am J Infect Control* 2001; 29: 152–157.
16. Banerjee SN, Grohskopf LA, Sinkowitz-Cochran RL, Jarvis WR. National Nosocomial Infections Surveillance System; Pediatric Prevention Network.Incidence of pediatric and neonatal intensive care unit-acquired infections. *Infect Control Hosp Epidemiol* 2006; 27:561–570.
17. Tita AT, Andrews WW. Diagnosis and management of clinical chorioamnionitis. *Clin Perinatol* 2010; 37:339–354.
18. Shatrov JG, Birch SC, Lam LT, Quinlivan JA, McIntyre S, Mendz GL. Chorioamnionitis and cerebral palsy: a meta-analysis. *Obstet Gynecol* 2010; 116:387–392.
19. Hartling L, Liang Y, Lacaze-Masmonteil D. Chorioamnionitis as a risk factor for bronchopulmonary dysplasia: a systematic review and meta-analysis. *Arch Dis Child Fetal Neonatal Ed* 2012; 97:F8–F17.

20. Kenyon S, Boulvain M, Neilson JP. Antibiotics for preterm rupture of membranes. *Cochrane Database Syst Rev* 2010, (Issue 8). Art. No.: CD001058. doi:10.1002/14651858.cd001058.pub2.
21. Kenyon SL, Taylor DJ, Tarnow-Mordi W, ORACLE Collaborative Group. Broad-spectrum antibiotics for preterm, prelabour rupture of fetal membranes: the ORACLE 1 randomised trial. *Lancet* 2001; 357:979–988.
22. Benitz WE, Gould JB, Druzin ML. Risk factors for early-onset group B streptococcal sepsis: estimation of odds ratios by critical literature review. *Pediatrics* 1999; 103:e77.
23. Puopolo KM, Draper D, Wi S, et al. Estimating the probability of neonatal early-onset infection on the basis of maternal risk factors. *Pediatrics* 2011; 128:e1155–e1163.
24. Bhutta ZA, Yusuf K. Early-onset neonatal sepsis in Pakistan: a case control study of risk factors in a birth cohort. *Am J Perinatol* 1997; 14:577–581.
25. Didier C, Streicher MP, Chognot D, et al. Late-onset neonatal infections: incidences and pathogens in the era of antenatal antibiotics. *Eur J Pediatr* 2012; 171(4):681–687.
26. Goldenberg RL, Culhane JF, Iams JD, Romero R. Epidemiology and causes of preterm birth. *Lancet* 2008; 371:75–84.
27. Zaidi AK, Huskins WC, Thaver D, Bhutta ZA, Abbas Z, Goldmann DA. Hospital-acquired neonatal infections in developing countries. *Lancet* 2005; 365:1175–1188.
28. Downey LC, Smith PB, Benjamin DK. Risk factors and prevention of late-onset sepsis in premature infants. *Early Hum Dev* 2010; 86(Supp. 1):7–12.
29. Benjamin DK, DeLong E, Cotton CM, Garges HP, Steinbach WJ, Clark RH. Mortality following blood culture in premature infants: increased with gram-negative bacteremia and candidemia, but not gram-positive bacteremia. *J Perinatol* 2004; 24:175–180.
30. Karlowicz MG, Buescher ES, Surka AE. Fulminant late-onset sepsis in a neonatal intensive care unit, 1988-1997, and the impact of avoiding empiric vancomycin therapy. *Pediatrics* 2000; 107:1387–1390.
31. Stoll B, Hansen N, Fanaroff AA, et al. Late-onset sepsis in very low birth weight neonates: the experience of the NICHD Neonatal Research Network. *Pediatrics* 2002; 110:285–291.
32. Gordon A, Isaacs D. Late onset Gram-negative bacillary infection in Australia and New Zealand, 1992-2002. *Pediatr Infect Dis J* 2006; 25:25–29.
33. Flidel-Rimon O, Friedman S, Lev E, Juster-Reicher A, Amitay M, Shinwell ES. Early enteral feeding and nosocomial sepsis in very low birthweight infants. *Arch Dis Child Fetal Neonatal Ed* 2004; 89:F289–F292.
34. Graham 3rd PL, Begg MD, Larson E, Della-Latta P, Allen A, Saiman L. Risk factors for late onset gram-negative sepsis in low birth weight infants hospitalized in the neonatal intensive care unit. *Pediatr Infect Dis J* 2006; 25:113–117.
35. Samanta S, Farrer K, Breathnach A, Heath PT. Risk factors for late onset gram-negative infections: a case-control study. *Arch Dis Child Fetal Neonatal Ed* 2011; 96:F15–F18.
36. Schelonka RL, Maheshwari Carlo WA, et al. T cell cytokines and the risk of blood stream infection in extremely low birth weight infants. *Cytokine* 2011; 53:249–255.
37. Bizzarro MJ, Jiang Y, Hussain N, Gruen JR, Bhandari V, Zhang H. The impact of environmental and genetic factors on neonatal late-onset sepsis. *J Pediatr* 2011; 158: 234–238.e1.
38. Smith KR, McCracken JP, Weber M, et al. Effect of reduction in household air pollution on childhood pneumonia in Guatemala (RESPIRE): a randomised controlled trial. *Lancet* 2011; 378:1717–1726.
39. Stoll BJ, Hansen NI, Adams-Chapman I, et al; National Institute of Child Health and Human Development Neonatal Research Network. Neurodevelopmental and growth impairment among extremely low-birth-weight infants with neonatal infection. *J Am Med Assoc* 2004; 292:2357–2365.

CHAPTER 3

Clinical manifestations

The clinical features of early-onset and late-onset neonatal septicaemia are generally non-specific and rarely indicate a specific bacteriologic or indeed microbiologic diagnosis.[1–9] A list derived from published studies of the clinical features, which differ little between early- and late-onset sepsis, is given in Table 3.1. The frequency of signs and symptoms varies somewhat with gestational age and between developing[1–4] and Western countries.[5–9]

In developing countries, two systematic reviews concluded that in young infants under 60 days old brought to a health-care facility, the most valuable signs and symptoms of sepsis were feeding difficulty, convulsions, fever or hypothermia, change in level of activity, tachypnoea, severe chest in-drawing, grunting and cyanosis.[8, 9] Pallor and poor capillary return were also positively associated with sepsis. These data help community health-care workers decide about hospital referral of sick infants.

In Western countries, septic infants usually present earlier with less florid signs. In a large US study of very low birth-weight infants the positive predictive value for most clinical signs varied from 14% to 20%, while hypotension had a positive predictive value of 31% but only occurred in 5% of babies.[1]

A minority of septicaemic babies has a focal infection, for example, skin abscess or swollen joint, which will not only provide a strong diagnostic indicator but also a likely focus for biopsy and hence a microbiologic diagnosis.

Simple laboratory tests may yield clues to sepsis: 10% of very low birth-weight infants with sepsis had hypoglycaemia and 11% had metabolic acidosis (see Chapter 4).[1]

3.1 Fever or hypothermia

Rectal temperatures measured with a mercury thermometer are the traditional 'gold standard' for temperature measurement in newborns. In one study, axillary temperatures were consistently about 0.27°C (SD 0.20°C) lower than rectal temperatures,[10] but another study using the same electronic device found significant differences between axillary and rectal temperatures.[11] An infrared skin thermometer gave similar readings to a rectal mercury thermometer below 37°C, but concordance was only 74% for readings ≥37°C.[12] Most of these studies study mainly afebrile infants, yet febrile infants are the major clinical concern.

The incidence of fever and hypothermia is gestation-dependent and also differs somewhat between early- and late-onset sepsis. Full-term infants are far more likely to respond to infection with fever than pre-term infants while pre-term infants are more likely to develop hypothermia. In a study of infants with early-onset GBS bacteraemia, 12% of full-term infants had fever at the time of admission compared with only 1% of pre-term infants, whereas the figures for hypothermia were 3% and 13%, respectively.[3] Significantly, about 85% of both full-term and pre-term infants with GBS sepsis had normothermia on admission.[3]

In late-onset sepsis, the reported onset of fever is nearer 50%, while 10–15% of septic infants have hypothermia.[1]

Evidence-Based Neonatal Infections, First Edition. David Isaacs.

Table 3.1 Clinical manifestations of neonatal septicaemia and approximate frequency.

Clinical manifestation	Early-onset sepsis	Late-onset sepsis
Apnoea	+++	+++
Fever	++	+++
Respiratory distress	+++	+++
Hypoxia	++	++
Poor feeding	++	++
Lethargy	++	++
Irritability	++	++
Hypothermia	+	++
Change in level of activity	++	++
Hypotension	+	+
Vomiting	+	+
Diarrhoea	+	+
Jaundice	0	+
Meconium-stained liquor	+	0
Convulsions	+	+
Cyanosis	+	+

Source: Data from References 1–9.

Key:

0	<1%
+	5–10%
++	10–25%
+++	25–55%

Note: The frequency of signs varies with disease severity and between Western and developing countries (see text) but these are the approximate frequencies derived from a literature search.

Question: How significant is fever?

Clearly, the presence of fever or hypothermia may indicate infection, but it may also be due to poor temperature regulation in pre-term infants, in infants with cerebral insults and possibly in dehydration.

Of 100 US infants who developed fever in the first 4 days, 10 had proven bacterial infection, 8 had other signs of infection.[13] Infants were only investigated if fever recurred; the 35 with a single episode of fever remained well. Newborns with temperature ≥39°C had a significantly higher incidence of bacterial infection than newborns with temperature <39°C, but low-grade fever did not exclude infection.[13]

Appleton and Foo described a febrile, full-term, breastfed infant aged 3 days with tachycardia and irritability who had hypernatraemia. The baby fed ravenously from a bottle and the fever resolved. They called this 'dehydration fever'.[14] A retrospective case-control study of 122 Israeli infants aged 1–4 days with fever but no other signs or symptoms of infection found only one infant had infection (GBS in urine culture) and the study reported an association between fever and weight loss, breastfeeding, caesarean section and high birth weight.[15]

Recommendations

- **Full-term infants aged 0–4 days with fever <39°C and no other symptoms can be monitored closely without commencing antibiotics.**
- **If fever resolves and does not recur, the infant should be observed but the risk is low.**
- **Fever ≥39°C is more likely to indicate serious bacterial infection.**
- **Any infant with fever plus one or more other clinical signs of infection should be cultured and treated with empiric antibiotics.**

3.2 Meconium

Meconium is usually sterile. There are two potential links between meconium and infection. Firstly, aspiration of thick meconium may cause airways obstruction and lung collapse, potentially complicated by bacterial pneumonia. There are no RCTs of antibiotics in meconium aspiration syndrome.[16] Secondly, meconium-stained liquor, uncommon in pre-term labour, was described in early-onset *Listeria monocytogenes* neonatal infection and postulated as being specific to listeriosis.[17, 18] Subsequent studies show that meconium-stained liquor can occur with infection due to other organisms and is not common in Listeria infection.[19, 20] Obstetric studies have reported culturing *Ureaplasma urealyticum*, streptococci, *Escherichia coli*, *Candida albicans* and *L. monocytogenes* from amniotic fluid in association with meconium-stained liquor in pre-term labour.[21, 22] In a UK case-control study, early-onset infection was no more common in pre-term babies born after meconium-stained liquor than in controls.[20] In Tanzania in contrast, meconium-stained liquor was an independent predictor of both early- and late-onset infection with *Staphylococcus aureus* and Gram-negative bacilli.[5]

It seems reasonable to conclude that meconium staining of the liquor in pre-term labour should alert the clinician to the possibility of infection with Listeria or other organisms and that empiric therapy if started should include ampicillin or penicillin to cover Listeria.

3.3 Jaundice

Jaundice is common in the first few days of life and likely to be physiologic or due to haemolysis. While it has been described in association with urinary tract infections it is debatable whether jaundice is a useful clinical sign in sepsis.

The two most pertinent clinical questions are:

Question 1: Is jaundice without other clinical features likely to be due to infection?

A highly selective case series from a tertiary Australian children's hospital found 9 of 22 babies (41%) referred with late jaundice had UTI.[23] In subsequent case series of babies with non-haemolytic jaundice, the incidence of UTI was 0 of 306 US babies <3 weeks,[24] 12 of 217 (5.5%) Taiwanese infants <8 weeks[25] and 12 of 160 (7.5%) afebrile jaundiced US infants <8 weeks, including 6 of 12 infants with onset of jaundice >8 days.[26]

A prospective Israeli cohort study found 3 of 93 full-term infants with unexplained jaundice <7 days without other features suggestive of sepsis had bacteraemia.[27]

In a Taiwanese cohort study 50 (2.3%) of 2128 infants with UTI had prolonged jaundice (28 unconjugated, 22 conjugated).[28] All infants >6 weeks had conjugated hyperbilirubinemia.

Recommendation: It is reasonable to perform blood cultures on infants with unexplained early jaundice and urine cultures on infants with late jaundice, but the risk of UTI is low.

Question 2: How likely is it that a septicaemic baby will be jaundiced?

The incidence of jaundice in babies with proven septicaemia was ≤30% in early studies, but this has not proved a consistent or useful clinical feature. In developing countries, jaundice is not common in neonatal sepsis, nor predictive of severe infection.[8] Jaundice was only present in 3–6% of septicaemic US babies[1, 29, 30] and the sole sign of infection in fewer than half.

Comment: Jaundice is rare in septicaemic infants.

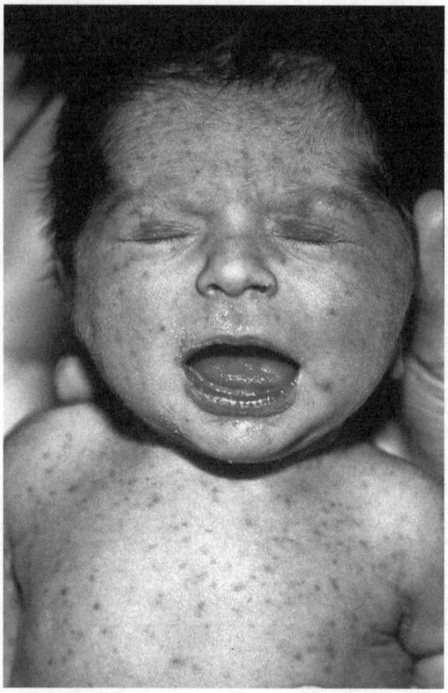

Figure 3.1 Granulomatous petechial rash of a newborn baby with *Listeria monocytogenes* infection. Reprinted with permission from Reference 31.

3.4 Rash

If a baby is born with a petechial rash, congenital infections with cytomegalovirus (CMV), rubella and toxoplasmosis should be considered, as well as non-infectious causes. However, babies born infected with Listeria can present with a clinically similar rash, which is actually an embolic, granulomatous rash (Figure 3.1). Other clinical features such as maternal fever, meconium staining of the liquor, hepatosplenomegaly and respiratory distress may help suggest the diagnosis of Listeria infection.[31] Later development of a petechial rash may be due to septicaemia, endocarditis or rarely meningococcal infection (see Section 14.4.1).

Pyogenic and septicaemia-associated skin lesions are considered in Chapter 13.

3.5 Respiratory signs or symptoms

3.5.1 Apnoea

Apnoea of prematurity occurs in most infants <30 weeks of gestation, in about 50% of babies 30–32 weeks and 10% of infants at 34 weeks.[29] The onset peaks between 5 and 7 days. Apnoea in a pre-term infant on the first day or after 2 weeks is unlikely to be physiologic and should trigger investigation and empiric treatment for sepsis.[32]

In full-term infants, apnoea is a more sinister sign of respiratory or central nervous system pathology or sepsis.[8, 9]

3.5.2 Respiratory distress

Symptoms and signs of respiratory distress include tachypnoea, grunting, chest wall or intercostal recession and cyanosis. Respiratory symptoms from birth in a pre-term baby may be due to hyaline membrane disease (surfactant deficiency), retained lung fluid (transient tachypnoea of the newborn) or sepsis. The radiographic appearance of pneumonia due to GBS or other bacterial pathogens can mimic hyaline membrane disease (see Chapter 8).

Later onset of respiratory distress may be due to bacterial pneumonia or viral or Chlamydial pneumonitis, but is also described in septic infants with normal chest radiographs.[8, 9] Tachypnoea can be due to acidosis or central stimulation in meningitis. The need for empiric treatment will depend on circumstances, but the usual low threshold applies.

References

1. Fanaroff AA, Korones SB, Wright LL, et al. Incidence, presenting features, risk factors and significance of late onset septicemia in very low birth weight infants. The National Institute of Child Health and Human Development Neonatal Research Network. *Pediatr Infect Dis J* 1998; 17:593–598.
2. Healy CM, Palazzi DL, Edwards MS, Campbell JR, Baker CJ. Features of invasive staphylococcal disease in neonates. *Pediatrics* 2004; 114:953–961.
3. Weisman LE, Stoll BJ, Cruess DF, et al. Early-onset group B streptococcal sepsis: a current assessment. *J Pediatr* 1992; 121:428–433.
4. Hamada S, Vearncombe M, McGeer A, Shah PS. Neonatal group B streptococcal disease: incidence, presentation, and mortality. *J Matern Fetal Neonatal Med* 2008; 21:53–57.
5. Kayange N, Kamugisha E, Mwizamholya DL, Jeremiah S, Mshana SE. Predictors of positive blood culture and deaths among neonates with suspected neonatal sepsis in a tertiary hospital, Mwanza-Tanzania. *BMC Pediatr* 2010; 10:39.
6. Weber MW, Carlin JB, Gatchalian S, Lehmann D, Muhe L, Mulholland EK; WHO Young Infants Study Group. Predictors of neonatal sepsis in developing countries. *Pediatr Infect Dis J* 2003; 22:711–717.
7. Young Infants Clinical Signs Study Group. Clinical signs that predict severe illness in children under age 2 months: a multicentre study. *Lancet* 2008; 371:135–142.
8. Opiyo N, English M. What clinical signs best identify severe illness in young infants aged 0-59 days in developing countries? A systematic review. *Arch Dis Child* 2011; 96:1052–1059.
9. Coghill JE, Simkiss DE. Which clinical signs predict severe illness in children less than 2 months of age in resource poor countries? *J Trop Pediatr* 2011; 57:3–8.
10. Voora S, Srinivasan G, Lilien LD, Yeh TF, Pildes RS. Fever in full-term newborns in the first four days of life. *Pediatrics* 1982; 69:40–44.
11. Hissink Muller PC, van Berkel LH, de Beaufort AJ. Axillary and rectal temperature measurements poorly agree in newborn infants. *Neonatology* 2008; 94:31–34.
12. Hutton S, Probst E, Kenyon C, Morse D, Friedman B, Arnold K, et al. Accuracy of different temperature devices in the postpartum population. *J Obstet Gynecol Neonatal Nurs* 2009; 38:42–49.
13. De Curtis M, Calzolari F, Marciano A, Cardilli V, Barba G. Comparison between rectal and infrared skin temperature in the newborn. *Arch Dis Child Fetal Neonatal Ed* 2008; 93:F55-F57.
14. Appleton RE, Foo CK. Dehydration fever in the neonate: a common phenomenon. *Arch Dis Child* 1989; 64:765–766.
15. Maayan-Metzger A, Mazkereth R, Kuint J. Fever in healthy asymptomatic newborns during the first days of life. *Arch Dis Child Fetal Neonatal Ed* 2003; 88:F312–F314.
16. Shivananda S, Murthy P, Shah PS. Antibiotics for neonates born through meconium stained amniotic fluid (Protocol). *Cochrane DB Syst Rev* 2006, (Issue 4). Art. No.: CD006183. doi:10.1002/14651858.CD006183
17. Halliday HL, Hirata T. Perinatal listeriosis: a review of twelve patients. *Am J Obstet Gynecol* 1979; 133:405–410.
18. Lennon D, Lewis B, Mantell C, et al. Epidemic perinatal listeriosis. *Pediatr Infect Dis* 1984; 3:30–34.
19. Scott H, Walker M, Gruslin A. Significance of meconium-stained amniotic fluid in the preterm population. *J Perinatol* 2001; 21:174–177.
20. Tybulewicz AT, Clegg SK, Fonfé GJ, Stenson BJ. Preterm meconium staining of the amniotic fluid: associated findings and risk of adverse clinical outcome. *Arch Dis Child Fetal Neonatal Ed* 2004; 89:F328–F330.
21. Mazor M, Furman B, Wiznitzer A, Shoham-Vardi I, Cohen J, Ghezzi F. Maternal and perinatal outcome of patients with preterm labor and meconium-stained amniotic fluid. *Obstet Gynecol* 1995; 86:830–833.
22. Romero R, Hanaoka S, Mazor M, et al. Meconium-stained amniotic fluid: a risk factor for microbial invasion of the amniotic cavity. *Am J Obstet Gynecol* 1991; 164:859–862.
23. Rooney J, Hill DJ, Danks DM. Jaundice associated with bacterial infection in the newborn. *Am J Dis Child* 1971; 122:39–41.
24. Maisels MJ, Kring E. Risk of sepsis in newborns with severe hyperbilirubinemia. *Pediatrics* 1992; 90:741–743.

25. Chen HT, Jeng MJ, Soong WJ, et al. Hyperbilirubinemia with urinary tract infection in infants younger than eight weeks old. *J Chin Med Assoc* 2011; 74:159–163.
26. Gracia FJ, Nagel AL. Jaundice as an early diagnostic sign of urinary tract infection in infancy. *Pediatrics* 2002; 109:846–851.
27. Linder N, Yatsiv I, Tsur M, et al. Unexplained neonatal jaundice as an early diagnostic sign of septicaemia in the newborn. *J Perinatol* 1988; 8:325–327.
28. Lee HC, Fang SB, Yeung CY, Tsai JD. Urinary tract infections in infants: comparison between those with conjugated vs unconjugated hyperbilirubinaemia. *Ann Trop Paediatr* 2005; 25:277–282.
29. Chavalitdhamrong PO, Escobedo MB, Barton LL, Zarkowsky H, Marshall RE. Hyperbilirubinaemia and bacterial infection in the newborn. A prospective study. *Arch Dis Child* 1975; 50:652–654.
30. Escobedo MB, Barton LL, Marshall RE, Zarkowsky H. The frequency of jaundice in neonatal bacterial infections. *Clin Pediatr* 1974; 13:656–657.
31. Isaacs D, Moxon ER. *Handbook of Neonatal Infections: A Practical Guide.* London: WB Saunders, 1999.
32. Henderson-Smart DJ, Steer PA. Caffeine versus theophylline for apnoea in preterm infants. *Cochrane DB Syst Rev* 2010, (Issue 1). Art. No.: CD000273. doi:10.1002/14651858.CD000273.pub2

CHAPTER 4
Laboratory tests

4.1 Microbiology

It is effectively impossible to practise good neonatal intensive care without reliable microbiology. If clinicians cannot or do not rely on microbiology results they will have insufficient guidance on antimicrobial use, inevitably leading to poor prescribing practices.

4.1.1 Blood cultures

The most important microbiologic test is the blood culture. Blood cultures should always be taken before starting empiric therapy and repeated if the infant does not improve or deteriorates.

Buttery reviewed the use of blood cultures in newborns and older children, concluding that they are sensitive and reliable, although more data are needed about blood volumes.[1]

Since 2000, the advent of automated systems for continuous blood-culture monitoring has improved efficiency, but cultures are rarely positive <12–24 hours.

4.1.1.1 Blood volume in blood cultures

Paediatric blood culture bottle manufacturers recommend using 1 mL of blood, but a UK study found 0.3–0.66 mL was sent.[1] Quantitative blood culture data show bacteraemic newborns have high levels of bacteraemia, particularly with Gram-negative bacilli such as *Escherichia coli*, but also with CoNS.[1] For CoNS, quantitative blood cultures show high-level bacteraemia in clinically infected babies but low-level bacteraemia when CoNS are thought clinically to be contaminants.[2,3] Quantitative blood cultures are expensive and primarily a research tool. Time to positive blood cultures is a useful surrogate measure of level of bacteraemia (Section 4.1.1.3).

An important Mexican study compared 'paired' blood cultures from 173 newborns and 291 infants.[4] A 2.2 mL venous blood sample was divided into 2 mL and 0.2 mL aliquots and inoculated into broth. The 2 mL blood culture was positive on 153 occasions and the microculture on 151 (sensitivity of 0.2 mL microculture compared to 2 mL culture 95%, specificity 99%).[4]

Conclusions for clinicians:
Even low volumes of blood detect neonatal bacteraemia reliably.
Most negative blood cultures are true negatives.

4.1.1.2 Multiple-site blood cultures

North American epidemiologic studies often define true CoNS bacteraemia as two or more positive blood cultures from different sites. In Europe and Australia, multiple-site blood cultures are rarely performed. A retrospective study of 460 newborns with suspected sepsis reported that paired cultures from different sites were helpful in confirming infection in eight infants and excluding it in 10 infants, but the retrospective nature casts doubt on the study's validity.[5] A prospective Canadian study found discordant blood cultures for CoNS in 5 of 100 paired cultures,[5] but the study design has been criticized.[6] In a prospective US study of 216 neonates with suspected sepsis, 269 paired blood cultures (≥1 mL) were taken from different sites. There was one early-onset Listeria infection and 22 late-onset infections, seven with CoNS.[6] Blood cultures were completely concordant for culture-negative and culture-positive infants, for both early- and late-onset sepsis and for all organisms. The authors conclude that two blood cultures from different sites are no more

Evidence-Based Neonatal Infections, First Edition. David Isaacs.

accurate than one blood culture of at least 1 mL volume for detecting neonatal infection.[6]

Blood cultures from central lines are prone to contamination, so simultaneous peripheral blood cultures should also be sent.

4.1.1.3 Time to positive blood cultures

At least 96% of positive blood cultures considered clinically significant grow within 48 hours and 97–99% within 72 hours; organisms which took >72 hours to grow are almost always contaminants.[3,7–15] The higher the level of bacteraemia, the quicker the blood cultures grow, so Gram-negative bacilli grow quicker in blood cultures than Gram-positive organisms.[2,7,15,16] Thus the time to positivity of blood cultures is a clinically useful surrogate measure of the level of bacteraemia and hence the likelihood of true infection.

4.1.1.4 Polymicrobial blood cultures

Polymicrobial paediatric blood cultures are usually but not always contaminated. However, a review of 15 episodes of polymicrobial blood or CSF cultures (3.9% of all culture-proven sepsis) found a significantly higher mortality associated with late-onset polymicrobial sepsis (7 of 10; 70%) than with late-onset monomicrobial sepsis (86 of 370; 23%). Group D streptococci were recovered in eight cases (53%). Five of 10 infants with late-onset polymicrobial infection had gastrointestinal foci; four of five with early-onset infection had prolonged rupture of membranes.[17] A larger study compared 105 episodes of polymicrobial bacteraemia in 102 infants (10% of all neonatal bacteraemia) with episodes of bacteraemia due to a single organism, mainly CoNS.[18] Infants with polymicrobial bacteraemia presented later (mean 37.5 vs. 24 days; $p < 0.001$) and were more likely to have a severe underlying condition and prolonged central venous catheterization. There was no difference in outcome or mortality.[18]

It is potentially hazardous to assume polymicrobial cultures are contaminants. The nature of the organisms isolated may give an important clue to their origin. Gram-negative bacilli suggest bowel or urinary tract origin. Exclusive skin organisms (e.g. CoNS, particularly multiple strains, α-haemolytic streptococci, micrococci, diphtheroids), increase the likelihood of contamination. GBS, Gram-negative bacilli or Candida grown in polymicrobial blood cultures should always be treated. Similarly, an infant with severe gastrointestinal pathology who grows one or more enteric organisms should always be treated. Repeated polymicrobial blood cultures may indicate genuine pathology, but should also raise the sinister possibility of factitious infection (Munchhausen syndrome by proxy).

4.1.2 Surface cultures

The term 'surface cultures' can be confusing. Some use it to mean only cultures from skin (e.g. ear, umbilicus) while some also include mucosal cultures (e.g. nose, nasopharynx, rectum).

Surface cultures can guide decisions regarding antibiotic cessation in suspected early sepsis. Ear and/or umbilical swab cultures may indicate the need for continuing antibiotic therapy in blood-culture-negative infants with suspected early-onset sepsis who are heavily colonized with GBS or Listeria (see Section 5.5.1). Negative surface and systemic cultures effectively exclude early-onset sepsis.

The use of surface cultures for routine surveillance is considered in Chapter 20.

4.1.3 Lumbar puncture

This section considers whether or not to perform lumbar puncture (LP) in suspected or proven sepsis. CSF fluid microscopy, biochemistry and culture interpretation is covered in Chapter 7.

Reasons for performing an immediate LP at the time of a 'septic screen' include the following.

- LP is a ' biopsy': a rapid Gram stain test often alters empiric antibiotic choice
- Infants with meningitis may have negative blood cultures, so delaying LP and only doing LP if blood cultures are positive will miss some infants with meningitis

Arguments for not performing an immediate LP include the following.

- Neonatal meningitis is rare
- LP is potentially harmful, for example, respiratory compromise from manipulating the infant,[19] bleeding, infection
- Delaying LP, treating empirically and only doing LP on infants with positive blood cultures minimizes harms from LP

Question: Is LP necessary in suspected early neonatal sepsis?

Critical questions are LP in respiratory distress syndrome (RDS) and whether delayed LP is a reasonable approach.

A literature search of LP in suspected early-onset sepsis found one non-systematic literature review[20] and 11 observational studies.[21–31] The review,[20] which covered pre-term and full-term infants noted studies did not always distinguish asymptomatic from symptomatic infants.[21–26] The reported incidence of meningitis varied from 0.25 to 1 per 1000 live births.[21–26]

Pre-term infants with respiratory distress from birth are much more likely to have hyaline membrane disease than sepsis. Two US studies evaluated LP in pre-term infants with RDS. In a retrospective study, 1495 (69%) of 2156 newborns admitted with respiratory distress on the first day of life had an LP. Four infants had meningitis (2.2 per 1000 infants with RDS and 2.7 per 1000 of those who had an LP).[21] A small prospective study of 203 consecutive infants with RDS found no cases of meningitis.[22]

In a retrospective US study, 10 (1.6%) of 644 newborns with maternal risk factors and **clinical signs** had meningitis, 3 (2.1%) of 145 with signs but no risk factors and none of 284 with risk factors alone.[22]

A retrospective 5-year US study reported 43 infants <72 hours old with meningitis out of a total population of 169 849 (0.25 per 1000 live births). The authors claimed a **delayed approach** to LP would have missed or delayed the diagnosis of meningitis in 16 infants (37% of all meningitis), including five pre-term infants with RDS (the total RDS population was not given).[24] In two large US studies the proportion of infants with meningitis who had negative blood cultures was 28% of infants (12 of 43) in one[25] and 38% (35 of 92) of infants >33 weeks of gestation (early- and late-onset not differentiated) in another.[26]

Conclusions:

- **Symptomatic infants <72 hours old: immediate LP is strongly recommended, because the incidence of meningitis is 1–2% and about a third of infants with meningitis have negative blood cultures**
- **Pre-term infants with RDS and no other clinical signs of infection: LP debatable as the risk of meningitis is low, but not zero, and blood cultures do not reliably identify infants with meningitis**
- **Developing countries: the risk of early-onset meningitis is probably high although the data are inconclusive**
- **If blood cultures are positive with an organism that causes meningitis and LP was not done, we recommend LP to guide the duration of therapy**

Question: Is LP necessary in suspected late-onset neonatal sepsis?

A literature search found one non-systematic literature review[27] and eight observational studies.[19,22–25,28–30] Neonatal meningitis is relatively rare in Western countries. CoNS which cause >50% of late-onset sepsis almost never cause meningitis. The review found 1.3–3.5% of infants with late sepsis has meningitis. The incidence of late-onset sepsis and the incidence of meningitis both increase with decreasing gestational age.[27] The review estimated that between 30 and 90 infants being investigated for sepsis would need an LP to detect one with meningitis.[27] However, the clinical diagnosis of neonatal meningitis is unreliable and relying on blood cultures in suspected late-onset sepsis, will cause clinicians to miss infants with meningitis.

The rate of negative blood cultures was 34% (45 of 134) of infants <1500 g with late-onset meningitis in a large US multicentre study[24] and, in two studies in which early- and late-onset meningitis were not clearly differentiated, 28% (8 of 29) in Ireland[31] and 38% (35 of 92 infants >33 weeks of gestation) in a US multicentre study.[25]

The incidence of late-onset meningitis in developing countries is unknown: very limited data suggests that meningitis occurs in 3–4% of neonates with late-onset sepsis.[22, 23] In one study, 8 (27%) of 30 infants with late-onset septicaemia who were not initially lumbar punctured were diagnosed later with meningitis.[30]

Conclusions:

- **Routine LP is strongly recommended in the evaluation of infants with suspected late-onset sepsis, because the incidence of meningitis is 1.3–4% and about a third of infants with meningitis have negative blood cultures**
- **In developing countries, the risk of late-onset meningitis is probably high, although data are scanty**

- **LP is strongly recommended for infants with late-onset sepsis and blood cultures positive with an organism that causes meningitis who had no LP, to guide the duration of therapy and prognosis**

4.1.4 Urine culture

Neonatal UTI is primarily a late-onset infection. In early-onset sepsis positive urine cultures are rare and usually reflect concomitant bacteraemia with presumed embolic renal spread, rather than primary UTI.[32] Urine culture is not routinely recommended in suspected early-onset sepsis.

In contrast, urine culture should be routine when evaluating infants for suspected late-onset sepsis. The incidence of neonatal UTI is 0.1–1% and may be up to 10% in low birth-weight infants. Concomitant bacteraemia is relatively uncommon, so UTI will be missed if urine culture is omitted and empiric antibiotics given. This will delay the diagnosis of any associated structural urinary tract abnormalities.

Question: What is the optimum method for collecting urine?

Bag specimens are only useful to rule out UTI when antibiotics are not being started, for example, a clinically well infant with prolonged jaundice. They are too easily contaminated to be useful in suspected sepsis when empiric antibiotics are started.

We found two randomized controlled trials (RCTs) comparing suprapubic bladder aspiration (SPA) with urethral catheterization. In one study, urethral catheterization successfully obtained ≥2 mL of urine from all 50 infants <6 months old randomized, and also from 27 infants who failed SPA. Suprapubic aspiration was only 46% successful.[33] In a small neonatal study, SPA was successful in 11 of 17 (65%) and catheter in 13 of 16 or 81% attempts ($p > 0.05$).[34] Observational studies report higher contamination rates with catheter specimens, but no difference was found in these small RCTs.

Two RCTs blindly assessed pain on a visual analogue scale or by brow-bulging in full-term and pre-term infants undergoing SPA or catheterization. Pain was greater for full-term or pre-term infants with SPA.[35, 36]

The combined success rate in obtaining urine from the three RCTs is 44 of 69 (63.8%) by SPA and 51 of 63 (81%) by catheter ($p = 0.03$, Fisher exact).[34–36]

Recommendation: Urethral catheterization is less painful and more effective than suprapubic aspiration for both pre-term and full-term infants and is the collection method of choice for suspected late-onset sepsis.

4.1.5 Gastric aspirates

Gastric aspirate microscopy for pus cells and/or bacteria has a low sensitivity (71–89%) and specificity (49–87%) for rapid diagnosis of early sepsis.[37] An infant with early-onset respiratory distress whose gastric aspirate is negative for pus cells and bacteria on microscopy is at low risk for early-onset infection, which is potentially useful for deciding not to treat with empiric antibiotics. Often, however, timeliness in obtaining the microscopy result to help clinical decision-making is a problem, particularly outside normal laboratory working hours.

4.1.6 Tracheal aspirates

Question: Are tracheal aspirate microscopy and cultures useful in guiding antibiotic therapy?

Bacteria seen on tracheal secretion Gram stain in neonates <12 hours old had 74% sensitivity and 47% predictive accuracy for bacteraemia in a 1984 US study.[32] The specificity was 98%. This suggests limited usefulness in guiding management of possible early sepsis.

Regarding late sepsis, a positive tracheal aspirate does not predict that an infant on long-term ventilation will develop sepsis: a well baby is as likely to be colonized as a sick one.[32,38–46] Furthermore, the organisms grown from tracheal aspirates correlate poorly with those in blood cultures.[39, 40]

However, routine respiratory tract cultures may identify particularly virulent colonizing organisms, for example, Pseudomonas, and particularly multi-resistant organisms for infection control purposes and to guide antibiotic use if the infant develops suspected sepsis (see Section 20.1.1).

A baby without pneumonia should not be treated merely because of a positive tracheal aspirate culture (see Chapter 8). Treat infection, not colonization.

Recommendation: Selective use of tracheal aspirates can be valuable to monitor colonization.

There is research interest in identifying the biomarkers of neutrophil activation in tracheal aspirates to predict which mechanically ventilated infants will develop sepsis.[41]

4.2 Rapid tests for sepsis

Various haematologic, biochemical and microbiologic tests have been studied or are being developed in order to identify rapidly infants with neonatal sepsis and also to identify non-infected infants.

A reliable abnormal test result can be used as a basis to '**rule in**' sepsis and start empiric antibiotics. A reliable normal test can be used to '**rule out**' sepsis.

The danger of over-reliance on a normal test result to rule out sepsis is that septic babies may be missed and treatment delayed. In clinical practice, the clinician can only afford to rely on a test or combination of tests with 100% sensitivity (i.e. identifies every infected infant) and none has been described.

There is often a trade-off between sensitivity and specificity: more sensitive tests are less specific. Combining tests as a **'sepsis screen'** increases sensitivity at the cost of decreased specificity. Many authors have reported using sepsis screens to decrease antibiotic use by improving identification of uninfected babies. However, sepsis screens are expensive.

An arguably safer and more cost-effective approach is to start many infants on antibiotics but stop them after 48–72 hours if systemic cultures are negative (see Section 5.5.1).

4.3 Haematologic tests

4.3.1 White cell counts

Manroe's seminal study of peripheral blood white cell counts identified early-onset neutropenia and the immature to total (I:T) neutrophil ratio as the two best predictors of neonatal infection.[42] The risk of bacterial infection in an infant <72 hours old with respiratory distress without asphyxia was 84% for neutropenia and 82% for an I:T ratio ≥0.2 (Figure 4.1).[42]

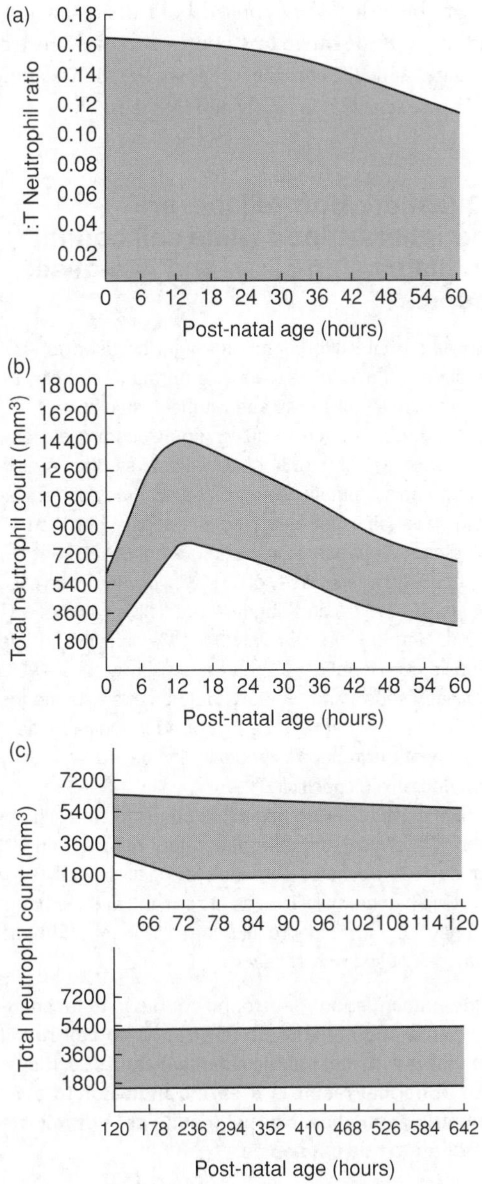

Figure 4.1 Reference ranges for normal white cell parameters in healthy neonates (normal ranges shaded). (a) Immature to total (I:T) ratio; (b) total neutrophil count to 60 hours; (c) total neutrophil count from 60 hours to 28 days. Adapted from Reference 42.

Manroe's values have been evaluated for both early- and late-onset sepsis and for pre-term as well as full-term infants. A Texas group developed new reference ranges, but when they applied both their new range and the Manroe range to 192 pre-term and full-term neonates with 202 episodes of sepsis, the Manroe range was more sensitive for early and late sepsis.[43]

Question: How reliable are peripheral blood white cell counts in diagnosing early- and late-onset sepsis?

An abnormal white cell count might be used to start antibiotics ('rule in' sepsis) or a normal count can be used to 'rule out' sepsis and withhold antibiotics.

A literature search found two non-Cochrane systematic reviews[43, 44] and 34 observational studies. A non-Cochrane systematic review of the accuracy of haematologic variables for early and late sepsis identified 12 studies.[43] Neutropenia in the first 72 hours had sensitivity of 63–89%, specificity of 68–98%, positive predictive value of 11–67% and negative predictive value of 88–99%. Neutropenia was only 33–44% sensitive in late sepsis. An I:T ratio $\geq$0.2 had a sensitivity of 86–90% for early sepsis and 18–90% for late sepsis. Using the presence of either neutropenia or neutrophilia to identify infants with sepsis modestly increased sensitivity but decreased specificity.[43]

Serial white cell counts might be useful, in conjunction with clinical and other laboratory results. In a US study 1539 neonates screened for possible early sepsis who had normal I:T ratios at zero and at 8–12 hours all had negative blood cultures at 24 hours and none was diagnosed with sepsis.[45]

Recommendation: Neutrophil counts to detect neutropenia and immature:total (I:T) white cell ratios are tests with reasonable sensitivity and specificity. An abnormal result is a strong indicator to start empiric antibiotics. Normal results are not reliable enough to rule out sepsis.

4.3.1.1 Neutropenia

Neutropenia in the first few days of life may be due to overwhelming infection. In very low birth-weight infants, however, neutropenia is usually secondary to growth retardation or maternal pre-eclampsia. In a retrospective cohort study, 38% of 338 babies <1000 g had one or more neutrophil counts <1000/μL.[46] Neutropenia lasted <1 day in 57% and 1–7.5 days in the rest.

Neutropenia age <3 days was associated with infection in only 6% of infants and 68% were either small for gestational age (<10th percentile) or had pregnancy-induced hypertension. In contrast 31% of infants with neutropenia >3 days had necrotizing enterocolitis (NEC) and 19% had bacterial infection.[46]

Only 9 (5.5%) of 162 infants <1500 g with proven bloodstream infection in one study were neutropenic, 6 of 30 (20%) with Gram-negative sepsis, 3 of 113 (2.6%) and none of 19 with fungal infection.[47]

4.3.2 Thrombocytopenia

Early thrombocytopenia (platelets $<150 \times 10^9$/L) is more common than late thrombocytopenia.[41] Early thrombocytopenia is usually a reflection of impaired fetal megakaryocytopoiesis associated with placental insufficiency, for example, growth restriction, maternal hypertension. The commonest causes of severe early-onset thrombocytopenia (platelets $<50 \times 10^9$/L) are immune thrombocytopenia, congenital infections (see Chapter 18) and perinatal asphyxia. In contrast, about 90% of cases of severe thrombocytopenia presenting after the first few days of life are due to late-onset bacterial sepsis, NEC, or both.[41]

Thrombocytopenia is relatively uncommon in sepsis,[36, 48] so its absence is not a useful basis to rule out infection. In contrast, presence of late thrombocytopenia, particularly if severe ($<50 \times 10^{9/}$/L), is a strong indicator of probable infection or NEC.

Question: Can the presence of thrombocytopenia help predict the organism causing sepsis?

In an Italian study of septic infants <1500 g, thrombocytopenia $<80 \times 10^{9/}$/L occurred in 16% of infants with Gram-negative, 18% with Gram-positive (16% of CoNS) and 20% with fungal infections.[48] In a US study of infants <1500 g, a higher proportion of infants with Gram-negative or fungal sepsis had thrombocytopenia compared to those with Gram-positive infection, but because Gram-positive bacteria caused 76% of all infections, the distinction was not clinically useful.[49] In India, however, Gram-negative sepsis predominates and the incidence of thrombocytopenia is high. In one study of infected infants <1500 g, 67% had thrombocytopenia, which was more common in infants with Gram-negative (71% of total) and fungal (9%)

infections.[50] In another Indian study, Klebsiella caused 62.5% of 200 nosocomial infections, and 60% of the infants had thrombocytopenia. However, thrombocytopenia was even more common (90%) in 31 infants with concurrent bacterial and fungal infections, whereas it was present in 33% of infants with CoNS infection.[51]

Thus thrombocytopenia can occur with CoNS, Gram-negative and fungal infection and the relative likelihood depends on local epidemiology and on individual infant factors such as gestational age and prior antibiotic use.

Recommendation: Late, severe thrombocytopenia is a strong indication to start antimicrobials but both Gram-negative and Gram-positive covers are essential, while empiric antifungals should be considered in high-risk infants.

4.4 Biochemical and immunologic tests

4.4.1 Acute phase reactants

4.4.1.1 Serum C-reactive protein

C-reactive protein (CRP) is a protein produced by the liver in response to infectious and non-infectious inflammatory processes. It is a non-specific, acute phase reactant synthesized within 6–8 hours of tissue damage with a half-life of 19 hours. The serum CRP is known to rise after perinatal asphyxia, surgery and other causes of inflammation as well as infection.[52, 54]

Question: Is a normal serum CRP level a reliable enough test to rule out infection in infants with suspected early- or late-onset neonatal infection?

A literature search found three non-Cochrane reviews of diagnostic tests for neonatal sepsis which included CRP.[36, 44, 54] When early and late sepsis were clearly differentiated, the sensitivity of CRP for early sepsis ranged from 43% to 90% and for late sepsis from 57% to 80%, while the specificity was 61–87% and 48–61%, respectively.[36] The negative predictive value varied from 38% to 98% but was mostly 85–95%.

A US paper reported that infants with three serial daily CRP measurements were very unlikely to have proven infection. By this time culture results will be negative, so serial CRP measurements are not clinically useful in this context.[55]

We conclude that CRP is insufficiently sensitive to be used as a stand-alone 'rule-out' diagnostic test for early- or late-onset sepsis.

The use of CRP in conjunction with other tests as a sepsis screen is considered below (Section 4.4.3).

Recommendation: A normal serum CRP cannot be used as the sole test to rule out early- or late-onset neonatal infection because the test sensitivity is too low.

Question: Can an abnormal serum CRP level be used as a reliable basis to start or continue antibiotics?

There is little value in measuring CRP in infants who will be treated with antibiotics anyway. CRP might be most useful to 'rule in' sepsis in infants with possible sepsis. The positive predictive value (the proportion of subjects with a positive test result who truly have sepsis) for CRP in one systematic review varied from 13% to 100% but was mostly around 50% for both early and late sepsis.[36] Using an abnormal CRP as a basis to decide which patients to treat will therefore mean that many infants without infection will be treated with antibiotics. The harm can be minimized by stopping antibiotics after 48–72 hours if cultures are negative.

Recommendation 1: Do not measure serum CRP unless the result will influence care. For an infant with possible sepsis, an abnormal serum CRP result is reasonable grounds for starting antibiotics.

Measuring serum CRP to determine when to stop antibiotics is widely preached and practiced. It replaces the gold standard for infection (a positive blood or CSF culture) with CRP as the new gold standard without evidence. Indeed elevated CRP is known to be non-specifically stimulated by many non-infectious inflammatory stimuli.

In a German study, infants with negative blood cultures at 48 hours but with a serum CRP >10 mg/L were designated as 'probably infected' (without reporting clinical features) and randomized to receive five additional days of antibiotics or to stop antibiotics when the daily CRP returned to normal.[52] As will be discussed in Chapter 5, studies suggest it is safe to stop antibiotics at 48 hours if systemic cultures are negative and the infant well.[56] Measuring the CRP at 48–72 hours in infants with negative blood and/or CSF cultures can only prolong antibiotic duration, not shorten it, with no added benefit.

Recommendation 2: Serum CRP should not be used to decide when to stop antibiotics in infants with negative blood and/or CSF cultures.

4.4.1.2 Procalcitonin

Procalcitonin is a peptide precursor of calcitonin, a hormone involved with calcium homoeostasis. Its physiologic function in infection is unknown. It is produced by parafollicular cells of the thyroid and by neuroendocrine cells in the lung and the intestine.[57] Procalcitonin serum levels rise rapidly in response to inflammatory stimuli, including endotoxin and other bacterial products, and it has been investigated as a marker of bacterial infections, including neonatal infection.[57] Procalcitonin can be detected in the plasma of volunteers within 2 hours of an endotoxin injection.[58]

Question: Is serum procalcitonin a useful test in the diagnosis of infants with suspected neonatal infection?

A literature search found two non-Cochrane systematic reviews with meta-analyses[53, 59] and 40 studies that measured procalcitonin levels in sepsis.

A systematic review and meta-analysis included 22 studies with adequate data to evaluate the sensitivity and specificity of procalcitonin in neonatal sepsis.[53] A big weakness is that most studies included culture-negative infants with 'clinical sepsis'.[53] Umbilical cord blood procalcitonin had 69–88% sensitivity and 72–98% specificity for early-onset sepsis in three studies which all included infants with clinical sepsis. The sensitivity of serum procalcitonin in early-onset sepsis varied widely from 53% to 100% and specificity from 72% to 100%.[53]

The sensitivity in proven late-onset sepsis was 44–100% (mostly around 80%) and sensitivity 37–100% (mostly 80–90%).[53]

In one review, procalcitonin was somewhat more sensitive than CRP in diagnosing late-onset infection (pooled sensitivity 72% vs. 55%).[59]

In conclusion, as with CRP, there should be good grounds for performing a test, and the value of procalcitonin is far from clear. A normal calcitonin level cannot be used to exclude sepsis and most infants with suspected sepsis will be started on antibiotics regardless of the procalcitonin (or CRP) level.

Recommendations: Routine procalcitonin measurement is not recommended in suspected sepsis. However, for an infant with possible sepsis, an abnormal serum procalcitonin result is strong grounds for starting antibiotics.

4.4.2 Cytokines

Many different cytokines have been evaluated as potential tests for neonatal infection, including interleukins IL-1β, Il-6, IL-8, IL-10 and IL-12, tumour necrosis factor (TNF)-α and newer cytokines such as resistin, visfatin and calprotectin.[54, 60, 61–65]

4.4.2.1 Interleukin-6 (IL-6)

IL-6 has been evaluated in early and late sepsis. The sensitivity for detecting culture-positive early sepsis in a German study was 67% and specificity 78%.[65] In a Hong Kong study, IL-6 had a higher sensitivity (89%) and negative predictive value (91%) in late-onset sepsis than other markers.[60] The sensitivity and specificity do not warrant using IL-6 alone, but it has been used in combination with CRP and other tests to improve sensitivity.

4.4.3 Cell surface markers

Advances in flow cytometry have enabled researchers to study the expression of cell surface markers, particularly CD64 and CD11b, in neonates.[66] Neutrophil CD64 was reported to have 96% sensitivity for clinical early-onset infection[67] and 95% sensitivity for proven late-onset infection.[68] The need for expensive specialist equipment severely limits the usefulness of these tests.

4.4.4 Combinations of tests as a sepsis screen

Two systematic reviews examined the reliability of combinations of one or more tests in suspected neonatal sepsis.[36, 54] One review found seven studies of combinations of haematologic tests and CRP in early and/or late sepsis.[36] Sensitivity was only 23–73% and specificity 45–98%. A subsequent review reported sensitivities of 81–97% and specificity of 93% for the combination of IL-6, CRP and the neutrophil cell surface marker CD64, of 93% and 88–96% respectively for IL-6 and/or CRP and 80% and 87% for IL-8 and/or CRP.[54] Combining CRP, IL-6 and procalcitonin gave a sensitivity for detecting late-onset sepsis of 98.3% and negative predictive value of 98.6%, so a baby that has all three tests negative has a 1.4% risk of being infected.[69] The costs of the tests may outweigh the benefits.

4.5 Molecular assays

Cultures suffer from some delay in diagnosis. New molecular assays can potentially give results within 12 hours. However, claims that molecular assays may be more sensitive than culture need to be weighed against the possibility that they are so sensitive they are detecting contaminants.

Molecular assays to detect pathogens are based on hybridization or amplification. Hybridization-based methods (e.g. fluorescence *in situ* hybridization or FISH) have not been evaluated formally in the diagnosis of neonatal sepsis, but amplification methods such as the polymerase chain reaction (PCR) have been studied. PCR is used to amplify specific target regions in the microbial genome. Broad-range PCR targets the 16S ribosomal RNA gene, a gene preserved in all bacteria, with conserved and variable regions. The initial PCR targets the conserved region. If positive, the species can be identified by targeting the variable regions using genus- or species-specific assays.[70]

The different amplification methods evaluated in the diagnosis of neonatal sepsis are the following.

- Broad-range PCR: PCR amplification strategies targeting conserved regions, for example, 16S rRNA in bacteria
- Real-time PCR: amplification of the template is monitored in real time
- PCR followed by post-PCR sequencing or hybridization
- Multiplex PCR: amplification directed against multiple organisms simultaneously
- Species- and genus-specific assays: bacterial and fungal PCR assays.[68]

Question: In infants with suspected sepsis are molecular assays compared with conventional culture reliable for the diagnosis of infection?

A systematic review of molecular assays assessed whether they have sufficient sensitivity (specified as >0.98) and specificity (>0.95) to replace microbial cultures in the diagnosis of neonatal sepsis.[70] The review of 23 eligible studies found the mean sensitivity was 0.90 (95% CI: 0.78–0.95%) and specificity 0.96 (95% CI: 0.94–0.97%), which did not meet the pre-specified criteria. Real-time PCR and broad-range conventional PCR were more sensitive and specific than other assays. There were insufficient data to evaluate whether results varied depending on gestational age or the organisms causing sepsis.[70]

Recommendation: Currently molecular assays are not sufficiently sensitive and specific for routine use in diagnosing neonatal infection.

4.6 Proteomics and gene expression profiling

Several novel tests are not yet ready for general clinical use, but show promise for early detection of infected infants. The most promising are new combinations of biomarkers identified by proteomics-based research and the use of gene expression profiling to detect infected infants.[71]

References

1. Buttery JP. Blood cultures in newborns and children: optimising an everyday test. *Arch Dis Child Fetal Neonatal Ed* 2002; 87:F25–F28.
2. St Geme III JW, Bell LM, Baumgart S, D'Angio CT, Harris CM. Distinguishing sepsis from blood culture contamination in young infants with blood cultures growing coagulase-negative staphylococci. *Pediatrics* 1990; 86:157–162.
3. Sabui T, Tudehope DI, Tilse M. Clinical significance of quantitative blood cultures in newborn infants. *J Paediatr Child Health* 1999; 35:578–581.
4. Solorzano-Santos F, Miranda-Novales MG, Leanos-Miranda B, Diaz-Ponce H, Palacios-Saucedo G. A blood micro-culture system for the diagnosis of bacteremia in pediatric patients. *Scand J Infect Dis* 1998; 30:481–483.

5. Wiswell TE, Hachey WE. Multiple site blood cultures in the initial evaluation for neonatal sepsis during the first week of life. *Pediatr Infect Dis J* 1991; 10:365–369.
6. Struthers S, Underhill H, Albersheim S, Greenberg D, Dobson S. A comparison of two versus one blood culture in the diagnosis and treatment of coagulase-negative staphylococcus in the neonatal intensive care unit. *J Perinatol* 2002; 22:547–549.
7. Sarkar S, Bhagat I, DeCristofaro JD, Wiswell TE, Spitzer AR. A study of the role of multiple site blood cultures in the evaluation of neonatal sepsis. *J Perinatol* 2006; 26: 18–22.
8. Guerti K, Devos H, Ieven MM, Mahieu LM. Time to positivity of neonatal blood cultures: fast and furious?. *J Med Microbiol* 2011; 60:446–453.
9. Jardine L, Davies MW, Faoagali J. Incubation time required for neonatal blood cultures to become positive. *J Paediatr Child Health* 2006; 42:797–802.
10. Kumar Y, Qunibi M, Neal T, Yoxall C. Time to positivity of neonatal blood cultures. *Arch Dis Child Fetal Neonatal Ed* 2001; 85:F182–F186.
11. Hurst MK, Yoder BA. Detection of bacteremia in young infants: is 48 hours adequate? *Pediatr Infect Dis J* 1995; 14:711–713.
12. Kurlat I, Stoll BJ, McGowan Jr JE. Time to positivity for detection of bacteremia in neonates. *J Clin Microbiol* 1989; 27:1068–1071.
13. Pichichero MD, Todd JK. Neonatal bacteremia. *J Pediatrics* 1979; 94:958–960.
14. Janjindamai W, Phetpisal S. Time to positivity of blood culture in newborn infants. *Southeast Asian J Trop Med Public Health* 2006; 37:171–176.
15. Garcia-Prats JA, Cooper TR, Schneider VF, Stager CE, Hansen TN. Rapid detection of microorganisms in blood cultures of newborn infants utilizing an automated blood culture system. *Pediatrics* 2000; 105:523–527.
16. Gaur AH, Flynn PM, Giannini MA, Shenep JL, Hayden RT. Difference in time to detection: a simple method to differentiate catheter-related from non-catheter-related bloodstream infection in immunocompromised pediatric patients. *Clin Infect Dis* 2003; 37:469–475.
17. Faix RG, Kovarik SM. Polymicrobial sepsis among intensive care nursery infants. *J Perinatol* 1989; 9:131–136.
18. Bizzarro MJ, Dembry LM, Baltimore RS, Gallagher PG. Matched case-control analysis of polymicrobial bloodstream infection in a neonatal intensive care unit. *Infect Control Hosp Epidemiol* 2008; 29:914–920.
19. Visser VE, Hall RT. Lumbar puncture in the evaluation of suspected neonatal sepsis. *J Pediatr* 1980; 96:1063–1067.
20. Fielkow S, Reuter S. Gotoff SP. Cerebrospinal fluid examination in symptom free infants with risk factor for infection. *J Pediatr* 1991; 119:971–973.
21. Ajayi OA. Mokuolu OA. Evaluation of neonates with risk factor for infection/suspected sepsis: is lumbar puncture necessary in the first 72 hours of life? *Trop Med Int Health* 1997; 2:284–288.
22. Kumar P, Sarkar S, Narang A. Role of routine lumbar puncture in neonatal sepsis. *J Paediatr Child Health* 1995; 31: 8–10.
23. Shiva F, Mosaffa N, Khabbaz R, Padyab M. Lumbar puncture in neonates under and over 72 hours of age. *J Coll Physicians Surg Pak* 2006; 16:525–528.
24. Stoll BJ, Hansen N, Fanaroff AA, et al. To tap or not to tap: high likelihood of meningitis without sepsis among very low birth weight infants. *Pediatrics* 2004; 113:1181–1186.
25. Garges HP, Moody MA, Cotten CM, et al. Neonatal meningitis: what is the correlation among cerebrospinal fluid cultures, blood cultures, and cerebrospinal fluid parameters? *Pediatrics* 2006; 117:1094–1100.
26. Isaacs D, Barfield C, Grimwood K, McPhee AJ, Minutillo C, Tudehope DI. Systemic bacterial and fungal infections in infants in Australian neonatal units. Australian Study Group for Neonatal units. *Med J Aust* 1995; 162:198–201.
27. Malbon K, Mohan R, Nicholl R. Should a neonate with possible late onset infection always have a lumbar puncture? *Arch Dis Child* 2006; 91:75–76.
28. Hristeva L, Bowler I, Booy R, King A, Wilkinson AR. Value of cerebrospinal fluid examination in the diagnosis of meningitis in the newborn. *Arch Dis Child* 1992; 69:514–517.
29. Schwersenski J, McIntyre L, Bauer C. Lumbar puncture frequency and cerebrospinal fluid analysis in the neonate. *Am J Dis Child* 1991; 145:54–58.
30. Hoque MM, Ahmed AS, Chowdhury MA, Darmstadt GL, Saha SK. Septicemic neonates without lumbar puncture: what are we missing? *J Trop Pediatr* 2006; 52:63–65.
31. Bell AH, Brown D, Halliday HL, McClure G, McReid M. Meningitis in the newborn – a 14 year review. *Arch Dis Child.* 1989; 64:873–874.
32. Sherman MP, Chance KH, Goetzman BW. Gram's stains of tracheal secretions predict neonatal bacteremia. *Am J Dis Child* 1984; 138:848–850.
33. Pollack Jr CV, Pollack ES, Andrew ME. Suprapubic bladder aspiration versus urethral catheterization in ill infants: success, efficiency and complication rates. *Ann Emerg Med* 1994; 23:225–230.
34. Tobiansky R, Evans N. A randomized controlled trial of two methods for collection of sterile urine in neonates. *J Pediatr Child Health* 1998; 34:460–462.
35. Kozer E, Rosenbloom E, Goldman D, Lavy G, Rosenfeld N, Goldman M. Pain in infants who are younger than 2 months during suprapubic aspiration and transurethral bladder catheterization: a randomized, controlled study. *Pediatrics* 2006; 118:e51–e56.
36. El-Naggar W, Yiu A, Mohamed A, et al. Comparison of pain during two methods of urine collection in preterm infants. *Pediatrics* 2010; 125:1224–1229.
37. Fowlie PW, Schmidt B. Diagnostic tests for bacterial infection from birth to 90 days – a systematic review. *Arch Dis Child Fetal Neonatal Ed* 1998; 78:F92–F98.
38. Lau YL, Hey E. Sensitivity and specificity of daily tracheal aspirate cultures in predicting organisms causing bacteremia

in ventilated neonates. *Pediatr Infect Dis J* 1991; 10:290–294.

39. Webber S, Lindsell D, Wilkinson AR, Hope PL, Dobson SR, Isaacs D. Neonatal pneumonia. *Arch Dis Child* 1990; 65:207–211.
40. Slagle TA, Bifano EM, Wolf JW, Gross SJ. Routine endotracheal cultures for the prediction of sepsis in ventilated babies. *Arch Dis Child* 1989; 64:34–38.
41. Chakravorty S, Roberts I. How I manage neonatal thrombocytopenia. *Br J Haematol* 2012; 156:155–162.
42. Manroe BL, Weinberg AG, Rosenfeld CR, Browne R. The neonatal blood count in health and disease. I. Reference values for neutrophilic cells. *J Pediatr* 1979; 95: 89–98.
43. Engle WD, Rosenfeld CR, Mouzinho A, Risser RC, Zeray F, Sanchez PJ. Circulating neutrophils in septic preterm neonates: comparison of two reference ranges. *Pediatrics* 1997; 99:E10.
44. Da Silva O, Ohlsson A, Kenyon C. Accuracy of leukocyte indices and C-reactive protein for diagnosis of neonatal sepsis: a critical review. *Pediatr Infect Dis J* 1995; 14:362–366.
45. Murphy K, Weiner J. Use of leukocyte counts in evaluation of early-onset neonatal sepsis. *Pediatr Infect Dis J* 2011; 31:16–19.
46. Christensen RD, Henry E, Wiedmeier SE, Stoddard RA, Lambert DK. Low blood neutrophil concentrations among extremely low birth weight neonates: data from a multihospital health-care system. *J Perinatol* 2006; 26:682–687.
47. Sarkar S, Bhagat I, Hieber S, Donn SM. Can neutrophil responses in very low birth weight infants predict the organisms responsible for late-onset bacterial or fungal sepsis? *J Perinatol* 2006; 26:501–505.
48. Manzoni P, Mostert M, Galletto P, et al. Is thrombocytopenia suggestive of organism-specific response in neonatal sepsis? *Pediatr Int* 2009; 51:206–210.
49. Guida JD, Kunig AM, Leef KH, McKenzie SE, Paul DA. Platelet count and sepsis in very low birth weight neonates: is there an organism-specific response? *Pediatrics* 2003; 111:1411–1415.
50. Bhat MA, Bhat JI, Kawoosa MS, Ahmad SM, Ali SW. Organism-specific platelet response and factors affecting survival in thrombocytopenic very low birth weight babies with sepsis. *J Perinatol* 2009; 29:702–708.
51. Charoo BA, Iqbal JI, Iqbal Q, Mushtaq S, Bhat AW, Nawaz I. Nosocomial sepsis-induced late onset thrombocytopenia in a neonatal tertiary care unit: a prospective study. *Hematol Oncol Stem Cell Ther* 2009; 2:349–353.
52. Ehl S, Gering B, Bartmann P, Högel J, Pohlandt F. C-reactive protein is a useful marker for guiding duration of antibiotic therapy in suspected neonatal bacterial infection. *Pediatrics* 1997; 99:216–221.
53. Yu Z, Liu J, Sun Q, Qiu Y, Han S, Guo X. The accuracy of the procalcitonin test for the diagnosis of neonatal sepsis: a meta-analysis. *Scand J Infect Dis* 2010; 42:723–733.
54. Mishra UK, Jacobs SE, Doyle LW, Garland SM. Newer approaches to the diagnosis of early onset neonatal sepsis. *Arch Dis Child Fetal Neonatal Ed* 2006; 91:F208–F212.
55. Benitz WE, Han MY, Madan A, Ramachandra P. Serial serum C-reactive protein levels in the diagnosis of neonatal infection. *Pediatrics* 1998; 102:E41.
56. Saini SS, Dutta S, Ray P, Narang A. Short course versus 7-day course of intravenous antibiotics for probable neonatal septicemia: a pilot, open-label, randomized controlled trial. *Indian Pediatr* 2011; 48:19–24.
57. van Rossum AM, Wulkan RW, Oudeslys-Murphy AM. Procalcitonin as an early marker of infection in neonates and children. *Lancet Infect Dis* 2004; 4 620–630.
58. Dandona P. Nix D, Wilson MF, et al. Procalcitonin increase after endotoxin injection in normal subjects. *J Clin Endocrinol Metab* 1994; 79:1605–1608.
59. Vouloumanou EK, Plessa E, Karageorgopoulos DE, Mantadakis E, Falagas ME. Serum procalcitonin as a diagnostic marker for neonatal sepsis: a systematic review and meta-analysis. *Intensive Care Med* 2011; 37:747–762.
60. Ng PC, Cheng SH, Chui KM, et al. Diagnosis of late onset neonatal sepsis with cytokines, adhesion molecule, and C-reactive protein in preterm very low birth weight infants. *Arch Dis Child Fetal Neonatal Ed* 1997; 77:F221–F227.
61. Chiesa C, Pellegrini G, Panero A, et al. C-reactive protein, interleukin-6, and procalcitonin in the immediate postnatal period: influence of illness severity, risk status, antenatal and perinatal complications, and infection. *Clin Chem* 2003; 49:60–68.
62. Cekmez F, Canpolat FE, Cetinkaya M, et al. Diagnostic value of resistin and visfatin, in comparison with C-reactive protein, procalcitonin and interleukin-6 in neonatal sepsis. *Eur Cytokine Netw* 2011; 22:113–117.
63. Terrin G, Passariello A, Manguso F, et al. Serum calprotectin: an antimicrobial peptide as a new marker for the diagnosis of sepsis in very low birth weight newborns. *Clin Dev Immunol* 2011; 2011:291085. Epub 2011 May 30.
64. Sherwin C, Broadbent R, Young S, et al. Utility of interleukin-12 and interleukin-10 in comparison with other cytokines and acute-phase reactants in the diagnosis of neonatal sepsis. *Am J Perinatol* 2008; 25:629–636.
65. Buck C, Bundschu J, Gallati H, Bartmann P, Pohlandt F. Interleukin-6: a sensitive parameter for the early diagnosis of neonatal bacterial infection. *Pediatrics* 1994; 93: 54–58.
66. Genel F, Atlihan F, Gulez N, et al. Evaluation of adhesion molecules CD64, CD11b and CD62L in neutrophils and monocytes of peripheral blood for early diagnosis of neonatal infection. *World J Pediatr* 2012; 8:72–75.
67. Ng PC, Li G, Chui KM, et al. Neutrophil CD64 is a sensitive diagnostic marker for early-onset neonatal infection. *Pediatr Res* 2004; 56:796–803.
68. Ng PC, Li K, Wong RP, Chui KM, Wong E, Fok TF. Neutrophil CD64 expression: a sensitive diagnostic marker for

late-onset nosocomial infection in very low birthweight infants. *Pediatr Res* 2002; 51:296–303.
69. Bohnhorst B, Lange M, Bartels DB, Bejo L, Hoy L, Peter C. Procalcitonin and valuable clinical symptoms in the early detection of neonatal late-onset bacterial infection. *Acta Paediatr* 2012; 101:19–25.
70. Pammi M, Flores A, Leeflang M, Versalovic J. Molecular assays in the diagnosis of neonatal sepsis: a systematic review and meta-analysis. *Pediatrics* 2011; 128:e973–e985.
71. Srinivasan L, Harris MC. New technologies for the rapid diagnosis of neonatal sepsis. *Curr Opin Pediatr* 2012; 24:165–171.

CHAPTER 5
Rational antibiotic use

Newborn infants with sepsis usually have a non-specific clinical presentation and can deteriorate rapidly if not treated. One of the most important principles of management of neonatal infection, therefore, is to **start antibiotics early** if there is any clinical suspicion of sepsis and indeed sometimes if the baby is asymptomatic but there are significant risk factors for sepsis. This sort of management approach is not amenable to randomized clinical trials, which would be unethical because of the high risk of death or disability of untreated infants. However, widespread empiric therapy risks selection of antibiotic-resistant bacteria. A rational approach to try to minimize antibiotic resistance is given in Table 5.1.

5.1 Choice of antibiotics for suspected early-onset sepsis

5.1.1 Choice of antibiotics for suspected early-onset sepsis

The rational choice of antibiotics for suspected early-onset sepsis depends on the likely organisms causing sepsis and their antibiotic susceptibility which may vary over time and within countries and differs particularly between Western countries and developing countries. However, all countries surveyed report early-onset infections with both Gram-positive cocci and Gram-negative bacilli, so empiric regimens need to cover both. While anaerobes occasionally cause early-onset sepsis, fulminant anaerobic infection is sufficiently rare that most regimens do not include antibiotics that specifically target anaerobes.

Possible regimens, in order from the narrowest to the broadest spectrum, include the following.

(1) Penicillin or ampicillin to cover most Gram-positive cocci plus an aminoglycoside (e.g. gentamicin, netilmicin, tobramycin, amikacin) to cover Gram-negative bacilli;

(2) A cephalosporin, for example cephalothin, to cover Gram-positive cocci including *Staphylococcus aureus* plus an aminoglycoside (e.g. gentamicin, netilmicin, tobramycin, amikacin) to cover Gram-negative bacilli;

(3) A β-lactam antibiotic such as a third generation cephalosporin (e.g. cefotaxime, ceftriaxone, ceftazidime) or an extended-spectrum penicillin with Pseudomonas activity (e.g. piperacillin, ticarcillin) used alone or with an aminoglycoside;

(4) An extended spectrum penicillin combined with a β-lactamase inhibitor (e.g. piperacillin–tazobactam, ticarcillin–clavulanate) as monotherapy; or

(5) A carbapenem, for example meropenem, to cover Gram-positive cocci and extended-spectrum β-lactamase (ESBL) producing Gram-negative bacilli.

Use the narrowest spectrum regimen possible. Although doctors often think that the broader the spectrum the better, this is a fallacy. The broader the spectrum, the more likely it is that an antibiotic will select for highly resistant organisms. Some antibiotic classes, such as third generation cephalosporins, are more potent resistance promoters than other classes with similar or even broader spectra of activity, such as aminoglycosides. Regimens (3), (4) and (5) should never be used as empiric regimens for early-onset sepsis, unless local sensitivity data mean that a narrower spectrum regimen would put infants at great risk. Even then, it may be possible to use a regimen such as penicillin (or cephalothin to cover *S. aureus*) plus amikacin if local ESBL-producing Gram-negative bacilli causing proven early-onset sepsis are sensitive to amikacin.

Because of the variation in causative organisms and susceptibilities, it is not surprising that there are almost no scientific studies comparing different antibiotic regimens in suspected early-onset sepsis. A Cochrane

Evidence-Based Neonatal Infections, First Edition. David Isaacs.

Table 5.1 Ten point plan to reduce antibiotic resistance in neonatal units.

(1) Always take cultures of blood (and perhaps cerebrospinal fluid and/or urine) before starting the infant on antibiotics.
(2) Use the narrowest spectrum antibiotics possible, almost always a penicillin (e.g. benzylpenicillin, flucloxacillin, piperacillin, ticarcillin) and an aminoglycoside (e.g. gentamicin, netilmicin, amikacin).
(3) Do not start treatment, as a general rule, with a third generation cephalosporin (e.g. cefotaxime, ceftazidime) or a carbapenem (e.g. imipenem, meropenem).
(4) Develop local and national antibiotic policies to restrict the use of expensive, broad spectrum antibiotics.
(5) Trust the microbiology laboratory: rely on the blood-culture results.
(6) Do not believe that abnormal results for a non-specific test, such as a raised serum C-reactive protein, mean that the baby is definitely septic.
(7) If blood cultures are negative at 2–3 days, it is almost always safe and appropriate to stop antibiotics.
(8) Try not to use antibiotics for long periods.
(9) Treat sepsis, but not colonisation.
(10) Do your best to prevent nosocomial infection, by reinforcing infection control, particularly hand washing.

Source: Adapted from Reference 15

Review, not updated since 2004,[1] found only two small RCTs comparing empiric monotherapy with therapy using two agents, given to a total of only 127 babies. One study of 45 babies compared ceftazidime with benzylpenicillin plus gentamicin; there were no deaths.[2] The other study of 72 babies compared ticarcillin–clavulanic acid with piperacillin and gentamicin for both early- and late-onset sepsis and found no significant difference in mortality.[3] Neither study found any difference in treatment failure or antibiotic resistance.

A later RCT compared ampicillin plus gentamicin with penicillin plus gentamicin in 283 babies with suspected early-onset sepsis.[4] Proven infection developed in 4.9% of infants and there were no differences in any parameter studied.[4] The spectrum of activity of ampicillin and penicillin is very similar and it would be surprising to find any differences in a relatively small study. Ampicillin is slightly less active than penicillin against most Gram-positive bacteria, but slightly more active against *Enterococcus faecalis*, but the clinical significance of these differences is probably unimportant.[5] Both are active against Listeria.[5]

An important study by de Man used a cross-over design to compare 'narrow spectrum' with 'broad spectrum' antibiotic regimens on two similar neonatal intensive care units.[6] The defined narrow spectrum regimen used penicillin G plus tobramycin as empiric therapy for possible early-onset sepsis and flucloxacillin plus tobramycin for possible late-onset sepsis, and used no broad-spectrum β-lactam antibiotics, such as amoxicillin and cefotaxime. The broad spectrum regimen used intravenous amoxicillin plus cefotaxime as empiric therapy for early or late sepsis. After 6 months of the study the units exchanged regimens. Weekly surveillance was by rectal and respiratory cultures.[6] Three babies treated with penicillin–tobramycin became colonized with Gram-negative bacilli resistant to the empirical therapy used compared with 41 neonates treated with amoxicillin–cefotaxime ($p < 0.001$). The relative risk for colonization with strains resistant to the empirical therapy was 18 times higher for the amoxicillin–cefotaxime regimen than for penicillin–tobramycin (95% CI 5.6–58). *Enterobacter cloacae* was the main organism isolated from babies receiving amoxicillin–cefotaxime, while *E. coli* predominated in babies on penicillin–tobramycin. These data provide strong evidence that a narrow spectrum penicillin–aminoglycoside regimen is less likely to be associated with the selection of resistant bacteria than an early-onset regimen incorporating amoxicillin and a third-generation cephalosporin. The strength of the observation was considerably strengthened by the finding that the resistance patterns were reversed when the units exchanged antibiotic policies after 6 months (Figure 5.1.)[6]

A large retrospective multi-centre US cohort study examined early antibiotic use in inborn neonates: 104 803 were treated with ampicillin plus gentamicin, while 24 111 were treated with ampicillin and cefotaxime.[7] Only 2% of babies treated had proven early-onset sepsis. After adjusting for possible confounders, neonates treated with ampicillin plus cefotaxime were more likely to die (4.7%) than neonates treated with ampicillin plus gentamicin (2.3%), (adjusted OR 1.5, 95% CI 1.4–1.7) and less likely to be discharged from hospital. The increased mortality occurred in both preterm and full-term babies. Different units used different regimens, so these results do not prove that cefotaxime increases mortality, but the size of the study and the degree of the difference in mortality led the authors to conclude that cefotaxime use in the first 3 days after birth, compared with gentamicin, is a

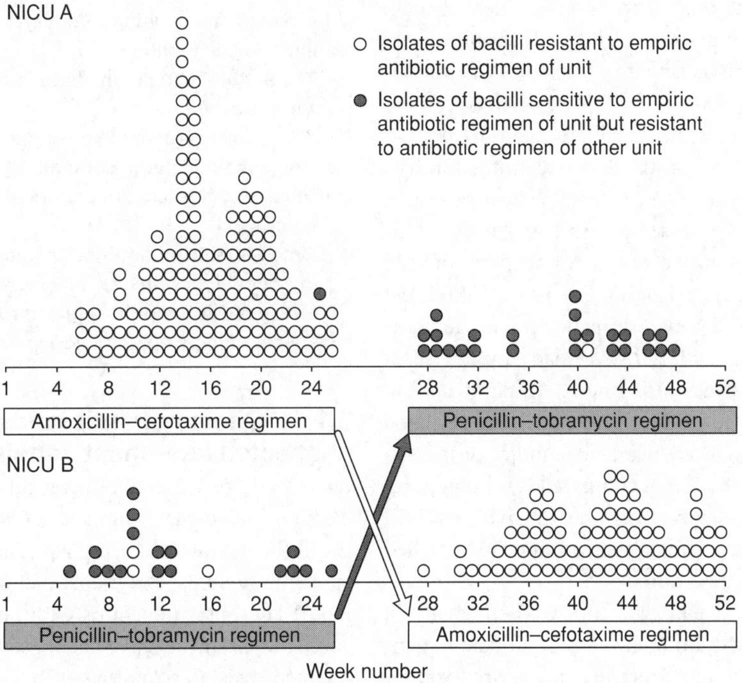

Figure 5.1 Distribution of colonising Gram-negative bacilli according to antibiotic regimen. (Adapted from Reference 6)

surrogate for an unrecognized factor or is itself associated with an increased risk of death.[7]

As discussed in Chapter 16, broad spectrum antibiotics, particularly third generation cephalosporins, are associated with an approximate doubling of the risk of neonatal candidiasis, which is a particular problem for low birth-weight infants and babies with predisposing gastro-intestinal abnormalities.[8]

Listeria and enterococci (faecal streptococci), which can both cause early-onset infection, are inherently resistant to third generation cephalosporins, so even if it is decided to use a third generation cephalosporin as empiric therapy for early-onset sepsis, it should be used in conjunction with an agent like ampicillin to which these organisms are sensitive.

The disadvantages of using aminoglycosides are predominantly concerns about toxicity and the need to monitor drug levels. Drug levels are monitored to make sure therapeutic levels are achieved and/or to avoid accumulation. If the baby stops antibiotics after 48–72 hours, drug levels are unnecessary because toxicity is cumulative and associated with prolonged aminoglycoside use.

Hearing loss in low birth-weight babies could be due to aminoglycoside toxicity, but other possible causes are genetic factors unrelated to aminoglycosides and environmental factors such as perinatal asphyxia, post-natal hypoxia, acidosis, bilirubin toxicity and noise. It is difficult to assess the relative contribution of aminoglycoside toxicity to neonatal deafness, particularly in pre-term infants. We could find no RCTs comparing hearing in babies who did and did not receive aminoglycosides. A Cochrane systematic review of 11 studies of 574 neonates treated with once daily or multiple daily doses of aminoglycosides reported minimal ototoxicity and nephrotoxicity with either regimen.[9] A 5-year New Zealand study compared hearing tested by otoacoustic emissions (OAE) in infants managed in a neonatal intensive care unit who received gentamicin and/or vancomycin (a glycopeptide antibiotic, not an aminoglycoside). Somewhat surprisingly, they found that babies who received gentamicin but no vancomycin had a significantly lower risk of OAE failure than babies who received neither antibiotic, while vancomycin use increased the risk of OAE failure.[10]

Aminoglycoside ototoxicity has been described in association with mutations of the mitochondrial 12s rRNA genes, which occur with a frequency of approximately one in 500 Europeans.[11] However, in a prospective case-cohort US neonatal study, four of 378 neonates exposed to gentamicin had mitochondrial mutations, but only one failed the initial hearing test.[12]. A German study addressed possible gentamicin ototoxicity with two approaches.[13] A cohort study of 8333 children examined for hearing disorders, found 134 (1.6%) had received previous treatment with gentamicin, and only eight of 134 (6%) had any degree of sensorineural hearing impairment. All eight had an alternative cause for hearing loss, such as perinatal asphyxia, acidosis, severe neonatal jaundice or meningitis. In addition, the author compared vestibular function in 30 children with normal hearing who received gentamicin in the neonatal period and 30 matched controls and found no difference.[13]

There are insufficient data to say whether any of the frequently used aminoglycosides, amikacin, gentamicin, netilmicin and tobramycin, is more toxic for neonates than the others, but there is most safety data for gentamicin.[8–13] Aminoglycosides accumulate in renal tissue and in the perilymph of the inner ear causing progressive toxicity, so it is recommended not to use them for longer than 7 days, if possible.

Antibiotics select for organisms that carry ancient resistance genes.[14] Antibiotic resistance is an example of Darwinian selection. The term 'unnatural selection' emphasizes the iatrogenic nature of rapid selection of resistant organisms from misusing broad spectrum antibiotics.[15] To minimize resistance, narrow spectrum antibiotics should always be preferred if the choice does not jeopardize babies.[15]

On the basis of the above data suggesting possible increased mortality with third generation cephalosporins and relatively reassuring data about aminoglycoside toxicity, the following recommendations are suggested:

Recommendations for choice of empiric antibiotics for possible early-onset sepsis

- **The empiric antibiotics for babies with possible early-onset neonatal infection should be based on the organisms causing infections locally and their antibiotic susceptibility.**
- **The antibiotic regimen should be as narrow spectrum as possible.**
- **A penicillin (ampicillin or penicillin) and an aminoglycoside (e.g. gentamicin) is the regimen of choice if this covers the local organisms adequately.**
- **Broad-spectrum antibiotics such as third generation cephalosporins and meropenem should not be included in empiric regimens unless essential because of local epidemiology.**

5.1.2 Choice of antibiotics for suspected late-onset sepsis

As for early-onset sepsis, the rational choice of antibiotics for possible late-onset sepsis should be based on the likely organisms causing sepsis and their antibiotic susceptibility. Like early sepsis, all countries surveyed report late-onset infections with both Gram-positive cocci and Gram-negative bacilli, so empiric antibiotic regimens need to cover these groups of organisms.

Possible regimens, in order from the narrowest to the broadest spectrum, include the following.

(1) A semi-synthetic penicillin with anti-staphylococcal activity, for example, cloxacillin, flucloxacillin, methicillin, nafcillin, oxacillin, to cover Gram-positive cocci plus an aminoglycoside (e.g. gentamicin, netilmicin, tobramycin) to cover Gram-negative bacilli;

(2) Penicillin or ampicillin to cover Gram-positive cocci plus an aminoglycoside to cover Gram-negative bacilli if staphylococcal infections are very rare;

(3) A broad spectrum β-lactam antibiotic such as a third generation cephalosporin (e.g. cefotaxime, ceftriaxone, ceftazidime) or an extended-spectrum penicillin with Pseudomonas activity (e.g. piperacillin, ticarcillin) used alone or with an aminoglycoside;

(4) A broad-spectrum carbapenem, for example, meropenem, as monotherapy to cover ESBL-producing Gram-negative bacilli; or

(5) A combination of an extended spectrum penicillin with a β-lactamase inhibitor (e.g. piperacillin–tazobactam, ticarcillin–clavulanate) as monotherapy. Specific anti-anaerobic cover is not used empirically in general.

A Cochrane systematic review failed to find any studies that effectively compared different antibiotic regimens,[16] with the exception of the study already quoted which compared ticarcillin–clavulanic acid with piperacillin and gentamicin for both early- and late-onset sepsis and found no difference in mortality.[3]

Continuing surveillance of late-onset infections is needed to monitor for changes in prevailing organisms and/or their susceptibility.[17]

In Western industrialized countries, the major need in empiric treatment of possible late-onset sepsis is to cover against fulminant infections, which are usually caused by Gram-negative bacilli or *S. aureus* (methicillin-sensitive *S. aureus* (MSSA) or methicillin-resistant *S. aureus* (MRSA)). Although CoNS are the most common single organism associated with late-onset sepsis, it is extremely rare for CoNS septicaemia to cause fulminant infection.[18, 19]

The mortality from Pseudomonas septicaemia is 52–74%, compared with 10–25% for other Gram-negative bacilli,[19–21] so empiric regimens should cover Pseudomonas, particularly if babies on the neonatal unit are known to be colonized.[22]

There is strong evidence that broad-spectrum antibiotics, as in regimens (3), (4) and (5) above, are major drivers of the emergence of antibiotic-resistant Enterobacteriaceae, particularly ESBL-producing Gram-negative bacilli.[23–26] Their use should be avoided if possible. In some developing countries, however, ESBL-producing Gram-negative bacilli circulate as community organisms as well as in hospital, and are an important cause of both early- and late-onset neonatal infection.[27, 28] In Kolkata, for example, more than half of all early- and late-onset neonatal infections were caused by multi-resistant Gram-negative bacilli.[28]

Question: For Gram-positive cover, should empiric regimens for suspected late sepsis in Western countries include vancomycin?

In a 10-year multicentre study from Australia and New Zealand, four of 1281 babies (0.3%) with CoNS infections died, and CoNS may have contributed to the deaths of 20 other babies (1.6%).[18] A 10-year study in a single US neonatal unit reported a total of 49 episodes of fulminant sepsis (lethal within 48 hours), of which 34 (69%) were caused by Gram-negative bacilli and only four by CoNS.[19] There were 277 episodes of CoNS infection, so the proportion of fatal CoNS infections was 1.4%. During the study, a decision was made after 6.7 years to change the empiric regimen for suspected late-onset sepsis from vancomycin plus cefotaxime to oxacillin plus gentamicin. When vancomycin was used for Gram-positive cover there were 141 episodes of CoNS sepsis, of which two were fulminant. For the remaining period when oxacillin was used, there were 136 episodes and two were fulminant.[19]

The main reason for changing from vancomycin was to avoid selecting for vancomycin-resistant enterococci (VRE).[19, 29] There are a number of reasons that oxacillin and gentamicin was apparently no less safe than vancomycin and cefotaxime. First, even for supposedly fulminant CoNS infections, the baby may be dying from an unrelated cause and the CoNS is a contaminant. While this is difficult to prove or disprove, neonatal clinicians will understand the argument. Second, some CoNS will respond to oxacillin or flucloxacillin. Third, central line-associated CoNS infections often respond to removal of the central line, so if the line is removed, the choice of antibiotic may be less critical. Finally, although aminoglycosides are not recommended to treat staphylococcal infections, they do have some anti-staphylococcal activity, so it is possible that gentamicin provides some additional cover.

The glycopeptide antibiotic vancomycin provides broad cover against Gram-positive organisms, but there are concerns about the selection of VRE[29] about possible ototoxicity,[10] and also concerns that vancomycin use actually predisposes to Gram-negative sepsis.[30] In a Dutch case-control study of 105 children (39 of them neonates) with Gram-negative bacteraemia, the strongest association was with prior use of vancomycin (OR 8.1; 95% CI 3.1–20.9). In a multiple logistic regression model, the use of vancomycin remained positively and strongly associated with Gram-negative bacteraemia (OR 3.9; 95% CI 1.3–11.2).[30] *S. aureus*, MSSA or MRSA, are intermediate in virulence between CoNS and Gram-negative bacilli, although there is strain-to-strain variability in MRSA virulence.[31] If MRSA is prevalent on a neonatal unit, the empiric late-onset regimen probably needs to include vancomycin, but if not the use of a semi-synthetic penicillin is much preferable.

Teicoplanin is a complex of five glycopeptides with a similar spectrum to vancomycin. It was mainly used in the 1990s in parts of Europe and has been suggested to have a better safety profile than vancomycin.[32, 33] However, it is less active than vancomycin against some CoNS, especially *Staphylococcus haemolyticus*.[34] A search found only one small comparative study in neonates of low-dose prophylactic teicoplanin and vancomycin, which showed no difference in toxicity or efficacy.[35] Although teicoplanin might be as effective as vancomycin, the limited pharmacologic data in neonates and concerns about antibiotic spectrum mean that it has been used rarely and cannot be advised as a suitable alternative to vancomycin for empiric regimens.

Recommendation: Vancomycin only needs to be included in the empiric antibiotic regimen for late-onset sepsis in neonatal units with a significant risk of MRSA infection.

Question: For Gram-negative cover in Western countries, what is the preferred regimen?

As discussed for early-onset sepsis above, there are theoretical concerns about the safety of aminoglycosides but the limited evidence available suggests they do not cause significant ototoxicity or nephrotoxicity in neonates. Aminoglycoside levels only need to be measured if they are continued for longer than 2–3 days. Aminoglycosides accumulate in the ears and kidneys causing progressive toxicity, so it is recommended not to use them for longer than 7 days, if possible. However, their use is preferred to broad-spectrum antibiotics, which are associated with the selection of multi-resistant organisms.[15, 36, 37]

If a strain of Gram-negative bacillus that is resistant to the aminoglycoside recommended in the empiric regimen becomes prevalent colonizing and/or infecting babies on a neonatal unit, one possibility is to change to another aminoglycoside to which the organism is sensitive. For example, when a gentamicin-resistant strain of Klebsiella colonized a number of babies and caused episodes of sepsis in a neonatal unit, a temporary change to netilmicin as empiric aminoglycoside of choice was successful, before returning to gentamicin.[38]

Recommendations for choice of empiric antibiotics for possible late-onset sepsis

- **The empiric antibiotics for babies with possible late-onset neonatal infection should be based on the organisms causing infections locally and their antibiotic susceptibility.**
- **The antibiotic regimen should be as narrow spectrum as possible.**
- **A semi-synthetic penicillin with anti-staphylococcal activity (e.g. cloxacillin, dicloxacillin, flucloxacillin, methicillin, nafcillin, oxacillin) and an aminoglycoside (e.g. gentamicin) is the regimen of choice if this covers the local organisms adequately.**
- **Vancomycin and an aminoglycoside (e.g. gentamicin) should be the chosen empiric regimen if there is a high prevalence of MRSA.**
- **Broad-spectrum antibiotics such as third generation cephalosporins and meropenem should not be included in empiric regimens unless essential because of local epidemiology.**

5.1.3 Antibiotics for suspected community-acquired sepsis in developing countries

The WHO currently recommends ampicillin or penicillin G plus gentamicin to treat suspected community-acquired late-onset sepsis in developing countries. However, a non-Cochrane systematic review and meta-analysis of 19 studies from 13 countries found resistance or reduced susceptibility to ampicillin/penicillin and gentamicin and equally commonly to third generation cephalosporins in up to 40% of cases.[39] An editorial on combating antimicrobial resistance subtitled 'The war against error' counselled against 'one size fits all' antibiotic recommendations and recommended tailoring antibiotic regimens to local epidemiology. The editorial also emphasized that bacteria have evolved resistance genes over millions of years, so escalating use of ever broader spectrum antibiotics is doomed to failure and alternative strategies to prevent infection are needed.[40]

5.1.4 Antibiotic rotation

Rotation of antibiotic regimens in neonatal units might reduce the selection of resistant strains by reducing antibiotic pressure. An adult surgical intensive care unit reported an improvement in antibiotic susceptibility of some Gram-negative bacilli following the introduction of an antibiotic rotation protocol, while the susceptibilities did not improve in the adjoining medical intensive care unit which did not introduce antibiotic rotation.[41] An adult intensive care unit which introduced antibiotic rotation reported a reduced incidence of ventilator-associated pneumonia but no significant change in antibiotic susceptibilities.[42] In contrast, two adult intensive care units reported that antibiotic rotation had no measurable effect on antibiotic susceptibility patterns.[43, 44]

A systematic review published in 2005 found 11 studies of antibiotic rotation. Only four had attempted to evaluate the effects and there were considerable methodological problems, both in the reviews and implementation. The authors advised against the use of antibiotic rotation to attempt to reduce antibiotic resistance rates.[45]

Only one NICU study is reported.[46] The unit was divided into two similar populations of babies. The empiric antibiotic regimen for suspected Gram-negative sepsis for one population (rotation team) was rotated monthly through gentamicin, piperacillin–tazobactam and ceftazidime. The other control team used an unrestricted choice of antibiotic according to the choice of the attending physician. After 1 year, 10.7% of infants in the rotation team and 7.7% of controls were colonized with resistant Gram-negative bacilli ($p > 0.05$).[46]

5.2 Prophylactic antibiotics

Prophylactic antibiotic use is when antibiotics are given to an uninfected baby with risk factors for infection to prevent the baby developing infection. Prophylaxis means prevention. This is different from empiric antibiotic use which means giving antibiotics to babies who may already be infected.

Question: Do prophylactic antibiotics compared with no prophylactic antibiotics improve outcome for any group of neonates?

All infants: An Italian RCT compared one with 3 days of ampicillin plus netilmicin for 130 infants admitted consecutively to the NICU. There was no difference in incidence of late-onset sepsis.[47]

Central venous catheters: We found a Cochrane systematic review[48] and a separate non-Cochrane systematic review,[49] both of which identified three small RCTs. Two studies used vancomycin and one used amoxicillin. Prophylactic vancomycin was associated with a statistically significant reduction in the incidence of bacteraemia but there was no change in mortality and no data on neurodevelopmental outcome. There was documented change in antibiotic susceptibility, although the methods for determining these were not robust. Both sets of authors cautioned that the routine use of prophylactic antibiotics for neonates with central venous catheters cannot be recommended because of concerns about the long-term safety.

Umbilical artery catheters: A Cochrane systematic review found only two small quasi-randomized trials and concluded there was insufficient evidence to recommend or advise against the use of prophylactic antibiotics.[50]

Umbilical venous catheters: A Cochrane systematic review found only one small trial which showed no effect of a short 3-day course of prophylactic antibiotics.[51]

Mechanical ventilation: A Cochrane systematic review found only one trial of fair quality which showed no effect of prophylactic antibiotics in any outcome, although bacteraemia rates were not reported.[52]

Neutropenia: As discussed in Chapter 4, neutropenia in the first few days of life may be due to overwhelming infection, but particularly in low birth-weight infants is much more commonly secondary to growth retardation or maternal pre-eclampsia.[53] Neutropenia at birth (defined as <2.2 neutrophils<1000/μL) was associated with a risk of 14% of proven or presumed early-onset sepsis (<48 hours) compared with 2% in non-neutropenic babies.[52] Sepsis was proven in 6% of neutropenic babies.[54]

Several studies have examined whether neutropenia is a risk factor for developing late-onset sepsis. Two studies which compared neutropenic babies of hypertensive mothers with neutropenic babies of normotensive mothers found highly significant differences. In an Australian study, late-onset infection developed in 55% of babies <1500 g of hypertensive mothers but only 12% of babies <1500 g of normotensive mothers.[55] In another study, 29% of neutropenic babies <2000 g born to hypertensive mothers developed sepsis compared to 5% of neutropenic babies <2000 g whose mothers were normotensive.[56] In contrast, other studies which included more mature babies have found that about 15% of neutropenic babies develop late-onset sepsis, that the neutropenic babies were less mature and of lower birth-weight, and infection was not more common than in matched controls.[57, 58]

'Late-onset neutropenia' developing after 3 weeks or more appears to be a benign condition in stable, growing very low birth-weight (VLBW) babies <1500 g. In a study of 51 VLBW babies who became neutropenic (defined as <1500/μL) after 3 weeks of age, neutropenia lasted 1–3 weeks and no baby developed sepsis.[59]

The evidence suggests that early neutropenia in VLBW babies is associated with a high risk of late-onset infection, particularly when the mother was hypertensive. This risk varies from 15% to 55% and increases with decreasing birth weight and gestation. If the baby is sick, empiric antibiotics should be started after taking cultures. If well, we recommend prophylactic antibiotics to cover against infection with *S. aureus* and Gram-negative bacilli until the neutropenia resolves, which is virtually always in less than a week.[53]

Recommendation: It is recommended to give prophylactic antibiotics with activity against staphylococci and Gram-negative bacilli (e.g. vancomycin and gentamicin) to VLBW babies <1500 g with neutropenia in the first 3 days, particularly if their mother is hypertensive. The antibiotics should be stopped when the neutropenia resolves, or after a week if it persists.

5.3 Which babies to treat?

5.3.1 Early-onset sepsis

The major maternal risk factors for early-onset neonatal sepsis in Chapter 2 (see Section 2.2.3) are prematurity, particularly if the onset of labour is spontaneous (the risk of sepsis increasing with decreasing gestation), prolonged rupture of the membranes, maternal fever and colonisation with or a previous baby infected with GBS.[60, 61] Gestation >42 weeks is also a risk factor. These risks are cumulative, so if more than one is present, the risk is greatly increased.[60, 61]

Whether or not to start empiric antibiotics depends on a balance of risks and benefits. This in turn depends on the baseline risk. For example, the risk that a full-term baby of a mother with membranes ruptured for 36 hours will develop early-onset infection is increased more than sevenfold, but the absolute risk is about two per 1000 live births, far less than for a 26-week gestation baby. Nevertheless, because the risks of missing sepsis are so great, we recommend that if there is one or more maternal risk factor, empiric antibiotics should be started after cultures have been taken.

Recommendation: Empiric antibiotics from birth are recommended if there is one or more maternal risk factors (spontaneous pre-term onset of labour, prolonged rupture of membranes >18 hours, maternal fever >38°C, post-maturity >42 weeks, known GBS colonisation or past baby with GBS without intrapartum antibiotics).

In addition, antibiotics should be given to any baby where there is a reasonable clinical suspicion that the baby is infected, such as a baby with unexpected early respiratory distress, with fever or with unexplained lethargy or feeding difficulties.

5.3.2 Late-onset sepsis

As with early-onset sepsis, it is so important not to miss sepsis that a very low threshold is recommended. This particularly applies to babies most likely to develop sepsis, such as the most premature babies receiving invasive respiratory support and artificial feeds.

5.4 Common clinical scenarios

5.4.1 Mother received intrapartum antibiotics

It is not uncommon that the mother has received intrapartum antibiotics. The US Centers for Disease Control (CDC) and the American Academy of Pediatrics (AAP) have both issued guidelines on a number of occasions. The AAP has endorsed the most recent CDC guidelines (Figure 5.2)[62] although we recommend searching for more recent AAP and/or CDC guidelines.

The basis for these guidelines is that: (i) there is no significant difference in the clinical presentation of early-onset GBS disease between infants exposed to intrapartum antibiotics and those not exposed;[63–67] (ii) clinical assessment is more reliable than laboratory tests in assessing sepsis;[64] and (iii) the risk of neonatal GBS infection is reduced from 29% to 46% if antibiotics are given less than 2 hours before delivery to 2.9% if given at 2–4 hours and to 1.2% if given more than 4 hours before delivery.[68, 69]

5.4.2 Full-term baby with early respiratory distress

A pre-term baby with early respiratory distress should almost always be started on empiric antibiotics because the baby will fulfil one or more of the risk factors in

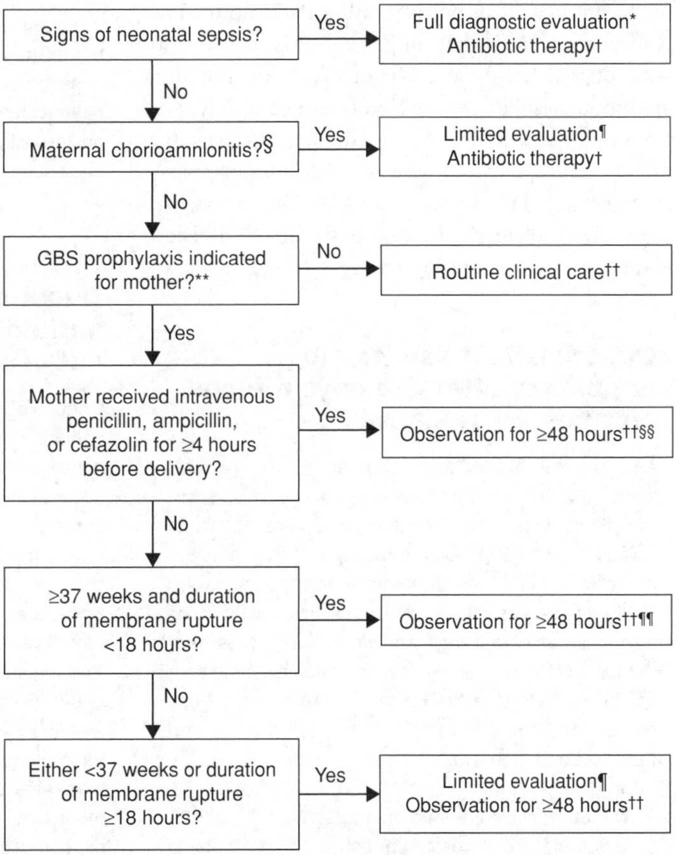

Figure 5.2 Algorithm for secondary prevention of early-onset group B streptococcal (GBS) disease among newborns. (Adapted from reference 62)
*Blood culture, full blood count, chest radiograph (if respiratory distress), and lumbar puncture (if stable). †Antibiotic therapy for early-onset sepsis, taking into account local antibiotic resistance patterns. §Consultation with obstetricians recommended. ¶Includes blood culture at birth and full blood count with differential and platelets (at birth and/or at 6–12 hours). **See http://www.cdc.gov/groupbstrep/guidelines/guidelines.html for indications for intrapartum GBS prophylaxis. ††If signs of sepsis develop, do a full diagnostic evaluation and start empiric antibiotic therapy. §§If ≥37 weeks of gestation, observation may occur at home after 24 hours, if safe. ¶¶Some experts recommend a full blood count with differential and platelets at age 6–12 hours.

Section 5.3.1 and because the risk of sepsis increases with decreasing gestational age.

Respiratory distress is less common in full-term babies. It may occur following elective Caesarean section due to retained lung fluid. The radiographic appearance of early-onset pneumonia can resemble 'wet lung' as well as hyaline membrane disease. If the mother has been screened for GBS, this may inform the decision about whether or not to start empiric antibiotics in a full-term baby with respiratory distress. However, because hyaline membrane disease is highly unlikely, the possibility of early-onset sepsis should always be considered in a full-term baby with early respiratory distress.

5.5 Duration of antibiotics

Advisedly, neonatologists have a low threshold for starting antibiotics empirically. The duration of antibiotics for babies with radiographic pneumonia, babies with urinary tract infection and babies with meningitis will be considered separately in the relevant chapters. The duration of antibiotics for babies with positive blood cultures will be considered in Section 5.2.2. However, the great majority of babies have negative blood cultures and the duration of antibiotics for these babies is not without controversy.

5.5.1 Antibiotic duration for blood-culture-negative babies

If there is a policy of starting antibiotics early, on the slightest suspicion of sepsis, the great majority of treated babies, usually >95%, will have negative blood cultures. A corollary of starting antibiotics early on suspicion is that, in general, they should be stopped early if blood cultures are negative, the baby is well and there are no other reasons to continue antibiotics. Again, this is not readily amenable to RCTs, so the evidence is from observational studies.

The data on blood volume and on time for positive cultures to grow suggest that most true positive blood cultures will be positive within 48–72 hours. The clinical corollary is that, in general, it is safe to stop antibiotics after 2–3 days. Arguments against stopping antibiotics despite negative blood cultures mainly centre around the difficulty in excluding false negative blood cultures and the wish to use laboratory measurements, usually serum acute phase reactants like C-reactive protein (CRP), as a basis for the decision about when to stop antibiotics.

Question: Is it safe to stop antibiotics after 2–3 days if blood cultures are negative?

A search of PubMed Clinical Queries found no relevant systematic reviews and only one small randomized controlled pilot trial.[70] The trial from India enrolled infants >1000 g and >30 weeks of gestation who presented with clinical signs consistent with late sepsis and raised CRP, were treated with empiric antibiotics and had negative cultures after 2 days and were well. Babies were randomized to stop antibiotics (short course) or to continue to a total of 7 days. Three of 26 babies in the 7-day course but none of 26 in the short-course group had recurrence of signs within 15 days of stopping antibiotics.[70]

The other evidence for stopping antibiotics after 2–3 days if blood cultures are negative and the baby is well comes from observational studies. A UK study compared outcomes from suspected sepsis before and after introduction of an early form of antibiotic stewardship programme.[70] The programme, to stop antibiotics after 2–3 days if cultures were negative and the chest X-ray normal, resulted in a >40% decrease in antibiotic use, found no increase in morbidity or mortality from early- or late-onset sepsis and no relapses after antibiotics were stopped within 2–3 days.[71] A longitudinal US study reported that 98% of positive blood cultures were detected within 48 hours, that seven of eight cultures that were positive after 48 hours were due to CoNS, and that discontinuing antibiotics after 48 hours for neonates with possible late-onset sepsis and negative blood cultures had become standard policy and was safe.[72] A longitudinal study from Switzerland documented a progressive and significant reduction in the duration of antibiotics for blood-culture-negative babies with no increase in mortality.[73]

These observational studies constitute only weak evidence in favour of early discontinuation of antibiotics. In all of them, the baby was assessed clinically as being well, and babies with radiographic pneumonia in the UK study were treated for 7–10 days. The question of whether antibiotics should be continued if a baby with possible early-onset sepsis was heavily colonized with GBS or Listeria will be considered later in this section.

Question: Is it safe to continue antibiotics after 2–3 days if blood cultures are negative?

Continuing antibiotics despite negative blood cultures could be harmful because of iatrogenic disease (e.g. adverse effects of antibiotics, complications of venous access) and because of the risk of selecting for resistant organisms.

An important observational US multicentre study examined antibiotic use in 4039 low birth-weight infants who received empiric antibiotic therapy, survived for more than 5 days and had negative blood cultures.[74] The median duration of antibiotics for culture-negative babies was 5 days (range 1–36 days) and 53% received antibiotics for 5 or more days, which the authors defined as 'prolonged therapy'. The authors compared babies who received 5 or more days (prolonged therapy) with those who received less than 5 days. As might be expected, the babies who received 5 or more days were different: less mature, with lower Apgar scores and more likely to be black. In multivariate analyses which allowed for known confounding factors, however, prolonged therapy was associated with a 46% increased risk of dying (95% CI 19–78) and a 30% increased risk of necrotizing enterocolitis (NEC) (95% CI 10–54). The increased mortality was not a result of NEC, so the two risks were apparently independent. Each additional day of empirical antibiotics was associated with increased odds of death and of NEC.[74]

This is an observational study, the two groups are clearly not comparable; the multivariate analysis can only allow for known confounding factors, so there is still a possibility that the increased mortality and increased incidence of NEC are not caused by the prolonged antibiotics. However, a case-control study of 124 babies with NEC found a significant association with prior antibiotics and the risk of NEC increased significantly with the duration of antibiotic exposure.[75]

The mechanism whereby antibiotics predispose to NEC and independently to death is unclear. However, a meta-analysis of RCTs of probiotics shows that they are not only associated with a 65% reduction in the incidence of NEC, but also with a 58% reduction in all-cause mortality which is not due to fewer deaths from NEC.[76] It is conceivable that prolonged antibiotics are having a profound effect on the intestinal flora of low birth-weight babies, resulting in an increased risk of NEC and of dying, and that probiotics are able to correct the adverse effects of prolonged antibiotics.

A subsequent US study of 365 low birth-weight babies again used multivariate analysis to allow for confounders and again found that babies given 5 or more days of empiric antibiotics in the first week after birth despite negative blood cultures had a significantly increased risk of developing late-onset sepsis, OR 2.45 (95% CI 1.28–4.67) and of one or more of late-onset sepsis, NEC or death, OR 2.66 (95% CI 1.1–6.3).[77]

These studies, despite their methodological problems, report a large increase in serious outcomes associated with giving low birth-weight babies prolonged empiric antibiotic therapy despite negative blood cultures. An RCT is unlikely for ethical and logistic reasons. The weight of evidence suggests that it may not be safe to continue antibiotics in babies <1500 g and that risk increases with increasing duration of antibiotics.

There seems little reason to continue empiric antibiotics in full-term babies if they are well and cultures are negative after 2–3 days. What happens in practice? In one study from a large US health maintenance organization, 998 full-term babies admitted to neonatal units and treated for suspected early-onset sepsis had negative blood cultures. After 24 hours they were all clinically well, had no respiratory signs and were feeding well orally. Over a quarter (28.7%) were treated with antibiotics for more than 3 days, 17% of them for 4–6 days and 11.6% for 7–10 days.[78] Most babies stayed in hospital for more than 4 days, showing that there was a considerable human cost as well as a financial cost.

Recommendation: It is recommended to stop antibiotics after 2–3 days if the infant is clinically well or stable and blood cultures are negative.

Question: Does the use of serum CRP help decide when to stop antibiotics in culture-negative babies?

A paper from Germany described the use of serum CRP to guide when to stop antibiotics.[79] The CRP was determined 24–48 hours after starting antibiotics in 176 babies >1500 g who had no central lines and were not mechanically ventilated and had negative blood cultures. Antibiotics were stopped in 94 babies because CRP was normal, but continued in 82 babies (46.5%) with CRP >10 mg/L. These 82 infants were called 'probably infected'; no clinical features were reported. Serum CRP was measured daily in 39 of the 82 babies and stopped when it became normal, whereas the remaining 43 babies completed at least 5 days of antibiotics. One baby in each group had a 'relapse' without positive cultures. The authors argued that "CRP could be a key parameter for guiding the duration of antibiotic treatment" and "would allow considerably shorter courses of antibiotic therapy".[79] Unfortunately this paper seems to have been quite influential and many clinicians use CRP measurements to guide when to stop antibiotics, even in developing countries.[80]

We have described large studies in the United Kingdom, United States and Switzerland which reported that it was safe to stop antibiotics after 2–3 days if blood cultures were negative and the baby was not severely unwell.[70–72] If it is safe to stop antibiotics after 2–3 days, then the practice of measuring the CRP and continuing antibiotics if the CRP is raised will inevitably lead to increased duration of antibiotics. In the German study, this comprised 46.5% of all babies started on antibiotics for possible late-onset sepsis.[79]

Never measuring CRP on culture-negative babies, merely stopping antibiotics after 2–3 days, would avoid the cost of measuring CRP and of giving antibiotics, remove the antibiotic pressure driving selection of resistant organisms and avoid iatrogenic disease due to antibiotics.

Recommendation: Routine measurement of serum CRP to guide duration of antibiotics should be avoided.

The use of acute phase reactants in general is considered in detail in Chapter 4.

Question: Should surface cultures guide continuing antibiotic treatment?

In general, surface cultures represent colonization, whereas treatment should be guided by systemic cultures, not surface cultures. However, blood cultures are a laboratory test and no laboratory test is 100% reliable.

While we have argued that for well babies with negative blood cultures and normal chest radiographs it is safe to stop antibiotics after 2–3 days, the same does not apply if the baby remains very unwell or if there is radiographic pneumonia.

Although intrapartum prophylaxis has reduced the incidence of early-onset neonatal GBS infection, some colonized mothers only receive prophylaxis shortly before delivery or not at all. Studies of babies born to GBS-positive mothers show that for every baby with proven GBS septicaemia, there is one baby born with positive surface swabs but negative systemic cultures who has clinical and hematologic and possibly radiographic features suggestive of infection. These babies have been referred to as having probable early-onset GBS infection (see also Chapters 8 and 14).[81, 82]

A similar situation can arise with early-onset Listeria infection when there may be clinical features suggestive of congenital infection and positive surface swabs, but negative systemic cultures of blood and CSF. The frequency of this situation is not reported. Because of concern about meningitis, we treat such babies as if for Listeria septicaemia (see Chapter 14). Occasionally, a similar clinical presentation may occur with a gram-negative bacillus such as *E. coli*, *Streptococcus pneumoniae*, untypable *Haemophilus influenzae* or another organism and an individual decision may be needed on whether or not to continue antibiotics.

If the baby is not colonized with any organism, it seems illogical to postulate early-onset infection. If a baby with early signs and symptoms consistent with infection remains unwell at 2–3 days but has negative surface and systemic infections, other diagnoses should be sought, for example congenital viral infection or non-infectious causes.

5.5.2 Duration of antibiotics for proven bacteraemia

There are very few studies on the duration of antibiotics for proven neonatal sepsis. Indeed, it has been suggested that the chosen duration is usually based on 'magic numbers' which are multiples of 5 or 7 days.[83] We could find only two RCTs, both of which were from India and both of which conformed to the magic numbers rule. One study compared 7 with 14 days of antibiotics in 69 infants with culture-proven sepsis but with meningitis excluded.[84] The only difference in outcome was in *S. aureus* infection: four of seven infants failed 7 days' treatment compared with zero of seven who received 14 days. Treatment failure was defined clinically and, although none of the infants had focal signs, osteomyelitis was not excluded (see Chapter 9). The other study compared 10 with 14 days of antibiotics in infants with proven bacteraemia who were well with normal CRP levels at 7 days of antibiotics. Not surprisingly, they found no difference; one infant had a clinical relapse in each group.[85]

It is usually recommended that, if meningitis has been excluded, the duration of antibiotics for proven neonatal bacteraemia should be 7–14 days. The scanty evidence suggests that infants who are well after 7 days can probably safely stop antibiotics, but for infants with *S. aureus* bacteraemia, especially if bone scan is not available, it may be safer to continue to 14 days. If bone scan is available, osteomyelitis should be excluded in infants with *S. aureus* bacteraemia (see Chapter 9: Osteomyelitis and septic arthritis).

5.5.3 Persistently positive blood cultures

Occasionally, despite apparently appropriate antibiotics, infants have persistently positive blood cultures, usually but not always associated with symptoms such as persistent fever or feed intolerance, but not necessarily with other major clinical signs of sepsis.[86, 87] In such cases, every attempt should be made to exclude an infected vascular catheter, endocarditis or another source of infection such as an abscess or thrombophlebitis. If a central line is present, the infecting organism will determine whether or not it is essential or advisable to remove the line, as discussed in Chapter 6 (see Section 6.9). Treatment will have to be individualized, but it is usual practice to continue antibiotics until the bacteraemia resolves.

References

1. Mtitimila EI, Cooke RWI. Antibiotic regimens for suspected early neonatal sepsis. Cochrane Database of Systematic Reviews 2004, Issue 4. Art. No.: CD004495. doi: 10.1002/14651858.CD004495.pub2.
2. Snelling S, Hart CA, Cooke RW. Ceftazidime or gentamicin plus benzylpenicillin in neonates less than forty-eight hours old. *J Antimicrob Chemother* 1983; 12:353–356.
3. Miall-Allen VM, Whitelaw AGL, Darrell JH. Ticarcillin plus clavulanic acid (Timentin) compared with standard antibiotic regimes in the treatment of early and late neonatal infection. *Brit J Clin Practice* 1988; 42: 273–279.

4. Metsvaht T, Ilmoja ML, Parm U, Maipuu L, Merila M, Lutsar I. Comparison of ampicillin plus gentamicin vs. penicillin plus gentamicin in empiric treatment of neonates at risk of early onset sepsis. *Acta Paediatr* 2010; 99:665–672.
5. Bush K. β-lactam antibiotics. In: *Antibiotic and Chemotherapy*. (eds RG Finch, D Greenwood, SR Norrby, RJ Whitley). 9th edn. Edinburgh: Churchill Livingstone, 2011. 200–225.
6. de Man P, Verhoeven BA, Verbrugh HA, Vos MC, van den Anker JN. An antibiotic policy to prevent emergence of resistant bacilli. *Lancet* 2000; 355:973–978.
7. Clark RH, Bloom BT, Spitzer AR, Gerstmann DR. Empiric use of ampicillin and cefotaxime, compared with ampicillin and gentamicin, for neonates at risk for sepsis is associated with an increased risk of neonatal death. *Pediatrics* 2006; 117:67–74.
8. Benjamin Jr DK, Stoll BJ, Gantz MG, et al. Neonatal candidiasis: epidemiology, risk factors and clinical judgment. *Pediatrics* 2010; 126:e865–e873.
9. Rao SC, Srinivasjois R, Hagan R, Ahmed M. One dose per day compared to multiple doses per day of gentamicin for treatment of suspected or proven sepsis in neonates. Cochrane Database of Systematic Reviews 2011, Issue 11. Art. No.: CD005091. doi: 10.1002/14651858.CD005091.pub3.
10. Vella-Brincat JW, Begg EJ, Robertshawe BJ, Lynn AM, Borrie TL, Darlow BA. Are gentamicin and/or vancomycin associated with ototoxicity in the neonate? A retrospective audit. *Neonatology* 2011; 100:186–193.
11. Guan MX. Mitochondrial 12S rRNA mutations associated with aminoglycoside ototoxicity. *Mitochondrion* 2011; 11:237–245.
12. Johnson RF, Cohen AP, Guo Y, Schibler K, Greinwald JH. Genetic mutations and aminoglycoside-induced ototoxicity in neonates. *Otolaryngol Head Neck Surg* 2010; 142:704–707.
13. Aust G. Vestibulotoxicity and ototoxicity of gentamicin in newborns at risk. *Int Tinnitus J* 2001; 7:27–29.
14. D'Costa VM, King CE, Kalan L, et al. Antibiotic resistance is ancient. *Nature* 2011; 477:457–461.
15. Isaacs D. Unnatural selection: reducing antibiotic resistance in neonatal units. *Arch Dis Child Fetal Neonatal Ed* 2006; 91:F72–F74.
16. Gordon A, Jeffery HE. Antibiotic regimens for suspected late onset sepsis in newborn infants. Cochrane Database of Systematic Reviews 2005, Issue 3. Art. No.: CD004501. doi: 10.1002/14651858.CD004501.pub2.
17. Gray JW. Surveillance of infection in neonatal intensive care units. *Early Human Development* 2007; 83:157–163.
18. Isaacs D. Australasian Study Group for Neonatal Infections. A ten-year multi-centre study of coagulase negative staphylococcal infections. *Arch Dis Child Fetal Neonatal Ed* 2003; 88:F89–F93.
19. Karlowicz MG, Buescher ES, Surka AE. Fulminant late onset sepsis in a neonatal intensive care unit, 1988–1997, and the impact of avoiding empiric vancomycin therapy. *Pediatrics* 2000; 107:1387–1390.
20. Stoll B, Hansen N, Fanaroff AA, et al. Late onset sepsis in very low birth weight neonates: the experience of the NICHD Neonatal Research Network. *Pediatrics* 2002; 110:285–291.
21. Gordon A, Isaacs D. Australasian Study Group for Neonatal Infections. Late onset Gram negative bacillary infections in Australia and New Zealand, 1992-2002. *Pediatr Infect Dis J* 2006: 25:25–29.
22. Gordon A, Isaacs D. Late-onset infection and the role of antibiotic prescribing policies. *Curr Opinion in Infect Dis* 2004; 17:231–236.
23. Zaoutis TE, Goyal M, Chu JH, et al. Risk factors for and outcomes of bloodstream infection caused by extended-spectrum beta-lactamase-producing Escherichia coli and Klebsiella species in children. *Pediatrics* 2005; 115:942–949.
24. Skippen I, Shemko M, Turton J, Kaufmann ME, Palmer C, Shetty N. Epidemiology of infections caused by extended-spectrum beta-lactamase-producing Escherichia coli and Klebsiella spp.: a nested case-control study from a tertiary hospital in London. *J Hosp Infect* 2006; 64:115–123.
25. Pitout JD, Laupland KB. Extended-spectrum beta-lactamase-producing Enterobacteriaceae: an emerging public-health concern. *Lancet Infect Dis* 2008; 8:159–166.
26. Falagas ME, Karageorgopoulos DE. Extended-spectrum beta-lactamase-producing organisms. *J Hosp Infect* 2009; 73:345–354.
27. Tiskumara R, Fakharee S-H,Liu C-Q, et al. Neonatal infections in Asia. *Arch Dis Child Fetal Neonatal Ed* 2009; 94:F144–F148.
28. Viswanathan R, Singh AK, Basu S, Chatterjee S, Sardar S, Isaacs D. Multi-drug resistant Gram negative bacilli causing early neonatal sepsis in India. *Arch Dis Fetal Neonatal Ed* 2012; 97: F182–F187.
29. Centers for Disease Control and Prevention. Preventing the spread of vancomycin resistance - a report from the Hospital Infection Control Practice Advisory Committee prepared by the Subcommittee on Prevention and Control of Antimicrobial-Resistant Microorganisms in Hospitals. *Federal Register* 1994; 59:22758–22763.
30. Van Houten MA, Uiterwaal CS, Heesen GJ, Arends JP, Kimpen JL. Does the empiric use of vancomycin in pediatrics increase the risk for Gram-negative bacteremia? *Pediatr Infect Dis J* 2001; 20:171–177.
31. Isaacs D, Fraser S, Hogg G, Li HY. *Staphylococcus aureus* infections in Australasian neonatal nurseries. *Arch Dis Child Fetal Neonatal Ed* 2004; 89:F331–F335.
32. Möller JC, Nelskamp I, Jensen R, Gatermann S, Iven H, Gortner L. Teicoplanin pharmacology in prophylaxis for coagulase-negative staphylococcal sepsis of very low birth-weight infants. *Acta Paediatr* 1996; 85:638–639.
33. Fanos V, Kacet N, Mosconi G. A review of teicoplanin in the treatment of serious neonatal infections. *Eur J Pediatr* 1997; 156:423–427.
34. Woodford N. Glycopeptides. In: *Antibiotic and Chemotherapy*. (eds RG Finch, D Greenwood, SR Norrby, RJ Whitley. 9th edn. Edinburgh: Churchill Livingstone, 2011. 265–271.
35. Möller JC, Nelskamp I, Jensen R, et al. Comparison of vancomycin and teicoplanin for prophylaxis of sepsis with coagulase negative staphylococci (CONS) in very low birth weight (VLBW) infants. *J Perinat Med* 1997; 25:361–367.

36. Russell AB, Sharland M, Heath PT. Improving antibiotic prescribing in neonatal units: time to act. *Arch Dis Child Fetal Neonatal Ed* 2010; published online Oct 30, 2010 doi:10.1136/adc.2007.120709.
37. Smith PB, Benjamin Jr DK. Choosing the right empirical antibiotics for neonates. *Arch Dis Child Fetal Neonatal Ed* 2011; 96:F2–F3.
38. Isaacs D, Catterson J, Hope PL, Wilkinson AR, Moxon ER. Factors influencing colonisation with gentamicin-resistant Gram negative organisms in the neonatal unit. *Arch Dis Child* 1988; 63:533–535.
39. Downie L, Armiento R, Subhi R, et al. Community acquired infant and neonatal sepsis in developing countries: efficacy of WHO's currently recommended antibiotics: a systematic review and meta-analysis. *Arch Dis Child* 2013;98:146–154.
40. Isaacs D, Andresen D. Combating antibiotic resistance: the war on error. *Arch Dis Child* 2013; 98:90–91.
41. Bennett KM, Scarborough JE, Sharpe M, et al. Implementation of antibiotic rotation protocol improves antibiotic susceptibility profile in a surgical intensive care unit. *J Trauma* 2007; 63:307–311.
42. Gruson D, Hilbert G, Vargas F, et al. Strategy of antibiotic rotation: long-term effect on incidence and susceptibilities of Gram-negative bacilli responsible for ventilator-associated pneumonia. *Crit Care Med* 2003; 31:1908–1914.
43. Warren DK, Hill HA, Merz LR, et al. Cycling empirical antimicrobial agents to prevent emergence of antimicrobial-resistant Gram-negative bacteria among intensive care unit patients. *Crit Care Med* 2004; 32:2450–2456.
44. Merz LR, Warren DK, Kollef MH, Fridkin SK, Fraser VJ. The impact of an antibiotic cycling program on empirical therapy for gram-negative infections. *Chest* 2006; 130:1672–1678.
45. Brown EM, Nathwani D. Antibiotic cycling or rotation: a systematic review of the evidence of efficacy. *J Antimicrob Chemother* 2005; 55:6–9.
46. Toltzis P, Dul MJ, Hoyen C, et al. The effect of antibiotic rotation on colonization with antibiotic-resistant bacilli in a neonatal intensive care unit. *Pediatrics* 2002; 110:707–711.
47. Auriti C, Ravà L, Di Ciommo V, Ronchetti MP, Orzalesi M. Short antibiotic prophylaxis for bacterial infections in a neonatal intensive care unit: a randomized controlled trial. *J Hosp Infect* 2005; 59:292–298.
48. Jardine LA, Inglis GDT, Davies MW. Prophylactic systemic antibiotics to reduce morbidity and mortality in neonates with central venous catheters. Cochrane Database of Systematic Reviews 2008, Issue 1. Art. No.: CD006179. doi: 10.1002/14651858.CD006179.pub2.
49. Lodha A, Furlan AD, Whyte H, Moore AM. Prophylactic antibiotics in the prevention of catheter-associated bloodstream bacterial infection in preterm neonates: a systematic review. *J Perinatol* 2008; 28:526–533.
50. Inglis GDT, Jardine LA, Davies MW. Prophylactic antibiotics to reduce morbidity and mortality in neonates with umbilical artery catheters. Cochrane Database of Systematic Reviews 2007, Issue 4. Art. No.: CD004697. doi: 10.1002/14651858.CD004697.pub3.
51. Inglis GDT, Davies MW. Prophylactic antibiotics to reduce morbidity and mortality in neonates with umbilical venous catheters. Cochrane Database of Systematic Reviews 2005, Issue 4. Art. No.: CD005251. doi: 10.1002/14651858.CD005251.pub2.
52. Inglis GDT, Jardine LA, Davies MW. Prophylactic antibiotics to reduce morbidity and mortality in ventilated newborn infants. Cochrane Database of Systematic Reviews 2007, Issue 3. Art. No.: CD004338. doi: 10.1002/14651858.CD004338.pub3.
53. Christensen RD, Henry E, Wiedmeier SE, Stoddard RA, Lambert DK. Low blood neutrophil concentrations among extremely low birth weight neonates: data from a multihospital health-care system. *J Perinatol* 2006; 26:682–687.
54. Doron MW, Makhlouf RA, Katz VL, Lawson EE, Stiles AD. Increased incidence of sepsis at birth in neutropenic infants of mothers with preeclampsia. *J Pediatr* 1994; 125:452–458.
55. Gray PH, Rodwell RL. Neonatal neutropenia associated with maternal hypertension poses a risk for nosocomial infection. *Eur J Pediatr* 1999; 158:71–73.
56. Cadnapaphornchai M, Faix RG. Increased nosocomial infection in neutropenic low birth weight (2000 grams or less) infants of hypertensive mothers. *J Pediatr* 1992; 121:956–961.
57. Mouzinho A, Rosenfeld CR, Sanchez PJ, Risser R. Effect of maternal hypertension on neonatal neutropenia and risk of nosocomial infection. *Pediatrics* 1992; 90:430–435.
58. Teng RJ, Wu TJ, Garrison RD, Sharma R, Hudak ML. Early neutropenia is not associated with an increased rate of nosocomial infection in very low-birth-weight infants. *J Perinatol* 2009; 29:219–224.
59. Omar SA, Salhadar A, Wooliever DE, Alsgaard PK. Late-onset neutropenia in very low birth weight infants. *Pediatrics* 2000; 106:e55.
60. Benitz WE, Gould JB, Druzin ML. Risk factors for early-onset group B streptococcal sepsis: estimation of odds ratios by critical literature review. *Pediatrics* 1999; 103:e77.
61. Puopolo KM, Draper D, Wi S, et al. Estimating the probability of neonatal early-onset infection on the basis of maternal risk factors. *Pediatrics* 2011; 128:e1155–e1163.
62. Centers for Disease Control and Prevention. Prevention of perinatal Group B streptococcal disease. *MMWR Recommendations and Reports* 2010; 59(RR-10):1–32. Link: http://www.cdc.gov/mmwr/pdf/rr/rr5910.pdf.
63. Bromberger P, Lawrence JM, Braun D, Saunders B, Contreras R, Petitti DB. The influence of intrapartum antibiotics on the clinical spectrum of early-onset group B streptococcal infection in term infants. *Pediatrics* 2000; 106: 244–250.
64. Escobar GJ, Li DK, Armstrong MA, et al. Neonatal sepsis workups in infants >/=2000 grams at birth: a population-based study. *Pediatrics* 2000; 106:256–263.
65. Pinto NM, Soskolne EI, Pearlman MD, Faix RG. Neonatal early-onset group B streptococcal disease in the era of intrapartum chemoprophylaxis: residual problems. *J Perinatol* 2003; 23:265–271.
66. Pulver LS, Hopfenbeck MM, Young PC, Stoddard GJ, Korgenski K, Daly J, et al. Continued early onset group B

streptococcal infections in the era of intrapartum prophylaxis. *J Perinatol* 2009; 29:20–25.
67. Puopolo KM, Madoff LC, Eichenwald EC. Early-onset group B streptococcal disease in the era of maternal screening. *Pediatrics* 2005; 115:1240–1246.
68. Lin FY, Brenner RA, Johnson YR, et al. The effectiveness of risk-based intrapartum chemoprophylaxis for the prevention of early-onset neonatal group B streptococcal disease. *Am J Obstet Gynecol* 2001; 184:1204–1210.
69. de Cueto M, Sanchez MJ, Sampedro A, Miranda JA, Herruzo AJ, Rosa-Fraile M. Timing of intrapartum ampicillin and prevention of vertical transmission of group B Streptococcus. *Obstet Gynecol* 1998;91:112–114.
70. Saini SS, Dutta S, Ray P, Narang A. Short course versus 7-day course of intravenous antibiotics for probable neonatal septicemia: a pilot, open-label, randomized controlled trial. *Indian Pediatr* 2011;48:19–24.
71. Isaacs D, Wilkinson AR, Moxon ER. Duration of antibiotic courses for neonates. *Arch Dis Child* 1987; 62:727–728.
72. Kaiser J, Cassat J, Lewno M. Should antibiotics be discontinued at 48 hours for negative late-onset evaluations in the neonatal intensive care unit? *J Perinatol* 2002; 22:445–447.
73. Zingg W, Pfister R, Posfay-Barbe KM, Huttner B, Touveneau S, Pittet D. Secular trends in antibiotic use among neonates: 2001-2008. *Pediatr Infect Dis J* 2011; 30:365–370.
74. Cotten CM, Taylor S, Stoll B, et al. Prolonged duration of initial empirical antibiotic treatment is associated with increased rates of necrotizing enterocolitis and death for extremely low birth weight infants. *Pediatrics* 2009; 123:58–66.
75. Alexander VN, Northrup V, Bizzarro MJ. Antibiotic exposure in the newborn intensive care unit and the risk of necrotizing enterocolitis. *J Pediatr* 2011; 159:392–397.
76. Deshpande G, Rao S, Patole S, Bulsara M. Updated meta-analysis of probiotics for preventing necrotizing enterocolitis in preterm neonates. *Pediatrics* 2010; 125:921–930.
77. Kuppala VS, Meinzen-Derr J, Morrow AL, Schibler KR. Prolonged initial empirical antibiotic treatment is associated with adverse outcomes in premature infants. *J Pediatr* 2011; 159:720–725.
78. Spitzer AR, Kirkby S, Kornhauser M. Practice variation in suspected neonatal sepsis: a costly problem in neonatal intensive care. *J Perinatol* 2005; 25:265–269.
79. Ehl S, Gering B, Bartmann P, Högel J, Pohlandt F. C-reactive protein is a useful marker for guiding duration of antibiotic therapy in suspected neonatal bacterial infection. *Pediatrics* 1997; 99:216–221.
80. Bomela HN, Ballot DE, Corey BJ, Cooper PA. Use of C-reactive protein to guide duration of empiric antibiotic therapy in suspected early neonatal sepsis. *Pediatr Infect Dis J* 2000; 19:531–535.
81. Webber S, Lindsell D, Wilkinson AR, et al. Neonatal pneumonia. *Arch Dis Child* 1990; 65:207–211.
82. Carbonell-Estrany X, Figueras-Aloy J, Salcedo-Abizanda S, de la Rosa-Fraile M, Castrillo Study Group. Probable early-onset group B streptococcal neonatal sepsis: a serious clinical condition related to intrauterine infection. *Arch Dis Child Fetal Neonatal Ed* 2008; 93:F85–F89.
83. Isaacs D. Magical numbers. *J Paediatr Child Health* 2012;48:189.
84. Chowdhary G, Dutta S, Narang A. Randomized controlled trial of 7-Day vs. 14-Day antibiotics for neonatal sepsis. *J Trop Pediatr* 2006; 52:427–432.
85. Gathwala G, Sindwani A, Singh J, Choudhry O, Chaudhary U. Ten days vs. 14 days antibiotic therapy in culture-proven neonatal sepsis. *J Trop Pediatr* 2010; 56:433–435.
86. Chapman RL, Faix RG. Persistent bacteremia and outcome in late onset infection among infants in a neonatal intensive care unit. *Pediatr Infect Dis J* 2003;22:17–21.
87. Khashu M, Osiovich H, Henry D, Al Khotani A, Solimano A, Speert DP. Persistent bacteremia and severe thrombocytopenia caused by coagulase-negative Staphylococcus in a neonatal intensive care unit. *Pediatrics* 2006; 117:340–348.

CHAPTER 6
Adjunctive treatment

A search of the literature on different adjunctive treatments found two systematic reviews of different modalities for the prevention or treatment of neonatal infections (Table 6.1).[17,18] Perhaps putting the cart after the horse, prevention will be considered in Chapter 23.

6.1 Resuscitation

Infants with severe sepsis usually need to be resuscitated with intravenous fluids and often with cardiopulmonary support in the form of artificial ventilation and possibly inotropes.[19] Hypoglycaemia should always be corrected.[19] Acidosis may need to be corrected if present and convulsions treated. Anaemia or thrombocytopenia may require transfusions of blood or platelets. There is evidence from observational data that early resuscitation of shocked neonates improves outcomes.[20]

There is very little evidence on which fluids to use in suspected neonatal sepsis and how much to give. There is strong evidence, summarized in a Cochrane systematic review of 65 studies, that the mortality of critically ill adults is no different whether crystalloids or colloids are used for fluid resuscitation.[21] The optimal volume of fluid for fluid resuscitation in septic children has been thrown into question by a study (the FEAST study) which found that rapid boluses of intravenous fluids increased mortality compared with standard fluid resuscitation for shocked, febrile East African children.[22] The significance of the FEAST study for shocked children in Western countries and for neonates in developing and Western countries remains to be evaluated.

6.2 Intravenous immunoglobulin

The full-term newborn infant is relatively poor at producing antibodies, particularly IgA and IgG, but is protected against many common infections by selective transplacental transfer of maternal antibodies. IgG is detectable in the foetus by 17 weeks and reaches half of the maternal IgG level by about 30 weeks of gestation. The foetus does not synthesize IgG until about 24 weeks of gestation.

Intravenous immunoglobulin (IVIG) is prepared from the purified, pooled plasma of blood donors and contains polyclonal IgG antibodies but no IgA or IgM antibodies. IVIG has been used both for prophylaxis and the treatment of neonatal infections.[1,23] The rationale for its use is that IgG can opsonize organisms, activate complement, bind to cell surface receptors, mediate antibody-dependent cytotoxicity and enhance neutrophil chemiluminescence and hence organism killing. IVIG also has many immunomodulatory effects on the cytokine cascade, it can down-regulate IL1, block Fc receptors on phagocytic cells and modulate Fc-receptor expression. It has a cytoprotective effect on TNF-α induced fibroblast cell death and can also reduce C3 activation and complement mediated inflammation.[24] High-dose polyclonal IVIG is used in the treatment of several inflammatory disorders of the central nervous system in adults and children. Bloodstream infections in extremely preterm infants, including CoNS infections, are associated with significant long-term neurodevelopmental impairment,[25,26] so efficacy studies of IVIG should assess neurodevelopmental impairment and disability-free survival.

Evidence-Based Neonatal Infections, First Edition. David Isaacs.

Table 6.1 Adjunctive interventions in treatment of sepsis (adapted from reference 1 with permission)

Intervention	Level of evidence	No. of infants	Summary of outcomes	Conclusions
IVIG (polyclonal):	Cochrane systematic review of IVIG for suspected or proven neonatal infection[1]	378	Mortality reduced in clinically suspected infection	Larger RCT needed
		262	Mortality reduced in proven infection	Larger RCT needed
	Cochrane systematic review of IVIG for sepsis and septic shock: neonatal studies[2]	174	No reduction in mortality with polyclonal IgG	Larger RCT needed
		164	No reduction in mortality with IgM-enriched IgG	Larger RCT needed
	One large RCT (INIS trial)[3]	3493	No significant difference in death or disability overall or in any sub-group	Strong evidence that IVIG does not improve outcome in neonatal sepsis and is not recommended.
Granulocyte transfusion	Cochrane systematic review of three small therapeutic RCTs[4]	44	No difference in mortality or sepsis	Not recommended. More RCTs needed.
Colony-stimulating factors (G-CSF or GM-CSF)	Cochrane systematic review of seven therapeutic RCTs[5]	257	No difference in mortality or sepsis	More RCTs needed
	Subgroup analysis of three therapeutic RCTs[5]	97	GM-CSF improves survival in sepsis with neutropenia:[6]	Insufficient data. More RCTs needed.
Exchange transfusion	One RCT[7] and two quasi-randomised RCTs[8, 9]	158	Exchange transfusion may improve survival in scleremic babies with Gram-negative sepsis.	Not recommended. More RCTs needed.
Activated protein C	No RCTs in neonates[10]		Ineffective in older children. Risk of bleeding including intraventricular haemorrhage.	Strong recommendation against use in neonates.
Pentoxifylline	Cochrane systematic review of four small RCTs[11]	227	Pentoxifylline appears to improve survival in proven sepsis.	Not recommended. More RCTs needed.
Lactoferrin	Cochrane systematic review[12]	0	No RCTs	Not recommended.
Melatonin	No RCTs in newborns. One observational study[13]		Non-significant effect on mortality. Insufficient data.	Not recommended. RCTs needed.
Central catheter removal	CoNS: two cohort studies[14, 15]	203	Catheter preserved in 46–51% of cases, but risk of complications increased with prolonged bacteraemia	Can often preserve central catheter in CoNS infection, but should remove it if bacteraemia persists
	S. aureus: one cohort study[14]	11	Very high complication rate (70%)	Catheter should be removed immediately in *S. aureus* infection
	Gram-negative bacilli: two cohort studies[14, 16]	95	High complication rate	Recommend immediate catheter removal in Gram-negative bacillary infection
	Enterococcus: one cohort study[14]	14	High complication rate	Recommend immediate catheter removal in enterococcal infection
	Candida: two cohort studies[14, 15]		Increased mortality with delayed removal	Strongly recommended to remove catheter in Candida infection

Question: Does IVIG given at the time of presentation with suspected sepsis improve outcome? Is there any sub-group of infants or infections for which IVIG is beneficial?

A search found two recent Cochrane systematic reviews[1, 2] and one large RCT published after the reviews.[3]

A Cochrane systematic review of IVIG for suspected or proven neonatal infection included 10 studies of variable quality.[1] Mortality was reduced in infants with clinically suspected infection given IVIG (seven studies, $n = 378$); typical relative risk RR 0.58 (95% CI; 0.38, 0.89); number needed to treat to save one life NNT = 10 (95% CI; 6, 33). Mortality was also reduced in infants with subsequently proven infection given IVIG (7 studies, $n = 262$); typical RR 0.55 (95% CI; 0.31, 0.98). Because of concerns about study quality, the authors felt there was insufficient evidence to support routine IVIG for infants with suspected or proven neonatal infection, and urged clinicians to wait for the results of the very large International Neonatal Immunotherapy Study (INIS trial) discussed below.[3]

A systematic review of IVIG to treat sepsis, severe sepsis and septic shock at any age found seven neonatal studies of polyclonal IVIG in 338 neonates with sepsis.[2] In a sub-analysis, polyclonal IVIG did not reduce mortality (RR 0.70; 95% CI 0.45–1.09). Two trials used IgM-enriched IVIG, but there was no significant reduction in mortality with standard polyclonal IVIG (RR 0.90; 95% CI 0.46–1.76; $n = 174$) or IgM-enriched polyclonal IVIG (RR 0.57; 95% CI 0.31–1.04; $n = 164$).[2]

The multi-centre, randomized placebo-controlled INIS trial enrolled 3493 infants being treated with antibiotics for suspected or proven serious infection and randomized them to two infusions of polyvalent IVIG (500 mg/kg) or placebo 48 hours apart.[3] There was no significant difference in the major outcome, death or disability, in 686 of 1759 infants (39%) who received IVIG and 677 of 1734 infants (39%) who received placebo (RR 1.00; 95% CI 0.92–1.08). There were no significant differences in rates of major or non-major disability at 2 years. Importantly, sub-group analysis could not identify any group, whether a patient group (e.g. extremely low birth-weight infants or infants with early- vs late-onset sepsis) or a particular group of organisms (e.g. infections with Gram-negative bacilli) for which IVIG improved outcome.[3] This is an important, unequivocally negative outcome from a very large RCT. IVIG is an expensive and limited resource, which should no longer be used to treat neonates with suspected or proven infection.

Recommendation: Intravenous immune globulin has no effect on the outcome of infants with suspected or proven neonatal sepsis and should not be used for this indication.

The use of prophylactic IVIG using polyclonal immunoglobulin and specific anti-staphylococcal immunoglobulin preparations to prevent neonatal infection will be considered in Chapter 23 on Prevention.

6.3 Granulocyte transfusions

Neonates, particularly pre-term neonates, have defective humoral and phagocytic immunity, predisposing them to bacterial and fungal infections. Neutropenia is common in growth-restricted infants and predisposes to sepsis (see Chapter 4). In pre-term infants, immature granulopoiesis results in a low neutrophil cell mass and a reduced capacity for increasing progenitor cell proliferation, so neutropenia commonly occurs in response to sepsis. Neutropenic septic infants, particularly those with early-onset sepsis, have a higher mortality than septic infants without neutropenia.[27, 28]

Granulocyte transfusions require finding a donor and performing leukopheresis, which often takes several hours. Buffy coats, prepared by centrifugation of whole blood, are easier to prepare but contain a lower dose of granulocytes and are less effective in reducing mortality in septic, neutropenic adults than granulocyte concentrates obtained by leukapheresis.[4]

A non-randomized study compared outcome in neonates with blood-culture proven sepsis, mainly antibiotic-resistant Klebsiella infections, who did or did not receive granulocyte transfusions. The mortality was 2 (10%) of 20 who received granulocyte transfusions and 13 (72%) of 18 infants cared for over the same period for whom granulocyte transfusion was not available. The beneficial effect was greater in infants <1500 g (mortality 10% vs 91%).[29] In a second study, 23 consecutive infants were treated with supportive care with or without granulocyte transfusions.[27] The selection process was not randomized and was not made clear. None of 13 transfused but four of 10 non-transfused comparison infants died

($p = 0.02$).[30] These two studies which are convincing at first glance, illustrate nicely the hazards of non-randomized studies with potential inherent biases, for example infants who receive granulocyte transfusions need to have survived for several hours to be able to receive the transfusions so may be have a pre-existing survival advantage compared with controls.

Granulocyte transfusions are expensive and have potential severe complications, notably fluid overload, transmission of blood-borne infection, graft-versus-host disease (GVHD) caused by lymphocytes in the transfusion, pulmonary complications secondary to leukocyte aggregation and sequestration, and sensitization to donor erythrocyte and leukocyte antigens.[4]

A Cochrane systematic review found four small RCTs.[4] A total of 44 infants with sepsis and neutropenia were randomized in three trials to receive granulocyte transfusions or placebo/supportive care.[6, 31, 32] In another trial, 35 infants with sepsis and neutropenia on antibiotics were randomized to granulocyte transfusion or IVIG.[33] Granulocyte transfusion did not improve 'all-cause mortality' compared with placebo or no transfusion, (typical RR 0.89, 95% CI 0.43–1.86).

In the study which compared granulocyte transfusion with IVIG, there was a reduction in 'all-cause mortality' of borderline statistical significance (RR 0.06, 95% CI 0.00–1.04).[33]

The only adverse effects reported in all the trials reviewed in the Cochrane review were pulmonary complications in trials that used buffy coat transfusions.[2]

There is inconclusive evidence to support or refute the routine use of granulocyte transfusions in neutropenic, septic neonates. An adequately powered multi-centre trial is needed.

6.4 Colony-stimulating factors

Granulocyte-macrophage colony stimulating factor (GM-CSF) and granulocyte colony stimulating factor (G-CSF) are naturally occurring cytokines that stimulate the production and anti-bacterial function of neutrophils and monocytes. They are routinely used to accelerate neutrophil recovery in adults and children receiving chemotherapy, where they cause only minor adverse events, such as low-grade fever. CSFs could potentially be used therapeutically to treat infants with suspected or proven sepsis with or without neutropenia, or prophylactically to prevent sepsis.

A Cochrane systematic review of G-CSF or GM-CSF in neonates[5] found seven treatment studies including 257 infants with suspected systemic bacterial infection and three prophylaxis studies with 359 neonates. The prophylactic use of CSFs will be considered in Chapter 23.

The treatment studies showed that G-CSF or GM-CSF added to antibiotic therapy in pre-term infants with suspected systemic infection did not reduce 'all-cause mortality': (typical RR 0.71, 95% CI 0.38, 1.33). The studies were all small with only 60 infants in the largest study. A sub-group analysis of 97 infected infants from three treatment studies with clinically significant neutropenia ($<1.7 \times 10^9$/L) at trial entry, did show a significant reduction in mortality by day 14 (RR 0.34, 95% CI 0.12–0.92, NNT 6, 95% CI 3–33).

The authors of the Cochrane review concluded that there is currently insufficient evidence that using G-CSF or GM-CSF to treat established systemic neonatal infection reduces mortality.[5]

6.5 Exchange transfusion

The rationale for exchange transfusion using adult blood to treat sepsis is to remove from the circulation toxic bacterial products such as endotoxins, to remove cytokines, to improve perfusion and tissue oxygenation, to replace clotting factors, to enhance humoral and cellular inflammatory responses and to correct neutropenia, if present. Exchange transfusion has predominantly been used as a salvage measure to treat overwhelming sepsis. There are no RCTs, only anecdotal reports, often of poor quality. An Indian paper reported 10 septic infants with sclerema who had not responded to antibiotics, treated with up to four exchange transfusions each. Seven infants were reported to have improved immediately and survived.[34] This sort of study is subject to considerable selection bias: an infant who survives long enough to have more than one exchange transfusion might have survived with antibiotics alone. In a quasi-RCT of exchange transfusion in 30 septic infants with neutropenia in India, mortality was 35% (7 of 20) in the transfusion group and 70% (7 of 10) in the controls ($p = 0.07$).[8] An RCT from the same institution randomly assigned culture-positive septic neonates with sclerema (mostly with Gram-negative sepsis) to exchange transfusion or no exchange transfusion. Ten of 20 babies (50%) in the study group died and 19 of 20 controls (95%), ($p = 0.003$).[7]

In contrast, a quasi-randomized study from Turkey, 7 (21%) of 33 babies of 32 to <37 weeks of gestation treated with exchange transfusion died, compared with nine (27%) of 33 who received IVIG and nine (41%) of 22 controls ($p > 0.05$).[9]

There is insufficient evidence to support exchange transfusion in neonatal sepsis.

6.6 Activated protein C

Bacteria produce endotoxins and other products which can activate the host immune system including complement, inflammatory, and coagulation cascades. The host pro-inflammatory response to infection can occasionally be excessive and lead to apoptosis, organ failure and death. Activation of the host anticoagulation process may lead to microvascular thrombus formation and disseminated intravascular coagulation. Thrombomodulin, an endothelial cell glycoprotein, combines with thrombin, converting protein C to its activated form. Activated protein C (APC) promotes fibrinolysis and blocks the production of tumour necrosis factor-α (TNF-α). APC has a short half-life. In sepsis, conversion to the activated form is reduced and the circulating pool of protein C is rapidly depleted, which can lead to increased inflammation, disseminated intravascular coagulation and multi-organ failure.

An initial RCT of adults with severe sepsis[35] found that recombinant human APC (drotrecogin-alfa) reduced 28 day all-cause mortality from 30.8% to 24.7%. Serious bleeding complications occurred significantly more often in the treatment group (3.5%) than the placebo group (2%).[35, 36] However, a later Cochrane systematic review found APC did not reduce mortality in adults (pooled RR 0.92, 95% CI 0.72–1.18) but increased bleeding.[37] APC did not reduce mortality in a RCT of 477 children with severe sepsis (RR 0.98, 95% CI 0.66–1.46), although bleeding was not increased.[10]

Neonates with or without sepsis are at increased risk for haemorrhage, including intraventricular haemorrhage, and APC is potentially harmful to them. There are no RCTs of APC in neonates.[10] APC should not be used in neonatal infection.

6.7 Pentoxifylline

The xanthine derivative pentoxifylline is a phosphodiesterase inhibitor that activates adenyl cyclase to increase cellular cyclic AMP concentration and suppress TNF-α production. Pentoxifylline improves endothelial cell function and reduces coagulopathy in sepsis. In adults with sepsis, pentoxifylline improves renal blood flow and reduces acute lung injury from chronic endotoxemia.[11, 38] Pentoxifylline reduced the incidence and severity of necrotizing enterocolitis (NEC) in a rat model.[39]

A Cochrane systematic review of pentoxifylline as an adjunct to antibiotics for treatment of suspected or confirmed late onset (>7 days) sepsis or NEC in neonates identified three small RCTs and one quasi-RCT.[11] Pentoxifylline therapy significantly decreased "all cause" mortality compared to placebo ($n = 227$, typical RR 0.40, 95% CI 0.20–0.77; NNT 7, 95% CI 4–20). In sub-group analyses mortality was significantly reduced in pre-term infants, infants with confirmed sepsis and infants with Gram-negative sepsis. Pentoxifylline treatment decreased the length of hospital stay by an average of 11 days, but not the development of NEC in neonates with sepsis. No adverse effects due to pentoxifylline were reported. Two of the studies were by the same research team in Poland and one each was in Egypt and India. The Cochrane reviewers commented that the evidence is weakened by methodologic deficiencies in the included studies.[11] They also noted that pentoxifylline is not licensed for use in neonates in many countries.

6.8 Lactoferrin

Lactoferrin is a naturally occurring glycoprotein found in high concentration in human colostrum and in lower concentrations in human milk, tears, saliva, seminal fluid and neutrophils. It is part of the innate immune response, with broad-spectrum antimicrobial activity against bacteria, fungi, viruses and protozoa, resulting from its ability to sequester iron or because of a direct lytic effect on microbial cell membranes.[40] Proteolysis of lactoferrin under acid conditions, for example in the stomach or in the neutrophil phagolysosomes, produces peptides called lactoferricins with enhanced antimicrobial activity.[13] Oral bovine lactoferrin has been used prophylactically (see Section 23.4.4).

A Cochrane systematic review found no RCTs of the use of lactoferrin to treat suspected or proven infection[12] and a literature search did not find any subsequent published trials. Randomized trials of lactoferrin in suspected or established infection are planned and the use of lactoferrin for this indication should be restricted to trials.

6.9 Melatonin

Melatonin reduces oxidative stress from toxic free radicals in animal models and thus might be helpful in sepsis.[41] Melatonin has been used in one neonatal non-randomized clinical trial of neonatal sepsis: 10 septic neonates given oral melatonin all survived, compared with seven of 10 control septic babies ($p > 0.05$).[42] Septic infants had higher serum levels of lipid peroxidation products than non-infected babies, but the levels were reduced to normal in septic infants treated with melatonin.[42] There are no RCTs of melatonin in neonates with infection.

6.10 Central line removal: if and when to pull the line

Approximately 5% of central venous catheters become infected,[43] at a rate that is usually between 4.4 and 12.1 per 1000 line days.[14,44–46] Whether or not it is critical to remove the central line as well as treat with antimicrobials is controversial. Neonatologists would often like to preserve precious central catheters for vascular access. The specific infecting organism is an important determinant of the risk from not removing the central catheter.[14,44–46] A Cochrane systematic review found no RCTs,[15] but there is some evidence from cohort studies to guide clinical practice.

6.10.1 Central line removal in coagulase-negative staphylococcus bacteraemia

Focal suppurative complications are less common in central line-associated infections due to CoNS than other organisms.[16,47] A US cohort study of infants with central venous catheters and CoNS bacteraemia compared early (≤3 days) with late removal of central catheters (>3 days) in addition to IV vancomycin. There was no significant difference in recurrence of bacteraemia or mortality between 56 infants with early and 63 with late removal, but bacteraemia lasted >3 days in 13% and 43%, respectively.[48] Of the infants with late removal, the success rate for treating successfully without removal was 79% for bacteraemia lasting 1–2 days, 44% if 3–4 days, but none of 19 with bacteraemia >4 days. A retrospective cohort study of central-line associated bacteraemia included 84 infants with CoNS infection.[16] Line sterilization using per catheter antibiotics was not attempted in 12 of the infants. Of the remaining 72, the catheter was salvaged without complications in 37 (51%) but 7 (10%) were judged to have developed end-organ damage (abscess two, endocarditis two, meningitis three) and one died. Neonates who had multiple positive blood cultures were more likely to have end-organ damage, which occurred in one infant with one positive blood culture, one with three positives and five with four or more positive cultures.[16] Central line salvage is successful in about half of all CoNS infections but central lines should be removed if bacteraemia persists.

6.10.2 Central line removal in *Staphylococcus aureus* bacteraemia

In a retrospective cohort study,[16] 11 infants had *S. aureus* bacteraemia. Line sterilization was attempted in 10, but was successful in only one. Nine had complicated bacteraemia (defined as organ damage, multiple positive blood cultures or death). Four had multiple sites of end-organ damage, including abscess (2), osteomyelitis (2), and endocarditis (1) and two died. One positive blood culture for *S. aureus* warrants central line removal.

6.10.3 Central line removal in Gram-negative bacteraemia

A retrospective cohort study[16] divided infants with Gram-negative bacteraemia into those infected with enteric Gram-negative and those with non-enteric Gram-negative bacilli (Pseudomonas, Alcaligenes and Stenotrophomonas). Catheter sterilization was unsuccessful in all five infants with non-enteric Gram-negative bacilli in whom it was attempted. Three infants had end-organ damage and three died. With enteric Gram-negative bacilli, 10 (34%) of 29 infants retained their catheters without complications, seven developed persistent bacteraemia, five end-organ damage, three meningitis and one died.[16] Another US retrospective cohort study compared instant with delayed (>2 days) catheter removal in Enterobacteriaceae (enteric Gram-negative bacillary) bacteraemia.[49] Although 17 (45%) of 38 were treated successfully without catheter removal, 16 (42%) had prolonged bacteraemia, two had recurrent bacteraemia and success was only 24% if bacteraemia persisted for more than 1 day. One infant developed meningitis and two died. The authors concluded that it might be possible to salvage some central catheters in infants with bacteraemia due to enteric Gram-negative bacilli, but not if bacteraemia persisted for more than 1 day. In practice, culture results are not back for 1–2 days, so if sterilization is attempted, this recommendation will mean keeping the catheter in for 2–3 days. In general the catheter should be removed in an infant with catheter-associated Gram-negative bacillary bacteraemia unless vascular access is otherwise impossible.

6.10.4 Central line removal in enterococcal bacteraemia

A retrospective cohort study[16] reported outcome in infants infected with enterococci (faecal streptococci). Sterilization was successful in 5 (42%) of 12 infants. Two babies developed end-organ failure, two had persistent bacteraemia, one developed endocarditis and one meningitis.

6.10.5 Central venous catheter removal in candidemia

A US retrospective cohort study compared outcome in 21 candidemic infants in whom their central catheter was removed immediately in 13 and retained in 8.[50] Persistent candidemia developed in 2 of 13 infants with early catheter removal and six of eight where the catheter was retained. Two early catheter removal infants developed new complications of candidiasis and none died. In contrast, persistent candidemia only resolved after catheter removal in three of eight infants where the catheter was retained, new complications developed in 3, and two died from systemic Candida infection.[50] A subsequent retrospective US cohort study compared early removal (≤3 days) with late removal (>3 days) in candidemic infants.[51] None of 21 infants in the early removal group died compared with 9 (34%) of 23 in the late removal group.[51] While these data may be confounded if catheters are only left in place in the sickest infants with the most difficult venous access, they nonetheless suggest that any central venous catheter in place should be removed and replaced with a peripheral cannula as soon as Candida is grown from blood.

6.11 Prophylactic antimicrobials

The use of prophylactic antibiotics is considered in Chapter 5 and of prophylactic antifungals in Chapter 16.

References

1. Ohlsson A, Lacy J. Intravenous immunoglobulin for suspected or subsequently proven infection in neonates. *Cochrane Database Syst Rev* 2010, (Issue. 3). Art. No.: CD001239. doi:10.1002/14651858.
2. Alejandria MM, Lansang MAD, Dans LF, Mantaring III JB. Intravenous immunoglobulin for treating sepsis, severe sepsis and septic shock. *Cochrane Database Syst Rev* 2002, (Issue. 1). Art. No.: CD001090. doi:10.1002/14651858.
3. INIS Collaborative Group, Brocklehurst P, Farrell B, King A, et al. Treatment of neonatal sepsis with intravenous immune globulin. *N Engl J Med* 2011; 365:1201–1211.
4. Pammi M, Brocklehurst P. Granulocyte transfusions for neonates with confirmed or suspected sepsis and neutropenia. *Cochrane Database Syst Rev* 2011, (Issue. 10). Art. No.: CD003956. doi:10.1002/14651858.
5. Carr R, Modi N, Doré CJ. G-CSF and GM-CSF for treating or preventing neonatal infections. *Cochrane Database Syst Rev* 2003, (Issue. 3). Art. No.: CD003066. doi:10.1002/14651858.
6. Christensen RD, Rothstein G, Anstall HB, Bybee B. Granulocyte transfusions in neonates with bacterial infection, neutropenia and depletion of mature marrow neutrophils. *Pediatrics* 1982; 70:1–6.
7. Sadana S, Mathur NB, Thakur A. Exchange transfusion in septic neonates with sclerema: effect on immunoglobulin and complement levels. *Indian Pediatrics* 1997; 34:20–25.
8. Vain NE, Mazlumian JR, Swarner OW, Cha CC. Role of exchange transfusion in the treatment of severe septicemia. *Pediatrics* 1980; 66:693–697.
9. Gunes T, Koklu E, Buyukkayhan D, Kurtoglu S, Karakukcu M, Patiroglu T. Exchange transfusion or intravenous immunoglobulin therapy as an adjunct to antibiotics for neonatal sepsis in developing countries: a pilot study. *Ann Trop Paediatr* 2006; 26:39–42.
10. Kylat RI, Ohlsson A. Recombinant human activated protein C for severe sepsis in neonates. *Cochrane Database Syst Rev* 2006, (Issue. 2). Art. No.: CD005385. doi:10.1002/14651858. CD005385.PUB2.
11. Haque KN, Pammi M. Pentoxifylline for treatment of sepsis and necrotizing enterocolitis in neonates. *Cochrane*

Database Syst Rev 2011, (Issue. 10). Art. No.: CD004205. doi:10.1002/14651858.CD004205.PUB2.

12. Pammi M, Abrams SA. Oral lactoferrin for the treatment of sepsis and necrotizing enterocolitis in neonates. *Cochrane Database Syst Rev* 2011, (Issue. 10). Art. No.: CD007138. doi:10.1002/14651858.CD007138.pub3.
13. Gifford JL, Hunter HN, Vogel HJ. Lactoferricin: a lactoferrin-derived peptide with antimicrobial, antiviral, antitumor and immunological properties. *Cell Molec Life Sciences* 2005; 62:2588–2598.
14. Mahieu LM, De Muynck AO, Ieven MM, De Dooy JJ, Goossens HJ, Van Reempts PJ. Risk factors for central vascular catheter-associated bloodstream infections among patients in a neonatal intensive care unit. *J Hosp Infect* 2001; 48:108–116.
15. Vasudevan C, McGuire W. Early removal versus expectant management of central venous catheters in neonates with bloodstream infection. *Cochrane Database Syst Rev* 2011, (Issue. 8). Art. No.: CD008436. doi: 10.1002/14651858. CD008436.pub2.
16. Benjamin Jr DK, Miller W, Garges H, et al. Bacteremia, central catheters, and neonates: when to pull the line. *Pediatrics* 2001; 107:1272–1276.
17. Tarnow-Mordi W, Isaacs D, Dutta S. Adjunctive immunologic interventions in neonatal sepsis. *Clin Perinatol* 2010; 37:481–499.
18. Cohen-Wolkowiez M, Benjamin Jr DK, Capparelli E. Immunotherapy in neonatal sepsis: advances in treatment and prophylaxis. *Curr Opin Pediatr* 2009; 21:177–181.
19. Kissoon N, Orr RA, Carcillo JA. Updated American College of Critical Care Medicine–pediatric advanced life support guidelines for management of pediatric and neonatal septic shock: relevance to the emergency care clinician. *Pediatr Emerg Care* 2010; 26:867–869.
20. Han YY, Carcillo JA, Dragotta MA, et al. Early reversal of pediatric-neonatal septic shock by community physicians is associated with improved outcome. *Pediatrics* 2003; 112:793–799.
21. Perel P, Roberts I. Colloids versus crystalloids for fluid resuscitation in critically ill patients. *Cochrane Database Syst Rev* 2011, (Issue. 3). Art. No.: CD000567. doi:10.1002/14651858.cd000567.pub4.
22. Maitland K, Kiguli S, Opoka RO, et al., for the FEAST Trial Group. Mortality after fluid bolus in African a. *N Engl J Med* 2011; 364:2483–2495.
23. Ohlsson A, Lacy J. Intravenous immunoglobulin for preventing infection in preterm and/or low birth weight infants. *Cochrane Database Syst Rev* 2004, (Issue. 1). Art. No.: CD000361. doi:10.1002/14651858.
24. Mohan PV, Tarnow-Mordi W, Stenson B, et al. Can polyclonal intravenous immunoglobulin limit cytokine mediated cerebral damage and chronic lung disease in preterm infants?. *Arch Dis Child Fetal Neonatal Ed* 2004; 89:F5–F8.
25. Stoll BJ, Hansen NI, Adams-Chapman I, et al. Neurodevelopmental and growth impairment among extremely low-birth-weight infants with neonatal infection. *J Am Med Assoc*2004; 292:2357–2365.
26. Adams-Chapman I, Stoll BJ. Neonatal infection and long-term neurodevelopmental outcome in the preterm infant. *Curr Opin Infect Dis* 2006; 19:290–297.
27. Rodwell RL, Taylor KM, Tudehope DI, Gray PH. Hematologic scoring system in early diagnosis of sepsis in neutropenic newborns. *Pediatric Infectious Disease Journal* 1993; 12:372–376.
28. Christensen RD, Henry E, Wiedmeier SE, Stoddard RA, Lambert DK. Low blood neutrophil concentrations among extremely low birth weight neonates: data from a multihospital health-care system. *J Perinatol* 2006; 26:682–687.
29. Cairo MS, Rucker R, Bennetts GA, et al. Improved survival of newborns receiving leukocyte transfusions for sepsis. *Pediatrics* 1984; 74:887–892.
30. Laurenti F, Ferro R, Isacchi G, et al. Polymorphonuclear leukocyte transfusion for the treatment of sepsis in the newborn infant. *J Pediatr* 1981;98:118–123
31. Baley JE, Stork EK, Warkentin PI, Shurin SB. Buffy coat transfusions in neutropenic neonates with presumed sepsis: A prospective randomized trial. *Pediatrics* 1987; 80:712–719.
32. Wheeler JG, Chauvenet AR, Johnson CA, Block SM, Dillard R, Abramson JS. Buffy coat transfusions in neonates with sepsis and neutrophil storage pool depletion. *Pediatrics* 1987; 79:422–425.
33. Cairo MS, Worcester CC, Rucker RW, et al. Randomized trial of granulocyte transfusions versus intravenous immune globulin therapy for neonatal neutropenia and sepsis. *Journal of Pediatrics* 1992; 120:281–285.
34. Mathur NB, Subramanian BK, Sharma VK, Puri RK. Exchange transfusion in neutropenic septicemic neonates: effect on granulocyte functions. *Acta Paediatrica* 1993; 82:939–943.
35. Bernard GR, Vincent JL, Laterre PF, et al. Efficacy and safety of recombinant human activated protein C for severe sepsis. *N Engl J Med* 2001; 344:699–709.
36. Bernard GR, Margolis BD, Shanies HM, et al. Extended evaluation of recombinant human activated protein C United States Trial (ENHANCE US): a single-arm, phase 3B, multicenter study of drotrecogin alfa (activated) in severe sepsis. *Chest* 2004; 125:2206–2216.
37. Nadel S, Goldstein B, Williams MD, et al. Drotrecogin alfa (activated) in children with severe sepsis: a multicentre phase III randomised controlled trial. *Lancet* 2007; 369:836–843.
38. Michetti C, Coimbra R, Hoyt DB, Loomis W, Junger W, Wolf P. Pentoxifylline reduces acute lung injury in chronic endotoxemia. *J Surg Res* 2003; 115:92–99.
39. Travadi J, Patole S, Charles A, Dvorak B, Doherty D, Simmer K. Pentoxifylline reduces the incidence and severity of necrotizing enterocolitis in a neonatal rat model. *Pediatr Res* 2006; 60:185–189.
40. Valenti P, Antonini G. Lactoferrin: an important host defence against microbial and viral attack. *Cell Molec Life Sciences* 2005; 62:2576–2587.
41. Gitto E, Pellegrino S, Gitto P, Barberi I, Reiter RJ. Oxidative stress of the newborn in the pre- and postnatal period and the clinical utility of melatonin. *J Pineal Res* 2009; 46:128–139.

42. Gitto E, Karbownik M, Reiter RJ, et al. Effects of melatonin treatment in septic newborns. *Pediatr Res* 2001;50:756–760.
43. Cartwright D. Central venous lines in neonates: a study of 2186 catheters. *Arch Dis Child Fetal Neonatal Ed* 2004; 89:F504–F508.
44. Chien LY, Macnab Y, Aziz K, Andrews W, McMillan DD, Lee SK; Canadian Neonatal Network. Variations in central venous catheter-related infection risks among Canadian neonatal intensive care units. *Pediatr Infect Dis J* 2002; 21:505–511.
45. Mahieu LM, De Dooy JJ, Lenaerts AE, Ieven MM, De Muynck AO. Catheter manipulations and the risk of catheter-associated bloodstream infection in neonatal intensive care unit patients. *J Hosp Infect* 2001; 48:20–26.
46. Olsen AL, Reinholdt J, Jensen AM, Andersen LP, Jensen ET. Nosocomial infection in a Danish Neonatal Intensive Care Unit: a prospective study. *Acta Paediatrica* 2009; 98:1294–1299.
47. Chapman RL, Faix RG. Persistent bacteremia and outcome in late onset infection among infants in a neonatal intensive care unit. *Pediatr Infect Dis J* 2003; 22:17–21.
48. Karlowicz MG, Furigay PJ, Croitoru DP, Buescher ES. Central venous catheter removal versus in situ treatment in neonates with coagulase-negative staphylococcal bacteremia. *Pediatr Infect Dis J* 2002; 21:22–27.
49. Nazemi KJ, Buescher ES, Kelly Jr RE, Karlowicz MG. Central venous catheter removal versus in situ treatment in neonates with enterobacteriaceae bacteremia. *Pediatrics* 2003; 111:e269–e274.
50. Eppes SC, Troutman JL, Gutman LT. Outcome of treatment of candidemia in children whose central catheters were removed or retained. *Pediatr Infect Disease J* 1989; 8:99–104.
51. Karlowicz MG, Hashimoto LN, Kelly Jr RE, Buescher ES. Should central venous catheters be removed as soon as candidemia is detected in neonates?. *Pediatrics* 2000; 106:E63.

CHAPTER 7
Bacterial meningitis

7.1 Epidemiology

Bacterial meningitis is more common in the neonatal period than at any other age.[1–3] A review of the epidemiology of neonatal bacterial meningitis found two non-Cochrane reviews of neonatal meningitis in Western countries[1, 2] and one in developing countries.[3] This chapter will concentrate on bacterial meningitis (see Chapter 16 for fungal meningitis, Chapter 17 for viral meningitis and Chapter 18 for tuberculous meningitis).

7.1.1 Incidence

The reported incidence of neonatal meningitis varies with diagnostic practice, changes in prevalent organisms, rates of prematurity and the use of intrapartum maternal antibiotic chemoprophylaxis to reduce GBS infection. In the United Kingdom, the rate of neonatal meningitis was 0.4–0.5 cases/1000 in the 1970s,[4, 5] but fell to 0.21–0.25/1000 live births in the 1980s and 1990s.[6–8] A US study reported a similar incidence of 0.25 cases/1000 live births from 1988–1992.[9] In Australia in the 1980s, the reported rate was 0.17 cases/1000 live births.[10]

Reports do not always distinguish early- from late-onset meningitis. The rate of early-onset meningitis in Australia from 1992–2002 was 0.11 per 1000 live births, but was 1.1 per 1000 infants <1500 g.[11] The proportion of US infants <1500 g who survived at least 3 days and developed late-onset meningitis was 1.4%.[12] High-risk populations may have an even higher incidence even if not so premature: 1% of neonates >34 weeks managed on US neonatal intensive care units developed meningitis, presumably because the population included infants with other risk factors.[13]

The incidence in developing countries is almost certainly higher than in Western countries but the data are subject to considerable uncertainty. As pointed out by the authors of a systematic review,[3] studies may define the 'neonatal period' as up to 30, 60 or 90 days. Because most births in developing countries occur at home and deaths are under-reported, the true incidence and mortality of neonatal meningitis is probably a lot higher than reported. A review of evidence from community-based studies in developing countries found a reported incidence of neonatal meningitis that varied from 0.8 per 1000 live births in the first week of life to 6.1 per 1000 live births overall.[14]

The population incidence of neonatal meningitis is arguably mainly of academic interest to the practicing neonatologist. It may help to plan services and to decide whether investigations like lumbar puncture (LP) should be performed routinely (see Section 4.1.3) to know whether meningitis is rare or common. However, the clinician's concern is whether the baby being examined at that moment has meningitis. Because the signs of meningitis are non-specific, the more helpful clinical statistic is the proportion of babies with meningitis. As discussed in Chapter 4, about 1 in every 500 pre-term babies with early-onset respiratory distress in the United States has meningitis.[15] On the other hand, around 10–30% of babies with proven early-onset bacteraemia have meningitis, although the proportion is falling with time. In an Australian study, 9.2% of 852 babies with early-onset sepsis from 1992–2002 had proven meningitis.[11] The proportion of babies with early-onset sepsis who develop meningitis depends partly on the infecting organism, because some organisms are more likely to lead to meningitis, and on the infant's gestational age, because the risk increases with falling gestation.

Evidence-Based Neonatal Infections, First Edition. David Isaacs.

The proportion of babies with late-onset sepsis in Western countries who have meningitis is usually reported to be lower than for early-onset sepsis, particularly since CoNS became responsible for more than half of all late-onset infections.[16] CoNS rarely cause meningitis: 0.4% of infants with CoNS sepsis in one study had meningitis.[17] In a large US study of infants <1500 g, 5.5% of bacteraemic infants were diagnosed with late-onset meningitis.[12] In an Australian study, a similar proportion of 5.9% of babies with late-onset sepsis had meningitis.[11]

There are few data from developing countries. A Kenyan cross-sectional study reported bacterial meningitis in 17.9% of infants with suspected neonatal sepsis.[18]

Around a third of all babies with meningitis has a negative blood culture at the time of meningitis (see Section 4.1.3),[13, 19] so treating an infant with suspected sepsis empirically with antibiotics without an LP, and basing decisions on blood cultures risks missing cases of meningitis.

7.1.2 Morbidity and mortality

Mortality depends on the organism (e.g. Gram-negative bacillary meningitis has a higher mortality[20]), the host (e.g. gestation, perinatal asphyxia, intraventricular haemorrhage, etc.) and the environment (e.g. time to diagnosis and treatment). The reported mortality rate from neonatal meningitis in Western countries is around 10–20%,[1, 11, 21, 22] whereas in developing countries it is nearer 40–60% (range 25–67%).[3]

Studies in Western countries show that about 20% of survivors of neonatal meningitis have moderate-to-severe disability, 10% severe and 10% moderate.[22–24]

In one study, 13 of 101 infants with neonatal meningitis died and 17 had moderate or severe disability at 1 year of age.[22] Important predictors of adverse outcome already present at 12 hours and at 96 hours were seizures, coma, use of inotropes, and leukopenia.[22] An abnormal EEG was a stronger predictor of adverse outcome and repeat EEGs improved the predictive accuracy.[25]

7.2 Pathogenesis

Most cases of neonatal meningitis are thought to result from bacteraemia. The evidence for this statement comes from animal models: infant rats inoculated intranasally with *Haemophilus influenzae* type b (Hib) develop intranasal colonization, then bacteraemia, then meningitis.[26, 27] Foetal scalp electrodes can rarely cause CSF leaks but have not been reported to result in meningitis.[28, 29] Although an infected scalp lesion or infected cephalhaematoma can lead to osteomyelitis and direct spread of organisms to the meninges,[30] this route of infection is extremely rare. An open meningomyelocoele will usually lead to meningitis if not closed, although when it is elected not to treat an infant with severe spina bifida and meningomyelocoele, it is commonly several days before the baby develops meningitis.[31–33]

As with all infectious diseases, the reason one baby gets meningitis and not another depends on a combination of host, organism and environmental factors. Interestingly, if one twin develops late-onset GBS meningitis there is a high likelihood that the other twin will also develop late-onset GBS infection (see Chapter 14). This could be due to the genetic factors (the host), virulence of the organism (the organism) or exposure to GBS in breast milk (the environment).

Factors that predispose to bacteraemia also predispose to meningitis, including host factors (prematurity, reduced immunity, perinatal asphyxia, hypoxia, acidosis) and invasive interventions such as mechanical ventilation, central venous catheterization and parenteral nutrition (see Section 2.2).

Environmental factors that predispose to early-onset meningitis include maternal risk factors: chorioamnionitis, maternal fever, prolonged rupture of membranes and colonization with virulent organisms, particularly GBS (see Chapter 2).

Organism factors are a major determinant of whether or not a baby gets bacterial meningitis. Some organisms which are common causes of bacteraemia almost never cause meningitis, e.g. *Staphylococcus aureus*[34] and CoNS.[17] Other organisms clearly have a greater predilection to invade the meninges. GBS is an important cause of early-onset neonatal meningitis, and its incidence can be reduced markedly by using intrapartum antibiotic chemoprophylaxis.[11] However, late-onset GBS infections, including meningitis, are not prevented by intrapartum chemoprophylaxis. Like the three major organisms causing infant meningitis, namely Hib, *Streptococcus pneumoniae* and *Neisseria meningitidis*, GBS has a polysaccharide (sugar) capsule which is an important

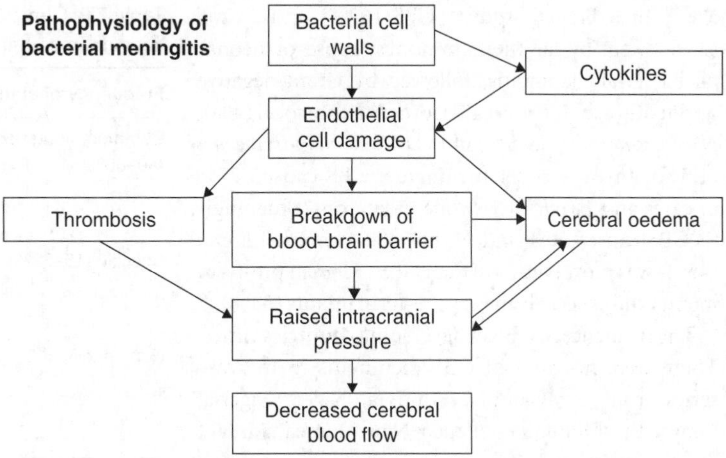

Figure 7.1 Pathophysiology of bacterial meningitis.

determinant of virulence. So, too, do about 80% of *Escherichia coli* strains causing meningitis: the K1 capsular antigen possessed by these *E. coli* is closely related to *N. meningitidis* group B capsular polysaccharide.[35] However, most Gram-negative bacilli are not encapsulated but are an important cause of neonatal meningitis, and tend to cause marked inflammation with ventriculitis.

Late-onset GBS meningitis is usually caused by serotype III, although this serotype causes only about a third of early-onset GBS infection. This implies that serotype III has other virulence determinants favouring colonization and later invasion (see Chapter 14).

Some organisms have a greater predilection for invasion of brain tissue to cause brain abscesses. Although neonatal brain abscesses have been described with different organisms including GBS, *S. pneumoniae*, *S. aureus*, anaerobes and Gram-negative bacilli, they are particularly commonly reported with *Citrobacter, Enterobacter sakazakii (Cronobacter sakazakii)* and *Proteus*.[36–38]

Bacterial meningitis does not usually involve direct invasion of the brain, yet results in major morbidity and mortality. The mechanisms underlying damage are summarized in Figure 7.1. Toxins such as endotoxin in the cell walls of Gram-negative bacilli and peptidoglycans and teichoic acid in Gram-positive cocci damage the vascular endothelium leading to breakdown of the blood–brain barrier with vascular leak, thrombosis, cerebral oedema and eventual impaired cerebral perfusion.

7.3 Organisms

In most Western countries, the most common organisms causing neonatal bacterial meningitis are GBS, *E. coli*, other Gram-negative bacilli, *S. pneumoniae* and Listeria[1, 2, 21, 39] (Table 7.1). In a US study which only reported cases of meningitis in infants <2 months due to GBS, *H. influenzae*, *S. pneumoniae*, *N. meningitidis* and Listeria, GBS caused 86.1% of cases and Listeria

Table 7.1 Organisms causing neonatal meningitis in Western countries[a].

Frequency of occurrence	Organisms
Common (>10%)*	Group B streptococcus (GBS) *Escherichia coli*
Uncommon (1–10%)	Other Gram-negative enteric bacilli *Listeria monocytogenes* *Streptococcus pneumoniae* Enterococci (faecal streptococci) Other streptococci
Rare (<1%)	Coagulase-negative staphylococci *Staphylococcus aureus* *Haemophilus influenzae* (usually untypeable) *Neisseria meningitidis* Anaerobes

[a]The exact proportions vary from country to country, with time, and with the use of intrapartum chemoprophylaxis.

5%.[39] In a French study,[21] GBS (59%) and *E. coli* (28%) were by far the commonest cause of neonatal bacterial meningitis, followed by Gram-negative bacilli other than *E. coli* (4%), other streptococci (4%), *N. meningitidis* (3%), and *Listeria monocytogenes* (1.5%). In early-onset meningitis, GBS caused 77% of cases and *E. coli* 18%, while in late-onset meningitis GBS caused 50% and *E. coli* 33%. However, *E. coli* (45%) was more common than GBS (32%) in pre-term infants and especially in very pre-term infants (54%).[21]

The incidence of GBS in developing countries varies. There were no cases of GBS meningitis in the case series from the Gambia, Ethiopia, Niger, Nigeria, Kenya, the Philippines, Papua New Guinea, Jordan, Saudi Arabia and Panama, summarized in a systematic review.[3] However, GBS was the most commonly reported organism causing meningitis in case series from Qatar, the United Arab Emirates, Malawi, Zimbabwe, South Africa and Trinidad, West Indies and was an important cause in case series from Thailand and Kenya.[3] It is difficult to know if these differences are because of variations in laboratory techniques or represent genuine differences in incidence (Table 7.2).

Table 7.2 Organisms causing neonatal meningitis in developing countries.

Frequency of occurrence	Organisms
Common (>10%)[a]	Klebsiella species *E. coli* Serratia species Acinetobacter species Salmonella (non-typhoidal) [a]GBS [a]*S. aureus*
Uncommon (1–10%)	Pseudomonas species Enterobacter species Other Gram-negative enteric bacilli [b]*S. pneumoniae* Enterococci (faecal streptococci) Other streptococci
Rare (<1%)	Coagulase-negative staphylococci *S. aureus* *H. influenzae* (usually untypeable) *N. meningitidis* Anaerobes

[a]Reported from some countries but not others.
[b]Can be <1 month, but more common at age 1–3 months.

Table 7.3 Clinical signs and estimated frequency in neonatal meningitis.

Frequency of signs	Clinical signs
Common, non-specific (40–60%)	Abnormal temperature (fever or hypothermia) Abnormal behaviour: lethargy or irritability
Specific (15–33%)	Bulging fontanelle (33%) Seizures (30%) Neck stiffness (15%)
Non-specific (15–40%)	Respiratory symptoms (tachypnoea, distress) Jaundice Vomiting or diarrhoea

Gram-negative enteric bacilli, particularly Klebsiella species, cause early- and late-onset meningitis worldwide. Non-typhoidal salmonellae and *S. aureus* are reported in some countries but not others. *S. pneumoniae* is more likely to cause post-neonatal infant meningitis but can also cause neonatal meningitis particularly in Africa.[3]

7.4 Clinical manifestations

The clinical signs in bacterial meningitis are mostly non-specific (Table 7.3).[1–7] However, a bulging fontanelle occurs in about 33% of infants with meningitis, seizures in 30% and neck stiffness in 15%. Opisthotonus (Figure 7.2) is a late and sinister sign.

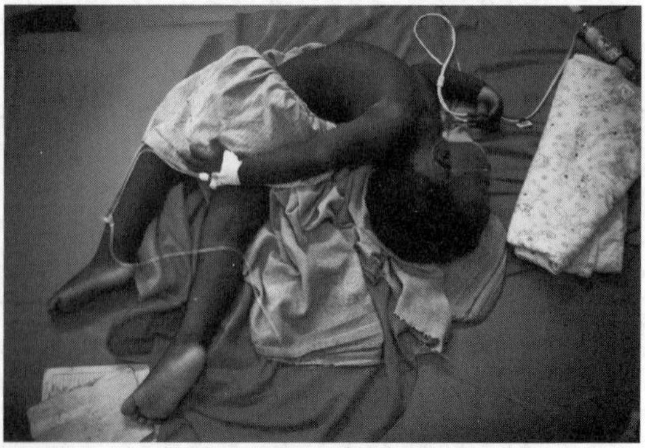

Figure 7.2 Bacterial meningitis causing severe opisthotonus (photo reproduced courtesy of Olivia Swann).

7.5 Diagnosis

The rationale for immediate LP in suspected sepsis is discussed in Chapter 4 (see Section 4.1.3). The common practice of starting empiric antibiotics without performing an LP and relying on the blood culture result to diagnose meningitis is dangerous: 28–38% of neonates with bacterial meningitis have a negative blood culture.[13, 19] The risk of LP causing respiratory compromise can be reduced by performing the LP with the infant in a sitting or modified lateral position.[40]

One paper described the interpretation of CSF results as both art and science, noting that in the second century Galen described CSF as a vaporous humour produced in the ventricles that provided energy to the rest of the body and commenting wryly "such theories have not been universally replaced by rationale."[41] The interpretation of neonatal CSF results is complicated by problems defining normal ranges, problems defining meningitis, interpretation of blood-stained CSF and influence of extraneous factors.

One barrier to defining normal ranges is an ethical problem. Although one 1966 South African study performed LPs on well full-term infants in the first day after birth,[41] it is not now considered ethical to LP a normal baby. Therefore in deciding that a baby who received an LP, usually for suspected sepsis, is in fact 'normal,' it is imperative to exclude viral or other occult infection, which is impossible in practice. Additionally, CSF parameters vary by gestational age and post-natal age.

The problem defining meningitis relates mainly to growth of possible CSF contaminants and situations where the blood culture grows an organism but the CSF does not, with or without changes in CSF microscopy or biochemistry.

7.5.1 Cerebrospinal fluid white cell count

A summary of CSF white cell counts from selected studies[13,42–48] is given in Table 7.4. There is quite good concordance between the mean or median white cell counts in the studies, which do not seem to vary greatly with gestation. A US study of infants <1500 g found no correlation between gestational age and CSF white count in infants who had an LP at birth. However, CSF white count decreased with increasing age.[49] This information is not useful to the clinician managing an infant with possible meningitis who wants to know "given the CSF findings, is this infant likely to be infected or can I withhold antibiotics?"

The clinician has a number of questions about CSFs.

Table 7.4 Normal values for CSF total white cell count ($\times 10^6$/L or per mm^3) from selected studies.

Study	Population (n)	Age (days)	Mean (SD)	Median	Range
Roberts (1925)[43]	Full-term (n = 423)	1	6.3		2–17
Naidoo (1968)[42]	Full-term well (n = 135)	1	5 (11.5)		0–90
Sarff (1976)[44]	Full term (n = 87)	1–10	8.2 (7.1)	5	0–32
	'Pre-term' (n = 30)		9.0 (8.2)	6	0–29
Rodriguez (1970)[45]	VLBW <1500 g (n = 71)	0–28	5		0–44
Ahmed (1996)[46]	Full-term (n = 108)	0–28	7.3 (14)	4	0–130
Bonadio (1992)[47]: review of 5 studies	Pre-term	0–28	9		0–29
	Term	1	8.2		0–22
	Term	1–28	11		0–50
Garges (2005)[13]	>34 weeks culture-negative (n = 8912)	0–28		6 [IQR 2–15]	0–90,000
Kestenbaum (2010)[48]	Full-term (n = 380) ill, enterovirus negative	0–28	4.8	3 (+2 SD = 19)	0–78

VLBW, very low birth weight; IQR, interquartile range (25th–75th centile); SD, standard deviation.

Question 1: Is there a safe cerebrospinal fluid white cell count to withhold antibiotics or a critical cerebrospinal fluid white cell count at which antibiotics should always be given?

There is considerable overlap between CSF white cell counts in uninfected infants (the normal reference ranges) and infants with meningitis. For example, in one study the range of CSF white cell counts in children with negative CSF cultures was 0–90 000.[13] No one would withhold antibiotics from an infant with a CSF white cell count of 90 000 and almost everyone would treat such an infant empirically with a full course of antibiotics for presumed bacterial meningitis, even if cultures were negative. However, does a CSF white cell count of 20 or 30 or higher indicate likely meningitis, should antibiotics be started and should they be continued if blood and CSF cultures are negative? The literature is not very helpful with these difficult clinical decisions.

A cohort study of neonates <34 weeks gestation assessed the reliability of CSF parameters in diagnosing meningitis by determining the area under the receiver operating characteristic (ROC) curves.[50] These were 0.80 for CSF white cell count, 0.63 for CSF glucose and 0.72 for CSF protein, which prompted the authors to urge caution in interpreting CSF parameters in pre-term neonates and stressed the importance of reliable CSF cultures.[51]

There are some outlier infants in most studies whose cultures are negative and who do not appear to have meningitis, but who nevertheless have CSF white cell counts as high as 50–90 cells/μL (Table 7.4).[42, 47, 48] An individualized approach is recommended, weighing up risks and benefits of stopping or continuing antibiotics.

Neonatal meningitis is rare. The vast majority of infants with CSF white counts in the 'reference range', whether defined as the mean plus 2 SD or the interquartile range around the median, will be uninfected. However, there is overlap and a very small number of babies with CSF counts within the reference range will have bacterial meningitis. Very occasionally a neonate with meningitis will have no white cells on initial CSF microscopy: this was the case in one of 119 infants in one study[44] and in 2 of 95 in another (while a further 8 of the 95 had CSF white counts of 1–8 cells).[13]

The clinician has to weigh the risks and benefits of withholding or starting antibiotics for any given infant. If antibiotics are started and CSF cultures are negative, but the CSF white count is ambiguous, say 20–30, the clinician will need to decide whether or not it is safe to stop antibiotics.

Conclusion: The overlap between CSF white cell counts in infants with meningitis and uninfected infants means the balance of risks and benefits needs to be considered for each individual infant regarding whether or not to start antibiotics and whether to continue antibiotics once started.

Question 2: Is the presence of cerebrospinal fluid neutrophils always abnormal?

Some authorities say that the presence of any neutrophils in the CSF suggest bacterial meningitis. However, studies report that neutrophils comprise 2–61% of the total CSF white cell count in apparently non-infected neonates.[41, 44] A review of five papers reported a mean absolute CSF neutrophil count of 0.4 (range 0–7) in non-infected term infants aged 0–28 days.[47] Another group reported that 5% of non-infected term infants had a neutrophil count >1,[41] while another study reported a mean neutrophil count of 2.8 (SD 4.9) in uninfected newborns.[50]

Conclusion 2: Finding two or three neutrophils in the CSF is common in uninfected newborns and not necessarily abnormal.

CSF microscopy often shows large numbers of red cells, either as a result of a traumatic LP or of intraventricular haemorrhage. It is common practice to correct for the presence of red cells in CSF on the basis of the ratio between red and white cells in peripheral blood. This ratio is about 500–1000 to 1 so, if the red cell count is reported as 30 000 say, the clinician 'allows' 30–60 white cells as being introduced into the CSF from the blood, not infection.

Question 3: For traumatic lumbar punctures, should clinicians correct for the number of red cells?

A review of neonatal LPs found that 2519 (39.5%) of 6374 were traumatic, defined as 500 or greater red cells/μL, and 114 infants had meningitis, including 50 with traumatic taps.[52] CSF white blood counts were adjusted downward using several commonly used methods and the authors calculated sensitivity, specificity, likelihood ratios and area under the ROC curves for predicting meningitis in neonates with traumatic LPs. The area under the ROC curve was similar for unadjusted or adjusted white cell counts. The authors conclude that adjustment of CSF white cell counts for increased red cells can result in decreased sensitivity with marginal gain in specificity and discouraged correction.

Recommendation 3: CSF white cell counts should not be adjusted for the presence of CSF red cells.

Question 4: How do previous antibiotics affect lumbar puncture culture results?

Clearly, prior antibiotics may sometimes sterilize the CSF. In a US cohort study repeat CSF cultures from 26 (22%) of 118 infants with culture-proven neonatal meningitis, taken after at least 24 hours of antibiotics to monitor disease activity and response to therapy, were positive.[53] A study of children with bacterial meningitis examined the effect of the interval between antibiotic administration and CSF culture in infants and children started on empiric parenteral antibiotics. GBS cultures remained positive through the first 8 hours after parenteral antibiotics.[54]

Answer 4: Prior antibiotics can sterilize the CSF but GBS cultures remain positive for at least 8 hours after parenteral antibiotics and repeat positive cultures are common in neonates.

Question 5: Does delay in processing affect cerebrospinal fluid parameters?

A prospective cohort study measured parameters in CSF from neonates with suspected sepsis within 30 minutes of LP and then again at 2 and 4 hours.[54] The mean CSF white count fell from 36 (SD 45) cells/μL at baseline to 28.6 (38) at 2 hours and 23.8 (34) at 4 hours. CSF glucose also fell with time (from a mean of 41 mg/dL to 38.3 at 2 and 36.2 at 4 hours).[55]

Answer 5: A delay of 2–4 hours can lead to a clinically important fall in CSF white count and glucose.

7.5.2 Cerebrospinal fluid protein

Normal CSF protein levels are considerably higher in neonates than in older children and adults. Furthermore, the normal CSF protein level is much higher in pre-term infants and falls with increasing post-natal age (Table 7.5).[49, 56] CSF protein is less reliable than CSF white count in the diagnosis of meningitis.[51]

7.5.3 Cerebrospinal fluid glucose

Normal neonatal CSF glucose levels are lower in neonates than in older children and adults, due to lower blood glucose levels, immature glucose exchange mechanisms, and increased permeability from an immature blood–brain barrier.[41] CSF glucose levels vary less with gestation than CSF protein. A review of five studies reported a mean CSF glucose level of 50 mg/dL (2.8 mmol/L), range 24–63, for pre-term infants, 52 mg/dL (2.9 mmol/L), range 34–119, for term infants on day 1 and 46 mg/dL (2.6 mmol/L), range 36–61, for term infants at 1–30 days. A study of 43 non-infected infants <1500 g found a mean CSF glucose level of 60 mg/dL (3.3 mmol/L), range 29–217.[47]

The CSF:blood glucose ratio is sometimes used to assess the likelihood of meningitis. In the above review, the mean ratio and range for pre-term infants was 0.74 (0.55–1.05) and for full-term infants was 0.81 (0.44–2.48).[47]

CSF glucose is not a reliable test in the evaluation of infants with possible meningitis.[51]

7.6 Antibiotic therapy

Antibiotic therapy for suspected neonatal meningitis should be guided whenever possible by CSF microscopy (Gram stain) which, as previously pointed out, is a form of tissue biopsy allowing rapid diagnosis and often indicating the likely organism. Gram-positive cocci are usually GBS but could be pneumococci, enterococci or occasionally staphylococci or other streptococci. Gram-negative rods could be *E. coli*, Klebsiella, Enterobacter, Proteus, Serratia, Pseudomonas or other Gram-negative bacilli. Gram-negative diplococci are usually *N. meningitidis*, while Gram-positive rods are usually Listeria. Gram stains are sometimes misleading, so empiric antibiotics should cover likely organisms until culture is confirmed.

Table 7.5 Normal values for CSF protein ([a]mg/dL) from selected studies.

Study	Population	Mean (±2 SD)	Range
Rodriguez (1970)[45]	VLBW <1500 g (n = 71):		
	<1000 g, age 1–7 days	162 (88–236)	
	<1000 g, age 8–30 days	159 (15–313)	
	1000–1500 g, age 1–7 days	136 (66–206)	
	1000–1500 g, age 8–30 days	137 (45–219)	
Sarff (1976)[44]	Full-term (n = 87)	90	20–170
	'Pre-term' (n = 30)	115	65–150
Bonadio (1992)[47]: review of five studies	Pre-term, age 0–28 days	115 (65–150)	
	Term, age 1 day	90 (20–170)	
	Term, age 1–28 days	84 (35–189)	
Ahmed (1996)[46]	Full-term, age 0–30 days (n = 108)	64 (16–112)	
Biou (2000)[57]	Full-term, age 1–8 days (n = 26)	71 (33–108)	26–135
	Full-term, 8–30 days (n = 76)	59 (31–90)	26–115
Saeedeh (2011)[50]	Full-term, 0–30 days (n = 48)	78 (25–131)	

[a]To convert to g/L, divide by 100

Factors guiding empiric antibiotic choice include gestation, age, known colonizing organisms, and local epidemiology. Table 7.6 gives some hopefully helpful hints.

When there is little antibiotic resistance of Gram-negative bacilli, and when staphylococci and Pseudomonas are unlikely, penicillin (or ampicillin) and cefotaxime, with or without an aminoglycoside, is reasonable empiric therapy. The penicillin or ampicillin is needed to cover Listeria and enterococci while the cefotaxime is needed to cover Gram-negative bacilli. Cefotaxime has a very similar spectrum to ceftriaxone but is preferred in neonates because ceftriaxone can displace bilirubin from albumin and can cause gall-bladder sludge. Cefotaxime has no activity against Pseudomonas, so if the baby is colonized with Pseudomonas or colonization is common in the unit, ceftazidime is preferred.

Table 7.6 Helpful hints on antibiotics for meningitis.

- Listeria are inherently resistant to third generation cephalosporins
- Enterococci (faecal streptococci) are inherently resistant to third generation cephalosporins
- Pseudomonas are resistant to cefotaxime and ceftriaxone
- Most Gram-negative bacilli are resistant to ampicillin
- Penicillin or ampicillin is the treatment of choice for penicillin-sensitive organisms
- Aminoglycosides cross inflamed meninges

When culture results are back, the antibiotic regimen should be rationalized to use the most effective narrow-spectrum regimen to treat the organism isolated. For example, GBS are invariably sensitive to penicillin or ampicillin, so using cefotaxime or ticarcillin to treat GBS meningitis risks selecting resistant organisms for no clinical advantage.

Pneumococcal meningitis is rare in the neonatal period but, when it does occur, it is important to determine sensitivities because of the emergence of strains with decreased susceptibility to penicillin, which are preferentially treated with a combination of vancomycin and a third generation cephalosporin (if sensitive).

Where antibiotic resistance is widespread it may be necessary to use broad spectrum antibiotics empirically until culture results are back. Consultation with a microbiologist or paediatric infectious disease specialist is strongly advised.

7.6.1 Duration of antibiotics for meningitis

The recommended duration of antibiotics for proven neonatal meningitis is empiric. Experienced clinicians report that treating Gram-negative bacillary meningitis for less than 3 weeks often results in relapse. On the other hand, around 10% of infants with Gram-negative bacillary or GBS meningitis relapse after apparently successful treatment.[1,2] Relapses can occur despite completely normal CSF parameters after stopping an antibiotic course of the recommended duration.[58] In addition neonates with meningitis who are well but have persisting CSF abnormalities can usually stop antibiotics successfully.[59] These two observations suggest LP is unnecessary at the end of treatment for bacterial meningitis if the clinical response is good (Section 7.7).[59]

Gram-negative meningitis commonly results in ventriculitis, with a high ventricular CSF white count and high CSF protein. Ventriculitis can be shown by ventricular tap, which can lead to sequelae such as cerebral cysts, or non-invasively by showing fibrous strands on cerebral ultrasound. Ventriculitis impairs CSF sterilization in Gram-negative meningitis, and persistent infection with repeat positive CSF cultures is associated with increased morbidity and mortality.[53,59] It is recommended to continue parenteral antibiotics for at least 3 weeks for Gram-negative meningitis.[1]

For GBS meningitis, 2 weeks is usually considered sufficient, but when GBS causes ventriculitis it may be prudent to continue antibiotics for 3 weeks.

Listeria is an intracellular organism and may be more difficult to treat. It is usually recommended to treat Listeria meningitis for at least 2 weeks.[1]

7.6.2 Intrathecal or intraventricular antibiotics

Because persistence of Gram-negative bacilli is associated with increased morbidity and mortality,[53] researchers have attempted to improve CSF antibiotic delivery. A RCT found that adding intrathecal antibiotics did not reduce morbidity or mortality compared with parenteral antibiotics alone.[60] An RCT of intraventricular antibiotics was stopped early because the mortality of infants treated with intraventricular antibiotics was significantly higher than controls treated with parenteral antibiotics alone.[61,62] Clinicians sometimes feel obliged to use intraventricular antibiotics when experiencing difficulty sterilizing CSF,[63] but as the only RCT suggests intraventricular antibiotics are harmful, the final neurologic outcome may be better if persistent parenteral antibiotics eventually succeed in sterilizing the CSF.

7.7 Repeat lumbar punctures

A repeat LP is sometimes recommended 24–48 hours into antibiotic therapy for Gram-negative meningitis to document sterilization of the CSF.[1] Persistence of CSF infection may indicate the need for cerebral imaging to look for a focus of infection such as obstructive ventriculitis or a collection. Persistence of infection might also be because of a resistant organism, so the choice of antibiotics should be reviewed. Delayed sterilization is associated with increased morbidity and mortality and has prognostic implications.[53,59]

A review of 27 cases of childhood bacterial meningitis (nine neonates) which recurred or relapsed concluded that routine LP was not routinely indicated at the end of apparently successful therapy, because a normal CSF did not exclude relapse and an abnormal CSF did not reliably predict relapse.[59]

7.8 Neuroimaging

There are no studies on the value of neuroimaging in neonatal meningitis. Magnetic resonance imaging (MRI) scan can show meningeal enhancement in neonatal meningitis, which may sometimes be helpful diagnostically, but neuroimaging should not be used instead of LP to diagnose meningitis. On the other hand, different modalities can detect intracerebral complications of meningitis, including hydrocephalus and sub-dural or intracerebral collections. Ultrasound is the least invasive and usually does not require sedation. Computerized tomography (CT) or MRI may require deep sedation or general anaesthetic.

7.9 Dexamethasone

There is some evidence that corticosteroids can be beneficial as adjunctive therapy for bacterial meningitis in children and adults. There is clear evidence of improved neurologic outcome in Hib meningitis, no evidence of either harm or benefit in meningococcal meningitis and disputed evidence about the benefits in pneumococcal meningitis.[64]

One clinical trial of 52 full-term neonates with bacterial meningitis allocated alternate infants to dexamethasone 0.15 mg/kg 6 hourly, started 10–15 minutes before the first dose of antibiotics and given for 4 days as adjunctive therapy or standard antibiotics.[65] Mortality and neurological sequelae were not significantly different between treatment and control groups.[65]

There are safety concerns about adverse neurologic outcomes including cerebral palsy from early[66] or late[67] use of post-natal corticosteroids to prevent or treat chronic lung disease. Corticosteroids are not recommended in neonatal meningitis.

7.10 Shunt infections

The incidence of CSF shunt infections depends on gestational age, comorbidities and the indication for CSF shunting. In one recent study of 58 pre-term infants <1500 g with CSF shunts for post-haemorrhagic hydrocephalus, 15.5% developed CSF shunt infections in the first 3 months.[68]

A study compared CSF parameters in uninfected and infected neonates with parameters in neonates without shunts.[69] Uninfected shunted neonates compared with uninfected neonates without shunts had higher CSF red cell counts, higher CSF protein levels and lower glucose levels but CSF white cell counts were no different. An upper limit of normal of 20 white cells/μL used as a cut-off had a sensitivity of 67% and a specificity of 62% for culture-proven infection in a neonate with a CSF shunt.[69] White cell counts in shunt infections are unreliable. Culture is as important for diagnosing shunt infections as for diagnosing meningitis in infants without shunts.

A study from 1975 reported that 78 (27%) of 289 patients with CSF shunts for hydrocephalus developed infections, half with CoNS and a quarter with *S. aureus*.[70] Infections rarely resolved when treated with parenteral antibiotics alone without removing the shunt. The rate of shunt infection has fallen considerably since then. Some adults and older children have had CoNS shunt infections successfully treated with parenteral and intraventricular antibiotics without shunt removal, but *S. aureus* infections were too problematic.[71] This practice has not been evaluated in neonates and the toxicity of intraventricular antibiotics shown by the randomized trial of their use in neonatal meningitis[61] should not be forgotten. In addition neonates given intravenous vancomycin have much higher CSF vancomycin levels than older children and adults[72, 73] so intraventricular vancomycin is less likely to be necessary to sterilize the CSF in a shunt infection.

The incidence of shunt infections can be halved by using prophylactic antibiotics at the time of shunt insertion.[74] This supports the theory that most shunt infections result from organisms introduced during neurosurgery. A Cochrane meta-analysis of 17 trials in 2134 patients found that 24 hours of prophylactic antibiotics significantly reduced shunt infections regardless of the patient's age and the type of shunt used (OR 0.52, 95% CI 0.36–0.74).[74] A single RCT of antibiotic-impregnated shunt tubing which did not include neonates showed a significant reduction in infections (OR 0.21, 95% CI 0.08–0.55).[75] Observational studies on antibiotic-impregnated shunt catheters in children are promising[76, 77] but neonatal trials are needed.

References

1. Heath PT, Nik Yusoff NK, Baker CJ. Neonatal meningitis. *Arch Dis Child Fetal Neonatal Ed* 2003; 88:F173–F178.
2. Berardi A, Lugli L, Rossi C, et al. Infezioni da Streptococco B Della Regione Emilia Romagna. Neonatal bacterial meningitis. *Minerva Pediatr* 2010; 62(3 Suppl 1):51–54.
3. Furyk JS, Swann O, Molyneux E. Systematic review: neonatal meningitis in the developing world. *Trop Med Int Health* 2011; 16:672–679.
4. Goldacre MJ. Acute bacterial meningitis in chuildhood. *Lancet* 1976; i:28–31.
5. Bell AH, Brown D, Halliday HL, McClure G, Reid MM. Meningitis in the newborn – a 14 year review. *Arch Dis Child* 1989; 64:873–874.
6. de Louvois J, Blackbourn J, Hurley R, et al. Infantile meningitis in England and Wales: a two year study. *Arch Dis Child* 1991; 66:603–607.
7. Holt DE, Halket S, de Louvois J, et al. Neonatal meningitis in England and Wales: 10 years on. *Arch Dis Child Fetal Neonatal Ed* 2001; 84:F85–F89.
8. Hristeva L, Booy R, Bowler I, et al. Prospective surveillance of neonatal meningitis. *Arch Dis Child* 1993; 69:14–18.
9. Wiswell TE, Baumgart S, Gannon CM, Spitzer AR. No lumbar puncture in the evaluation for early neonatal sepsis: will meningitis be missed? *Pediatrics* 1995; 95:803–806.
10. Francis BM, Gilbert GL. Survey of neonatal meningitis in Australia: 1987–1989. *Med J Aust* 1992; 156:240–243.
11. May M, Daley A, Donath S, Isaacs D, Australasian Study Group for Neonatal Infections. Early-onset neonatal meningitis in Australia and New Zealand, 1992–2002. *Arch Dis Child Fetal Neonatal Ed* 2005; 90:F324–F327.
12. Stoll BJ, Hansen N, Fanaroff AA, et al. To tap or not to tap: high likelihood of meningitis without sepsis among

very low birth weight infants. *Pediatrics* 2004; 113:1181–1186.

13. Garges HP, Moody MA, Cotten CM, et al. Neonatal meningitis: what is the correlation among cerebrospinal fluid cultures, blood cultures, and cerebrospinal fluid parameters? *Pediatrics* 2006; 117:1094–1100.
14. Thaver D, Zaidi AKM. Burden of neonatal infections in developing countries. A review of evidence from community-based studies. *Pediatr Infect Dis J* 2009; 28:S3–S9.
15. Eldadah M, Frenkel LD, Hiatt IM, et al. Evaluation of routine lumbar punctures in newborn infants with respiratory distress syndrome. *Paediatr Infect Dis J* 1987; 6:243–246.
16. Malbon K, Mohan R, Nicholl R. Should a neonate with possible late onset infection always have a lumbar puncture? *Arch Dis Child* 2006; 91:75–76.
17. Isaacs D, Australasian Study Group for Neonatal Infections. A ten-year multi-centre study of coagulase negative staphylococcal infections. *Arch Dis Child Fetal Neonatal Ed* 2003; 88:F89–F93.
18. Laving AM, Musoke RN, Wasunna AO, Revathi G. Neonatal bacterial meningitis at the newborn unit of Kenyatta National Hospital. *East Afr Med J* 2003; 80:456–462.
19. Fielkow S, Reuter S, Gotoff SP. Cerebrospinal fluid examination in symptom free infants with risk factor for infection. *J Paediatr* 1991; 119:971–973.
20. Franco SM, Cornelius VE, Andrews BF. Long-term outcome of neonatal meningitis. *Am J Dis Child* 1992; 146:567–571.
21. Gaschignard J, Levy C, Romain O, et al. Neonatal bacterial meningitis: 444 cases in 7 years. *Pediatr Infect Dis J* 2011; 30:212–217.
22. Klinger G, Chin CN, Beyene J, Perlman M. Predicting the outcome of neonatal bacterial meningitis. *Pediatrics* 2000; 106:477–482.
23. Stevens JP, Eames M, Kent A, Halket S, Holt D, Harvey D. Long term outcome of neonatal meningitis. *Arch Dis Child Fetal Neonatal Ed* 2003; 88:F179–F184.
24. de Louvois J, Halket S, Harvey D. Neonatal meningitis in England and Wales: sequelae at 5 years of age. *Eur J Pediatr* 2005; 164:730–734.
25. Klinger G, Chin CN, Otsubo H, Beyene J, Perlman M. Prognostic value of EEG in neonatal bacterial meningitis. *Pediatr Neurol* 2001; 24:28–31.
26. Moxon ER, Smith AL, Averill DR, Smith DR. *Haemophilus influenzae* meningitis in infant rats after intranasal inoculation. *J Infect Dis* 1974; 129:154–162.
27. Moxon ER, Ostrow PT. *Haemophilus influenzae* meningitis in infant rats: role of bacteremia in pathogenesis of age-dependent inflammatory responses in cerebrospinal fluid. *J Infect Dis* 1974; 135:303–307.
28. Sorokin Y, Weintraub Z, Rothschild A, Abramovici H, Iancu TC. Cerebrospinal fluid leak in the neonate–complication of fetal scalp electrode monitoring. Case report and review of the literature. *Isr J Med Sci* 1990; 26:633–635.
29. Nieburg P, Gross SJ. Cerebrospinal fluid leak in a neonate associated with fetal scalp electrode monitoring. *Am J Obstet Gynecol* 1983; 147:839–840.
30. Nakwan N, Nakwan N, Wannaro J, Dissaneevate P, Kritsaneepaiboon S, Chokephaibulkit K. Septicemia, meningitis, and skull osteomyelitis complicating infected cephalhematoma caused by ESBL-producing Escherichia coli. *Southeast Asian J Trop Med Public Health* 2011; 42:148–151.
31. Althouse R, Wald N. Survival and handicap of infants with spina bifida. *Arch Dis Child* 1980; 55:845–850.
32. Lorber J, Salfield SA. Results of selective treatment of spina bifida cystica. *Arch Dis Child* 1981; 56:822–830.
33. Shehu BB, Ameh EA, Ismail NJ. Spina bifida cystica: selective management in Zaria, Nigeria. *Ann Trop Paediatr* 2000; 20:239–242.
34. Isaacs D, Fraser S, Hogg G, Li HY. Staphylococcus aureus infections in Australasian neonatal nurseries. *Arch Dis Child Fetal Neonatal Ed* 2004; 89:F331–F335.
35. Robins JB, McCracken Jr GH, Gotschuch EC, et al. *Escherichia coli* K1 capsular polysaccharide associated with neonatal meningitis. *N Engl J Med* 1974; 290:1216–1220.
36. Graham DR, Band JD. Citrobacter diversus brain abscess and meningitis in neonates. *J Am Med Assoc* 1981; 245:1923–1925.
37. Kline MW. Pathogenesis of brain abscess caused by *Citrobacter diversus* or *Enterobacter sakazakii*. *Pediatr Infect Dis J* 1988; 7:891–892.
38. Messerschmidt A, Prayer D, Olischar M, Pollak A, Birnbacher R. Brain abscesses after Serratia marcescens infection on a neonatal intensive care unit: differences on serial imaging. *Neuroradiology* 2004; 46:148–152.
39. Thigpen MC, Whitney CG, Messonnier NE, et al; Emerging Infections Programs Network. Bacterial meningitis in the United States, 1998–2007. *N Engl J Med* 2011; 364:2016–2025.
40. Weisman LE, Merenstein GB, Steenbarger JR. The effect of lumbar puncture position in sick neonates. *Am J Dis Child* 1983; 137:1077–1079.
41. Connell T, Curtis N. How to interpret a CSF – the art and the science. In: *Hot Topics in Infection and Immunity in Children* (eds AJ Pollard, A Finn). New York, Springer, 2005. pp 199–216.
42. Naidoo BT. The cerebrospinal fluid in the healthy newborn infant. *South Afr Med J* 1968; 42:473–477.
43. Roberts MH. The spinal fluid in the newborn with especial reference to intracranial hemorrhage. *J Am Med Assoc* 1925; 85:500–503.
44. Sarff LD, Platt LH, McCracken Jr GH. Cerebrospinal fluid evaluation in neonates: comparison of high-risk infants with and without meningitis. *J Pediatr* 1976; 88:473–477.
45. Rodriguez AF, Kaplan SL, Mason Jr EO. Cerebrospinal fluid values in the very low birth weight infant. *J Pediatr* 1990; 116:971–974.

46. Ahmed A, Hickey SM, Ehrett S, et al. Cerebrospinal fluid values in the term neonate. *Pediatr Infect Dis J* 1996; 15:298–303.
47. Bonadio WA. The cerebrospinal fluid: physiologic aspects and alterations associated with bacterial meningitis. *Pediatr Infect Dis J* 1992; 11:423–431.
48. Kestenbaum LA, Ebberson J, Zorc JJ, Hodinka RL, Shah SS. Defining cerebrospinal fluid white blood cell count reference values in neonates and young infants. *Pediatrics* 2010; 125:257–264.
49. Mhanna MJ, Alesseh H, Gori A, Aziz HF. Cerebrospinal fluid values in very low birth weight infants with suspected sepsis at different ages. *Pediatr Crit Care Med* 2008; 9:294–298.
50. Saeedeh TE, Hossain N, Mojgan BM, et al. Comparing cerebrospinal fluid values in newborns and infants until two months old with or without meningitis. *Pediatr Int* 2011. doi:10.1111/j.1442-200X.2011.03551.x.
51. Smith PB, Garges HP, Cotton CM, Walsh TJ, Clark RH, Benjamin Jr DK. Meningitis in preterm neonates: importance of cerebrospinal fluid parameters. *Am J Perinatol* 2008; 25:421–426.
52. Greenberg RG, Smith PB, Cotten CM, Moody MA, Clark RH, Benjamin Jr DK. Traumatic lumbar punctures in neonates: test performance of the cerebrospinal fluid white blood cell count. *Pediatr Infect Dis J* 2008; 27:1047–1051.
53. Greenberg RG, Benjamin Jr DK, Cohen-Wolkowiez M, et al. Repeat lumbar punctures in infants with meningitis in the neonatal intensive care unit. *J Perinatol* 2011; 31:425–429.
54. Kanegaye JT, Soliemanzadeh P, Bradley JS. Lumbar puncture in pediatric bacterial meningitis: defining the time interval for recovery of cerebrospinal fluid pathogens after parenteral antibiotic pretreatment. *Pediatrics* 2001; 108:1169–1174.
55. Rajesh NT, Dutta S, Prasad R, Narang A. Effect of delay in analysis on neonatal cerebrospinal fluid parameters. *Arch Dis Child Fetal Neonatal Ed* 2010; 95:F25–F29.
56. Shah SS, Ebberson J, Kestenbaum LA, Hodinka RL, Zorc JJ. Age-specific reference values for cerebrospinal fluid protein concentration in neonates and young infants. *J Hosp Med* 2011; 6:22–27.
57. Biou D, Benoist JF, Houng CN, Morel P, Marchand M. Cerebrospinal fluid protein concentrations in children: age-related values in patients without disorders of the central nervous system. *Clin Chem* 2000; 46:399–403.
58. McCracken GH. The rate of bacteriologic response to antimicrobial therapy in neonatal meningitis. *Am J Dis Child* 1972; 123:547–553.
59. Schaad UB, Nelson JD, McCracken Jr GH. Recrudescence and relapse in bacterial meningitis of childhood. *Pediatrics* 1981; 67:188–195.
60. McCracken GH, Mize SG. A controlled study of intrathecal antibiotic therapy in gram-negative enteric meningitis of infancy. Report of the National Meningitis Cooperative Study Group. *J Pediatr* 1976; 89:66–72.
61. McCracken GH, Mize SG, Threlkeld N. Intraventricular gentamicin therapy in Gram-negative bacillary meningitis of infancy. *Lancet* 1980; 1:787–791.
62. Shah SS, Ohlsson A, Shah VS. Intraventricular antibiotics for bacterial meningitis in neonates. *Cochrane Database of Systematic Reviews* 2004, Issue 4. Art. No.: CD004496. doi: 10.1002/14651858.CD004496.pub2.
63. Alaoui SY, Nejmi SE, Chakir AA, Hmamouchi B, Chlilek A. Intraventricular colistin use in neonatal meningitis caused by Acinetobacter baumanii. *Ann Fr Anesth Reanim* 2011; 30(11):854–855. Epub 2011 Oct 5.
64. Brouwer MC, McIntyre P, de Gans J, Prasad K, van de Beek D. Corticosteroids for acute bacterial meningitis. *Cochrane Database of Systematic Reviews* 2010, Issue 9. Art. No.: CD004405. doi: 10.1002/14651858.CD004405.pub3.
65. Daoud AS, Batieha A, Al-Sheyyab M, Abuekteish F, Obeidat A, Mahafza T. Lack of effectiveness of dexamethasone in neonatal bacterial meningitis. *Eur J Pediatr* 1999; 158:230–233.
66. Halliday HL, Ehrenkranz RA, Doyle LW. Early (<8 days) postnatal corticosteroids for preventing chronic lung disease in preterm infants. *Cochrane Database of Systematic Reviews* 2010, Issue 1. Art. No.: CD001146. doi: 10.1002/14651858.CD001146.pub3.
67. Halliday HL, Ehrenkranz RA, Doyle LW. Late (>7 days) postnatal corticosteroids for chronic lung disease in preterm infants. *Cochrane Database of Systematic Reviews* 2009, Issue 1. Art. No.: CD001145. doi: 10.1002/14651858.CD001145.pub2.
68. Fulkerson DH, Vachhrajani S, Bohnstedt BN, et al. Analysis of the risk of shunt failure or infection related to cerebrospinal fluid cell count, protein level, and glucose levels in low-birth-weight premature infants with posthemorrhagic hydrocephalus. *J Neurosurg Pediatr* 2011; 7:147–151.
69. Lenfestey RW, Smith PB, Moody MA, et al. Predictive value of cerebrospinal fluid parameters in neonates with intraventricular drainage devices. *J Neurosurg* 2007; 107(Suppl):209–212.
70. Schoenbaum SC, Gardner P, Shillito J. Infections of cerebrospinal fluid shunts: epidemiology, clinical manifestations, and therapy. *J Infect Dis* 1975; 131:543–552.
71. Brown EM, Edwards RJ, Pople IK. Conservative management of patients with cerebrospinal fluid shunt infections. *Neurosurgery* 2008; 62(Suppl 2):661–669.
72. Schaad UB, Nelson JD, McCracken Jr GH. Pharmacology and efficacy of vancomycin for staphylococcal infections in children. *Rev Infect Dis* 1981; 3(suppl): S282–S288.
73. Reiter PD, Doron MW. Vancomycin cerebrospinal fluid concentrations after intravenous administration in premature infants. *J Perinatol* 1996; 16:331–335.
74. Ratilal BO, Costa J, Sampaio C. Antibiotic prophylaxis for surgical introduction of intracranial ventricular shunts. *Cochrane Database of Systematic Reviews* 2006, Issue 3. Art. No.: CD005365. doi: 10.1002/14651858.CD005365.pub2.

75. Govender ST, Nathoo N, van Dellen JR. Evaluation of an antibiotic-impregnated shunt system for the treatment of hydrocephalus. *J Neurosurg* 2003; 99:831–839.
76. Hayhurst C, Cooke R, Williams D, Kandasamy J, O'Brien DF, Mallucci CL. The impact of antibiotic-impregnated catheters on shunt infection in children and neonates. *Childs Nerv Syst* 2008; 24:557–562.
77. Thomas R, Lee S, Patole S, Rao S. Antibiotic-impregnated catheters for the prevention of CSF shunt infections: a systematic review and meta-analysis. *Br J Neurosurg* 2012; 26:175–184.

CHAPTER 8

Respiratory tract infections

8.1 Pneumonia

Pneumonia is inflammation of the lungs, which can be infectious or non-infectious (e.g. chemical). Foetal and neonatal pneumonia can be classified into congenital or intrauterine (transplacentally acquired), early-onset and late-onset.

8.1.1 Incidence and mortality of pneumonia

Pneumonia particularly affects infants in developing countries. In 2009, there were an estimated 1.32 million neonatal deaths in the world, almost in all developing countries.[1] Pneumonia contributed to the deaths of an estimated 15–38% of these babies,[2,3] or 200 000–500 000 newborn infants annually.[1–3] A separate analysis of global data came up with a similar estimate of 386 000 neonatal deaths in 2008 from pneumonia (95% CI 264 000–545 000).[4] The neonatal period is the greatest risk period for death from pneumonia.[5,6]

In Western countries, neonatal pneumonia occurs primarily as early-onset disease due to ascending infection from the maternal birth canal, for example, GBS pneumonia; as late-onset ventilator-associated pneumonia (VAP) in pre-term infants; or as late-onset viral, for example, respiratory syncytial virus or herpes simplex virus or chlamydial pneumonia. The incidence and mortality depend on factors such as intrapartum chemoprophylaxis and the gestational age of the pre-term patient population. Widespread use of artificial surfactant has permitted early extubation of almost all pre-term infants to nasal continuous positive airway pressure (CPAP) and reduced the incidence of VAP greatly.

The case fatality rate of neonatal pneumonia is higher for early-onset pneumonia than for late-onset pneumonia and higher in developing countries than Western countries. The reported case fatality rate for neonatal pneumonia from community and hospital-based studies in developing countries was 25% (range 8–48%).[2] The case fatality rate for early-onset pneumonia in one developing country study was 74% and for late-onset pneumonia 39%.[2] The case fatality rate for early-onset pneumonia, mainly due to GBS, in a UK teaching hospital was 29% and 2.4% for late-onset pneumonia.[8]

8.1.2 Pathology of pneumonia

8.1.2.1 Pathology of congenital or intrauterine pneumonia

The characteristic histopathologic feature of congenital or intrauterine pneumonia from autopsies of stillborn babies or early neonatal deaths is a diffuse neutrophil alveolar inflammatory infiltrate, often with squamous cells and vernix.[3–5] Bacteria are rarely seen or cultured and, unlike classical bacterial pneumonia, there is little or no pleural reaction, bronchopulmonary tissue involvement or fibrinous alveolar exudate. These features suggest that foetal asphyxia or hypoxia may be a more important cause of congenital or intrauterine pneumonia than infection. However, intrauterine pneumonia can also occur in the setting of maternal systemic infection in the mother, such as rubella, cytomegalovirus (CMV), syphilis, listeriosis, tuberculosis, and HIV.[1]

8.1.2.2 Pathology of early neonatal pneumonia

The histopathologic features of pneumonia acquired at or around the time of birth resemble childhood pneumonia with dense cellular pulmonary infiltrate

Evidence-Based Neonatal Infections, First Edition. David Isaacs.

and bacteria. GBS pneumonia can cause hyaline membranes, similar to those seen in hyaline membrane disease, due to surfactant deficiency or dysfunction.[9]

Early-onset pneumonia is an extremely common feature of early-onset sepsis which usually results from amniotic fluid infection followed by ascending infection of the foetal lung.

8.1.2.3 Pathology of late neonatal pneumonia

The histopathologic features of late-onset neonatal pneumonia are similar to early-onset pneumonia, although there may be organism-specific findings.[10] For example, pneumatocoeles tend to be seen in *Staphylococcus aureus* pneumonia, but also occasionally with Klebsiella, other Gram-negative bacilli and *Streptococcus pneumoniae.* Respiratory syncytial virus (RSV) pneumonitis is associated with giant cell formation while other viruses and Chlamydia cause mononuclear cell infiltrate without specific histopathologic features.[10]

8.1.3 Microbiology of pneumonia

8.1.3.1 Microbiology of congenital or intrauterine pneumonia

In autopsy studies bacteria could be cultured from the lungs of 55% of infants who were stillborn or died within 24 hours of birth, from 70% of infants who died at 1–7 days of age and from 100% of infants who died at 7–28 days of age.[10] However, bacteria could also be cultured from the lungs of many infants who died without pneumonia: 36% stillborn or <1 day, 53% at 1–7 days and 75% at 7–28 days.[10] This shows the caution that needs to be exercised when organisms are cultured from 'normally sterile sites.' The organisms cultured from the lungs of infants who died without pneumonia are either colonizing organisms or invaded after death. The relatively low proportion of stillborn infants and those dying <1 day with positive cultures is further evidence that some early pneumonia is due to asphyxial aspiration, not infection.

The organisms cultured in congenital or intrauterine pneumonia are those found in the maternal birth canal, mainly GBS, other streptococci and Gram-negative enteric bacilli such as *Escherichia coli,* Klebsiella, Proteus and Enterobacter.[10]

Table 8.1 Organisms isolated from endotracheal aspirate and/or blood in 35 cases of early-onset pneumonia (<48 hours), Oxford 1984–1987.

Organism	Number
Group B streptococcus	20 (57%)
Streptococcus pneumoniae	3 (9%)
Haemophilus influenzae	2 (6%)
Group F streptococcus	1 (3%)
No organism isolated	9 (26%)

Source: Reproduced from Reference 8 with permission from BMJ Publishing Group Ltd.

8.1.3.2 Microbiology of early neonatal pneumonia

In Western countries, the organisms causing early pneumonia are the same as those that cause early-onset sepsis (see Section 2.2.3) and come from the maternal genital tract. There are few published studies. In a UK study 27 (77%) of 35 cases of early-onset pneumonia (onset <2 days) had one or more maternal risk factors for sepsis, most commonly spontaneous onset of pre-term labour.[8] The study was performed before intrapartum chemoprophylaxis and 20 (57%) of the cases were due to GBS (Table 8.1). Sixteen (46%) of the babies had positive blood cultures.[8]

8.1.3.3 Microbiology of late neonatal pneumonia

The predominant organisms isolated from the nasopharynx (nasopharyngeal aspirate) or trachea (endotracheal aspirate) of babies with VAP in both developing countries[11] and Western settings[8] are Gram-negative bacilli (Pseudomonas, Klebsiella, Acinetobacter, *E. coli* and other coliforms) and staphylococci (*S. aureus* and CoNS). GBS is only rarely isolated from babies with late pneumonia[8] and thought to be a colonizing commensal, not a cause of late pneumonia. While routine endotracheal cultures predict poorly which babies will develop sepsis,[12] they do provide data on colonizing organisms which might be causing pneumonia, so inform empiric antibiotic choice.

Late-onset GBS pneumonia is a potentially dangerous diagnosis to make because of the danger of missing another treatable cause of late pneumonia such as HSV or Chlamydia. If a baby 3 days of age or older develops respiratory distress and pneumonic changes, strong consideration should be given to a diagnosis of

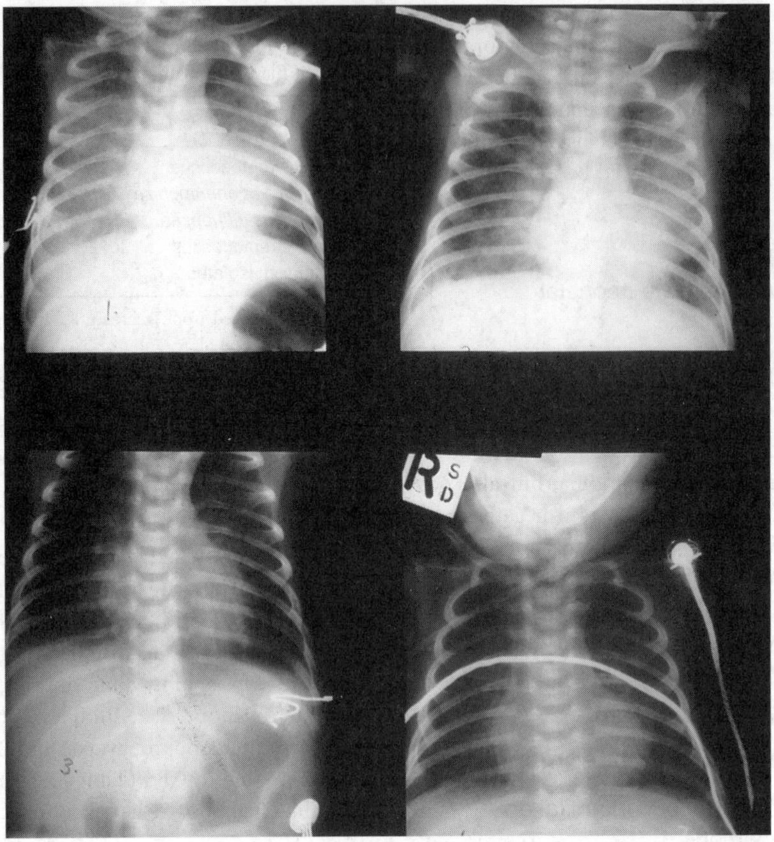

Figure 8.1 Chlamydia pneumonitis, age 14 days, showing perihilar changes and progressive clearing with treatment over 10 days with treatment.

Chlamydia pneumonitis (Figure 8.1) or of HSV pneumonitis (Figure 8.2), because both need special tests for diagnosis. Untreated HSV pneumonitis often leads to fatal disseminated HSV infection (see Chapter 17).[13]

In developing countries, there are few data on the organisms responsible for community-acquired pneumonia. In a Chinese study, 425 (56%) of 760 sputum samples from newborns with community-acquired pneumonia grew potential pathogens.[14] Gram-negative organisms, mostly *E. coli, Klebsiella pneumoniae* and *Haemophilus influenzae,* were responsible for 65%; the rest grew mainly *S. aureus* or CoNS.[14]

8.1.4 Clinical features of pneumonia

The clinical features of neonatal congenital or early-onset pneumonia are indistinguishable from hyaline membrane disease. Signs of respiratory distress may include grunting, chest recession or retraction, nasal flaring, tachypnoea, dyspnoea, apnoea and cyanosis. Systemic signs may include lethargy, poor feeding and hypo- or hyperthermia. The signs of late pneumonia are similar but usually less dramatic.

Around 95% of infants with early-onset GBS infection with respiratory involvement develop clinical signs within 24 hours of birth (see Chapter 14). Respiratory distress starting between days 2 and 7 is very unlikely to be GBS pneumonia or hyaline membrane disease: the differential diagnosis includes HSV pneumonitis which must not be missed, virus infections (e.g. RSV, rhinovirus, influenza), Chlamydia pneumonitis, aspiration pneumonia, cardiac and other non-infectious causes.

8.1.5 Radiology of pneumonia

The radiologic appearance in early-onset GBS pneumonia may show a granular pattern, indistinguishable from hyaline membrane disease (Figure 8.3a) or more focal consolidation (Figure 8.3b).

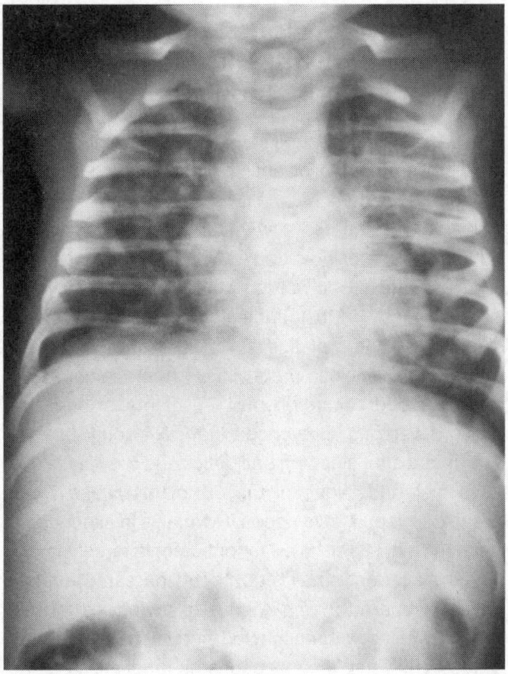

Figure 8.2 HSV pneumonitis: full-term infant with fast breathing aged 5 days; no history of maternal genital herpes; patchy pneumonitis; nasopharyngeal aspirate HSV-positive; infant recovered after acyclovir treatment.

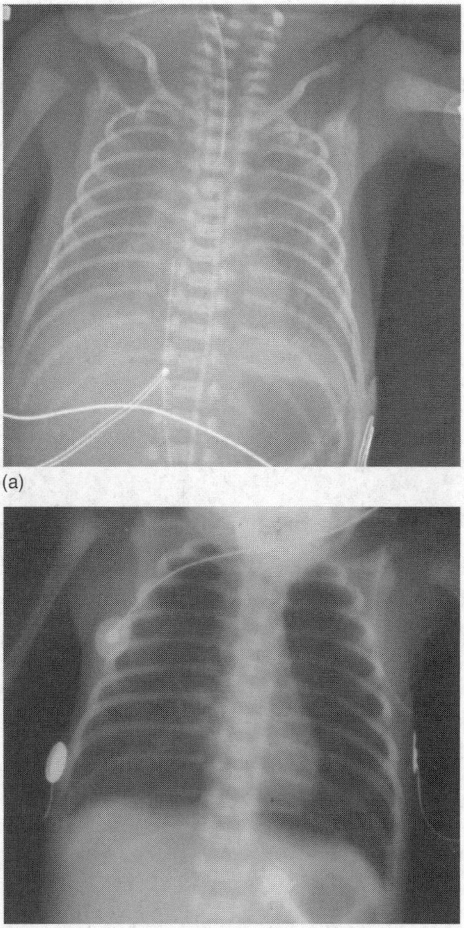

(a)

(b)

Figure 8.3 (a) Group B streptococcal pneumonia: granular appearance resembling hyaline membrane disease. (b) Group B streptococcal pneumonia: hyperinflation and patchy right lower lobe changes.

In a full-term infant, granular appearance (Figure 8.3a) is most likely to be due to bacterial pneumonia. In a pre-term infant, hyaline membrane disease is more likely, but bacterial pneumonia should be considered.

Ventilator-associated late-onset pneumonia can be difficult to distinguish from non-specific atelectasis. Persistent patchy consolidation is intuitively more likely to be due to bacterial infection, but there is no formal evidence.

Staphylococcal pneumonia can cause focal consolidation which may progress to pleural effusion (Figure 8.4a), pneumatocoele formation (Figure 8.4b) and empyema (Figure 8.4c). While these radiologic features suggest *S. aureus* infection, other organisms including Gram-negative bacilli such as Klebsiella[15] and *E. coli*[16] can also cause pneumatocoeles, so the empiric antibiotics for an infant with pneumatocoeles should include Gram-negative cover.

Viral and Chlamydial infections are reported to cause patchy infiltrates and often hyperinflation, but no studies have compared radiologic appearance in neonatal viral and bacterial pneumonia. Studies in older children suggest the 'classical' radiologic features of viral and bacterial pneumonia overlap, while children can have simultaneous viral and bacterial pneumonia. For this reason it is unsafe to withhold antibiotics for a diagnosis of viral pneumonia made solely on radiologic grounds.

8.1.6 Antibiotic treatment of pneumonia

8.1.6.1 Antibiotic treatment of early-onset pneumonia

The choice of antibiotics for suspected early-onset pneumonia, which results from organisms acquired

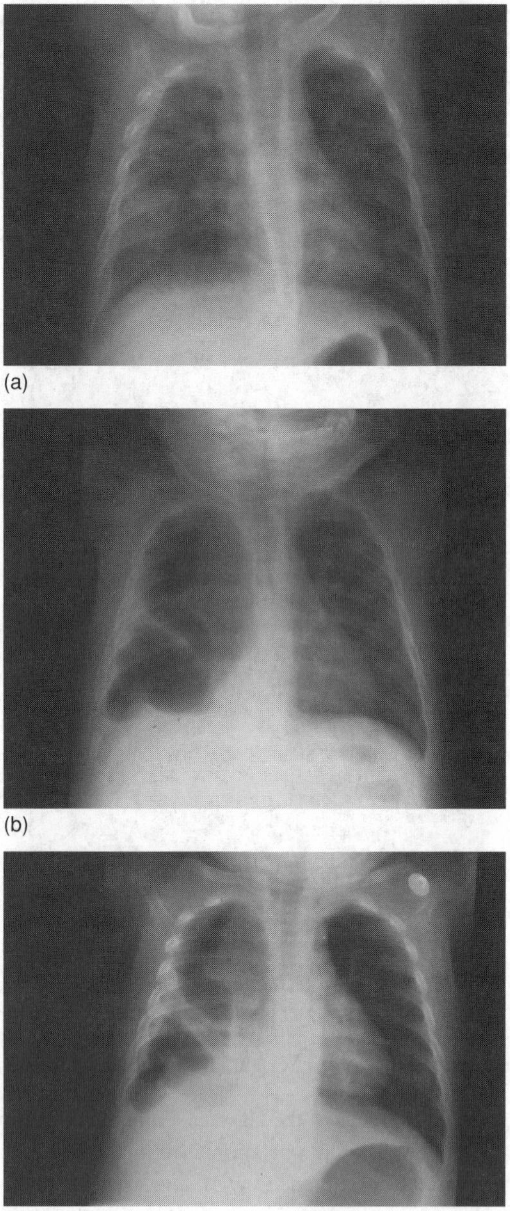

Figure 8.4 (a) Staphylococcal pneumonia; round pneumonia and right pleural collection. (b) Staphylococcal pneumonia; large right pneumatocoele and pleural collection with mediastinal shift to left. (c) Staphylococcal pneumonia; loculated empyema.

from the maternal birth canal, is the same as for early-onset sepsis (see Chapter 5) and depends on the likely pathogens based on local epidemiology.

Question: How long should antibiotics be given to treat early-onset pneumonia?

Two randomized controlled trials (RCTs) address the problem of duration of antibiotics for culture-negative early-onset pneumonia.

An RCT compared 4 with 7 days of antibiotics for full-term neonates admitted with pneumonia, not meconium aspiration, who were asymptomatic after 48 hours of antibiotics.[17] Most babies' respiratory symptoms began <24 hours of age. Over 90% of mothers had intrapartum antibiotic prophylaxis and no infant had a positive blood culture. Two of 35 infants in the 4-day group developed tachypnoea in the 24-hour observation period after stopping antibiotics and one had antibiotics restarted. None of the 38 infants in the 7-day group developed tachypnoea. No infants in either group needed re-hospitalization for pneumonia or sepsis.[17]

A subsequent small study from the same authors which compared 2 with 4 days of antibiotics for full-term neonates with suspected pneumonia was terminated early when 3 of 14 neonates randomized to the 2-day group had recurrence of symptoms after ceasing antibiotics.[18]

There are no data on the optimal duration of antibiotics for infants who remain symptomatic and no data on the optimal duration of antibiotics for culture-positive infants. Many guidelines recommend 7–10 days of antibiotics for GBS pneumonia, but this appears to be an example of the use of magical numbers[19] and not based on data. It may be best to base antibiotic duration on individual clinical response.

Recommendation: Four days plus a 24-hour observation period appears to be safe for most neonates with culture-negative early-onset pneumonia who are asymptomatic after 48 hours. For culture-positive infants there are no data although few relapse after 7 days of antibiotics.

8.1.6.2 Antibiotic treatment of late-onset pneumonia

Routine endotracheal aspirate cultures do not predict which infants on mechanical ventilation will develop sepsis, because colonization is equally likely in those who do and do not develop sepsis. However, if a ventilated baby develops late-onset pneumonia it is common sense to base the choice of antibiotics on known colonizing organisms, particularly if these are resistant to the unit policy antibiotics. For example, if a baby known to have endotracheal Pseudomonas colonization develops pneumonia, it would be foolish to use cefotaxime alone for Gram-negative cover, since Pseudomonas are inherently resistant to cefotaxime. Staphylococci, both *S. aureus* and CoNS, are common endotracheal colonizers. *S. aureus* is a well-recognized cause of neonatal pneumonia. It is controversial whether CoNS ever causes pneumonia or is merely a commensal. Nevertheless, it is recommended that empiric regimens for late-onset pneumonia, as for late-onset sepsis (see Chapter 5), include staphylococcal and Gram-negative cover.

The optimal duration of antibiotics for late-onset pneumonia has not been studied. Guidelines often recommend 7–10 days of antibiotics for late-onset pneumonia, another example of magical numbers[19] not based on data. As for early pneumonia, it may be best to base antibiotic duration on individual clinical response.

8.1.7 Adjunctive management of pneumonia

Any infant with pneumonia needs to be assessed clinically regarding the need for cardiorespiratory support and screened for hypoxemia. It has been estimated that between 1.5 and 2.7 million children with pneumonia present to health-care facilities in developing countries each year,[20] many of them neonates. Oximeters to assess oxygenation[21] and oxygen to treat hypoxemia are clearly needed. Most neonates with pneumonia in developing countries do not have ready access to mechanical ventilation.

8.1.8 Case management of neonatal pneumonia

In developing countries, poor access to health care is an important determinant of morbidity and mortality of neonatal pneumonia. Timely case management can save lives. Different strategies of case management include oral or injectable antibiotics, treatment at home or in first-level health facilities and inpatient treatment in hospital. A non-Cochrane meta-analysis of nine community-based studies of pneumonia case management in neonates, infants and older children reported a reduction in all-cause mortality of 27% (95% CI 18–35) and of pneumonia mortality of 42% (95% CI 22–57) in neonates compared to controls.[22] A subsequent non-Cochrane systematic review of the effect of different strategies on mortality of neonatal pneumonia identified seven studies.[23] A meta-analysis of four studies suggested oral antibiotics for neonatal pneumonia were associated with a 25% reduction in all-cause mortality (95% CI 11–36) and a 42% reduction (18–59%) in neonatal pneumonia-specific mortality.[23] Injectable antibiotics have not been studied to the same extent.

8.1.9 Prevention of neonatal pneumonia

It has long been known that neonatal and infant pneumonia is associated with air pollution, but an RCT comparing woodstoves with chimneys versus traditional open wood fires in Guatemala households was the first study to provide strong evidence that reducing pollution reduces pneumonia in children <18 months (Figures 8.5a and b).[24] The study was not powered to look at neonatal pneumonia and did not report ages of pneumonia cases.

There is a well-recognized association between passive exposure to tobacco smoke and pneumonia and other respiratory infections in infants and young children,[25] but no studies of whether reducing tobacco smoke exposure prevents neonatal pneumonia.

A non-Cochrane systematic review found some evidence that tight swaddling can reduce oxygen saturation and predispose to neonatal respiratory infection including pneumonia.[26]

An Israeli RCT found changing ventilator circuits daily, compared with every 3 days, reduced colonization but not VAP.[27] An observational study from Taiwan found no difference in incidence of VAP in neonates whose circuits were changed every 3 or 7 days.[28]

Tracheal suctioning without disconnection from the ventilator reduces the number of episodes of hypoxia by about half compared with disconnecting the infant to perform suction, but has not been shown to reduce the incidence of pneumonia.[29]

Primary prevention of pneumonia through immunization is considered in Chapter 23.

8.2 Otitis media

There is a paucity of data on neonatal otitis media.[30] Neonatal ears are not routinely examined in most

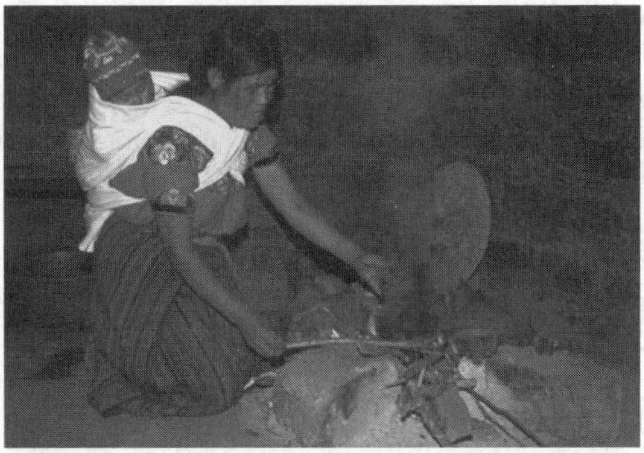

(a)

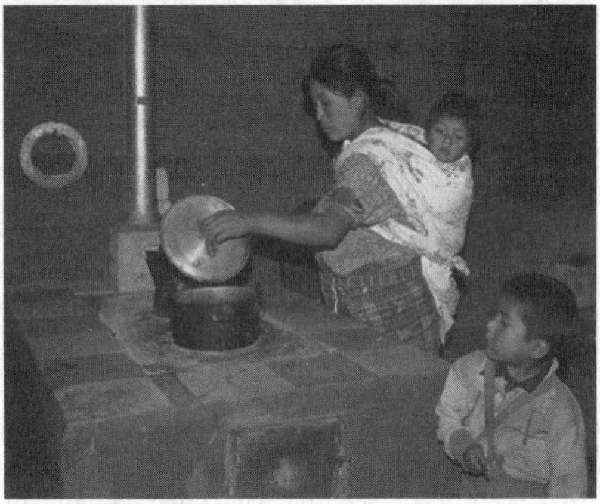

(b)

Figure 8.5 (a) Open wood fire in Guatemala. Reproduced from University of California, Berkeley. (b) Chimney reduced woodsmoke exposure by half in Guatemala. Reproduced from Reference 24 with permission from Elsevier. Copyright © 2011 Elsevier.

countries. The neonatal ear canal is narrow and ear examination is tricky. Autopsy examinations identified pathogens in the middle ear fluid of 10% of infants who died in the neonatal period, but all also had either pneumonia or meningitis.[31]

A study of 68 full-term, healthy infants using otoscopy, tympanometry and acoustic emissions found that all babies had fluid in both ears at 3 hours of age; the fluid had resolved by 3 days of age in 73% but was still present in 13% by otoscopy at 2 weeks of age.[32]

A cohort study of Australian Aboriginal infants found that they were often colonized with *S. pneumoniae*, untypeable *H. influenzae* and *Moraxella catarrhalis* in the neonatal period and 50% had documented otitis media by 30 days of age compared with only one of 17 non-Aboriginal infants.[33] The early bacterial colonization of Aboriginal infants was attributed to high rates of cross-infection due to overcrowding and poor hygiene.[33]

Other studies have also shown that *S. pneumoniae* and *H. influenzae* are the commonest isolates in neonatal otitis media, but Gram-negative enteric bacilli are sometimes isolated and Pseudomonas is a common isolate from chronic ear discharge. However, *S. aureus* and GBS may also be isolated from neonates with otitis media, showing the need for cultures. If a neonate develops discharging ears, the ear should be swabbed and antibiotic treatment directed to the causative organisms. *Mycobacterium tuberculosis* can cause chronic ear discharge, usually in association with maternal pulmonary TB, and should be suspected if there are risk factors for TB.

References

1. Oestergaard MZ, Inoue M, Yoshida S, et al., United Nations Inter-Agency Group for Child Mortality Estimation and the Child Health Epidemiology Reference Group. Neonatal mortality levels for 193 countries in 2009 with trends since 1990: a systematic analysis of progress, projections, and priorities. *PLoS Med* 2011; 8:e1001080.
2. Duke T. Neonatal pneumonia in developing countries. *Arch Dis Child Fetal Neonatal Ed* 2005; 90:F211–F219.
3. Davies PA, Aherne W. Congenital pneumonia. *Arch Dis Child* 1962; 37:598–602.
4. Black RE, Cousens S, Johnson HL, et al., Child Health Epidemiology Reference Group of WHO and UNICEF. Global, regional, and national causes of child mortality in 2008: a systematic analysis. *Lancet* 2010; 375:1969–1987.
5. Sazawal S, Black RE, Pneumonia Case Management Trials Group. Effect of pneumonia case management on mortality in neonates, infants, and preschool children: a meta-analysis of community-based trials. *Lancet Infect Dis* 2003; 3:547–556.
6. Zaidi AK, Ganatra HA, Syed S, et al. Effect of case management on neonatal mortality due to sepsis and pneumonia. *BMC Public Health* 2011; 11(Suppl. 3):S13.
7. Shakunthala SKV, Rao GM, Urmila S. Diagnostic lung puncture aspiration in acute pneumonia of newborn. *Indian Pediatr* 1978; 15:39–44.
8. Webber S, Wilkinson AR, Lindsell D, Hope PL, Dobson SRM, Isaacs D. Neonatal pneumonia. *Arch Dis Child* 1990; 65:207–211.
9. Herting E, Gefeller O, Land M, van Sonderen L, Harms K, Robertson B. Surfactant treatment of neonates with respiratory failure and group B streptococcal infection. Members of

the Collaborative European Multicenter Study Group. *Pediatrics* 2000; 106:957–964.
10. Barter RA, Hudson JA. Bacteriological findings in perinatal pneumonia. *Pathology* 1974; 6:223–230.
11. Petdachai W. Ventilator-associated pneumonia in a newborn intensive care unit. *Southeast Asian J Trop Med Public Health* 2004; 35:724–729.
12. Slagle TA, Bifano EM, Wolf JW, Gross SJ. Routine endotracheal cultures for the prediction of sepsis in ventilated babies. *Arch Dis Child* 1989; 64:34–38.
13. Campbell AN, O'Driscoll MC, Robinson DL, Read SE. A case of neonatal herpes simplex with pneumonia. *Can Med Assoc J* 1983; 129:725–726.
14. Wang H, Tang J, Xiong Y, Li X, Gonzalez F, Mu D. Neonatal community-acquired pneumonia: pathogens and treatment. *J Paediatr Child Health* 2010; 46:668–672.
15. Papageovgiou A, Bauer CR, Fletcher BD, Stern L. Klebsiella pneumonia with pneumatocele formation in a newborn infant. *Can Med Assoc J* 1973; 109:1217–1219.
16. Kunh JP, Lee SB. Pneumatoceles associated with *Escherichia coli* pneumonias in the newborn. *Pediatrics* 1973; 51:1008–1011.
17. Engle WD, Jackson GL, Sendelbach D, et al. Neonatal pneumonia: comparison of 4 vs 7 days of antibiotic therapy in term and near-term infants. *J Perinatol* 2000; 20:421–426.
18. Engle WD, Jackson GL, Sendelbach DM, et al. Pneumonia in term neonates: laboratory studies and duration of antibiotic therapy. *J Perinatol* 2003; 23:372–377.
19. Isaacs D. Magical numbers. *J Paediatr Child Health* 2012; 48:189.
20. Subhi R, Adamson M, Campbell H, et al.,Hypoxaemia in Developing Countries Study Group. The prevalence of hypoxaemia among ill children in developing countries: a systematic review. *Lancet Infect Dis* 2009; 9:219–227.
21. Duke T, Subhi R, Peel D, Frey B. Pulse oximetry: technology to reduce child mortality in developing countries. *Ann Trop Paediatr* 2009; 29:165–175.
22. Sazawal S, Black RE; Pneumonia Case Management Trials Group. Effect of pneumonia case management on mortality in neonates, infants, and preschool children: a meta-analysis of community-based trials. *Lancet Infect Dis* 2003; 3:547–556.
23. Zaidi AK, Ganatra HA, Syed S, et al. Effect of case management on neonatal mortality due to sepsis and pneumonia. *BMC Public Health* 2011; 11(Suppl. 3):S13.
24. Smith KR, McCracken JP, Weber M, et al. Effect of reduction in household air pollution on childhood pneumonia in Guatemala (RESPIRE): a randomised controlled trial. *Lancet* 2011; 378:1717–1726.
25. DiFranza JR, Lew RA. Morbidity and mortality in children associated with the use of tobacco products by other people. *Pediatrics* 1996; 97:560–568.
26. van Sleuwen BE, Engelberts AC, Boere-Boonekamp MM, Kuis W, Schulpen TW, L'Hoir MP. Swaddling: a systematic review. *Pediatrics* 2007; 120:e1097–e1106.
27. Makhoul IR, Kassis I, Berant M, Hashman N, Revach M, Sujov P. Frequency of change of ventilator circuit in premature infants: Impact on ventilator-associated pneumonia. *Pediatr Crit Care Med* 2001; 2:127–132.
28. Hsieh TC, Hsia SH, Wu CT, Lin TY, Chang CC, Wong KS. Frequency of ventilator-associated pneumonia with 3-day versus 7-day ventilator circuit changes. *Pediatr Neonatol* 2010; 51:37–43.
29. Taylor JE, Hawley G, Flenady V, Woodgate PG. Tracheal suctioning without disconnection in intubated ventilated neonates. *Cochrane Database Syst Rev* 2011; (12):CD003065. doi: 10.1002/14651858.CD003065.pub2.
30. Syggelou A, Fanos V, Iacovidou N. Acute otitis media in neonatal life: a review. *J Chemother* 2011; 23:123–126.
31. deSa DJ. Infection and amniotic aspiration of middle ear in stillbirth and neonatal deaths. *Arch Dis Child* 1973; 48:872–880.
32. Roberts DG, Johnson CE, Carlin SA, Turczyk V, Karnuta MA, Yaffee K. Resolution of middle ear effusion in newborns. *Arch Pediatr Adolesc Med* 1995; 149:873–877.
33. Leach AJ, Boswell JB, Asche V, Nienhuys TG, Mathews JD. Bacterial colonization of the nasopharynx predicts very early onset and persistence of otitis media in Australian aboriginal infants. *Pediatr Infect Dis J* 1994; 13:983–989.

CHAPTER 9

Osteomyelitis and septic arthritis

9.1 Epidemiology

Osteomyelitis and septic arthritis are rare infections in newborns.[1] *Staphylococcus aureus* is known to have a predilection for bones and joints and causes over 90% of osteoarticular infections in older children and adults. However, when neonatal and infant staphylococcal infections were common in the 1950s and 1960s, neonatal osteomyelitis and septic arthritis remained relatively uncommon.[1] A population-based study from Sweden reported rates of neonatal osteomyelitis of 0.3 cases per 1000 live births in the 1960s and 1970s.[2]

Neonatal intensive care using indwelling central lines and other invasive procedures has been associated with a modest increase in the incidence of neonatal osteomyelitis. Whereas pre-term infants are rarely reported in case series predating neonatal intensive care,[3,4] in an Australian case series of neonatal osteomyelitis, 57% were pre-term.[5]

9.2 Pathogenesis

Neonatal osteomyelitis is thought to be acquired through haematogenous (blood-borne) spread. The evidence comes from the clinical presentation, commonly with concomitant bacteraemia and multifocal osteomyelitis, and from experimental studies in animals. Evidence of the blood supply to bone comes mainly from a series of pioneering experiments using injection of blood vessels of tibial bones from children and mammals.[6,7] Neonatal osteomyelitis often affects long bones and experimental and pathologic studies suggest it starts in the vascular metaphysis (Figure 9.1). An intravenous injection of pathogenic bacteria localizes in the metaphyseal veins within 2 hours.[7] Spread from the metaphysis can occur through nutrient vessels that supply the growth plate.[6,7] The neonate is sometimes said, unlike older children and adults, to have transphyseal vessels which allow haematogenous spread from metaphysis to epiphysis across the growth plate (physis). However, the nutrient vessels would allow spread of organisms without needing to invoke transphyseal vessels. Transphyseal vessels are present in birds and it has been suggested that their presence might contribute to the frequent co-occurrence of osteomyelitis and septic arthritis in neonates.[8] However, the neonatal periosteum is thinner than in older children and a subperiosteal abscess is more likely to rupture into soft tissues. Indeed, this is probably the reason that neonatal osteomyelitis is often surprisingly indolent. The joint capsule of the neonate encompasses the metaphysis, so pus from the metaphysis can rupture through the periosteum directly into the joint and cause septic arthritis (Figure 9.1).

Other important routes of osteomyelitis include direct inoculation and extension from adjacent structures. Calcaneal osteomyelitis can result from direct inoculation when heel pricks are performed on the point of the heel overlying the calcaneus (Figure 9.2) instead of the recommended area of the fleshy pads to the side of the heel[10] (Figure 9.3). Other procedures that can cause osteomyelitis due to direct inoculation include scalp electrodes,[11] femoral punctures, radial arterial punctures and rarely lumbar puncture. Fracture and osteomyelitis may coexist; in some cases there may be evidence of the fracture coming first[12] but it may be difficult otherwise to distinguish pre-existing from pathologic fracture.

Skull osteomyelitis following infected cephalhaematoma[13] and osteomyelitis of the phalanx following paronychia are examples of direct spread from adjacent structures.

Evidence-Based Neonatal Infections, First Edition. David Isaacs.

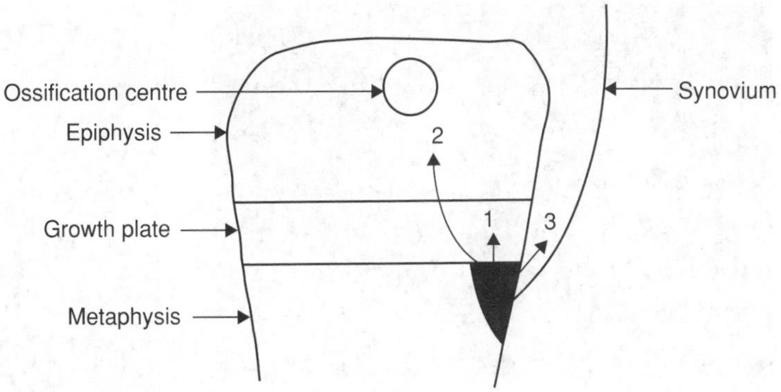

Figure 9.1 Schematic of spread of haematogenous osteomyelitis in neonatal long bone. Infection originates in vascular region in metaphysis (shaded) and can spread contiguously into growth plate (1) via transphyseal blood vessels into epiphysis (2) or rupture through thin periosteum into the joint causing septic arthritis (3). Reproduced with permission from Reference 9.

Antenatal and perinatal complications are described in up to a half of infants in a case series of neonatal osteomyelitis.[1]

Intravascular catheters are a potential source of infection which can disseminate to bone, although neonatal osteomyelitis remains rare despite the frequent use of catheters and is surprisingly rare as a complication of central-line-associated bacteraemia.

Transplacental spread occurs in syphilis and infants with congenital syphilis may have osteitis (Figure 18.9). However, transplacental spread is otherwise thought to be a rare cause of neonatal osteomyelitis.

9.3 Clinical

It has been recognized for over 100 years that neonatal osteomyelitis has two clinical presentations: benign and severe. In the pre-antibiotic era, the severe form was common and there was a recognized association with omphalitis, but in recent times over 80% of patients have had a benign presentation.[3,14–16]

Neonates who present with the benign form of osteomyelitis often appear remarkably well. They may be afebrile and feed well. The most common presentation is with swelling, tenderness and decreased movement.[3,14–16] Sometimes the neonate will not move a limb but otherwise does not seem to be in pain

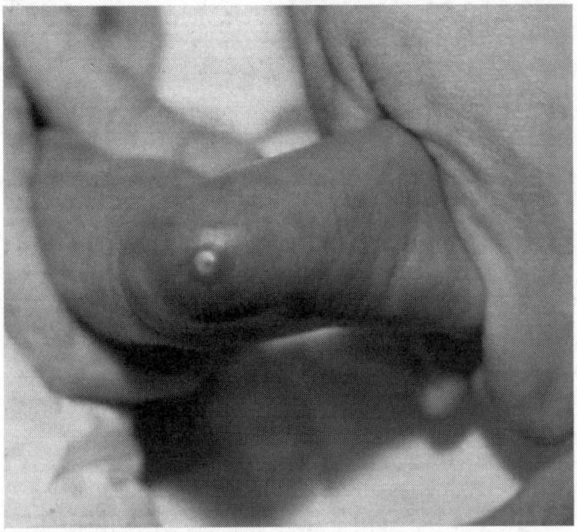

Figure 9.2 Abscess due to calcaneal osteomyelitis caused by a heel prick on the point of the heel overlying the os calcis, instead of the sides of the foot.

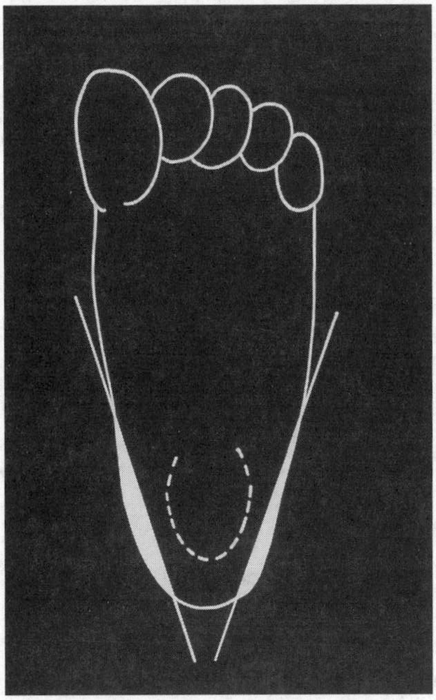

Figure 9.3 Correct site for heel pricks in fleshy part at side of foot (white shaded area). Reproduced with permission from Reference 9.

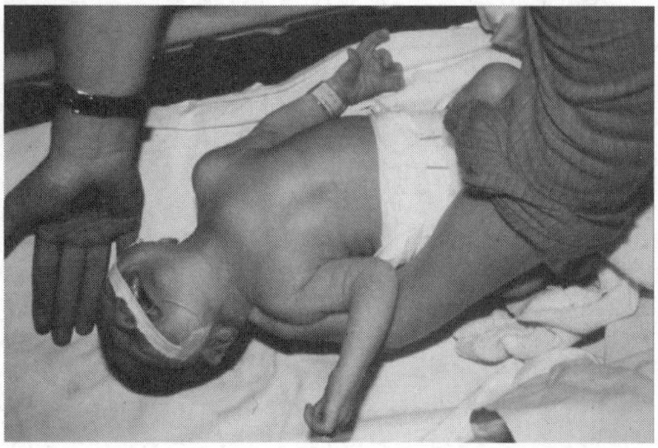

Figure 9.4 Baby with cleft lip and palate who stopped moving left arm. The Moro response (shown) was abnormal mimicking Erb's palsy. There was swelling overlying the left clavicle, blood cultures grew *S. aureus* and the diagnosis was confirmed as osteomyelitis of the clavicle. Reproduced with permission from Reference 16.

(pseudopalsy). If the immobile limb is an arm, the infant may be misdiagnosed as having Erb's palsy (Figure 9.4) and if a leg, misdiagnosed as foot-drop from sciatic nerve injury (Figure 9.5a).[16] Limb swelling may be due to an abscess from a ruptured bone abscess and can be apparently painless, at least at rest. Infants with the benign presentation have a low mortality, but may be left with bony complications. Progression to disseminated osteomyelitis has a worse prognosis for survival (Figure 9.5b).[16] Early diagnosis is important to limit damage and avoid dissemination. The possibility of underlying osteomyelitis should always be considered in an infant with cellulitis, with or without swelling. Neonatal maxillary cellulitis is well recognized, for example, to be associated with underlying osteomyelitis.[17] Similarly, limb swelling without discoloration or systemic symptoms should alert clinicians to possible osteomyelitis.

While the long bones are involved in over two-thirds of cases of neonatal osteomyelitis, almost any bone (and joint) can be involved. Neonatal vertebral osteomyelitis is notoriously difficult to diagnose, often not until an abscess ruptures through to the periphery or to the peritoneum.[18] The clavicle and ribs are other well-recognized sites, while pelvic, scapular, sternal, mandibular and phalangeal osteomyelitis are all described.[1] The joints associated with septic arthritis are classically those close to long

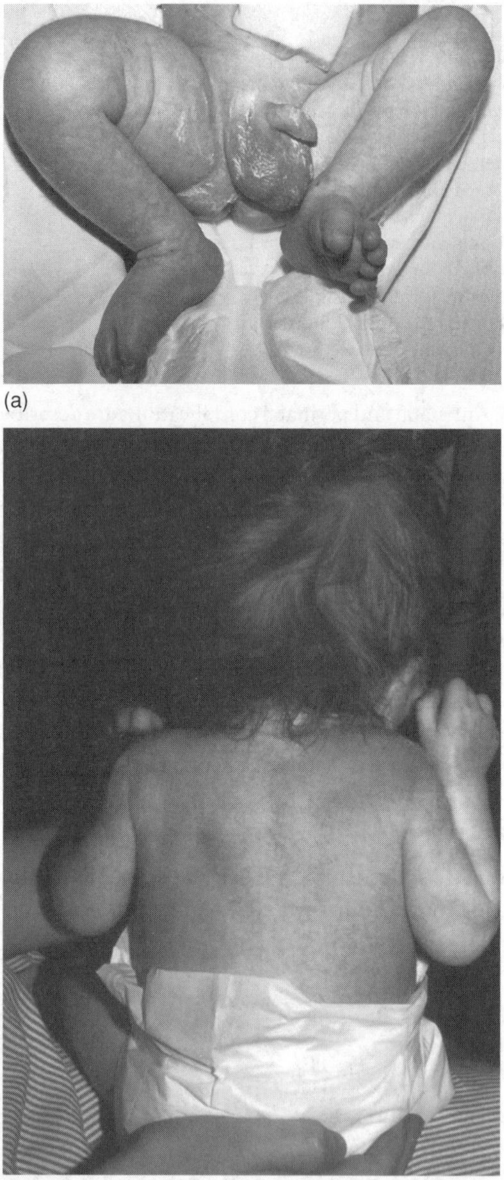

(a)

(b)

Figure 9.5 (a) Boy aged 2 weeks passed urine through umbilicus (patent urachus) and had foot-drop. Misdiagnosed as sciatic nerve damage from intramuscular injection. Note swelling of the right thigh.[16] (b) Same baby as (a) developed cellulitis over shoulder and wrist. Blood cultures grew *S. aureus.* Swelling in thigh aspirated 30 mL of pus. Necrosis of femoral head of femur secondary to septic arthritis of hip. Diagnosis: multifocal staphylococcal osteomyelitis and septic arthritis.[16]

bones, particularly hip, shoulder, knee, ankle and wrist joints.[1, 5,19–24]

In a case series of 94 neonates and infants <4 months old investigated for possible osteomyelitis, 30 babies were diagnosed with osteomyelitis or septic arthritis. Four (16%) of 27 babies investigated for *S. aureus* bacteraemia without focal signs or symptoms were diagnosed with osteomyelitis or septic arthritis by imaging.[5]

Routine bone scan and hip ultrasound scan should be considered for neonates who grow *S. aureus* in blood cultures, even in the absence of signs.

Between a third and a half of neonatal osteomyelitis is multifocal, including infants with a benign presentation.[1–5,13–15] GBS osteomyelitis and/or septic arthritis classically presents with a benign presentation at 2–4 weeks of age only involving one limb, usually humerus (Figure 9.5) or femur.[1, 16, 19] GBS osteomyelitis and arthritis are manifestations of late-onset infection and, like GBS meningitis and other forms of late-onset GBS disease, are usually caused by serotype III (Chapter 14). Early-onset GBS infection is virtually never associated with osteoarticular infection.[1, 19]

Pre-term infants are more likely to present early than full-term infants: in a study from Australia 5 of 17 pre-term infants (29.4%) presented in the first week of life but only 1 of 13 full-term infants.[5]

In severe osteomyelitis, the infant has signs of sepsis with lethargy, irritability, feeding problems, vomiting and abdominal distension, with or without fever. Symptoms or signs of osteomyelitis may be present concurrently or may develop later, even after appropriate antibiotics have been started.[3, 15, 16]

9.4 Organisms

Staphylococcus aureus, by far the most common cause of neonatal osteomyelitis and septic arthritis in pre-antibiotic times, remains a major pathogen in Western and developing countries (Table 9.1).[1–5] Since the 1970s, GBS sometimes outnumbered *S. aureus* in a case series from North America.[1, 4, 20]

In early reports of osteomyelitis, most *S. aureus* isolates were penicillin sensitive.[1, 3] Only about 10% of *S. aureus* are currently penicillin sensitive. Neonatal unit outbreaks of MRSA osteomyelitis and septic arthritis have been reported.[25, 26] Community-acquired neonatal MRSA osteoarticular infection is rarely reported.

Table 9.1 Organisms causing neonatal osteomyelitis and septic arthritis.

Staphylococcus aureus (including MRSA)
Group B streptococcus
Gram-negative bacilli (increasingly common in developing countries)
• *Klebsiella*
• *Escherichia coli*
• *Enterobacter*
• *Salmonella*
• *Pseudomonas*
• *Proteus*, etc.
Other Gram-positive cocci
• Coagulase-negative staphylococci
• Group A streptococcus
• *Streptococcus pneumoniae*
Fungi, particularly *Candida*
Neisseria gonorrhoeae
Treponema pallidum
Anaerobes

Gram-negative bacilli are rare causes of neonatal osteoarticular infection in Western countries, but have been increasingly reported to cause neonatal Gram-negative osteomyelitis and septic arthritis in developing countries,[23, 27] including infections caused by multi-resistant organisms including extended spectrum beta-lactamase (ESBL) producers.[13] *Klebsiella* predominates, but almost any Gram-negative bacillus has been reported at least once as causing osteoarticular infections (Table 9.1).[1, 23, 27]

Other organisms reported as causing neonatal osteoarticular infection include coagulase-negative staphylococci,[28] *Streptococcus pneumoniae* and group A streptococcus (Table 9.1).

Candida is increasingly reported as a cause of neonatal osteoarticular infection[29] (Chapter 16). *Neisseria gonorrhoeae* is well known to cause septic arthritis,[30] but gonococcal osteomyelitis is also well described.[1] Syphilis was an important cause of osteitis and osteochondritis prior to widespread maternal serologic screening and remains an important cause in disadvantaged populations, mainly but not exclusively in developing countries (Chapter 18).[1]

Anaerobes are rare causes of neonatal osteomyelitis or septic arthritis, usually in association with a previous anaerobic collection.[31]

9.5 Diagnosis

9.5.1 Radiology

The plain radiograph may be abnormal much earlier than in older children. In an Austrian study, plain radiography identified 13 (65%) of 20 infants with osteomyelitis, of whom only 4 had clinical signs. Bone scan (Figure 9.6) identified 18 (90%) infants.[32]

The later the presentation the more likely the radiograph will be abnormal. In an Australian case series, ≤6 of 9 plain radiographs were normal when symptoms had been present ≤3 days, but after 5 days the sensitivity was comparable to bone scan.[5]

An early study reported low sensitivity of bone scintigraphy using technetium Tc 99m diphosphonate bone scan in neonatal osteomyelitis.[33] However, whether because of improved technique or technology, subsequent studies have reported bone scan to be very sensitive. One small US study reported that bone scan correctly identified all 15 infected infants,[34] while case series from Australia[5] and Austria[32] reported 84% and 90% sensitivity, respectively. The specificity in the Australian study was 89% and negative predictive value 92%.[5]

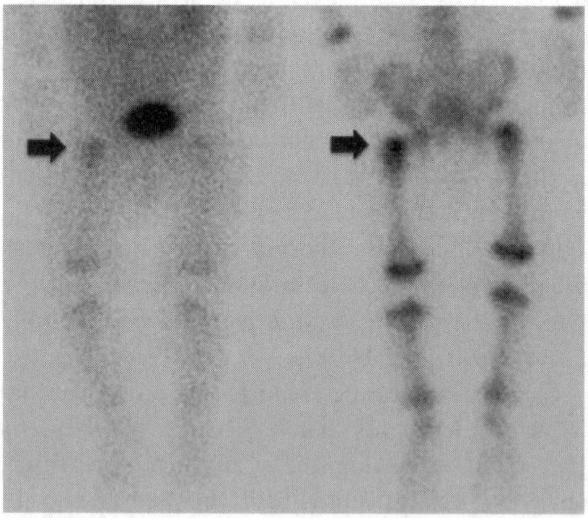

(a) (b)

Figure 9.6 Bone scan of 35-week gestation baby who presented at 3 weeks of age with fever but no bone or joint signs showing proximal right femoral osteomyelitis (courtesy of Prof. Rob Howman-Giles.) (a) early (b) delayed. Blood culture grew *S. aureus* and bone scan performed to exclude osteomyelitis. Scan shows focal increased uptake (see arrow). X-ray and hip ultrasound were normal.

Adding gallium scanning to bone scan in one study improved diagnostic sensitivity from 84% to 90%.[5] Computerized tomography (CT),[35] positive emission tomography (PET)[35] and magnetic resonance imaging (MRI) scans[36, 37] may help, but their sensitivity and specificity have not been formally evaluated.

Ultrasound is the modality of choice for diagnosing septic arthritis of the hip and of many other joints.[38] It is non-invasive and rapid. If a significant fluid collection is present in the hip joint, it is an indication for immediate drainage to prevent necrosis of the femoral head and long-term sequelae. Ultrasound may help diagnose osteomyelitis by identification of a subperiosteal collection.[39]

Hip ultrasound for septic arthritis should be performed on all infants with *S. aureus* bacteraemia and/or osteoarticular infection because this diagnosis is easily missed resulting in permanent deformity.

9.5.2 Laboratory parameters

Haematologic parameters are not helpful. The white cell count is often within normal limits.[1, 5, 15, 40] Serum acute phase reactants and erythrocyte sedimentation rate are usually abnormal in severe osteomyelitis but often normal in the benign form.[1, 15]

9.5.3 Needle aspiration

For septic arthritis, open incision and drainage are often indicated therapeutically and will yield specimens for microbiology. On the other hand, there are situations where needle aspiration is preferable. CT- or ultrasound-guided aspiration may be useful for deep collections.[1, 15]

9.6 Treatment

9.6.1 Antimicrobial treatment

There are no randomized controlled trials (RCTs) of antibiotic treatment of neonatal bacterial osteomyelitis. Whenever possible the choice of antimicrobial treatment should be based on microscopy and modified following culture and antimicrobial sensitivity results. Empiric therapy needs to cover *S. aureus*, and possibly MRSA, and Gram-negative organisms and local epidemiology may need consideration. If a baby is colonized with MRSA or multi-resistant Gram-negative bacilli it is advisable clearly to use an antibiotic regimen that covers these organisms.

Infants with severe osteomyelitis and/or septic arthritis may also have meningitis. If lumbar puncture cannot be performed, it may be necessary to use an empiric antibiotic regimen effective against meningitis.

Antibiotics should always be given parenterally. The combination of a semi-synthetic penicillin (e.g. flucloxacillin, dicloxacillin, nafcillin, oxacillin) or cephalosporin (e.g. cephalothin) with an aminoglycoside (e.g. gentamicin) will cover methicillin-sensitive *S. aureus*, GBS, other Gram-positives and almost all Gram-negative bacilli and is a reasonable empiric antibiotic regimen if MRSA and multi-resistant Gram-negative bacilli are unlikely. In severe sepsis, it is probably prudent to include vancomycin in any empiric regimen to cover MRSA septicaemia. Antibiotics should be modified in the light of positive cultures. Benzylpenicillin remains the antibiotic choice for bone or joint infections due to penicillin-sensitive *S. aureus*.

The route and duration of antibiotic treatment is controversial. Oral antibiotic absorption is less efficient in neonates than older children and in pre-term than full-term infants (Chapter 25). In older children with osteomyelitis[41] and/or septic arthritis[42] it is safe to give parenteral antibiotics for 3–7 days and complete a total of 3–4 weeks of antibiotics with oral therapy provided there is a good clinical response. Total duration of antibiotics <3 weeks in children is associated with unacceptably high rates of relapse, so 3 weeks is the absolute minimum duration. A similar approach was described in five full-term newborns who received 5–9 days of IV antibiotics followed by 6 weeks of oral dicloxacillin.[43] No infant needed readmission although one infant relapsed clinically after stopping oral antibiotics and continued oral antibiotics for 12 weeks.[43] While sequential intravenous–oral therapy has been used successfully for neonatal osteomyelitis when vascular access was problematic,[44] most experts feel this should only ever be done if therapy can be closely monitored. The usual recommendation for neonatal bacterial osteomyelitis is for at least 4 weeks of parenteral antibiotics.

Fungal osteomyelitis is discussed in Chapter 16.

9.6.2 Surgical treatment

Open incision and drainage are generally necessary for large joint collections and for some tissue collections. Radiologically guided aspiration followed by antimicrobials may suffice for some joint and soft tissue collections. In one retrospective study of infections involving large joints, growth disturbance was present in 20 of 36 foci when operation was not performed but only 4 of 19 operated foci.[45]

The risks and benefits of operating on bones to drain intramedullary collections are controversial.

9.7 Prognosis

The outcome of neonatal osteomyelitis and septic arthritis depends on a number of factors including prematurity, benign or severe presentation, speed of diagnosis, site and treatment.[46] The mortality is low except in the severe form but morbidity due to deformity is common. Infections of large joints need prompt surgical management and any delay in operating on infected hip joints is associated with significant morbidity due to necrosis of the femoral head and subsequent limb shortening and limp (Figure 9.7).[1, 15, 16, 45]

In a Swedish long-term follow-up study, early age of onset and failure to operate on large joints were associated with a worse prognosis regarding growth disturbance.[45] In a Brazilian study, 38% of infants with bone and/or joint infections had sequelae and hip involvement was associated with a worse outcome.[47]

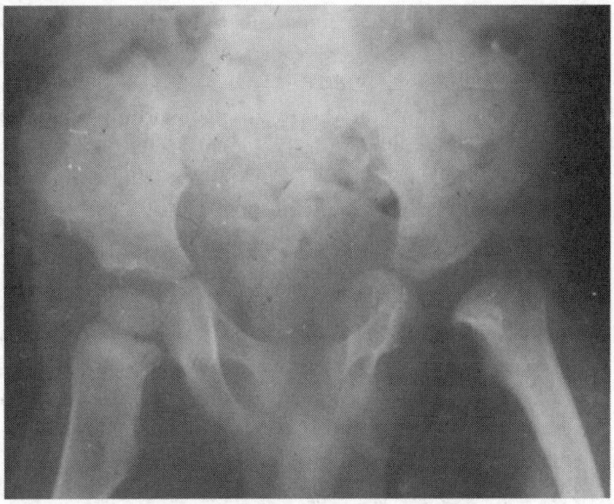

Figure 9.7 Necrotic destruction of left femoral head and dislocation of left hip secondary to delayed treatment of septic arthritis of the left hip.

The causative organism may also be a significant factor in outcome. Four Japanese neonates with MRSA septic arthritis of the hip who presented with sepsis and thigh swelling all had femoral head deformity and severe discrepancy in leg length on follow-up. In contrast, five neonates with methicillin-sensitive *S. aureus* hip arthritis had fewer sequelae with only low-grade deformity of the femoral head and no marked leg length discrepancy.[48]

References

1. Overturf GD. Bacterial infections of the bone and joints. In: *Infectious Diseases of the Fetus and Newborn Infant*, 7th edn (eds JS Remington, JO Klein, CB Wilson, V Nizet, Y Maldonado). Philadelphia: Elsevier, 2011. pp 296–309.
2. Bennet S, Bergdahl S, Eriksson M, Zetterstrom R. The outcome of neonatal septicaemia during 15 years. *Acta Paediatr Scand* 1989; 78:40–43.
3. Weissberg ED, Smith AL, Smith DH. Clinical features of neonatal osteomyelitis. *Pediatrics* 1974; 53:505–510.
4. Fox L, Sprunt K. Neonatal osteomyelitis. *Pediatrics* 1978; 62:535–542.
5. Wong M, Isaacs D, Howman-Giles R, Uren R. Clinical and diagnostic features of osteomyelitis occurring in the first three months of life. *Pediatr Infect Dis J* 1995; 14:1047–1053.
6. Trueta J, Morgan JD. The vascular contribution to osteogenesis. I. Studies by the injection method. *J Bone Joint Surg Br* 1960; 42-B:97–109.
7. Trueta J. The three types of acute haematogenous osteomyelitis. A clinical and vascular study. *J Bone Joint Surg Br* 1959; 41-B:671–680.
8. Alderson M, Speers D, Emslie K, Nade S. Acute haematogenous osteomyelitis and septic arthritis–a single disease. An hypothesis based upon the presence of transphyseal blood vessels. *J Bone Joint Surg Br* 1986; 68:268–274.
9. Isaacs D, Moxon ER. *A Handbook of Neonatal Infections: A Practical Guide.* London: Saunders, 1999.
10. Yüksel S, Yüksel G, Oncel S, Divanli E. Osteomyelitis of the calcaneus in the newborn: an ongoing complication of Guthrie test. *Eur J Pediatr* 2007; 166:503–504.
11. McGregor JA, McFarren T. Neonatal cranial osteomyelitis: a complication of fetal monitoring. *Obstet Gynecol* 1989; 73:490–492.
12. Valerio PG, Harmsen P. Osteomyelitis as a complication of perinatal fracture of the clavicle. *Eur J Pediatr* 1995; 154:497–498.
13. Nakwan N, Nakwan N, Wannaro J, Dissaneevate P, Kritsaneepaiboon S, Chokephaibulkit K. Septicemia, meningitis, and skull osteomyelitis complicating infected cephalhematoma caused by ESBL-producing *Escherichia coli. Southeast Asian J Trop Med Public Health* 2011; 42:148–151.
14. Brill PW, Winchester P, Krauss AN, Symchych P. Osteomyelitis in a neonatal intensive care unit. *Radiology* 1979; 131:83–87.
15. Dessì A, Crisafulli M, Accossu S, Setzu V, Fanos V. Osteo-articular infections in newborns: diagnosis and treatment. *J Chemother* 2008; 20:542–550.
16. Isaacs D, Bower B, Moxon ER. Lesson of the week: neonatal osteomyelitis presenting as nerve palsy. *BMJ* 1986; 292:1071.
17. Loh FC, Ling SY. Acute osteomyelitis of the maxilla in the newborn. *J Laryngol* 1993; 107:627–628.
18. Barton LL, Villar RG, Rice SA. Neonatal group B streptococcal vertebral osteomyelitis. *Pediatrics* 1996; 98:459–461.
19. Memon IA, Jacobs NM, Yeh TF, Lilien LD. Group B streptococcal osteomyelitis and septic arthritis. Its occurrence in infants less than 2 months old. *Am J Dis Child* 1979; 133:921–923.
20. Dan M. Neonatal septic arthritis. *Isr J Med Sci* 1983; 19:967–971.
21. Dan M. Septic arthritis in young infants: clinical and microbiologic correlations and therapeutic implications. *Rev Infect Dis* 1984; 6:147–155.
22. Kabak S, Halici M, Akcakus M, Cetin N, Narin N. Septic arthritis in patients followed-up in neonatal intensive care unit. *Pediatr Int* 2002; 44:652–657.
23. Deshpande SS, Taral N, Modi N, Singrakhia M. Changing epidemiology of neonatal septic arthritis. *J Orthop Surg (Hong Kong)* 2004; 12:10–13.
24. Pittard 3rd WB, Thullen JD, Fanaroff AA. Neonatal septic arthritis. *J Pediatr* 1976; 88:621–624.
25. Ish-Horowicz MR, McIntyre P, Nade S. Bone and joint infections caused by multiply resistant Staphylococcus aureus in a neonatal intensive care unit. *Pediatr Infect Dis J* 1992; 11:82–87.
26. Tan KW, Tay L, Lim SH. An outbreak of methicillin-resistant Staphylococcus aureus in a neonatal intensive care unit in Singapore: a 20-month study of clinical characteristics and control. *Singapore Med J* 1994; 35:277–282.
27. Adeyemo AA, Akindele JA, Omokhodion SI. Klebsiella septicaemia, osteomyelitis and septic arthritis in neonates in Ibadan, Nigeria. *Ann Trop Paediatr* 1993; 13:285–289.
28. Eggink BH, Rowen JL. Primary osteomyelitis and suppurative arthritis caused by coagulase-negative staphylococci in a preterm neonate. *Pediatr Infect Dis J* 2003; 22:572–573.
29. Yousefzadeh DK, Jackson JH. Neonatal and infantile candidal arthritis with or without osteomyelitis: a clinical and radiographical review of 21 cases. *Skeletal Radiol* 1980; 5:77–90.
30. Babl FE, Ram S, Barnett ED, Rhein L, Carr E, Cooper ER. Neonatal gonococcal arthritis after negative prenatal screening and despite conjunctival prophylaxis. *Pediatr Infect Dis J* 2000; 19:346–349.
31. Brook I. Infected neonatal cephalohematomas caused by anaerobic bacteria. *J Perinat Med* 2005; 33:255–258.
32. Aigner RM, Fueger GF, Ritter G. Results of three-phase bone scintigraphy and radiography in 20 cases of neonatal osteomyelitis. *Nucl Med Commun* 1996; 17:20–28.
33. Ash JM, Gilday DL. The futility of bone scanning in neonatal osteomyelitis: concise communication. *J Nucl Med* 1980; 21:417–420.

34. Bressler EL, Conway JJ, Weiss SC. Neonatal osteomyelitis examined by bone scintigraphy. *Radiology* 1984; 152:685–688.
35. Offiah AC. Acute osteomyelitis, septic arthritis and discitis: differences between neonates and older children. *Eur J Radiol* 2006; 60:221–232.
36. Martijn A, van der Vliet AM, van Waarde WM, van Aalderen WM. Gadolinium-DTPA enhanced MRI in neonatal osteomyelitis of the cervical spine. *Br J Radiol* 1992; 65:720–722.
37. Dormans JP, Drummond DS. Pediatric hematogenous osteomyelitis: new trends in presentation, diagnosis, and treatment. *J Am Acad Orthop Surg* 1994; 2:333–341.
38. Berberian G, Firpo V, Soto A, et al. Osteoarthritis in the neonate: risk factors and outcome. *Braz J Infect Dis* 2010; 14:413–418.
39. Rubin LP, Wallach MT, Wood BP. Radiological case of the month. Neonatal osteomyelitis diagnosed by ultrasound. *Arch Pediatr Adolesc Med* 1996; 150:217–218.
40. Frederiksen B, Christiansen P, Knudsen FU. Acute osteomyelitis and septic arthritis in the neonate, risk factors and outcome. *Eur J Pediatr* 1993; 152:577–580.
41. Peltola H, Pääkkönen M, Kallio P, Kallio MJ; Osteomyelitis-Septic Arthritis Study Group. Short- versus long-term antimicrobial treatment for acute hematogenous osteomyelitis of childhood: prospective, randomized trial on 131 culture-positive cases. *Pediatr Infect Dis J* 2010; 29:1123–1128.
42. Peltola H, Pääkkönen M, Kallio P, Kallio MJ; Osteomyelitis-Septic Arthritis (OM-SA) Study Group. Prospective, randomized trial of 10 days versus 30 days of antimicrobial treatment, including a short-term course of parenteral therapy, for childhood septic arthritis. *Clin Infect Dis* 2009; 48:1201–1210.
43. Cole WG, Dalziel RE, Leitl S. Treatment of acute osteomyelitis in childhood. *J Bone Joint Surg* 1982; 64:218–223.
44. Ecury-Goossen GM, Huysman MA, Verhallen-Dantuma JC, Man P. Sequential intravenous-oral antibiotic therapy for neonatal osteomyelitis. *Pediatr Infect Dis J* 2009; 28:72–73.
45. Bergdahl S, Ekengren K, Eriksson M. Neonatal hematogenous osteomyelitis: risk factors for long-term sequelae. *J Pediatr Orthop* 1985; 5:564–568.
46. Ekengren K, Bergdahl S, Eriksson M. Neonatal osteomyelitis. Radiographic findings and prognosis in relation to site of involvement. *Acta Radiol Diagn (Stockh)* 1982; 23(3B):305–311.
47. Berberian G, Firpo V, Soto A, et al. Osteoarthritis in the neonate: risk factors and outcome. *Braz J Infect Dis* 2010; 14:413–418.
48. Mortia M, Nakamura H, Kitano T. Comparison of clinical outcome after treatment of hip arthritis caused by MRSA with that caused by non-MRSA in infants. *J Pediatr Orthop B* 2009; 18:1–5.

CHAPTER 10
Urinary tract infections

10.1 Epidemiology

The term urinary tract infection (UTI) refers to infection of the kidney(s) and/or the bladder, so includes pyelonephritis and cystitis. Urine collection methods do not distinguish the site of infection which can sometimes be deduced from imaging. The reported incidence of neonatal UTI varies according to the method of urine collection (bag and clean catch specimens were commonly used in the 1950s until it was appreciated that they are frequently contaminated), the colony count used to define infection and the population studied.

10.1.1 Definition of urinary tract infection

The traditional definition of UTI is a pure growth of 100 000 (10^5) colony forming units (CFU)/mL, or 10^8 CFU/L, from a voided specimen. This figure is derived from studies comparing voided specimens from women who were about to be catheterized with their subsequent catheter specimens,[1] and its relevance in children is assumed but not proven. A lower number of organisms or of colonies is considered significant if grown from a newly inserted catheter or a urine collected by suprapubic aspiration (SPA), specimens less likely to be contaminated. Using the figure of 10^5/mL or 10^8/L as the reference value to define UTI, a comparative study of children with recurrent UTI suggested the figures in Table 10.1 as thresholds to define a UTI when urine is collected by different methods.[2] There are no similar data for neonates, so the clinical significance of growing lesser numbers of organisms or colonies from neonatal urine is unknown.

Bacteria grow rapidly, so specimens containing few introduced bacteria left at room temperature or greater for more than an hour can yield false-positive urine cultures.

10.1.2 Method of urine collection

Catheter urine collection is less painful and more likely to succeed than suprapubic aspirate[3–5] (see Section 4.1.4).

10.2 Pathogenesis

In neonates, it is not known whether kidney infection is primary with secondary spread to the bloodstream and even the meninges or occurs embolically secondary to septicaemia. The primary site of infection might be different in early-onset and late-onset UTI, with bacteraemic spread more likely in early sepsis and ascending infection from the urethra more likely in late UTI.

Urine cultures are sometimes positive in early-onset septicaemia and/or meningitis. In one study, 9 of 188 infants investigated for early-onset sepsis had bacteraemia and 1 also had a positive urine culture (with GBS).[6] Two babies had positive urine cultures with negative blood cultures. One grew *Escherichia coli* and was treated for UTI. The other baby grew *Staphylococcus epidermidis* from an SPA and recovered untreated, showing that SPA urines are not immune to contamination.

In the same study, 1 of 189 infants with suspected late-onset sepsis had *Klebsiella* grown from both blood and urine. Ten other babies had positive blood but negative urine cultures and 13 babies had positive urine cultures but negative blood cultures.[6]

Anatomic abnormalities of the urinary tract, particularly obstructive abnormalities such as posterior urethral valves, vesico-ureteric and pelvi-ureteric junction stenosis are associated with UTI. Reports suggest

Evidence-Based Neonatal Infections, First Edition. David Isaacs.

Table 10.1 Threshold diagnostic criteria of bacterial counts for acute urinary tract infection in children.

Method of urine collection	Minimum level of bacteriuria for diagnosis of UTI
Clean catch in girls	100 000 (10^5) CFU/mL (or 10^8/L)
Clean catch in boys	10 000 (10^4) CFU/mL (or 10^7/L)
New catheter	10 000 (10^4) CFU/mL (or 10^7/L)
Suprapubic aspiration	Gram-negative bacilli: any colonies Gram-positive cocci: 5000 CFU/mL (or 5×10^6/L)

Source: Reproduced with permission from Reference 47.
N.B. CFU/mL = colony-forming units per mL (or organisms/mL).

that 5–20% of neonates with UTI have an obstructive uropathy,[7] while half of all infants with an obstructive uropathy will present with UTI.[8]

The incidence of UTI increases with decreasing gestational age and birth weight. Fungal UTIs occur almost exclusively in babies <1500 g. Mature babies who develop fungal UTI are usually receiving parenteral nutrition for major congenital malformations, for example, gastrointestinal disease, or prolonged broad-spectrum antibiotics (see Chapter 16).[9]

In the first year of life, boys have double the incidence of UTI than girls,[10, 11] whereas girls predominate after the age of one. The reported incidence of UTI in retrospective studies was 0.1–0.2% for circumcised male infants, 0.4–0.6% for female infants, but 1.1–4.1% for uncircumcised male infants. Circumcision is protective against UTI in males (Section 10.6). Within 2 weeks of birth the prepuce is heavily colonized with *E. coli*.[12] Circumcision is associated with a reduction in periurethral carriage of *E. coli* and *Proteus*.[13, 14] These data support the theory that the prepuce is an important source of the uropathogens that cause UTI in boys.

While the above data suggest that host factors are a major determinant of susceptibility to UTI, organism factors are also important. There are many strains of *E. coli* in faeces, yet the strains that cause UTI are very different from diarrhoeal and non-pathogenic strains. Uropathogenic strains of *E. coli* have been extensively studied and carry genes for various virulence factors including adhesins such as P-fimbriae that facilitate adherence to uroepithelium, iron uptake systems and cytotoxins.[15–17]

Vesico-ureteric reflux (VUR) has been associated with UTI, but it remains controversial whether babies are born with VUR which predisposes to UTI or whether UTI can cause transient reflux and to what extent babies with UTI should be investigated for reflux[7] (Section 10.5).

10.3 Clinical

The clinical presentation of UTI is non-specific. In a US study, the symptoms of infants with bacteraemia did not differentiate them from those with bacteriuria.[6] Most of the data on the clinical presentation of neonatal UTI come from studies in the 1970s of relatively mature preterm and full-term infants.[7] In these studies, half the infants had an insidious presentation with failure to thrive with or without low-grade fever, feeding problems, vomiting, irritability, lethargy and jaundice.

Infants with UTI can also present acutely with signs of sepsis including fever, meningismus, abdominal distension and hepatosplenomegaly. Jaundice occurs in about 20% of patients with UTI but is an unreliable indicator of UTI (see Chapter 3).

10.4 Laboratory

10.4.1 Microscopy

Question: How useful is urine microscopy in diagnosing or excluding urinary tract infection?

A non-Cochrane meta-analysis of 26 studies of infants and children <12 years old with UTI found that any organisms seen on Gram stain had 93% sensitivity and 95% specificity for detecting UTI, so the presence of organisms on Gram stain strongly suggested UTI.[18] In contrast, pyuria was highly unreliable. One-third of children with UTI did not have >5 white blood cells per high-power field in a centrifuged urine sample, while 23% did not have >10 white blood cells/mm^3 in uncentrifuged urine. The false-positive rate for pyuria was 11–21%. This meta-analysis did not include enough neonatal or infant studies to do a subgroup analysis by age.

A subsequent non-Cochrane meta-analysis of 48 studies in infants and children used a different technique, receiver operator curves (ROC), to analyse a combination of sensitivity and specificity.[19] The authors concluded that urine specimens collected by catheter or SPA performed best, and the most reliable tests were pyuria (10 or more white cells per high-power field) and bacteriuria (any bacteria on Gram stain). This meta-analysis included a subgroup analysis of neonates and infants <6 months old and found no significant difference from older children in the ROC.[19]

In a small study, phase-contrast microscopy for bacteria was as sensitive as culture, although slightly less specific.[20]

For the clinician, normal urine microscopy does not exclude neonatal UTI reliably. A significant proportion of neonates with UTI have no white cells in the urine. Incidentally, many laboratories decline to perform urine Gram stains because culture results will be available only the next day and sick patients should already be receiving empiric therapy.

Answer: A positive Gram stain strongly suggests UTI but a negative Gram stain does not exclude UTI. Pyuria suggests UTI but up to a third of infants with UTI do not have any white cells in the urine.

10.4.2 Urinalysis

Question: How useful is urine dipstick testing in diagnosing or excluding urinary tract infection?

A non-Cochrane meta-analysis of 26 studies of infants and children <12 years old with UTI found that a dipstick test positive for both nitrite and leucocyte esterase had a sensitivity of 88% and a specificity of 93%.[18] These tests performed better than pyuria (defined as >10 white cells/mm^3), which was only 77% sensitive.[18]

A non-Cochrane systematic review found 39 studies which evaluated dipstick tests for detecting UTI in children <5 years old.[21] The review concluded that either a dipstick positive for both nitrite and leucocyte esterase or microscopy positive for both pyuria and bacteriuria made UTI extremely likely. Similarly, they concluded that a dipstick negative for both nitrite and leucocyte esterase or microscopy negative for both pyuria and bacteriuria made UTI unlikely.[21]

If rapid tests can identify children with UTI with a high degree of probability they can be used as a basis for choosing which children should start empiric therapy. The best specificity (98%) in the two meta-analyses was for nitrite.[18,21] If specificity is high, false positives are rare, so a positive nitrite could be used as a basis to start empiric therapy.

On the other hand, when using a test to decide which infants to rule out from empiric therapy, the sensitivity needs to be virtually 100% if the risk of not starting therapy is high. The sensitivity of nitrite and leucocyte esterase in the above studies was not sufficient to say that a negative urinalysis rules out UTI.[18,21]

Neither of the above meta-analyses did subgroup analyses by age. However, a more recent non-Cochrane systematic review compared the diagnostic performance of dipstick testing in infants with older children (>2 years old).[22] A meta-analysis of six studies found that urine dipstick testing performed significantly worse in infants and was unreliable in this age group for ruling out UTI.

Answer: A baby with a positive urinalysis for nitrites and/or leucocyte esterase is reasonably likely to have a UTI but a negative urinalysis does not exclude UTI. Urinalysis is less reliable in neonates than in children >2 years old.

10.4.3 Urine culture

Urine obtained by catheter or SPA should be cultured for bacteria and yeasts. The microbiology of UTI has changed with advances in neonatal intensive care. *E. coli* continues to be by far the most important cause of community-acquired UTI in most countries, although neonatal *Klebsiella* UTI is increasing in some developing countries (Table 10.2). The major shift, however, has been in neonatal intensive care units (NICUs), where CoNS have become responsible for up to 30% of UTIs.[7,23] In addition, yeasts are a major cause of UTI in high-risk infants (see Chapter 16).

There are increasing reports of UTI caused by multiresistant Gram-negative bacilli from many countries, including resource-rich and developing countries.[24–29] These include increasing reports of infections with Gram-negative bacilli producing extended-spectrum β-lactamases (ESBL).[24–29]

10.4.4 Blood culture

Blood cultures should always be performed in any infant with suspected UTI and certainly before empiric antibiotics are commenced. The blood culture is often

Table 10.2 Important causes of neonatal urinary tract infections.

Gram-negative bacilli
- *Escherichia coli*
- *Klebsiella* species
- *Enterobacter* species
- *Proteus* species
- *Pseudomonas* species
- Other Gram-negative bacilli

Gram-positive cocci
- Enterococci (faecal streptococci)
- Coagulase-negative staphylococci
- Group B streptococcus
- Other Gram-positive cocci

Fungal
- *Candida*
- Other fungi

positive in neonatal UTI, so the blood culture result may help with the interpretation of an equivocal urine culture result. Furthermore the signs of UTI are non-specific, so the infant with suspected UTI may be bacteraemic without having a UTI.

10.4.5 Lumbar puncture

UTI and bacteraemia may be complicated by meningitis and it is important to perform LP in sick babies with suspected early-onset or late-onset sepsis (see Section 4.1.3). Sterile CSF pleocytosis is well recognized in association with UTI. There is some dispute as to what proportion of infants with UTI has sterile pleocytosis, with estimates ranging from 0% to 8% (depending on definition) of infants age <60 days[30] to 18% of infants aged 1–3 months.[31] These studies do not distinguish neonates from older infants. In a study from Sweden, 9 of 31 (29%) untreated newborns with UTI had sterile CSF pleocytosis of 22–200 white cells/mm^3 at diagnosis.[32] More recent data are scarce, partly because LP is often not performed prospectively in infants with suspected UTI.

10.4.6 Haematology

The peripheral blood total and differential white blood cell count may be normal or abnormal and do not reliably distinguish uninfected infants from those with UTI.[7]

10.4.7 Acute phase reactants

A meta-analysis found a significant association between high-grade (Grade III or greater) VUR and serum procalcitonin, both as a continuous variable (VUR more likely the higher the procalcitonin) and as a binary variable.[33] However, the sensitivity of 83% means one in six infants with high-grade VUR will have a normal procalcitonin, while the specificity of 43% in a population where the incidence of high-grade VUR is low (about 2%[23]) means that a positive procalcitonin in a child with a first UTI has little or no practical value in management.

10.5 Radiology

Radiologic investigation of the urinary tract is important first during the investigation of an infant with possible UTI and second in the investigation of an infant with a proven UTI.

If antenatal ultrasound results are available, before embarking on new radiologic investigations it is recommended to check the ultrasound which may show important, relevant information.

One reason for radiologic investigation of a child with suspected UTI is to detect renal tract abnormalities, including enlarged or echogenic kidneys, abnormal collecting systems, or renal fungal or pyogenic abscesses. Another reason is to detect associated anomalies that require surgery, such as ureterocoele, bladder distension secondary to posterior urethral valves and stones. Ultrasound is the least invasive investigation and will identify most renal tract abnormalities reliably, although is not as sensitive for diagnosing pyelonephritis as technetium-99m-labelled dimercaptosuccinic acid (DMSA) scan and not as sensitive for VUR as cystourethrogram. However, it is rarely critical to diagnose either of these conditions urgently with such a high degree of certainty and the alternative tests are invasive.

Both ultrasound scans and voiding cystourethrography (VCU) used to be recommended in any neonate or infant with a proven UTI because high-grade VUR was thought to predispose to renal infection and a combination of UTI and reflux would lead to renal impairment and end-stage renal failure. However, most end-stage renal failure is now thought to occur in children with congenitally dysplastic kidneys, and the value of routine VCU is questioned.

Question: What radiologic investigations are indicated in a newborn with a proven urinary tract infection?

In a large retrospective study from Taiwan, 119 of 699 children who had VCU, ultrasound and DMSA scans performed had high-grade (III or greater) VUR.[34] Ultrasound was only 67% sensitive in identifying high-grade VUR compared to VCU. Technetium-99m-labelled DMSA scan had a similar sensitivity for identifying high-grade VUR of 65.5%, but combining both tests improved the sensitivity to 83%. The authors recommended reserving routine VCU for infants with abnormal ultrasound or DMSA scans.[34] A Belgian study of infants with first febrile UTI found that ultrasound had 97% sensitivity and 94% specificity for identifying clinically significant uropathies including high-grade VUR.[35]

Studies confined to NICU infants suggest even more strongly that VCU should not be performed routinely in UTI. A US retrospective cohort study reported the imaging results on NICU infants <2 months old who developed UTI.[36] A major abnormality was identified by imaging in 5 of 118 infants (4%) and ultrasound identified all 5 with abnormalities (4%).

Recommendation: Current evidence suggests that all newborns with UTI should be investigated by ultrasound (if available). DMSA scans add relatively little to ultrasound. Voiding cystourethrogram should be reserved for infants with abnormal ultrasounds and/or DMSA scans and not performed routinely.

10.6 Treatment

10.6.1 Antimicrobial therapy

The choice of empiric therapy for an infant with suspected UTI might be guided by urine or CSF microscopy. If the infant has organisms or white cells seen on CSF Gram stain, the choice will be as for empiric treatment of meningitis (see Chapters 5 and 7). If the urine Gram stain shows organisms and the CSF is normal, the antibiotics chosen should cover the likely uropathogens, taking into account colonizing organisms and local epidemiology. If the urine Gram stain shows Gram-negative bacilli, the clinician will need to decide whether to use two antibiotics with activity against Gram-negative bacilli and whether or not one of them must provide anti-staphylococcal and enterococcal cover. The severity of the infant's illness is likely to affect this choice. If no organisms are seen in urine or CSF, empiric therapy will be as for suspected late-onset sepsis (see Chapter 5). The combination of vancomycin to cover *Staphylococcus aureus*, including MRSA, CoNS and most Gram-positive organisms and an aminoglycoside to cover Gram-negative bacilli is commonly used. The parenteral route should always be used for empiric therapy because of the risk of bacteraemia.

If Gram-negative bacilli are seen in the urine, the infant probably has Gram-negative UTI and possibly Gram-negative bacteraemia and/or meningitis. An LP should be performed. Monotherapy is as effective as combination therapy except for *Pseudomonas aeruginosa* bacteraemia.[37, 38]

Renal abscesses may be caused by *S. aureus*, *Streptococcus milleri* or Gram-negative bacilli, so the choice of antibiotics should cover these possibilities in a baby with renal abscess until the cause is determined. Cefotaxime covers methicillin-sensitive *S. aureus*, but not MRSA, and also covers most Gram-negative bacilli except *Pseudomonas* and ESBL-producing organisms.

The optimal duration of parenteral antibiotics in neonatal UTI is unknown. Studies in older children should not be extrapolated uncritically to newborns.[39, 40] Absorption of antibiotics is relatively poor in newborns (see Chapter 24) and initial parenteral therapy is strongly recommended, in case the infant is bacteraemic. However, there is some evidence that it is possible to use IV followed by oral antibiotics to treat non-bacteraemic UTI. A large retrospective multi-centre cohort study of over 12 000 US infants <6 months with UTI found treatment failure rates of 1.6% with short-course IV (3 or fewer days) followed by oral antibiotics compared with 2.2% for 4 days or longer of IV antibiotics. Treatment failure was predicted by pre-existing urinary tract abnormalities but not by age.[41] It seems reasonable to recommend basing the duration of IV antibiotics on clinical response and urine culture results. If an infant is usually fed orally, is responding clinically and the urine is sterile after 2–4 days, it is reasonable to change to oral antibiotics to complete a total of 14 days of antibiotics.[7]

10.6.1.1 Asymptomatic bacteriuria

In a New Zealand study, 14 (1%) of 1460 infants investigated with clean catch urine cultures had bacteriuria confirmed by SPA, and 9 of the 14 were asymptomatic.[42] Five of the nine asymptomatic babies cleared their urine without antibiotics while four needed antibiotics. Thus asymptomatic bacteriuria really does occur in neonates, but is rare.

10.6.2 Adjunctive therapy

Babies with obstructive uropathy may become severely hyponatraemic. Careful monitoring of blood electrolytes and correction of electrolyte imbalance are important in UTI. Renal function (serum creatinine, urea and electrolytes) should be monitored acutely and after recovery.

Blood pressure should be monitored for acute hypotension with sepsis and for hypertension.

10.7 Prevention

10.7.1 Prophylactic antibiotics

A Cochrane systematic review of long-term antibiotics to prevent recurrence of UTI found five studies of 1069 children.[41] The primary analysis found no significant difference in UTI incidence (RR 0.75, 95% CI 0.36–1.53). However, if the analysis was confined to studies at low risk of bias, the difference was significant (RR 0.68, 95% CI 0.48–0.95) and was similar for children with and without VUR.[41]

The largest contributor to the Cochrane meta-analysis was a large Australian RCT of 576 children (median age 14 months) with VUR or first UTI randomized to trimethoprim–sulfamethoxazole or placebo for 1 year.[43] Antibiotics reduced the proportion of infants with UTI from 19% to 13%, an absolute difference of 6%, and the risk difference was similar across subgroups, including infants with VUR. The number needed to treat (NNT) is 16 infants, that is, 16 children with UTI need to be treated with prophylactic antibiotics for 1 year to prevent one child having a UTI. The authors conclude that decisions about prophylaxis should be made individually based on the benefits and risks of adverse events, inconvenience and antibiotic resistance.[43]

For children with abnormal urinary tracts, or those who have already had one recurrence, the risk of UTI is higher, the risk–benefit equation different and the threshold for starting prophylactic antibiotics lower.

10.7.2 Circumcision

If prophylactic antibiotic use is controversial, it pales into insignificance beside the controversy over circumcision. Opinions vary from advocates of routine neonatal circumcision to those who think neonatal circumcision is an assault and should be banned until the infant is old enough to make his own decision. Advocates of routine circumcision cite reduction in UTI and in HIV infection as primary reasons.

A non-Cochrane systematic review identified one RCT, four cohort studies and seven case-control studies of over 400 000 boys.[44] A meta-analysis of the studies found that circumcision reduced the risk of UTI significantly by 87% (OR 0.13, 95% CI 0.08–0.20). In the normal male population the background risk of UTI is 1%, so 111 normal boys would need to be circumcised to prevent one UTI.[44] Many argue that the risks of routine circumcision in Western countries outweigh the benefits. However, there may be reasons to promote circumcision in developing countries to prevent HIV.[45]

For a child with a high baseline risk of UTI (previous UTIs or urinary tract abnormalities), the risk–benefit equation is very different. For example, it has been calculated that only one boy with posterior urethral valves needs to be circumcised to prevent one UTI.[46]

References

1. Cohen SN, Kass EH. A simple method for quantitative urine culture. *N Engl J Med* 1967; 277:176–180.
2. Hellerstein S. Recurrent urinary tract infections in children. *Pediatr Infect Dis* 1982; 1:271–281.
3. Tobiansky R, Evans N. A randomized controlled trial of two methods for collection of sterile urine in neonates. *J Pediatr Child Health* 1998; 34:460–462.
4. Kozer E, Rosenbloom E, Goldman D, Lavy G, Rosenfeld N, Goldman M. Pain in infants who are younger than 2 months during suprapubic aspiration and transurethral bladder catheterization: a randomized, controlled study. *Pediatrics* 2006; 118:e51–e56.
5. El-Naggar W, Yiu A, Mohamed A, et al. Comparison of pain during two methods of urine collection in preterm infants. *Pediatrics* 2010; 125:1224–1229.
6. Visser VE, Hall RT. Urine culture in the evaluation of suspected neonatal sepsis. *J Pediatr* 1979; 94:635–638.

7. Long SS, Klein JO. Bacterial infections of the urinary tract. In: *Infectious Diseases of the Fetus and Newborn Infant*, 7th edn (eds JS Remington, JO Klein, CB Wilson, V Nizet, Y Maldonado). Philadelphia: Elsevier, 2011. pp 311–319.
8. Bensman A, Baudon JJ, Jablonski JP, Lasfargues G. Uropathies diagnosed in the neonatal period: symptomatology and course. *Acta Paediatr Scand* 1980; 69:499–503.
9. Rabalais GP, Samiec TD, Bryant KK, Lewis JJ. Invasive candidiasis in infants weighing more than 2500 grams at birth admitted to a neonatal intensive care unit. *Pediatr Infect Dis J* 1996; 15:348–352.
10. Wiswell TE, Smith FR, Bass JW. Decreased incidence of urinary tract infections in circumcised males. *Pediatrics* 1985; 75:901–903.
11. Wiswell TE, Roscelli JD. Corroborative evidence for the decreased incidence of urinary tract infections in circumcised male infants. *Pediatrics* 1986; 78:96–99.
12. Bollgren I, Winberg J. The periurethral aerobic flora bacterial flora in healthy boys and girls. *Acta Paediatr Scand* 1976; 65:74–80.
13. Wiswell TE, Miller GM, Gelston Jr HM, Jones SK, Clemmings AF. Effect of circumcision status on periurethral bacterial flora during the first year of life. *J Pediatr* 1988; 113:442–446.
14. Glennon J, Ryan PJ, Keane CT, Rees JP. Circumcision and periurethral carriage of Proteus mirabilis in boys. *Arch Dis Child* 1988; 63:556–557.
15. Fusel EN, Kaack B, Cherry R, Roberts JA. Adherence of bacteria to human foreskins. *J Urol* 1988; 140:997–1001.
16. Yamamoto S. Molecular epidemiology of uropathogenic Escherichia coli. *J Infect Chemother* 2007; 13:68–73.
17. Mahjoub-Messai F, Bidet P, Caro V, et al. *Escherichia coli* isolates causing bacteremia via gut translocation and urinary tract infection in young infants exhibit different virulence genotypes. *J Infect Dis* 2011; 203:1844–1849.
18. Gorelick MH, Shaw KN. Screening tests for urinary tract infection: a meta-analysis. *Pediatrics* 1999; 104:e54.
19. Huicho L, Campos-Sanchez M, Alamo C. Meta-analysis of urine screening tests for determining the risk of urinary tract infection in children. *Pediatr Infect Dis J* 2002; 21:1–11.
20. Coulthard MG, Nelson A, Smith T, Perry JD. Point-of-care diagnostic tests for childhood urinary-tract infection: phase-contrast microscopy for bacteria, stick testing, and counting white blood cells. *J Clin Pathol* 2010; 63:823–829.
21. Whiting P, Westwood M, Watt I, Cooper J, Kleijnen J. Rapid tests and urine sampling techniques for the diagnosis of urinary tract infection (UTI) in children under five years: a systematic review. *BMC Pediatr* 2005; 5:4.
22. Mori R, Yonemoto N, Fitzgerald A, Tullus K, Verrier-Jones K, Lakhanpaul M. Diagnostic performance of urine dipstick testing in children with suspected UTI: a systematic review of relationship with age and comparison with microscopy. *Acta Paediatr* 2010; 99:581–584.
23. Nowell L, Moran C, Smith PB, et al. Prevalence of renal anomalies after urinary tract infections in hospitalized infants less than 2 months of age. *J Perinatol* 2010; 30:281–285.
24. Akram M, Shahid M, Khan AU. Etiology and antibiotic resistance patterns of community-acquired urinary tract infections in J N M C Hospital Aligarh, India. *Ann Clin Microbiol Antimicrob* 2007; 6:4.
25. Kouassi-M'bengue A, Folquet-Amorissani M, Nassirou F, et al. Neonatal urinary tract infections in Abidjan: the problem of bacterial resistance. *Mali Med* 2008; 23:34–37. French.
26. Al Benwan K, Al Sweih N, Rotimi VO. Etiology and antibiotic susceptibility patterns of community- and hospital-acquired urinary tract infections in a general hospital in Kuwait. *Med Princ Pract* 2010; 19:440–446.
27. Díaz MA, Hernández-Bello JR, Rodríguez-Baño J, et al; Spanish Group for Nosocomial Infections (GEIH). Diversity of Escherichia coli strains producing extended-spectrum beta-lactamases in Spain: second nationwide study. *J Clin Microbiol* 2010; 48:2840–2845.
28. Topaloglu R, Er I, Dogan BG, et al. Risk factors in community-acquired urinary tract infections caused by ESBL-producing bacteria in children. *Pediatr Nephrol* 2010; 25:919–925.
29. Hsueh PR, Hoban DJ, Carmeli Y, et al. Consensus review of the epidemiology and appropriate antimicrobial therapy of complicated urinary tract infections in Asia-Pacific region. *J Infect* 2011; 63:114–123.
30. Shah SS, Zorc JJ, Levine DA, Platt SL, Kuppermann N. Sterile cerebrospinal fluid pleocytosis in young infants with urinary tract infections. *J Pediatr* 2008; 153:290–292.
31. Schnadower D, Kuppermann N, Macias CG, et al. Sterile cerebrospinal fluid pleocytosis in young febrile infants with urinary tract infections. *Arch Pediatr Adolesc Med* 2011; 165:635–641.
32. Bergstrom T, Larson H, Lincoln K, et al. Neonatal urinary tract infections. XII. Eighty consecutive patients with neonatal infection. *J Pediatr* 1972; 80:858–866.
33. Leroy S, Romanello C, Galetto-Lacour A, et al. Procalcitonin is a predictor for high-grade vesicoureteral reflux in children: meta-analysis of individual patient data. *J Pediatr* 2011; 159:644–651.
34. Lee MD, Lin CC, Huang FY, Tsai TC, Huang CT, Tsai JD. Screening young children with a first febrile urinary tract infection for high-grade vesicoureteral reflux with renal ultrasound scanning and technetium-99m-labeled dimercaptosuccinic acid scanning. *J Pediatr* 2009; 154:797–802.
35. Ismaili K, Wissing KM, Lolin K, et al. Characteristics of first urinary tract infection with fever in children: a prospective clinical and imaging study. *Pediatr Infect Dis J* 2011; 30:371–374.
36. Nowell L, Moran C, Smith PB, et al. Prevalence of renal anomalies after urinary tract infections in hospitalized infants less than 2 months of age. *J Perinatol* 2010; 30:281–285.
37. Paul M, Grozinsky S, Soares-Weiser K, Leibovici L. Beta lactam antibiotic monotherapy versus beta lactam-aminoglycoside antibiotic combination therapy for sepsis. *Cochrane Database Syst Rev* 2006; Issue 1. Art. No.: CD003344. doi: 10.1002/14651858.CD003344.pub2

38. Safdar N, Handelsman J, Maki DG. Does combination antimicrobial therapy reduce mortality in Gram-negative bacteraemia? A meta-analysis. *Lancet Infect Dis* 2004; 4:519–527.
39. Hodson EM, Willis NS, Craig JC. Antibiotics for acute pyelonephritis in children. *Cochrane Database Syst Rev* 2007; Issue 4. Art. No.: CD003772. doi: 10.1002/14651858.CD003772.pub3
40. Michael M, Hodson EM, Craig JC, Martin S, Moyer VA. Short versus standard duration oral antibiotic therapy for acute urinary tract infection in children. *Cochrane Database Syst Rev* 2003; Issue 1. Art. No.: CD003966. doi: 10.1002/14651858.CD003966
41. Williams G, Craig JC. Long-term antibiotics for preventing recurrent urinary tract infection in children. *Cochrane Database Syst Rev* 2011; Issue 3. Art. No.: CD001534. doi: 10.1002/14651858.CD001534.pub3
42. Abbott GD. Neonatal bacteriuria: a prospective study in 1,460 infants. *Br Med J* 1972; 1:267–269.
43. Craig JC, Simpson JM, Williams GJ, et al.; Prevention of Recurrent Urinary Tract Infection in Children with Vesicoureteric Reflux and Normal Renal Tracts (PRIVENT) Investigators. Antibiotic prophylaxis and recurrent urinary tract infection in children. *N Engl J Med* 2009; 361:1748–1759.
44. Singh-Grewal D, Macdessi J, Craig J. Circumcision for the prevention of urinary tract infection in boys: a systematic review of randomised trials and observational studies. *Arch Dis Child* 2005; 90:853–858.
45. Siegfried N, Muller M, Deeks JJ, Volmink J. Male circumcision for prevention of heterosexual acquisition of HIV in men. *Cochrane Database Syst Rev* 2009; Issue 2. Art. No.: CD003362. doi: 10.1002/14651858.CD003362.pub2
46. Mukherjee S, Joshi A, Carroll D, Chandran H, Parashar K, McCarthy L. What is the effect of circumcision on risk of urinary tract infection in boys with posterior urethral valves? *J Pediatr Surg* 2009; 44:417–421.
47. Isaacs D, Moxon ER. *Handbook of Neonatal Infections.* London: Saunders, 1999.

CHAPTER 11

Necrotizing enterocolitis and gastrointestinal infections

11.1 Necrotizing enterocolitis

Some authorities argue that NEC is an infectious disease, because intestinal bacteria are needed for NEC to occur,[1] but this does not show causation. All infants become colonized with intestinal bacteria and bowel wall necrosis predisposes to bloodstream invasion with intestinal bacteria.

11.1.1 Epidemiology of necrotizing enterocolitis

NEC is primarily a disease of prematurity and only 5–10% of cases occur in full-term infants. NEC was scarcely recognized as an entity until 50 years ago.

The incidence of NEC varies between different neonatal units and often varies within the same neonatal unit over time. Outbreaks of apparent NEC have been described in association with a number of intestinal pathogens, including Gram-negative bacilli (e.g. *Klebsiella*, *Enterobacter*, *Escherichia coli*, *Pseudomonas*), staphylococci and intestinal viruses (e.g. rotavirus, norovirus, coronaviruses, enteroviruses). No single organism is consistently associated with NEC, although outbreaks raise the possibility that NEC is a common end-point of different intestinal insults. An association has been described between NEC and detection of delta toxin, an exotoxin produced by some strains of CoNS[2] and by certain delta toxin-producing strains of *Staphylococcus aureus*[3] but delta toxin is not the sole cause of NEC.

Clostridium perfringens and *C. septicum* can cause an NEC-like illness in animals and pigbel is an NEC of New Guinea children caused by toxin-producing strains of *C. perfringens* in association with heavy protein meals. However, while Clostridia and clostridial toxin have been isolated from some neonates with NEC, this finding is not consistent and Clostridia and clostridial toxin can also be found in the stool of many normal infants.

NEC could be the final common pathway for factors causing gut ischaemia. Early studies reported that neonates with NEC had high rates of maternal and perinatal risk factors for gut ischaemia and a high incidence of conditions such as persistent ductus arteriosus (PDA). However, in case-control studies, many of these conditions, including PDA,[4] were as common in control infants. In addition, different studies sometimes report contradictory risk factors, perhaps because of the selection of controls. For example, one study reported a greater than sevenfold increase in the risk of NEC associated with antenatal maternal indomethacin for tocolysis,[5] whereas another found antenatal indomethacin was not associated with NEC and post-natal indomethacin was associated with a 35% reduction in NEC.[6]

The risk of NEC increases with decreasing gestation. In a US case-control study, the incidence of NEC was 6.5% of infants <1500 g, 1% for infants of 1500–2000 g, 0.3% for 2000–2500 g and 0.04% for infants admitted who weighed >2500 g.[4] In a multi-centre Canadian study of infants admitted to NICU, the incidence of NEC was 6.6% of infants <1500 g but 0.7% of infants >1500 g.[7] A US case-control study of over 15 000 preterm neonates admitted to intensive care, of whom 390 (2.6%) had NEC, found low birth weight was the most important "risk factor" associated with NEC.[8] Other associations included need for mechanical ventilator support and low Apgar score at 5 minutes.[8]

Evidence-Based Neonatal Infections, First Edition. David Isaacs.

An early Australian case-control study identified hypothermia on admission as the major risk factor for NEC, while polycythaemia was associated with more severe NEC.[9]

Finally, a US study of infants with NEC found no risk factors but breast milk was strongly protective, reducing the incidence by 91% (95% CI 44–98).[10] Although NEC almost never occurs until enteral feeds are introduced, it is simplistic to say enteral feeds cause NEC (Section 11.1.1.1).

Case-control studies may not identify relatively uncommon conditions predisposing to NEC. For example, children with cyanotic congenital heart disease are at increased risk of NEC, presumably on the basis of impaired gut perfusion or oxygenation, but in a case series of NEC few will have congenital heart disease. In a case series of infants with congenital heart disease admitted to a cardiac intensive care unit, 21 (3.3%) of 643 developed NEC.[11] Within the cohort, the risk was increased 3.8-fold for infants with hypoplastic left heart syndrome and 6.3-fold for truncus arteriosus or aorto-pulmonary window. NEC was associated with prematurity, highest dose of prostaglandin and episodes of shock or low cardiac output, all potentially ischemic insults.[11]

Risk factors for NEC are shown in Table 11.1. The most important avoidable risk factor is prolonged use of antibiotics. In a large observational US study of infants <1000 g with negative blood cultures at birth, those continued on antibiotics for 5 or more days had a 42% increase in risk of NEC and a 50% increase in all-cause mortality compared with infants whose antibiotics were stopped earlier.[12] A case-control study found that infants with NEC were less likely to have had respiratory distress and more likely to have reached full feeds than controls.[13] Infants with NEC were far more likely to have culture-proven sepsis. However, when infants with confirmed sepsis were excluded, there was a significant association between duration of antibiotics and risk of NEC, and infants who received >10 days of antibiotics had a nearly threefold increased incidence of NEC.[13] In another observational study, prolonged initial empiric antibiotics were associated with a 2.66-fold increased risk of late-onset sepsis, NEC or death.[14]

Table 11.1 Risk factors for necrotizing enterocolitis.

Prematurity[2,5,8]
Hypothermia[9]
Perinatal asphyxia[8]
Prolonged use of antibiotics from birth despite negative cultures[12–14]
Blood transfusion[15, 16]
Formula feeding[8]

A meta-analysis of 11 retrospective case-control studies and one cohort study found that recent blood transfusion was associated with NEC and that neonates with transfusion-associated NEC compared with neonates with NEC but no recent transfusion were younger, weighed less and were more likely to have PDA and to be receiving ventilator support.[15] A Canadian case-control study found that 15.5% of infants with NEC had been transfused in the previous 2 days compared with 7.7% of age-matched controls.[16] This suggests blood transfusion should be avoided if possible in ventilated infants with PDA.

Full-term infants almost always develop their NEC in the first week of life and while some have risk factors such as congenital heart disease around half have no identifiable risk factor.[17, 18]

11.1.1.1 Feeding and necrotizing enterocolitis

Breast milk protects against NEC. In a prospective multicenter study, NEC developed in 5.5% of 926 preterm infants and was 6–10 times more common in infants fed exclusively with formula than exclusively with breast milk and 3 times more common in those who received mixed formula and breast milk.[19] The increased risk of NEC with mixed feeding compared to breast milk alone suggests there is something harmful in formula feeds as well as protective in breast milk. In this study pasteurized donor breast milk was as protective as raw mother's milk.[19]

In a Cochrane systematic review and meta-analysis of data from five trials comparing donor breast milk with pre-term formula in pre-term infants, NEC was significantly increased in the formula-fed group (typical RR 2.5, 95% CI 1.2, 5.1; number needed to harm = 33, 95% CI 17, 100).[20]

In some epidemiologic case-control studies, infants with NEC were more likely to have reached full feeds than control infants,[10, 13] although other studies disagree.[5] However, increasing scientific evidence suggests delaying enteral feeds or increasing their volume slowly does not prevent NEC. A Cochrane systematic review and meta-analysis of five randomized controlled trials (RCTs) in 600 infants <1500 g found delayed introduction of enteral feeds to later than 5–7 days compared with ≤ 4 days after birth did not reduce NEC (typical RR 0.89, 95% CI 0.58–1.37) or all-cause mortality, but did delay the time to establish full enteral feeds.[21]

An RCT comparing minimal enteric feeds with advancing feeds in 141 pre-term infants was stopped early when 7 infants in the advancing group (10%) developed NEC compared with only one fed minimal volumes.[22] However, subsequent studies have not confirmed this association. A Cochrane systematic review and meta-analysis of four trials (496 infants) found that slow advancement of enteral feeds compared with faster rates of increase did not prevent NEC (typical RR 0.91, 95% CI 0.47–1.75) or reduce all-cause mortality but infants on slow advancement took longer to regain birth weight and to establish full enteral feeding.[23]

11.1.2 Pathogenesis of necrotizing enterocolitis

NEC is characterized histopathologically by extensive inflammation of the gut with ischaemia and necrosis of the intestinal epithelium. Even if ischaemia contributes to the necrosis, it does not explain the inflammation. The length and depth of the necrosis vary. The classical sites of NEC are the terminal ileum and caecum, which are the most common sites if perforation occurs,[24] but the whole bowel can be involved. The molecular and cellular mechanisms causing the pathologic changes are poorly understood. Various exogenous and endogenous mediators such as endotoxin (lipopolysaccharide), inflammatory cytokines, platelet activating factor and nitric oxide have been postulated to have a role in pathogenesis.[25] There is intense interest in molecular signalling in NEC: nitric oxide may play a significant role as a molecular signalling 'hub' in the failure of the gut barrier in NEC,[25] while activation of cyclooxygenase-2, a critical enzyme in the biosynthesis of prostanoids, may be a critical step in pathogenesis.[26]

11.1.3 Clinical presentation of necrotizing enterocolitis

Pre-term babies with NEC usually present between the second and eighth week after birth: in one study the median age of presentation was 13 days.[2, 5] In contrast, full-term babies almost always present in the first week, with a mean age of presentation around 4–5 days of age.[5, 17, 18]

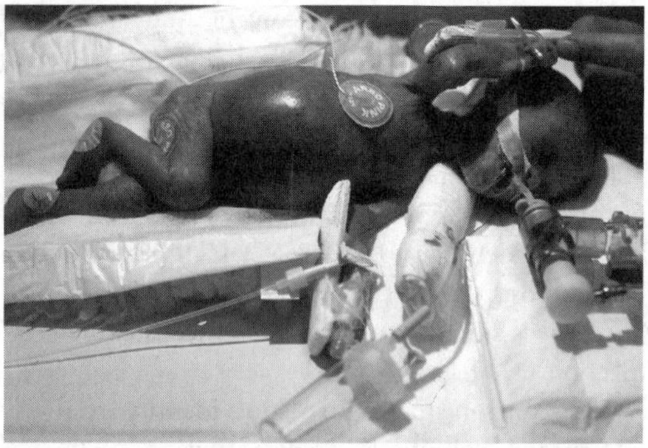

Figure 11.1 Red, shiny distended abdomen of infant with necrotizing enterocolitis.

The clinical presentation may be insidious or fulminant. The insidious presentation is with intolerance of enteral feeds, abdominal distension, tenderness to palpation and possibly with vomiting, apnoea, bradycardia, irritability or lethargy and temperature instability. The fulminant presentation is with gross abdominal distension and shock, with or without bloody diarrhoea. The abdomen may be tense, red and shiny as well as distended (Figure 11.1) Perforation causes signs of peritonism with a rigid abdomen as well as shock. In severe cases there may be oedema and induration of the abdominal wall. Abdominal crepitus is a rare, sinister sign.

A common clinical problem is assessing whether or not a pre-term infant who becomes intolerant of feeds with increasing gastric aspirates has NEC. If the abdomen is soft and non-tender, NEC is unlikely, whereas a tender distended abdomen is highly suspicious. In either case, the radiologic appearance may help, whereas blood tests are generally unhelpful.

11.1.4 Radiology of necrotizing enterocolitis

The early radiographic signs of NEC are non-specific, showing abdominal distension and generalized bowel dilatation, suggestive but not diagnostic of ileus. Later more overt radiographic signs of NEC may include bowel wall oedema, a fixed loop on repeated radiographs, an increasingly gasless abdomen, intramural

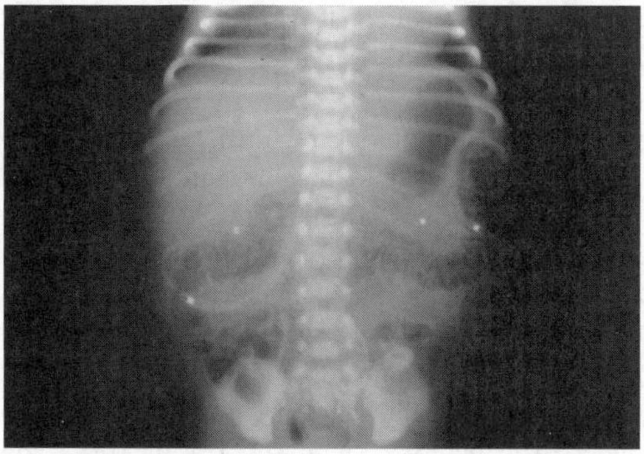

Figure 11.2 Necrotizing enterocolitis: extensive intramural gas throughout transverse colon and bowel wall oedema.

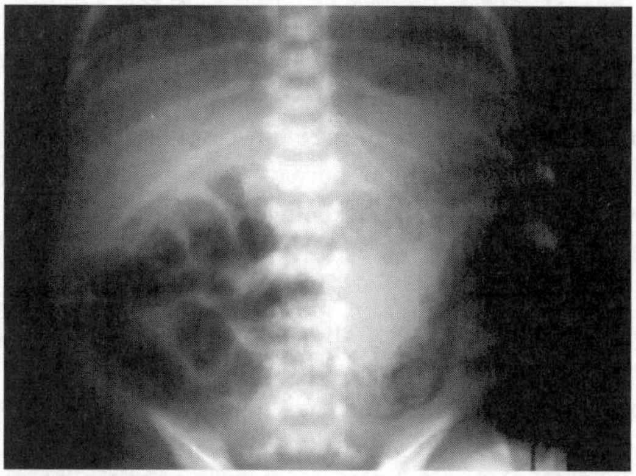

Figure 11.4 Necrotizing enterocolitis: intramural gas in descending colon and air in liver outlining biliary tree (portal venous gas).

gas (Figures 11.2 and 11.3), air in the biliary tree (Figure 11.4) and free air due to perforation (Figure 11.5) As with many radiographic investigations, there is relatively poor agreement between experts on the interpretation of radiographs[27, 28] and indeed, a radiologist who read the same radiographs twice 3–6 months apart, often interpreted them differently.[27] Reassuringly, trained experts fared better than in-training observers.[27]

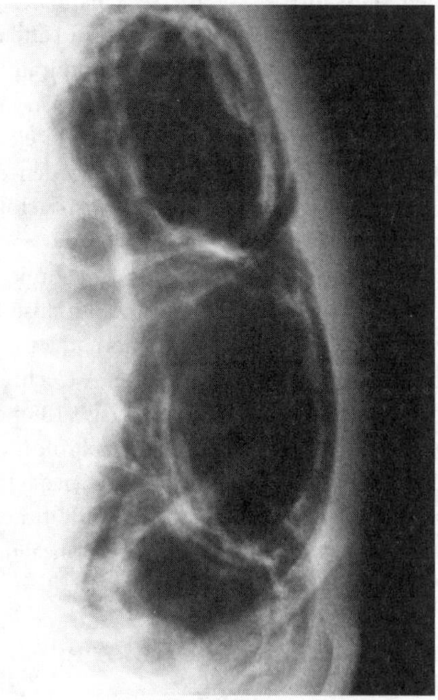

Figure 11.3 Close-up of left side of abdomen showing double shadow of intramural gas in descending colon.

Even more reassuringly, a Duke University study using a 10-point scoring scale to score radiographs found much better inter- and intra-observer agreement.[29] In a subsequent study, local experts used the scale to assign radiographic scores in a blinded fashion to radiographs from infants with suspected NEC, based on the presence or absence of fixed bowel loops, pneumatosis intestinalis (intramural gas) or portal venous gas.[30] Patients with higher scores were more likely to need surgery and the scale performed well when assessed by receiver-operating characteristic curve.

In a South Korean study, neonates with NEC and bowel distension without pneumatosis on plain radiograph had either echogenic dots or dense granular echogenicities in the bowel wall.[31] In a Canadian study, infants treated medically were less likely to have

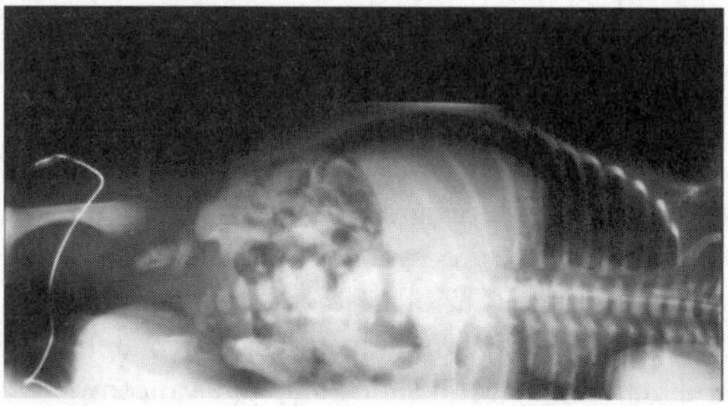

Figure 11.5 Lateral decubitus film showing free air above liver due to intestinal perforation.

abnormal ultrasound appearance than those treated surgically. An adverse outcome was associated with ultrasound findings of free gas, focal fluid collections or three or more of increased bowel wall echogenicity, absent bowel perfusion, portal venous gas, bowel wall thinning, bowel wall thickening, free fluid with echoes and intramural gas.[32]

Although NEC is the single most common cause of pneumoperitoneum, even in developing countries,[33] pneumoperitoneum can also occur due to isolated perforation of the bowel not caused by NEC.

11.1.5 Laboratory tests in necrotizing enterocolitis

Blood culture should always be performed in suspected NEC: up to a third of infants with NEC are bacteraemic. Meningitis occurs in about 1% of cases of NEC. LP should be considered prospectively and also considered retrospectively if blood cultures grow an organism likely to cause meningitis.

A full blood count will identify thrombocytopaenia and/or neutropoenia. Acute phase reactants, generally raised in NEC, do not distinguish NEC from other causes of inflammation or sepsis.

Stool microscopy may reveal multiple Gram-positive cocci in staphylococcal enterocolitis which can mimic NEC. Stool bacterial cultures in suspected NEC are of limited value except during a possible outbreak. *Clostridium difficile* toxin may be found in asymptomatic infants and should not be routinely sought. However, in an apparent outbreak of NEC, *C. difficile* toxin testing is advisable as are stool viral studies because of the infection control implications.

11.1.6 Treatment of necrotizing enterocolitis

The empiric antibiotic treatment of NEC is based on the need to cover bowel organisms. The most common organisms isolated from blood culture in case series of NEC are Gram-negative bacilli (*E. coli*, *Klebsiella*, *Pseudomonas* and *Enterobacter*),[8,34–36] but other important pathogens include *S. aureus*,[4] CoNS[3] and enterococci, while anaerobes are occasionally isolated.[8,34–36]

There are no RCTs of antibiotic treatment of NEC. A sequential study from Canada compared ampicillin and gentamicin with cefotaxime and vancomycin.[37] The incidence of culture-positive peritonitis and mortality in infants <2200 g was lower in the second study period, but the sequential nature of the study casts doubt on whether this was due to the different antibiotic regimens.[37]

The empiric antibiotic regimen for NEC is generally recommended to include anti-staphylococcal cover (vancomycin if MRSA is prevalent or the infant is colonized) and appropriate Gram-negative cover. Clindamycin and gentamicin are often used, clindamycin providing cover against Gram-positive and most anaerobic organisms and gentamicin against Gram-negative bacilli. Vancomycin and gentamicin are preferred if there is a significant risk of MRSA and many would add metronidazole to provide anaerobic cover. Local epidemiology may also inform the choice of antibiotics.

If meningitis is clinically suspected but LP not performed, empiric antibiotic cover should obviously include antibiotics that penetrate CSF.

If blood cultures are positive, the antibiotic regimen should be modified accordingly and the need for LP reconsidered carefully.

The optimal duration of antibiotic therapy for NEC has not been studied formally. It is usual to continue antibiotics until the infant is tolerating feeds again. Bacteraemia is treated for 7–10 days (see Chapter 5) and meningitis for 14–21 days (see Chapters 5 and 7).

Ancillary management includes careful attention to the need for circulatory and cardiorespiratory support, blood and platelet transfusions and monitoring and correcting abnormalities of fluid and electrolyte balance and blood sugar. There is no evidence for or against adjunctive treatment of NEC with lactoferrin[38] or any other immunomodulatory therapy.

A critical consideration is the need for surgical intervention; an early surgical opinion and close follow-up are important. The surgical alternatives are open laparotomy and peritoneal drainage. A Cochrane systematic review[39] found only two trials (185 patients) comparing peritoneal drainage and laparotomy. These found no difference in mortality or need for parenteral nutrition, although in one study time to full enteral feeds was prolonged in the peritoneal drainage group.[40,41]

11.1.7 Outcome of necrotizing enterocolitis

Mortality depends on severity, but is around 20–30% of severe cases, generally higher the lower the gestation, and higher for infants managed surgically than medically.[19,41–43] Interestingly, however, in a study of infants <1500 g who required surgery, the mortality was 25% in infants <1000 g and those 1000–1500 g. The only variables associated with increased mortality were pan-necrosis and the length of the segment of necrotic bowel.[44]

In a follow-up study of infants <1000 g, surgically but not medically managed infants with NEC had a significantly increased risk of periventricular leukomalacia, IQ <70, neurodevelopmental impairment and growth retardation than those without NEC.[45]

In a systematic review of 10 studies of infants 45% of infants with NEC were neurodevelopmentally impaired and they were significantly more likely than gestational age-matched controls to have impaired neurodevelopment (OR 1.6, 95% CI 1.3–2.0), cerebral palsy (OR 1.5, 95% CI 1.2–2.0), visual (OR 2.3, 95% CI 1.0–5.1), cognitive (OR 1.7, 95% CI 1.4–2.2) and psychomotor impairment (OR 1.7, 95% CI 1.3–2.2). The risk of disability increased with severity of NEC.[46]

Infants in the UK ORACLE study who developed NEC had an increased risk of all grades of impairment at age 7 years.[47] Children with NEC were four times more likely to suffer bowel problems (short bowel syndrome, strictures, fistulas and anastomotic leak, presence of stoma) than non-NEC children and had significant long-term motor, sensory and cognitive impairment.[47]

11.1.8 Prevention of necrotizing enterocolitis

Question: What are the best ways to prevent necrotizing enterocolitis?

Prevention of NEC is a high priority (Table 11.2). There is strong evidence that **breast milk** protects against NEC and that donor milk is as effective as maternal milk.[19,20]

Probiotics reduce the incidence of NEC, but their routine use is still controversial. A Cochrane systematic review of 16 trials (2842 infants) found probiotics were associated with a 65% reduction in the incidence of severe NEC (95% CI 48–76) and 60% reduction in all-cause mortality (95% CI 40–73).[53] A previous non-Cochrane systematic review using Cochrane methodology found a reduction in NEC incidence of at least 30%.[54] Two trials confined to exclusively breast-fed infants found a significant 71% reduction in NEC with probiotics (95% CI 34–87).[55,56] Some argue for routine probiotics because the evidence is too strong to ignore.[57] Others urge caution because many different probiotic preparations were used in relatively mature infants,[58] and some studies suggest possible increased risk of sepsis in extremely low birth-weight infants.[43] Additionally, the manufacture of most probiotic products is not subject to rigorous quality control.[43] A critical systematic review of the strength of the level of evidence using Oxford Centre for Evidence Based Medicine criteria found considerable 'clinical heterogeneity' in the 15 trials and concluded that there is insufficient evidence to recommend routine probiotics.[59] It is hoped that further studies will clarify the situation. The current balance of evidence suggests probiotics probably save lives and are unlikely to cause significant harm and it seems only a matter of time before they are recommended routinely. Evidence-based guidelines reviewing different preparations are helpful for anyone contemplating introducing probiotics.[60]

Because of the strong association between prolonged empiric antibiotics and NEC,[12–14] antibiotics should be stopped after 2–3 days if systemic cultures are negative. This recommendation is particularly important for extremely low birth-weight infants.

Table 11.2 Strategies to prevent necrotizing enterocolitis.

Strong evidence from meta-analyses of randomized controlled trials (RCTs)
Use breast milk (mother or donor) and avoid formula feeds[20]
Prophylactic oral probiotics[9] (Section 11.1.8)
Convincing evidence from large observational studies
Avoid continuing antibiotics >4 days if cultures are negative[12, 14] and do not use antibiotics for long periods without evidence of infection[13]
One RCT, more trials needed
Arginine supplementation[48]
Prophylactic oral lactoferrin[49, 50]
Evidence of efficacy but not recommended due to risk of resistance
Prophylactic enteral antibiotics[51]
Evidence that the intervention is ineffective
Oral immunoglobulins IgG and IgA[52]

Lactoferrin is a normal component of human colostrum, milk, tears and saliva and forms part of the host defences to infection (see Chapter 23). In an Italian RCT which randomized infants <1500 g to placebo, lactoferrin alone or lactoferrin plus the probiotic *Lactobacillus rhamnosus* GG, oral lactoferrin alone did not reduce the incidence of NEC significantly (RR 0.33, 95% CI 0.09–1.17) but the combination of lactoferrin and *L. rhamnosus* GG was associated with a significant reduction in NEC (RR 0.05, 95% CI 0.00–0.90).[49, 50] Further large studies of prophylactic lactoferrin are in progress.

One proposed mechanism of intestinal injury in NEC is that vascular dysfunction might result from altered nitric oxide synthase (NOS) activity leading to an imbalance between nitric oxide and superoxide production by the intestinal vascular endothelium.[61] **Arginine** can act as a tissue substrate for nitric oxide production and arginine supplementation can prevent NEC in animal models.[62] A Cochrane review[63] found only one RCT in which infants <1250 g or <32 weeks received arginine supplementation orally or in their parenteral nutrition in their first 28 days.[48] NEC developed in 21 of 77 infants in the placebo group (27%) but only 5 of 75 (7%) in the arginine group. There were no adverse effects of arginine during the trial or on follow-up.[48, 51] It is surprising there have not been more studies of arginine supplementation.

Prophylactic oral aminoglycosides (kanamycin and gentamicin) reduced NEC in some early trials but not others and were associated with aminoglycoside resistance.[64] Oral vancomycin reduced the incidence of NEC in an RCT from 27.5% to 12.7%, but vancomycin might predispose to Gram-negative organisms.[52] A Cochrane systematic review and meta-analysis of five RCTs found prophylactic enteral antibiotics reduced NEC in infants <1500 g by 53% (95% CI 22–72) with a number needed to treat of 10, but increased the risk of colonization with resistant organisms.[64] The authors urged caution because of the risk of resistance. Four of the studies in the Cochrane review were of aminoglycosides in the 1970s and the most recent trial of vancomycin was published in 1998. No further studies are planned and no authorities recommend prophylactic enteral antibiotics because of the risk of resistance and the availability of safer alternative methods of prevention.

A Cochrane systematic review of oral immunoglobulin preparations (IgG or combined IgG and IgA) found three trials and a total of 2095 infants. The incidence of NEC was not significantly reduced (typical RR 0.84, 95% CI 0.57–1.25).[65]

Recommendations: Breast milk, either maternal or donor milk, should be used whenever possible to reduce the risk of NEC. Empiric antibiotics for suspected early-onset sepsis should be stopped after 2–3 days if systemic cultures are negative and certainly not used longer than 4 days without strong reason. Antibiotics should not be used for prolonged periods except to treat proven sepsis. Prophylactic probiotics appear effective but further data are needed before a firm recommendation to use them routinely.

11.2 Neonatal diarrhoeal infections

Although oral rehydration,[66] improved hygiene,[67, 68] and increasing use of effective rotavirus vaccines[69] have decreased the mortality of diarrhoeal diseases in the neonatal period,[70] diarrhoeal diseases remain an important cause of morbidity, particularly in developing countries.[71] The incidence of neonatal diarrhoea is rarely reported separately from the incidence of diarrhoea in older infants. Much neonatal diarrhoea occurs in the home, making incidence data more difficult to collect.

11.2.1 Epidemiology of neonatal diarrhoeal infections

The incidence of diarrhoeal diseases in neonates is affected by various factors, notably the level of exposure to diarrhoeal organisms. Neonates may be exposed at birth to maternal organisms that can cause diarrhoea. Thereafter their siblings and contaminated water are important potential sources of diarrhoeal organisms.

Breastfeeding is highly protective against diarrhoeal disease. In a systematic review, not breastfeeding resulted in a more than 10-fold increased risk of diarrhoea mortality in comparison to exclusive breastfeeding among infants 0–5 months of age (RR = 10.52).[72] While the most dramatic benefits of breastfeeding are seen in developing countries, in a non-Cochrane systematic review of breastfeeding in industrialized countries six of eight studies found breastfeeding protected against diarrhoeal infections.[73] Breast milk contains IgA antibodies which protect against virulence antigens of enteropathogenic *E. coli* (EPEC) and *Shigella*, lipopolysaccharides of *Shigella* and *Vibrio cholera*, toxins produced by enterotoxigenic *E. coli* (ETEC) and *V. cholerae* and surface proteins of *Campylobacter* and *Giardia*.[74, 75] Breast milk also contains leucocytes, oligosaccharides that can block attachment of organisms, lactoferrin which degrades EPEC surface antigens and other complex molecules such as glycoconjugates with anti-infective and anti-inflammatory properties.[74, 75]

The neonate appears less likely to develop diarrhoeal illness in association with some pathogens than older children. For example, *C. difficile* toxin and rotavirus are often found in stool samples from asymptomatic neonates, whereas older children with either of these are commonly symptomatic. Transplacentally acquired maternal IgG antibodies may offer some protection, but it is also possible that diarrhoea is partly immune mediated and that the immaturity of the neonatal immune system sometimes protects against disease if not infection.

11.2.2 Microbiology of neonatal diarrhoeal infections

Some of the organisms that can cause neonatal diarrhoea are listed in Table 11.3. In Western countries, the most likely cause of neonatal diarrhoea is an enteric virus infection and rapid testing for enteric viruses, usually using PCR[76] or ELISA,[77] is recommended if available (see Chapter 17). There is no specific treatment for rotavirus, norovirus, enteric adenovirus, astrovirus or enterovirus infections. The main importance of diagnosis is for infection control purposes.

Bacterial stool cultures are of most importance in developing countries and, although often performed in Western countries, the yield is low unless the infant has diarrhoea with blood and/or mucus or unless there are other reasons to suspect bacterial infection. In developing countries, in contrast, neonatal diarrhoea is not infrequently bacterial in origin and the incidence of bacteraemia with diarrhoeal illness is higher in the neonatal period than at any other age,[78–80] so investigations should include bacterial cultures of stool and blood and of CSF if clinically indicated.

Table 11.3 Organisms responsible for neonatal diarrhea.

Bacteria
Escherichia coli
• Enteropathogenic *E. coli* (EPEC)
• Enterotoxigenic *E. coli* (ETEC)
• Enterohaemorrhagic *E. coli* (EHEC)
• Enteroinvasive *E. coli* (EIEC)
• Enteroaggregative *E. coli* (EAEC)
• Other *E. coli*
Salmonella
Shigella
Campylobacter
Aeromonas
Vibrio cholerae
Yersinia
Clostridium difficile
Parasites
Cryptosporidium
Entamoeba histolytica
Giardia
Viruses
Rotavirus
Norovirus
Astrovirus
Enteroviruses

11.2.3 Clinical features of neonatal diarrhoeal infections

Viral infections predominantly infect the small intestine causing watery diarrhoea or loose stools without blood in the stools. Asymptomatic rotavirus infection is well described. However, in a case series of neonates with bacterial diarrhoea, a highly variable proportion presents with watery diarrhoea, so bacterial culture of watery stools is still important. Neonatal cholera is fortunately rare and *V. cholerae* is another organism which seems to cause less neonatal disease than expected.

Blood and/or mucus in the stools suggest colonic involvement, most likely due to *Salmonella*, *Shigella* or *Campylobacter* infection. Yersinia infection of the newborn is very rarely described; infected infants present typically with watery diarrhoea or with mucus and flecks of blood.[81] Cryptosporidium infection of newborns has been described, typically causing watery diarrhoea without blood, but is rare. Bloody stools have been described in older children with cryptosporidiosis. Blood is only very rarely described in the stools of children with viral enteritis. Amoebic dysentery is rare in the neonatal period but has been described.

Systemic bacterial infection most commonly occurs with non-typhoidal *Salmonella*, *Shigella* and *Campylobacter* infections. Non-typhoidal *Salmonella* bacteraemia typically but not always causes high fever in older children but neonates are often afebrile.[78–80] Salmonellosis can cause signs and symptoms related to osteomyelitis, septic arthritis, meningitis and sometimes pneumonia. Rarer manifestations of salmonellosis include pericarditis, pyelonephritis, mastitis, cholecystitis, endophthalmitis and cutaneous abscesses.[78–80]

Shigella infections-acquired peripartum usually appear within 3 days of birth and can present with mild diarrhoea or severe colitis.[82] Abdominal tenderness is common in older children, but is not characteristically described in neonates. However, neonates are more likely than older children to have severe *Shigella* infection with dehydration, septicaemia, meningitis, toxic megacolon, colonic perforation and death.[82]

11.2.4 Management of neonatal diarrhoeal infection

The two primary concerns are to assess and correct dehydration and to decide whether or not to treat empirically for bacteraemia or meningitis. Correction of shock, if present, with intravenous fluids is the first priority. In older children, oral rehydration is safe and effective and only 1 in 25 children will not tolerate enteral fluids.[83] However, there are no useful data on best mode of rehydration in neonates, which will often be dictated by safety and availability. In older children evidence from one RCT[84] and observational studies[85–87] suggest normal saline is safer than hypotonic saline solutions for parenteral rehydration, but comparable data are not available for neonates. Medications such as anti-emetics and ondansetron should not be given to vomiting neonates because they are potentially harmful and their efficacy and safety has not been demonstrated.

In general, neonatal gastroenteritis should not be treated with antibiotics because there is no evidence that they shorten the disease and antibiotics are known to prolong carriage of *Salmonella*.[88] Parenteral antibiotics should be started if there is reasonable suspicion of systemic bacterial infection, after taking blood and possibly CSF for culture. The choice of antibiotics will be to cover enteric organisms taking into account local epidemiology and antibiotic sensitivities. However, diarrhoea can be a non-specific sign of systemic infection in neonates and the possibility of infection with non-enteric organisms such as *S. aureus* should also be considered.

Cefotaxime will cover *Salmonella* and *Shigella* infections in most parts of the world, as well as sensitive *S. aureus*, most other Gram-positive organisms and most Yersinia infections. *Campylobacter* species are generally resistant to β-lactams including cefotaxime, but *C. fetus* is sensitive to aminoglycosides. *C. jejuni* is most susceptible to macrolides such as azithromycin, but empiric therapy for *C. jejuni* infection is rarely needed. A combination of cefotaxime and an aminoglycoside is a reasonable combination for initial empiric antibiotic therapy of suspected severe enteric infection complicated by sepsis, if local organisms are susceptible. Other combinations may be needed where antibiotic resistance is a major problem. Antibiotic therapy should be reviewed in the light of cultures.

There is evidence from a Cochrane meta-analysis of 63 studies, 56 of them in infants and children, that therapeutic probiotics shorten the duration of infectious diarrhoea by about 1 day.[89] No study specifically addressed neonatal diarrhoea. Probiotics also reduce the duration of persistent diarrhoea by an average of 4 days.[90]

11.2.5 Prevention of diarrhoeal diseases

Good infection control is the primary method of preventing neonatal diarrhoeal disease. If an outbreak does occur on a neonatal unit, attention to improved hand-washing, screening both symptomatic and asymptomatic infants for the organism and cohorting of infected babies are an effective way of halting an outbreak.[91]

Probiotics have been shown to prevent antibiotic-associated diarrhoea in children[92] but there are no data about prevention of diarrhoeal infection in neonates.

11.2.5.1 Rotavirus vaccines

Rotavirus vaccines are highly effective in preventing rotavirus diarrhoea,[93] although the effectiveness is greater in Western countries[94, 95] than in developing countries.[96, 97] In countries that have introduced universal infant rotavirus vaccines, there has been a herd immune effect with a reduction in rotavirus diarrhoea at all ages.[93]

The only other vaccines against diarrhoeal diseases are against organisms that only very rarely cause neonatal diarrhoea, *V. cholerae* and *Salmonella typhi.* Studies from Mexico and Australia suggest a possible increase in the risk of intussusception in the 7 days after an infant receives rotavirus vaccine. Although the increased risk may be as much as fivefold in those 7 days, it is of very short duration and it is still not clear whether or not rotavirus vaccine merely causes intussusception to occur earlier in an infant already genetically predestined to develop intussusception. What is clear is that even in the United States the risk of intussusception causing an emergency department visit, hospitalization or even death is a minute fraction of the number of such cases prevented by a routine rotavirus immunization program.[98] In developing countries the benefits of rotavirus immunization are far greater and outweigh the risks many thousand-fold.

Pre-term infants are at increased risk for hospitalization from rotavirus during their early years of life.[99] The monovalent human live-attenuated oral rotavirus vaccine Rotarix and the live, pentavalent, human-bovine reassortant vaccine Rotateq are well tolerated and immunogenic in pre-term infants $\geq$27 to $<$37 weeks of gestation in clinical trials, with no increase in the risk of serious adverse events, compared with placebo.[99] Medically stable pre-term infants should be vaccinated according to the same schedule as full-term infants, starting at age 6–8 weeks.[99] The vaccine viruses are excreted in faeces, Rotarix for approximately 10 days and because of the theoretical risk of horizontal transfer of the vaccine virus to other infants, it is recommended to defer immunization of infants still hospitalized at 6 weeks of age until discharge.[99]

11.3 Peritonitis

NEC is the single most common cause of neonatal peritonitis in Western[100–103] and developing countries,[33] responsible for about half of all cases. Other causes of peritonitis include spontaneous perforation, perforation secondary to feeding tubes, meconium peritonitis usually secondary to cystic fibrosis, Hirschsprung enterocolitis, volvulus, perforated stricture and rarely appendicitis.[33,100–106]

Infants with spontaneous localized intestinal perforation weigh less than infants with NEC, have lower Apgar scores and present at a younger age.[107,108] In one study, 11 of 13 infants with spontaneous localized intestinal perforation had received indomethacin.[108]

The clinical presentation of spontaneous intestinal perforation not due to NEC is clinically indistinguishable from NEC. Infants develop feed intolerance or vomiting, hypotension, abdominal distension and blue or purple discoloration of the abdominal wall, emphasized by some authors as occurring significantly more often than in NEC.[105–108] The abdomen is often gasless and pneumatosis intestinalis is absent.[107]

The initial treatment of perforation is resuscitation with correction of shock and attention to circulation, fluid and electrolyte balance and cardiorespiratory status, including assessment of the need for artificial ventilation. An urgent surgical opinion should be sought to assess the need for immediate surgical correction of the cause of the perforation.

In a 1980 paper the most common isolates from peritoneal fluid were *E. coli* and Bacteroides, followed by Group D streptococci (enterococci).[104] Blood cultures were positive in 32%, mostly with *E. coli.* On the basis of their study, the authors recommended empiric therapy with ampicillin, clindamycin and gentamicin for neonatal peritonitis, with adjustment based on culture results.[104] Subsequent studies have reported a range of organisms in peritoneal fluid similar to NEC, with Gram-negative bacilli (e.g. *E. coli, Klebsiella, Enterobacter*) predominating, but Gram-positive organisms (enterococci, *S. aureus,* CoNS), anaerobes and *Candida* are also important isolates.[100–103,105–108] Candida peritonitis can mimic NEC (see Section 16.3.7). Unless fungal peritonitis is suspected from the clinical picture and from the Gram stain of peritoneal fluid, empiric antibiotic therapy should be as for NEC (Section 11.1.6). The duration of antibiotic therapy for peritonitis has not been formally studied.

References

1. Morowitz MJ, Poroyko V, Caplan M, Alverdy J, Liu DC. Redefining the role of intestinal microbes in the pathogenesis of necrotizing enterocolitis. *Pediatrics* 2010; 125:777–785.
2. Scheifele DW, Bjornson GL, Dyer RA, Dimmick JE. Delta-like toxin produced by coagulase-negative staphylococci is

associated with neonatal necrotizing enterocolitis. *Infect Immun* 1987; 55:2268–2273.
3. Overturf GD, Sherman MP, Scheifele DW, Wong LC. Neonatal necrotizing enterocolitis associated with delta toxin-producing methicillin-resistant Staphylococcus aureus. *Pediatr Infect Dis J* 1990; 9:88–91.
4. Stoll BJ, Kanto Jr WP, Glass RI, Nahmias AJ, Brann Jr AW. Epidemiology of necrotizing enterocolitis: a case control study. *J Pediatr* 1980; 96:447–451.
5. Sood BG, Lulic-Botica M, Holzhausen KA, et al. The risk of necrotizing enterocolitis after indomethacin tocolysis. *Pediatrics* 2011; 128:e54–e62.
6. Sharma R, Hudak ML, Tepas 3rd JJ, et al. Prenatal or postnatal indomethacin exposure and neonatal gut injury associated with isolated intestinal perforation and necrotizing enterocolitis. *J Perinatol* 2010; 30:786–793.
7. Sankaran K, Puckett B, Lee DS, et al; Canadian Neonatal Network. Variations in incidence of necrotizing enterocolitis in Canadian neonatal intensive care units. *J Pediatr Gastroenterol Nutr* 2004; 39:366–372.
8. Guthrie SO, Gordon PV, Thomas V, Thorp JA, Peabody J, Clark RH. Necrotizing enterocolitis among neonates in the United States. *J Perinatol* 2003; 23:278–285.
9. Yu VY, Joseph R, Bajuk B, Orgill A, Astbury J. Perinatal risk factors for necrotizing enterocolitis. *Arch Dis Child* 1984; 59:430–434.
10. Thompson A, Bizzarro M, Yu S, Diefenbach K, Simpson BJ, Moss RL. Risk factors for necrotizing enterocolitis totalis: a case-control study. *J Perinatol* 2011; 31:730–738.
11. McElhinney DB, Hedrick HL, Bush DM, et al. Necrotizing enterocolitis in neonates with congenital heart disease: risk factors and outcomes. *Pediatrics* 2000; 106:1080–1087.
12. Cotten CM, Taylor S, Stoll B, et al. Prolonged duration of initial empirical antibiotic treatment is associated with increased rates of necrotizing enterocolitis and death for extremely low birth weight infants. *Pediatrics* 2009; 123:58–66.
13. Alexander VN, Northrup V, Bizzarro MJ. Antibiotic exposure in the newborn intensive care unit and the risk of necrotizing enterocolitis. *J Pediatr* 2011; 159:392–397.
14. Kuppala VS, Meinzen-Derr J, Morrow AL, Schibler KR. Prolonged initial empirical antibiotic treatment is associated with adverse outcomes in premature infants. *J Pediatr* 2011; 159:720–725.
15. Mohamed A, Shah PS. Transfusion associated necrotizing enterocolitis: a meta-analysis of observational data. *Pediatrics* 2012; 129:529–540.
16. Stritzke AI, Smyth J, Synnes A, Lee SK, Shah PS. Transfusion-associated necrotising enterocolitis in neonates. *Arch Dis Child Fetal Neonatal Ed* 2013; 98:F10–F14.
17. Ostlie DJ, Spilde TL, St Peter SD, et al. Necrotizing enterocolitis in full-term infants. *J Pediatr Surg* 2003; 38:1039–1042.
18. Maayan-Metzger A, Itzchak A, Mazkereth R, Kuint J. Necrotizing enterocolitis in full-term infants: case-control study and review of the literature. *J Perinatol* 2004; 24:494–499.
19. Lucas A, Cole TJ. Breast milk and neonatal necrotising enterocolitis. *Lancet* 1990; 336:1519–1523.
20. Quigley M, Henderson G, Anthony MY, McGuire W. Formula milk versus donor breast milk for feeding preterm or low birth weight infants. *Cochrane Database Syst Rev* 2007; Issue 4. Art. No.: CD002971. doi: 10.1002/14651858.CD002971.pub2
21. Morgan J, Young L, McGuire W. Delayed introduction of progressive enteral feeds to prevent necrotising enterocolitis in very low birth weight infants. *Cochrane Database Syst Rev* 2011; Issue 3. Art. No.: CD001970. doi: 10.1002/14651858.CD001970.pub3
22. Berseth CL, Bisquera JA, Paje VU. Prolonging small feeding volumes early in life decreases the incidence of necrotizing enterocolitis in very low birth weight infants. *Pediatrics* 2003; 111:529–534.
23. Morgan J, Young L, McGuire W. Slow advancement of enteral feed volumes to prevent necrotising enterocolitis in very low birth weight infants. *Cochrane Database Syst Rev* 2011; Issue 3. Art. No.: CD001241. doi: 10.1002/14651858.CD001241.pub3
24. Bell MJ. Peritonitis in the newborn – current concepts. *Pediatr Clin N Am* 1985; 32:1181–1201.
25. Lugo B, Ford HR, Grishin A. Molecular signalling in necrotizing enterocolitis: regulation of intestinal COX-2 expression. *J Pediatr Surg* 2007; 42:1165–1171.
26. Upperman JS, Potoka D, Grishin A, Hackam D, Zamora R, Ford HR. Mechanisms of nitric oxide-mediated intestinal barrier failure in necrotizing enterocolitis. *Semin Pediatr Surg* 2005; 14:159–166.
27. Rehan VK, Seshia MM, Johnston B, Reed M, Wilmot D, Cook V. Observer variability in interpretation of abdominal radiographs of infants with suspected necrotizing enterocolitis. *Clin Pediatr (Phila)* 1999; 38:637–643.
28. Di Napoli A, Di Lallo D, Perucci CA, et al. Inter-observer reliability of radiological signs of necrotising enterocolitis in a population of high-risk newborns. *Paediatr Perinat Epidemiol* 2004; 18:80–87.
29. Coursey CA, Hollingsworth CL, Gaca AM, Maxfield C, Delong D, Bisset 3rd G. Radiologists' agreement when using a 10-point scale to report abdominal radiographic findings of necrotizing enterocolitis in neonates and infants. *Am J Roentgenol* 2008; 191:190–197.
30. Coursey CA, Hollingsworth CL, Wriston C, Beam C, Rice H, Bisset 3rd G. Radiographic predictors of disease severity in neonates and infants with necrotizing enterocolitis. *Am J Roentgenol* 2009; 193:1408–1413.
31. Kim WY, Kim WS, Kim IO, Kwon TH, Chang W, Lee EK. Sonographic evaluation of neonates with early-stage necrotizing enterocolitis. *Pediatr Radiol* 2005; 35:1056–1061.
32. Silva CT, Daneman A, Navarro OM, et al. Correlation of sonographic findings and outcome in necrotizing enterocolitis. *Pediatr Radiol* 2007; 37:274–282.
33. Khan TR, Rawat JD, Ahmed I, et al. Neonatal pneumoperitoneum: a critical appraisal of its causes and subsequent management from a developing country. *Pediatr Surg Int* 2009; 25:1093–1097.

34. Kliegman RM. Neonatal necrotizing enterocolitis : implications for an infectious disease. *Pediatr Clin N Am* 1979; 26:327–344.
35. Kliegman RM, Fanaroff AA. Necrotizing enterocolitis. *N Engl J Med* 1984; 310:1093–1103.
36. Stoll BJ. Epidemiology of necrotizing enterocolitis. *Clin Perinatol* 1994; 21:205–218.
37. Scheifele DW, Ginter GL, Olsen E, Fussell S, Pendray M. Comparison of two antibiotic regimens for neonatal necrotizing enterocolitis. *J Antimicrob Chemother* 1987; 20:421–429.
38. Pammi M, Abrams SA. Oral lactoferrin for the treatment of sepsis and necrotizing enterocolitis in neonates. *Cochrane Database Syst Rev* 2011; Issue 10. Art. No.: CD007138. doi:10.1002/14651858.CD007138.pub3
39. Rao SC, Basani L, Simmer K, Samnakay N, Deshpande G. Peritoneal drainage versus laparotomy as initial surgical treatment for perforated necrotizing enterocolitis or spontaneous intestinal perforation in preterm low birth weight infants. *Cochrane Database Syst Rev* 2011; Issue 6. Art. No.: CD006182. doi:10.1002/14651858.CD006182.pub2
40. Moss RL, Dimmitt RA, Barnhart DC, et al. Laparotomy versus peritoneal drainage for necrotizing enterocolitis and perforation. *N Engl J Med* 2006; 354:2225–2234.
41. Rees CM, Eaton S, Kiely EM, Wade AM, McHugh K, Pierro A. Peritoneal drainage or laparotomy for neonatal bowel perforation? A randomized controlled trial. *Ann Surg* 2008; 248:44–51.
42. Fitzgibbons SC, Ching Y, Yu D, et al. Mortality of necrotizing enterocolitis expressed by birth weight categories. *J Pediatr Surg* 2009; 44:1072–1075.
43. Neu J, Walker WA. Necrotizing enterocolitis. *N Engl J Med* 2011; 364:255–264.
44. Alexander F, Smith A. Mortality in micro-premature infants with necrotizing enterocolitis treated by primary laparotomy is independent of gestational age and birth weight. *Pediatr Surg Int* 2008; 24:415–419.
45. Hintz SR, Kendrick DE, Stoll BJ, et al; NICHD Neonatal Research Network. Neurodevelopmental and growth outcomes of extremely low birth weight infants after necrotizing enterocolitis. *Pediatrics* 2005; 115:696–703.
46. Rees CM, Pierro A, Eaton S. Neurodevelopmental outcomes of neonates with medically and surgically treated necrotizing enterocolitis. *Arch Dis Child Fetal Neonatal Ed* 2007; 92:F193–F198.
47. Pike K, Brocklehurst P, Jones D, et al. Outcomes at 7 years for babies who developed neonatal necrotising enterocolitis: the ORACLE Children Study. *Arch Dis Child Fetal Neonatal Ed.* 2012 Jan 20. [Epub ahead of print] PubMed PMID: 22267398.
48. Amin HJ, Zamora SA, McMillan DD, et al. Arginine supplementation prevents necrotizing enterocolitis in the premature infant. *J Pediatr* 2002; 140:425–431.
49. Pammi M, Abrams SA. Oral lactoferrin for the prevention of sepsis and necrotizing enterocolitis in preterm infants. *Cochrane Database Syst Rev* 2011; Issue 10. Art. No.: CD007137. doi:10.1002/14651858.CD007137.pub3
50. Manzoni P, Rinaldi M, Cattani S, et al. Bovine lactoferrin supplementation for prevention of late-onset sepsis in very low-birth-weight neonates: a randomized trial. *JAMA* 2009; 302:1421–1428.
51. Amin HJ, Soraisham AS, Sauve RS. Neurodevelopmental outcomes of premature infants treated with l-arginine for prevention of necrotising enterocolitis. *J Paediatr Child Health* 2009; 45:219–223.
52. Siu YK, Ng PC, Fung SC, et al. Double blind, randomised, placebo controlled study of oral vancomycin in prevention of necrotising enterocolitis in preterm, very low birthweight infants. *Arch Dis Child Fetal Neonatal Ed* 1998; 79:F105–F109.
53. AlFaleh K, Anabrees J, Bassler D, Al-Kharfi T. Probiotics for prevention of necrotizing enterocolitis in preterm infants. *Cochrane Database Syst Rev* 2011; Issue 3. Art. No.: CD005496. doi:10.1002/14651858.CD005496.pub3
54. Deshpande G, Rao S, Patole S, Bulsara M. Updated meta-analysis of probiotics for preventing necrotizing enterocolitis in preterm neonates. *Pediatrics* 2010; 125:921–930.
55. Lin HC, Su BH, Chen AC, et al. Oral probiotics reduce the incidence and severity of necrotizing enterocolitis in very low birth weight infants. *Pediatrics* 2005; 115:1–4.
56. Samanta M, Sarkar M, Ghosh P, Ghosh J, Sinha M, Chatterjee S. Prophylactic probiotics for prevention of necrotizing enterocolitis in very low birth weight newborns. *J Trop Pediatr* 2009; 55:128–131.
57. Tarnow-Mordi WO, Wilkinson D, Trivedi A, Brok J. Probiotics reduce all-cause mortality and necrotizing enterocolitis: it is time to change practice. *Pediatrics* 2010; 125:1068–1070.
58. Soll RF. Probiotics: are we ready for routine use? *Pediatrics* 2010; 125:1071–1072.
59. Mihatsch WA, Braegger CP, Decsi T, et al. Critical systematic review of the level of evidence for routine use of probiotics for reduction of mortality and prevention of necrotizing enterocolitis and sepsis in preterm infants. *Clin Nutr* 2012; 31:6–15.
60. Deshpande GC, Rao SC, Keil AD, Patole SK. Evidence-based guidelines for use of probiotics in preterm neonates. *BMC Med* 2011; 9:92.
61. Whitehouse JS, Xu H, Shi Y, et al. Mesenteric nitric oxide and superoxide production in experimental necrotizing enterocolitis. *J Surg Res* 2010; 161:1–8.
62. Akisu M, Ozmen D, Baka M, et al. Protective effect of dietary supplementation with L-arginine and L-carnitine on hypoxia/reoxygenation-induced necrotizing enterocolitis in young mice. *Biol Neonate* 2002; 81:260–265.
63. Shah PS, Shah VS. Arginine supplementation for prevention of necrotising enterocolitis in preterm infants. *Cochrane Database Syst Rev* 2007; Issue 3. Art. No.: CD004339. doi:10.1002/14651858.CD004339.pub3
64. Bury RG, Tudehope D. Enteral antibiotics for preventing necrotizing enterocolitis in low birthweight or preterm infants. *Cochrane Database Syst Rev* 2001; Issue 1. Art. No.: CD000405. doi:10.1002/14651858.CD000405

65. Foster JP, Cole MJ. Oral immunoglobulin for preventing necrotizing enterocolitis in preterm and low birth weight neonates. *Cochrane Database Syst Rev* 2004; Issue 1. Art. No.: CD001816. doi:10.1002/14651858.CD001816.pub2
66. Munos MK, Walker CL, Black RE. The effect of oral rehydration solution and recommended home fluids on diarrhoea mortality. *Int J Epidemiol* 2010; 39(Suppl 1):i75–i87.
67. Fewtrell L, Kaufmann RB, Kay D, Enanoria W, Haller L, Colford Jr JM. Water, sanitation, and hygiene interventions to reduce diarrhoea in less developed countries: a systematic review and meta-analysis. *Lancet Infect Dis* 2005; 5:42–52.
68. Cairncross S, Hunt C, Boisson S, et al. Water, sanitation and hygiene for the prevention of diarrhoea. *Int J Epidemiol* 2010; 39(Suppl 1):i193–i205.
69. Munos MK, Walker CL, Black RE. The effect of rotavirus vaccine on diarrhoea mortality. *Int J Epidemiol* 2010; 39(Suppl 1):i56–i62.
70. Black R, Cousens S, Johnson HL, et al. Global, regional, and national causes of child mortality in 2008: a systematic analysis. *Lancet* 2010; 375:1969–1987.
71. Boschi-Pinto C, Lanata CF, Black R. The global burden of diarrhea. *Matern Child Health* 2009; 3:225–243.
72. Lamberti LM, Fischer Walker CL, Noiman A, Victora C, Black RE. Breastfeeding and the risk for diarrhea morbidity and mortality. *BMC Public Health* 2011; 11(Suppl 3):S15.
73. Duijts L, Ramadhani MK, Moll HA. Breastfeeding protects against infectious diseases during infancy in industrialized countries. A systematic review. *Matern Child Nutr* 2009; 5:199–210.
74. Schack-Nielsen L, Michaelsen KF. Advances in our understanding of the biology of human milk and its effects on the offspring. *J Nutr* 2007; 137:503S–510S.
75. O'Ryan ML, Nataro JP, Cleary TG. Microorganisms responsible for neonatal diarrhea. In: *Infectious Diseases of the Fetus and Newborn Infant*, 7th edn (eds JS Remington, JO Klein, CB Wilson, V Nizet, Y Maldonado). Philadelphia: Elsevier, 2011. pp 359–418.
76. Feeney SA, Armstrong VJ, Mitchell SJ, Crawford L, McCaughey C, Coyle PV. Development and clinical validation of multiplex TaqMan® assays for rapid diagnosis of viral gastroenteritis. *J Med Virol* 2011; 83:1650–1656.
77. Kirby A, Gurgel RQ, Dove W, Vieira SC, Cunliffe NA, Cuevas LE. An evaluation of the RIDASCREEN and IDEIA enzyme immunoassays and the RIDAQUICK immunochromatographic test for the detection of norovirus in faecal specimens. *J Clin Virol* 2010; 49:254–257.
78. O'Dempsey TJ, McArdle TF, Lloyd-Evans N, et al. Importance of enteric bacteria as a cause of pneumonia, meningitis and septicaemia among children in a rural community in the Gambia. *Pediatr Infect Dis J* 1994; 13:122–128.
79. Berkley JA, Lowe BS, Mwangi I, et al. Bacteremia among children admitted to a rural hospital in Kenya. *N Engl J Med* 2005; 352:39–47.
80. Graham SM. Non-typhoidal salmonellosis in Africa. *Curr Opin Infect Dis* 2010; 23:409–414.
81. Paisley JW, Lauer BA. Neonatal Yersinia enterocolitica enteritis. *Pediatr Infect Dis J* 1992; 11:331–332.
82. Viner Y, Miron D, Gottfried E, Segal D, Luder A. Neonatal shigellosis. *Isr Med Assoc J* 2001; 3:964–966.
83. Hartling L, Bellemare S, Wiebe N, Russell KF, Klassen TP, Craig WR. Oral versus intravenous rehydration for treating dehydration due to gastroenteritis in children. *Cochrane Database Syst Rev* 2006; Issue 3. Art. No.: CD004390. doi:10.1002/14651858.CD004390.pub2
84. Neville KA, Verge CF, Rosenberg AR, O'Meara MW, Walker JL. Isotonic is better than hypotonic saline for intravenous rehydration of children with gastroenteritis: a prospective randomised study. *Arch Dis Child* 2006; 91:226–232.
85. Moritz ML, Ayus JC. Prevention of hospital-acquired hyponatremia: a case for using isotonic saline. *Pediatrics* 2003; 111:227–230.
86. Hoorn EJ, Geary D, Robb M, Halperin ML, Bohn D. Acute hyponatremia related to intravenous fluid administration in hospitalized children: an observational study. *Pediatrics* 2004; 113:1279–1284.
87. Neville KA, Verge CF, O'Meara MW, Walker JL. High antidiuretic hormone levels and hyponatremia in children with gastroenteritis. *Pediatrics* 2005; 116:1401–1407.
88. Aserkoff B, Bennett JV. Effect of antibiotic therapy in acute salmonellosis on the fecal excretion of salmonellae. *N Engl J Med* 1969; 281:636–640.
89. Allen SJ, Martinez EG, Gregorio GV, Dans LF. Probiotics for treating acute infectious diarrhoea. *Cochrane Database Syst Rev* 2010; Issue 11. Art. No.: CD003048. doi:10.1002/14651858.CD003048.pub3
90. Bernaola Aponte G, Bada Mancilla CA, Carreazo Pariasca NY, Rojas Galarza RA. Probiotics for treating persistent diarrhoea in children. *Cochrane Database Syst Rev* 2010; Issue 11. Art. No.: CD007401. doi:10.1002/14651858.CD007401.pub2
91. Isaacs D, Dobson SRM, Wilkinson AR, Hope PL, Eglin R, Moxon ER. Conservative management of an echovirus 11 outbreak on a neonatal unit. *Lancet* 1989; i:543–545.
92. Johnston BC, Goldenberg JZ, Vandvik PO, Sun X, Guyatt GH. Probiotics for the prevention of pediatric antibiotic-associated diarrhea. *Cochrane Database Syst Rev* 2011; Issue 11. Art. No.: CD004827. doi:10.1002/14651858.CD004827.pub3
93. Soares-Weiser K, MacLehose H, Bergman H, et al. Vaccines for preventing rotavirus diarrhoea: vaccines in use. *Cochrane Database Syst Rev* 2012; Issue 2. Art. No.: CD008521. doi:10.1002/14651858.CD008521.pub2
94. Vesikari T, Matson DO, Dennehy P, et al; Rotavirus Efficacy and Safety Trial (REST) Study Team. Safety and efficacy of a pentavalent human-bovine (WC3) reassortant rotavirus vaccine. *N Engl J Med* 2006; 354:23–33.
95. Vesikari T, Karvonen A, Prymula R, et al. Efficacy of human rotavirus vaccine against rotavirus gastroenteritis during the first 2 years of life in European infants: randomised, double-blind controlled study. *Lancet* 2007; 370:1757–1763.

96. Madhi SA, Cunliffe NA, Steele D, et al. Effect of human rotavirus vaccine on severe diarrhea in African infants. *N Engl J Med* 2010; 362:289–298.
97. Zaman K, Dang DA, Victor JC, et al. Efficacy of pentavalent rotavirus vaccine against severe rotavirus gastroenteritis in infants in developing countries in Asia: a randomised, double-blind, placebo-controlled trial. *Lancet* 2010; 376:615–623.
98. Desai R, Cortese MM, Meltzer MI, et al. Potential intussusception risk versus benefits of rotavirus vaccination in the United States. *Pediatr Infect Dis J* 2013; 32:1–7.
99. Centers for Disease Control and Prevention. Prevention of rotavirus gastroenteritis among infants and children. *MMWR Recomm Rep* 2009; 58(RR-02):1–24.
100. Zamir O, Shapira SC, Udassin R, Peleg O, Arad I, Nissan S. Gastrointestinal perforations in the neonatal period. *Am J Perinatol* 1988; 5:131–133.
101. Zorludemir U, Koca M, Olcay I, Yücesan S. Neonatal peritonitis. *Turk J Pediatr* 1992; 34:157–166.
102. Bell MJ. Peritonitis in the newborn – current concepts. *Pediatr Clin N Am* 1985; 32:1181–1201.
103. Bell MJ. Perforation of the gastro-intestinal tract and peritonitis in the neonate. *Surg Gynecol Obstet* 1985; 160:20–26.
104. Bell MJ, Ternberg JL, Bower RJ. The microbial flora and antimicrobial therapy of neonatal peritonitis. *J Pediatr Surg* 1980; 15:569–573.
105. Meyer CL, Payne NR, Roback SA. Spontaneous, isolated intestinal perforations in neonates with birth weight less than 1,000 g not associated with necrotizing enterocolitis. *J Pediatr Surg* 1991; 26:714–717.
106. Mintz AC, Applebaum H. Focal gastrointestinal perforations not associated with necrotizing enterocolitis in very low birth weight neonates. *J Pediatr Surg* 1993; 28:857–860.
107. Adderson EE, Pappin A, Pavia AT. Spontaneous intestinal perforation in premature infants: a distinct clinical entity associated with systemic candidiasis. *J Pediatr Surg* 1998; 33:1463–1467.
108. Pumberger W, Mayr M, Kohlhauser C, Weninger M. Spontaneous localized intestinal perforation in very-low-birth-weight infants: a distinct clinical entity different from necrotizing enterocolitis. *J Am Coll Surg* 2002; 195:796–803.

CHAPTER 12

Eye infections

12.1 Conjunctivitis

Conjunctivitis can vary from a benign illness with sticky eyes which respond to saline washes through to sight-threatening gonococcal infection and life-threatening HSV infection. It is critical to diagnose HSV infection promptly to institute antiviral treatment before the HSV spreads to the brain (HSV encephalitis) or disseminates widely. Other critical clinical considerations include diagnosing chlamydial conjunctivitis and orbital or periorbital cellulitis.

12.1.1 Epidemiology of neonatal conjunctivitis

Conjunctivitis is one of the commonest neonatal infections. The reported incidence varies by definition used and population studied. Severe conjunctivitis due to *Neisseria gonorrhoeae* or *Chlamydia trachomatis* may be selectively reported. Other causes of conjunctivitis are bacterial infection, viral infection and chemical, due to agents used for chemoprophylaxis.

In Western countries, the reported incidence of conjunctivitis is often quoted as from 1% to 12%, based on data from the 1970s and 1980s.[1–7] A later US neonatal intensive care unit (NICU)-based study reported an incidence of 5% for nosocomial conjunctivitis.[8] The reported incidence of conjunctivitis from developing countries is usually higher. A hospital-based study from Brazil reported nosocomial conjunctivitis in 17.7% of infants.[9] Community-based studies in Africa and other developing countries often report an incidence of neonatal conjunctivitis greater than 20%.[10–12]

12.1.2 Clinical

The clinical features of gonococcal and chlamydial conjunctivitis are sufficiently similar that they cannot be distinguished clinically with reliability.[1–3,13]

Gonococcal ophthalmia neonatorum classically presents with purulent eye discharge starting 2–5 days after birth (Figure 12.1a), often with bilateral eyelid oedema and chemosis. However, eyelid oedema is also a feature of severe chlamydial infection. Less commonly, purulent eye discharge may be present at birth if the baby has acquired intrauterine gonococcal infection (Figure 12.1b) or present later if infection is more sub-acute. Asymptomatic infection has been reported. Untreated gonococcal conjunctivitis can progress to corneal involvement with ulceration, perforation or endophthalmitis.[13]

Chlamydial conjunctivitis (sometimes called inclusion conjunctivitis of the newborn) usually presents at 5–14 days, but intrauterine infection can result in earlier presentation.[14] The severity can vary from mild conjunctival injection with minimal discharge to severe purulent conjunctivitis with chemosis and eyelid oedema, indistinguishable clinically from gonococcal conjunctivitis (Figure 12.2).[14] Inflammatory exudate can adhere to the conjunctiva and cause a pseudomembrane. Acute corneal involvement is very rarely described. In severe chronic infection, neovascularization of the cornea can result in pannus formation (corneal invasion by small blood vessels) and sight-threatening scarring as occurs in trachoma.[14]

Children with HSV conjunctivitis usually acquire infection perinatally and present typically before 7 days of age, although may present from 1 to 14 days, rarely

Evidence-Based Neonatal Infections, First Edition. David Isaacs.

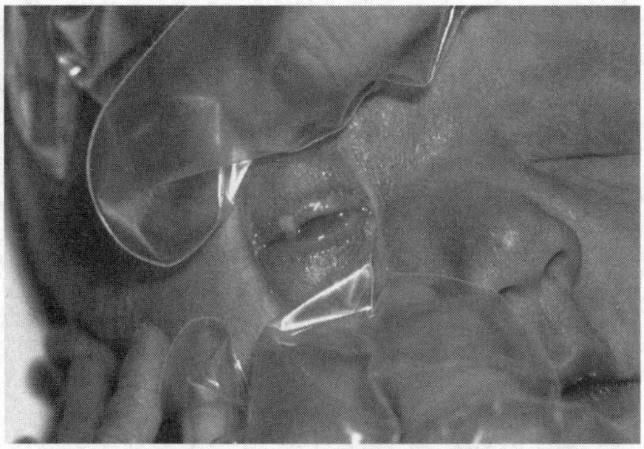

(a)

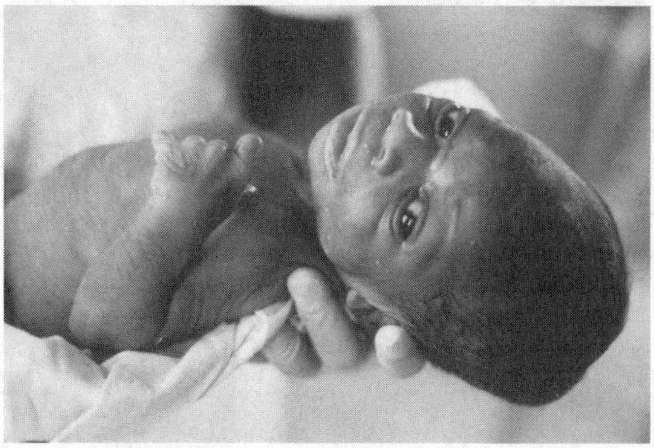

(b)

Figure 12.1 (a) Purulent eye discharge at 3 days of age due to *Neisseria gonorrhoeae*. (b) Purulent discharge at birth due to *in utero* gonococcal infection.

later (Figure 12.3a and 12.3b).[15, 16] As many as 90% of neonates with HSV conjunctivitis have discrete skin vesicles or bullous skin lesions which should alert the clinician to the diagnosis (see Chapter 17). Dendritic corneal ulceration is a characteristic but late sign of HSV infection (Figure 12.4). HSV may be localized to the skin, eye or mouth, so the baby's skin and oral cavity should be examined carefully for lesions.[15, 16] HSV can disseminate rapidly, so not only should the baby be examined to exclude hepatitis, DIC and encephalitis, but treatment should be instituted urgently to prevent dissemination.

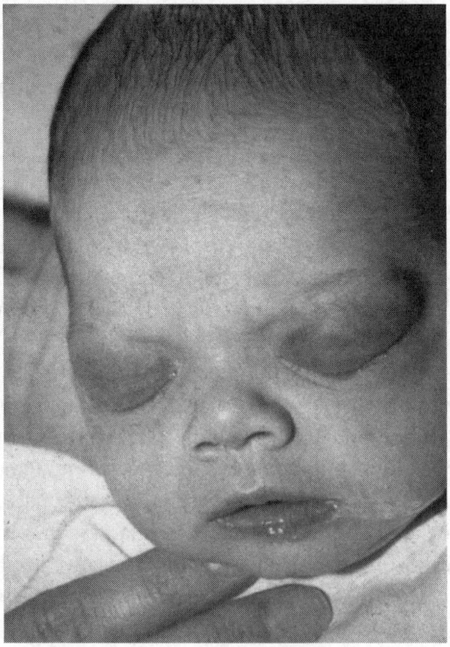

Figure 12.2 Infant aged 7 days with bilateral eyelid oedema and purulent discharge from *Chlamydia trachomatis* infection.

Pseudomonas conjunctivitis usually presents in the second or third week of life with purulent discharge and eyelid oedema and erythema. This can progress rapidly to involve the cornea and can result in perforation and panophthalmitis and be complicated acutely by septicaemia or meningitis and chronically by pannus formation.[17]

12.1.3 Diagnosis of neonatal conjunctivitis

The most important organisms are *N. gonorrhoeae*, *C. trachomatis* and HSV, which need completely different methods of identification.

A Gram stain of the exudate in gonococcal ophthalmia neonatorum usually reveals Gram-negative intracellular diplococci, although *Neisseria meningitidis*, a very rare cause of neonatal conjunctivitis, has the same appearance. Although culture is the 'gold standard' test, the organism is fastidious in its growth. Conjunctival swabs are preferably charcoal impregnated, calcium alginate or Dacron swabs, because other swabs inhibit growth. The specimen either needs to be inoculated onto culture media at the bedside or transported to the laboratory rapidly in suitable transport media.[18] No transport medium reliably supports gonococci for more than 24 hours. Gonococci need enriched media such as chocolate agar and 5% CO_2

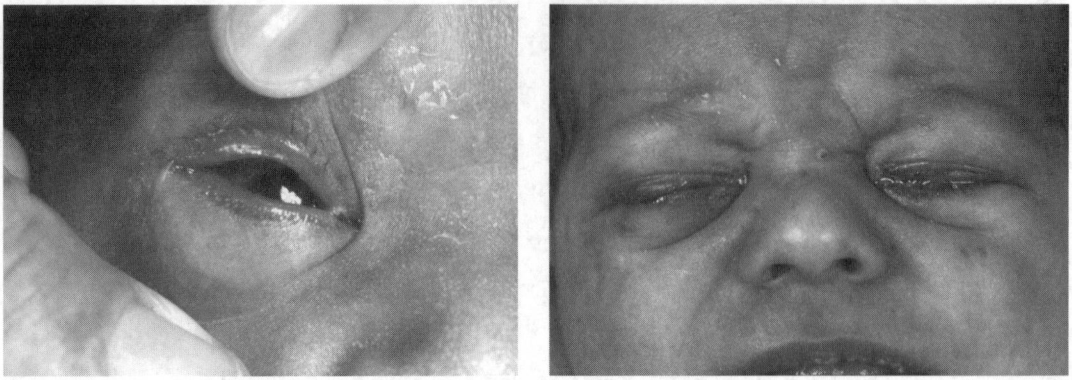

(a) (b)

Figure 12.3 (a) Neonatal herpes simplex virus (HSV) conjunctivitis with marked conjunctivitis but no skin lesions. (b) Bilateral exudative HSV conjunctivitis with isolated herpetic skin lesions.

for optimal growth. Non-culture detection of *N. gonorrhoeae* by nucleic acid hybridization or polymerase chain reaction (PCR) amplification used in many laboratories has acceptable sensitivity and specificity.[19, 20] Gonococcal ophthalmia comes from the mother, so the mother, her partner and other sexual contacts should be screened for gonorrhoea. In addition, gonococcal ophthalmia is often associated with chlamydial infection, so the infant and the parents should be screened for Chlamydia and other sexually transmitted infections not already excluded.

Culture for Chlamydia requires special media, is time-consuming and expensive and has been superseded by non-culture techniques. In Western countries, enzyme immunoassays, PCR and direct fluorescent antibody testing of eye and nasopharyngeal secretions have all been shown to have acceptable sensitivity and specificity.[20–23] In developing countries, if rapid tests are not available, Giemsa staining of conjunctival scrapings for intracytoplasmic inclusions has a sensitivity of 30–70% compared with culture or more sophisticated tests.[24, 25]

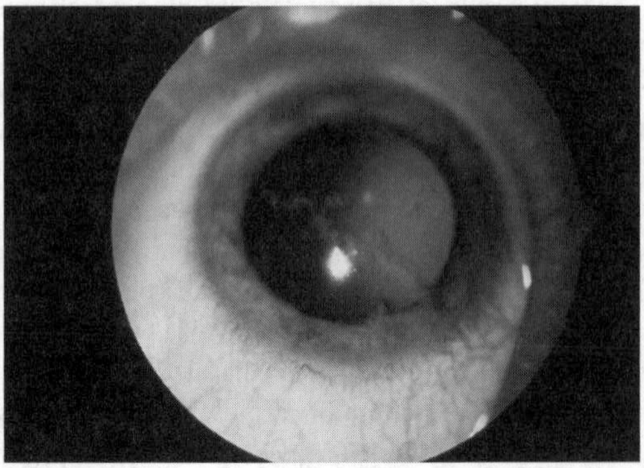

Figure 12.4 Dendritic (branching) ulcer of HSV infection.

If HSV is suspected, rapid diagnosis is important as a basis for early treatment. Conjunctival swabs and fluid from any skin vesicles should be tested using the best available rapid test. Tests with high sensitivity and specificity include PCR, ELISA and fluorescent antibody tests.[15, 16]

Bacterial eye culture may grow an organism, but this does not guarantee causation. In a prospective case-control study from Thailand, Chlamydia and *Staphylococcus aureus* were isolated significantly more often from infants with conjunctivitis, whereas CoNS, Acinetobacter, Pseudomonas and diphtheroids were at least as commonly isolated from controls.[26] This was a small study and Pseudomonas can undoubtedly be a serious ocular pathogen. There are occasional reports of Pseudomonas endopthalmitis but also of outbreaks of invasive Pseudomonas eye infection associated with fatal septicaemia.[17] A retrospective observational study from the United States of 65 NICU infants with culture-positive conjunctivitis found Gram-negative bacilli in 25 (38%), mostly Klebsiella, *Escherichia coli* or Serratia, and occasionally Pseudomonas or Enterobacter.[27] The interpretation of a positive eye culture with a potentially pathogenic organism depends on the clinical scenario.

Other organisms that can cause neonatal conjunctivitis include *Haemophilus influenzae* (both untypeable and type b), *Streptococcus pneumoniae*, *Mycoplasma hominis* and Candida (Section 12.2 and see Chapter 16).

12.1.4 Management of neonatal conjunctivitis

12.1.4.1 Gonococcal infection

Originally gonococcal conjunctivitis could be cured with penicillin, but penicillinase-producing strains of gonococcus are now common worldwide. Gonococcal ophthalmia is rare in Western countries and almost all recent studies have been conducted in developing countries. In an observational study in Kenya, none of 68 patients with gonococcal conjunctivitis failed treatment with a single dose of intramuscular (IM) kanamycin plus gentamicin eye ointment.[28] However, kanamycin followed by saline washes did not cure all patients[28] and also fails to eradicate oropharyngeal carriage in a proportion of infants.[29] An RCT in Kenya compared single-dose IM ceftriaxone plus 7 days of topical gentamicin with single-dose kanamycin plus 7 days of topical gentamicin or topical tetracycline.[29] There were no treatment failures in the 55 infants treated with ceftriaxone who returned for follow-up, although 6 infants did not return for follow-up. In contrast, 3 of 50 infants given kanamycin had persistent or recurrent gonococcal infection.[29] In a small study, single-dose ceftriaxone cured six infants with gonococcal ophthalmia, although a seventh did not return for follow-up and two needed treatment for Chlamydia conjunctivitis.[30] Ceftriaxone can displace bilirubin bound to albumin so may not be safe in jaundiced babies. Single-dose cefotaxime successfully treated ophthalmia and eradicated carriage in all 9 patients in a study in Rwanda.[31] In the United States, the recommended treatment of proven gonococcal ophthalmia is with a single IM or IV dose of ceftriaxone 25–50 mg/kg to a maximum of 125 mg or with a single IM or IV dose of cefotaxime 100 mg/kg, plus immediate and regular saline irrigation.[13, 32] Topical antibiotics are unnecessary if a third generation cephalosporin is used. If the infant has evidence of disseminated gonococcal infection with septic arthritis, bacteraemia or meningitis, 7 days of parenteral therapy is recommended using ceftriaxone 25–50 mg up to 125 mg once daily or cefotaxime 100–150 mg/kg/day given 8 hourly. Cefotaxime is preferred for infants, particularly pre-term, with hyperbilirubinaemia.[13,32–34] The evidence that single-dose therapy is effective is based on one RCT and observational studies with incomplete follow-up. The Australian Therapeutic Guidelines recommend 7 days of parenteral antibiotics for all babies with gonococcal ophthalmia and recommend adding empiric azithromycin pending investigations if there is a high risk of Chlamydia.[35] Single-dose therapy should be given empirically to infants born to mothers with active gonococcal infection, even if the infant is asymptomatic.[13,32–34]

In most Western countries notification of public health authorities is mandatory if an infant presents with gonococcal ophthalmia to enable contact tracing and investigation for other sexually transmitted diseases. There may even be child protection issues if infection is not clearly acquired perinatally.

12.1.4.2 Chlamydial infection

The standard treatment for chlamydial conjunctivitis is oral erythromycin 40 mg/kg/day in four divided doses (10 mg/kg/dose 6 hourly). Oral therapy is preferred to topical therapy which, although it has comparable efficacy, does not eradicate carriage.[36] Oral therapy is recommended to decrease the risk of subsequent Chlamydia pneumonitis, which develops in about 30% of untreated infants with nasopharyngeal Chlamydia.[14] About 10–20% of infants' conjunctivitis fails to resolve with oral erythromycin, necessitating further treatment.[14, 37]

In a small observational study of oral azithromycin 20 mg/kg once daily, two of five babies failed to respond to 1 day. However, 3 days of azithromycin 20 mg/kg once daily successfully treated seven infants, although one remained culture positive in the nasopharynx.[38]

In the absence of RCTs either erythromycin or azithromycin seems appropriate.

12.1.4.3 Herpes simplex virus conjunctivitis

HSV infection is considered in Chapter 17 (see Section 17.2). The dose of aciclovir for a neonate is 20 mg/kg/dose given IV 8 hourly, 14 days for localized disease and 21 days for encephalitis.[39]

12.1.4.4 Bacterial conjunctivitis

Topical antibiotics speed clinical and microbiologic recovery from bacterial conjunctivitis in older children and adults, although 65% of those on placebo resolve within 2–5 days.[40] There are no comparable data for neonates. If gonococcal and chlamydial infections are excluded, *S. aureus* is the main bacterium implicated. A review of 53 papers found that topical fusidic acid was as good as topical chloramphenicol for neonates presenting with sticky eyes.[41] Topical antibiotics apart from chloramphenicol and fusidic acid sometimes used to treat bacterial conjunctivitis include tetracyclines, quinolones, aminoglycosides, sulfonamides and polymyxin, but none has been studied systematically in newborns. Sticky eyes, which may also be due to chemical conjunctivitis secondary to prophylactic agents, often resolve with saline washes without topical antibiotics.

If the neonate with conjunctivitis has periorbital redness and/or swelling (Figure 12.5) this is a worrying sign of orbital cellulitis. Maxillary osteomyelitis (see Chapter 9), which is frequently misdiagnosed as orbital cellulitis, should be considered. Even if underlying osteomyelitis is unlikely, the neonate with orbital cellulitis merits careful assessment and probably systemic antibiotics because of the risk of bacteraemia with any cellulitis.

It is important to distinguish colonization with Pseudomonas from Pseudomonas conjunctivitis, but a neonate with purulent Pseudomonas conjunctivitis should be treated urgently with systemic antipseudomonal antibiotics after taking cultures of blood and CSF, because of the risk of systemic infection.[17] Pseudomonas are intrinsically resistant to cefotaxime and ceftriaxone, so the choice lies between an aminoglycoside, a synthetic penicillin with or without a β-lactamase inhibitor (e.g. piperacillin–tazobactam, ticarcillin–clavulanate) or a carbapenem.

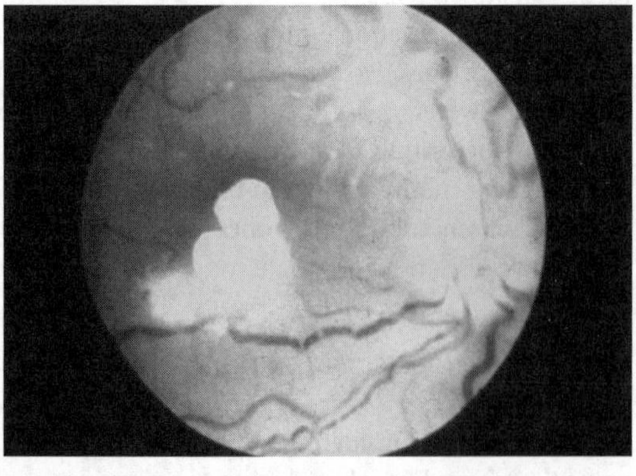

Figure 12.5 Candida chorioretinitis: the fluffy lesions in the vitreous are described as 'snowballs' and are typical of candidiasis.

12.1.5 Prevention

There are four approaches to prevention of neonatal eye infections: prevention of sexually transmitted diseases, antenatal screening of pregnant women for genital infection, ocular prophylaxis at birth and early diagnosis and treatment of ophthalmia neonatorum.[42] Prophylaxis against ophthalmia neonatorum dates from 1881 when Credé first introduced the practice of instilling a drop of 1% silver nitrate into the newborn's eyelids, dramatically reducing eye infections and blindness. The benefits and risks of ocular prophylaxis depend on the prevalence of gonococcal and chlamydial infection in the population, the efficacy and adverse effects of any prophylaxis and the ability to screen pregnant women for gonorrhoea and Chlamydia infection.

Silver nitrate is highly effective at preventing gonococcal ophthalmia neonatorum, but less effective in preventing chlamydial ophthalmitis or pneumonitis.[43–48] It is no longer used in Western countries because it causes chemical conjunctivitis in a high proportion of babies. It is not used in many developing countries because of expense. Gentamicin eye ointment has been shown to cause severe ocular ulcerative dermatitis.[49, 50] The alternatives are topical erythromycin, tetracycline, povidone–iodine or no prophylaxis.

In an RCT of prophylaxis for infants born to women who isolated Chlamydia from their cervix, 12 (33%) of 36 infants given silver nitrate developed Chlamydia conjunctivitis but none of 24 given topical erythromycin. Nasopharyngeal colonization developed in 10 (29%) given silver nitrate and 5 (21%) given erythromycin; 3 and 1 of these respectively developed Chlamydia pneumonia.[44]

A Kenyan study compared silver nitrate with tetracycline ointment in a population where the prevalence of maternal gonococcal infection was 6.4% and maternal Chlamydia 8.9%.[45] The incidence of gonococcal, chlamydial and other conjunctivitis after prophylaxis was 0.4%, 0.7% and 6.2%, respectively, for silver nitrate and 0.1%, 0.5% and 4.5%, respectively, for tetracycline.[45]

Silver nitrate ocular prophylaxis was compared with erythromycin and tetracycline in a US setting.[46] Only 8 (0.06%) of 12 431 babies had gonococcal opthalmitis, 7 of them born to women who received no antenatal care. There was no significant difference in the proportion of infants of Chlamydia-positive mothers who developed chlamydial conjunctivitis (20% silver nitrate, 14% erythromycin, 11% tetracycline).[46] A study from China used the same three agents but included a control group and showed none of the agents was superior to no prophylaxis in preventing Chlamydia conjunctivitis.[47]

In an RCT in Kenya, over 3000 newborns were randomized to receive topical 2.5% povidone–iodine, 1% silver nitrate or 0.5% erythromycin ointment.[48] Povidone–iodine was more effective than either of the other agents against Chlamydia and caused less non-infectious conjunctivitis, which was thought to be a chemical conjunctivitis.[48] However, in an Israeli study povidone–iodine caused chemical conjunctivitis in 5% of infants compared with none with tetracycline ointment and had a higher incidence of infective conjunctivitis than tetracycline (10.4% vs. 5.2%).[51]

A non-Cochrane meta-analysis of prophylactic agents found only eight studies, all with methodological problems. The authors concluded that all the agents used appear to be effective against gonococcal infection but that erythromycin and povidone–iodine are superior to silver nitrate for chlamydial infection.[52]

12.2 Endophthalmitis

Neonatal endophthalmitis is a rare but potentially devastating disease which is not only sight threatening, but also frequently associated with septicaemia and meningitis.[53] A large retrospective case series compared neonates with endophthalmitis in a US nationwide database with those without endophthalmitis and identified low birth-weight, bacteraemia, candidaemia, respiratory infection, blood transfusion and retinopathy of prematurity as 'risk factors' associated with developing neonatal endophthalmitis.[53] The reported incidence of neonatal endophthalmitis almost halved between 1998 (8.71 per 100 000) and 2006 (4.42 per 100 000).[53]

The most frequently reported organisms causing neonatal endophthalmitis are Candida,[54] Pseudomonas and GBS.

12.2.1 Candida endophthalmitis

Candida can cause fluffy exudates visible in the aqueous humor or retina (Figure 12.5 and see Chapter 16). A non-Cochrane systematic review and meta-analysis searched published papers on neonatal Candida infections for reported end-organ damage.[55] The median reported prevalence of endophthalmitis in Candida septicaemia was 3% (interquartile range 0–17%) but there may have been considerable under-reporting. In a case series of 24 cases of Candida septicaemia in Spanish neonatal units, two babies had ophthalmitis.[56]

12.2.2 Pseudomonas endophthalmitis

A review of neonatal bacterial endophthalmitis reported prematurity and colonization with *Pseudomonas aeruginosa* as the major risk factors for bacterial endophthalmitis.[57] Most cases of Pseudomonas endophthalmitis are isolated case reports, but there have been reports of small outbreaks of Pseudomonas endophthalmitis causing bacteraemia and meningitis with a very high mortality.[17, 58]

12.2.3 Group B streptococcal endophthalmitis

GBS endophthalmitis can complicate neonatal bacteraemia and, interestingly, endogenous endophthalmitis can also occur in adults in association with endocarditis, malignancy or diabetes. In neonates, there are only isolated case reports of GBS endophthalmitis and no reports of nosocomial outbreaks.[59–61]

12.3 Nasolacrimal duct obstruction and dacryocystitis

Congenital nasolacrimal duct obstruction is the commonest cause of chronic eye discharge in babies, affecting up to 20% of all newborns.[62–64] It causes epiphora (excessive tears), chronic or recurrent conjunctivitis, or eye discharge, which can progress to acute dacryocystitis (Figure 12.6).

Management approaches vary depending on severity: observation, simple probing, probing with silastic intubation and dacryocystorhinostomy. In an observational study, 964 of 4792 infants (20%) had defective

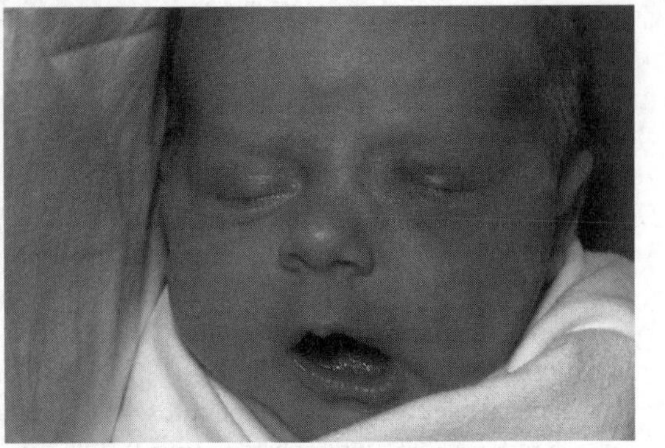

Figure 12.6 Conjunctivitis and orbital cellulitis secondary to nasolacrimal duct obstruction: left paranasal swelling and periorbital erythema.

lacrimal drainage documented by a fluorescein disappearance test and 95% of the 964 had symptoms of epiphora in the first month of life.[65] Spontaneous remission of epiphora occurred throughout the year, and 96% of cases had resolved before patients reached the age of 1 year.[65] Most babies with nasolacrimal duct obstruction can be treated with massage alone, although there are no RCTs of its efficacy.[63–66] More severe cases may need probing or saline irrigation by an ophthalmologist, which are equally effective.[67]

Maxillary osteomyelitis can be misdiagnosed as dacryocystitis or orbital cellulitis (see Chapter 9).[68]

12.4 Orbital abscess

Orbital abscess is rare in neonates.[69, 70] It should be considered in infants who present with orbital cellulitis (see Chapter 13), especially if complicated by proptosis, and is diagnosed by CT scan of the orbit.[69] It has been described in association with dacryocystitis (Figure 12.5)[70] and ethmoiditis.[69] *S. aureus* is the organism most frequently implicated, but empiric therapy should include Gram-negative cover, while drainage of the abscess should allow antibiotic treatment to be guided by Gram stain and culture results.

References

1. Jackson D, McKenna H. Bacteria in ophthalmia neonatorum. *Pathology* 1975; 7:199–201.
2. Prentice MJ, Hutchinson CR, Taylor-Robinson D. A microbiological study of neonatal conjunctivae and conjunctivitis. *Br J Ophthalmol* 1977; 61:601–607.
3. Pierce JM, Ward ME, Seal DV. Ophthalmia neonatorum in the 1980s: incidence, aetiology and treatment. *Br J Ophthalmol* 1982; 66:728–731.
4. Mølgaard IL, Nielsen PB, Kaern J. A study of the incidence of neonatal conjunctivitis and of its bacterial causes including Chlamydia trachomatis. Clinical examination, culture and cytology of tear fluid. *Acta Ophthalmol (Copenh)* 1984; 62:461–471.
5. Sandstrom I. Etiology and diagnosis of neonatal conjunctivitis. *Acta Paediatr Scand* 1987; 76:221–227.
6. Fransen L, van den Berghe P, Mertens A, et al. Incidence and bacterial aetiology of neonatal conjunctivitis. *Eur J Pediatr* 1987; 146:152–155.
7. Dannevig L, Straume B, Melby K. Ophthalmia neonatorum in northern Norway. I: Epidemiology and risk factors. *Acta Ophthalmol (Copenh)* 1992; 70:14–18.
8. Haas J, Larson E, Ross B, See B, Saiman L. Epidemiology and diagnosis of hospital-acquired conjunctivitis among neonatal intensive care unit patients. *Pediatr Infect Dis J* 2005; 24:586–589.
9. Brito DV, Brito CS, Resende DS, Moreira do Ó J, Abdallah VO, GontijoFilho PP. Nosocomial infections in a Brazilian neonatal intensive care unit: a 4-year surveillance study. *Rev Soc Bras Med Trop* 2010; 43:633–637.
10. Laga M, Plummer FA, Nzanze H, Namaara W, Brunham RC, Ndinya-Achola JO, et al. Epidemiology of ophthalmia neonatorum in Kenya. *Lancet* 1986; 2:1145–1149.
11. van Bogaert LJ. Ophthalmia neonatorum revisited. *Afr J Reprod Health* 1998; 2:81–86.
12. Fransen L, Klauss V. Neonatal ophthalmia in the developing world. Epidemiology, etiology, management and control. *Int Ophthalmol* 1988; 11:189–196.
13. Woods CR. Gonococcal infections in neonates and young children. *Semin Pediatr Infect Dis* 2005; 16:258–270.
14. Darville T. Chlamydia trachomatis infections in neonates and young children. *Semin Pediatr Infect Dis* 2005; 16:235–244.
15. Kimberlin DW. Herpes simplex virus infections in neonates and early childhood. *Semin Pediatr Infect Dis* 2005; 16:271–281.
16. Thompson C, Whitley R. Neonatal herpes simplex virus infections: where are we now? *Adv Exp Med Biol* 2011; 697:221–230.
17. Boyle EM, Ainsworth JR, Levin AV, Campbell AN, Watkinson M. Ophthalmic Pseudomonas infection in infancy. *Arch Dis Child Fetal Neonatal Ed* 2001; 85:F139–F140.
18. Jephcott AE, Bhattacharya MN, Jackson DH. Improved transport and culture system for the rapid diagnosis of gonorrhoea. *Br J Vener Dis* 1976; 52:250–252.
19. Koumans EH, Johnson RE, Knapp JS, St Louis ME. Laboratory testing for *Neisseria gonorrhoeae* by recently introduced non-culture tests: a performance review with clinical and public health considerations. *Clin Infect Dis* 1998; 27:1171–1180.
20. Cook RL, Hutchinson SL, Ostergaard L, Braithwaite RS, Ness RB. Systematic review: non-invasive testing for *Chlamydia*

trachomatis and *Neisseria gonorrhoeae. Ann Intern Med* 2005; 142:914–925.

21. Hammerschlag MR, Roblin PM, Gelling M, Tsumura N, Jule JE, Kutlin A. Use of polymerase chain reaction for the detection of Chlamydia trachomatis in ocular and nasopharyngeal specimens from infants with conjunctivitis. *Pediatr Infect Dis J* 1997; 16:293–297.
22. Yip PP, Chan WH, Yip KT, Que TL, Kwong NS, Ho CK. The use of polymerase chain reaction assay versus conventional methods in detecting neonatal chlamydial conjunctivitis. *J Pediatr Ophthalmol Strabismus* 2008; 45:234–239.
23. Sachdeva P, Patel AL, Sachdev D, Ali M, Mittal A, Saluja D. Comparison of an in-house PCR assay, direct fluorescence assay and the Roche AMPLICOR Chlamydia trachomatis kit for detection of C. trachomatis. *J Med Microbiol* 2009; 58:867–873.
24. Duggan MA, Pomponi C, Kay D, Robboy SJ. Infantile chlamydial conjunctivitis. A comparison of Papanicolaou, Giemsa and immunoperoxidase staining methods. *Acta Cytol* 1986; 30:341–346.
25. Madhavan HN, Rao SK, Natarajan K, Sitalakshmi G, Jayanthi I, Roy S. Evaluation of laboratory tests for diagnosis of chlamydial infections in conjunctival specimens. *Indian J Med Res* 1994; 100:5–9.
26. Sergiwa A, Pratt BC, Eren E, Sunona TC, Hart CA. Ophthalmia neonatorum in Bangkok: the significance of Chlamydia trachomatis. *Ann Trop Paediatr* 1993; 13:233–236.
27. Chen CJ, Starr CE. Epidemiology of gram-negative conjunctivitis in neonatal intensive care unit patients. *Am J Ophthalmol* 2008; 145:966–970.
28. Fransen L, Nsanze H, D'Costa L, Brunham RC, Ronald AR, Piot P. Single-dose kanamycin therapy of gonococcal ophthalmia neonatorum. *Lancet* 1984; 2:1234–1237.
29. Laga M, Naamara W, Brunham RC, et al. Single-dose therapy of gonococcal ophthalmia neonatorum with ceftriaxone. *N Engl J Med* 1986; 315:1382–1385.
30. Haase DA, Nash RA, Nsanze H, et al. Single-dose ceftriaxone therapy of gonococcal ophthalmia neonatorum. *Sex Transm Dis* 1986; 13:53–55.
31. Lepage P, Bogaerts J, Kestelyn P, Meheus A. Single-dose cefotaxime intramuscularly cures gonococcal ophthalmia neonatorum. *Br J Ophthalmol* 1988; 72:518–520.
32. American Academy of Pediatrics. Gonococcal infections. In: *Red Book: 2009 Report of the Committee on Infectious Diseases*, 28th edn (eds LK Pickering, CJ Baker, DW Kimberlin, SS Long). Elk Grove Village, IL: American Academy of Pediatrics, 2009. pp. 305–313.
33. Centers for Disease Control and Prevention (CDC). Sexually transmitted diseases treatment guidelines, 2010. *MMWR Recomm Rep* 2010; 59(RR-12):1–110.
34. Hammerschlag M. Chlamydial and gonococcal infections in infants and children. *Clin Infect Dis* 2011; 53(Supp 3):S99–S102.
35. Antibiotic Expert Group. *Therapeutic Guidelines: Antibiotic*, Version 14. Melbourne: Therapeutic Guidelines Limited, 2010. pp. 96–97.
36. Patamasucon P, Rettig PJ, Faust KL, Kusmiesz HT, Nelson JD. Oral v topical erythromycin therapies for chlamydial conjunctivitis. *Am J Dis Child* 1982; 136:817–821.
37. Hammerschlag MR, Chandler JW, Alexander ER, English M, Koustky L. Longitudinal studies of chlamydial infection in the first year of life. *Pediatr Infect Dis* 1982; 1:395–401.
38. Hammerschlag MR, Gelling M, Roblin PM, Kutlin A, Jule JE. Treatment of neonatal chlamydial conjunctivitis with azithromycin. *Pediatr Infect Dis J* 1998; 17:1049-1050.
39. Jones CA, Walker KS, Badawi N. Antiviral agents for treatment of herpes simplex virus infection in neonates. *Cochrane Database Syst Rev* 2009; Issue 3. Art. No.: CD004206. doi: 10.1002/14651858.CD004206.pub2
40. Sheikh A, Hurwitz B. Antibiotics versus placebo for acute bacterial conjunctivitis. *Cochrane Database Syst Rev* 2006; Issue 2. Art. No.: CD001211. doi: 10.1002/14651858.CD001211.pub2
41. Grayson A, Wylie K. Towards evidence-based emergency medicine: best BETs from the Manchester Royal Infirmary. BET 3: Fusidic acid or chloramphenicol for neonates with sticky eyes. *Emerg Med J* 2011; 28:634.
42. Foster A, Klauss V. Ophthalmia neonatorum in developing countries. *N Engl J Med* 1995; 332:600–601.
43. Silva LR, Gurgel RQ, Lima DRR, Cuevas LE. Current usefulness of Credé's method of preventing neonatal ophthalmia. *Ann Trop Pediatr* 2008; 28:45–48.
44. Hammerschlag MR, Chandler JW, Alexander ER, et al. Erythromycin ointment for ocular prophylaxis of neonatal chlamydial infection. *JAMA* 1980; 244:2291–2293.
45. Laga M, Plummer FA, Piot P, et al. Prophylaxis of gonococcal and chlamydial ophthalmia neonatorum. A comparison of silver nitrate and tetracycline. *N Engl J Med* 1988; 318:653–657.
46. Hammerschlag MR, Cummings C, Roblin PM, Williams TH, Delke I. Efficacy of neonatal ocular prophylaxis for the prevention of chlamydial and gonococcal conjunctivitis. *N Engl J Med* 1989; 320: 769–772.
47. Chen JY. Prophylaxis of ophthalmia neonatorum: comparison of silver nitrate, tetracycline erythromycin and no prophylaxis. *Pediatr Infect Dis J* 1992; 11:1026–1030.
48. Isenberg SJ, Apt L, Wood M. A controlled trial of povidone–iodine as prophylaxis against ophthalmia neonatorum. *N Engl J Med* 1995; 332:562–566.
49. Binenbaum G, Bruno CJ, Forbes BJ, et al. Periocular ulcerative dermatitis associated with gentamicin ointment prophylaxis in newborns. *J Pediatr* 2010; 156:320–321.
50. Nathawad R, Mendez H, Ahmad A, et al. Severe ocular reactions after neonatal ocular prophylaxis with gentamicin ophthalmic ointment. *Pediatr Infect Dis J* 2011; 30:175–176.
51. David M, Rumelt S, Weintraub Z. Efficacy comparison between povidone iodine 2.5% and tetracycline 1% in prevention of ophthalmia neonatorum. *Ophthalmology* 2011; 118:1454–1458.
52. Darling EK, McDonald H. A meta-analysis of the efficacy of ocular prophylactic agents used for the prevention of

gonococcal and chlamydial ophthalmia neonatorum. *J Midwifery Womens Health* 2010; 55:319–327.

53. Moshfeghi AA, Charalel RA, Hernandez-Boussard T, Morton JM, Moshfeghi DM. Declining incidence of neonatal endophthalmitis in the United States. *Am J Ophthalmol* 2011; 151:59–65.
54. Benjamin Jr DK, Poole C, Steinbach WJ, Rowen JL, Walsh TJ. Neonatal candidemia and end-organ damage: a critical appraisal of the literature using meta-analytic techniques. *Pediatrics* 2003; 112:634–640.
55. Baley JE, Ellis FJ. Neonatal candidiasis: ophthalmologic infection. *Semin Perinatol* 2003; 27:401–405.
56. Rodriguez D, Almirante B, Park BJ, et al; Barcelona Candidemia Project Study Group. Candidemia in neonatal intensive care units: Barcelona, Spain. *Pediatr Infect Dis J* 2006; 25:224–229.
57. Lohrer R, Belohradsky BH. Bacterial endophthalmitis in neonates. *Eur J Pediatr* 1987; 146:354–359.
58. Burns RP, Rhodes Jr DH. Pseudomonas eye infection as a cause of death in premature infants. *Arch Ophthalmol* 1961; 65:517–525.
59. Greene GR, Carroll WL, Morozumi PA, Ching FC. Endophthalmitis associated with group-B streptococcal meningitis in an infant. *Am J Dis Child* 1979; 133:752–753.
60. Berger BB. Endophthalmitis complicating neonatal group B streptococcal septicemia. *Am J Ophthalmol* 1981; 92:681–684.
61. McCourt EA, Hink EM, Durairaj VD, Oliver SC. Isolated group B streptococcal endogenous endophthalmitis simulating retinoblastoma or persistent fetal vasculature in a healthy full-term infant. *J AAPOS* 2010; 14:352–355.
62. Robb RM. Congenital nasolacrimal duct obstruction. *Ophthalmol Clin North Am* 2001; 14:443–446.
63. Tan AD, Rubin PA, Sutula FC, Remulla HD. Congenital nasolacrimal duct obstruction. *Int Ophthalmol Clin* 2001; 41:57–69.
64. MacEwen CJ, Young JDH. Epiphora during the first year of life. *Eye* 1991; 5:596–600.
65. Kushner BJ. Congenital nasolacrimal system obstruction. *Arch Ophthalmol* 1982; 100:597–600.
66. Kim YS, Moon SC, Yoo KW. Congenital nasolacrimal duct obstruction: irrigation or probing? *Korean J Ophthalmol* 2000; 14:90–96.
67. Young JD, MacEwen CJ, Ogston SA. Congenital nasolacrimal duct obstruction in the second year of life: a multicentre trial of management. *Eye* 1996; 10:485–491.
68. Loh FC, Ling SY. Acute osteomyelitis of the maxilla in the newborn. *J Laryngol* 1993; 107:627–628.
69. Cruz AA, Mussi-Pinhata MM, Akaishi PM, Cattebeke L, Torrano da Silva J, Elia Jr J. Neonatal orbital abscess. *Ophthalmology* 2001; 108:2316–2320.
70. Kikkawa DO, Heinz GW, Martin RT, Nunery WN, Eiseman AS. Orbital cellulitis and abscess secondary to dacryocystitis. *Arch Ophthalmol* 2002; 120:1096–1099.

CHAPTER 13
Skin and soft tissue infections

The skin may be involved as follows.
- The primary site of bacterial infection, as in cellulitis, impetigo, furunculosis, paronychia and staphylococcal scalded skin syndrome
- A manifestation or complication of underlying bacteraemia or fungaemia and rarely endocarditis, as with some pustular embolic rashes (Figure 3.1), subcutaneous abscesses, petechiae, purpura, ecchymoses or vasculitic lesions
- A complication of surgical procedures, as in wound infections
- A manifestation of congenital and viral infections (see Chapters 17 and 18).

Soft tissue infections can be primary or may be collections that drained from lymph nodes in pyogenic or mycobacterial infection, from bone in osteomyelitis (Figure 13.1b and see Chapter 9), from muscle in pyomyositis, or rarely from organs, such as a renal abscess.

13.1 Host and environmental factors

The neonate may be exposed to skin trauma during delivery, through mechanical pressure (e.g. cephalhaematoma) or instrumentation (e.g. forceps, ventouse, scalp electrodes). The skin of extremely pre-term neonates is fragile and easily damaged and a potential source of infection. The use of skin barrier therapy to prevent infections is discussed in Section 23.3.2. The umbilical cord represents a potential source of infection, preventable with good umbilical cord care (see Section 23.3.1). For infants needing neonatal intensive care, the skin barrier is broken for vascular access and sometimes for invasive procedures such as chest drains.

Surgical procedures including male circumcision can become infected. In the past, the *moel* who performed ritual Jewish circumcisions achieved haemostasis by sucking the end of the penis, which was not infrequently associated with transmission of *Mycobacterium tuberculosis*.[1] Tuberculosis of the penis associated with circumcision still occurs rarely.[2] Other infections associated with circumcision include bacterial infections due to *Staphylococcus aureus*, GBS, fungal infections[3] and acute infections with HSV and *Treponema pallidum*.[4–6] Interestingly, although HSV and syphilis were sometimes acquired at the time of circumcision historically, circumcision actually protects against the acquisition of HSV-2 infection and syphilis later in life.[7] Circumcision also protects against urinary tract infections (see Chapter 10),[8] HIV infection[9] and probably against human papillomavirus (HPV) infections.[10, 11]

Male newborn infants are more susceptible than female infants to colonization with *S. aureus* and to develop infections.[12, 13] A review of studies found that males were about 50% more likely than females to develop staphylococcal skin lesions.[13]

13.2 Organism factors

Some organisms have a predilection for causing skin and soft infections, of which the commonest by far is *S. aureus*.[14–16] MRSA is associated with skin and soft tissue infections in children and adults, notably the USA 300 clone in North America which has been associated with community-acquired MRSA infections.[17] Some reports suggest MRSA does not cause more skin and soft tissue infections than methicillin-sensitive *S. aureus* in neonates.[14–16] However, these studies were either under-powered or did not

Evidence-Based Neonatal Infections, First Edition. David Isaacs.

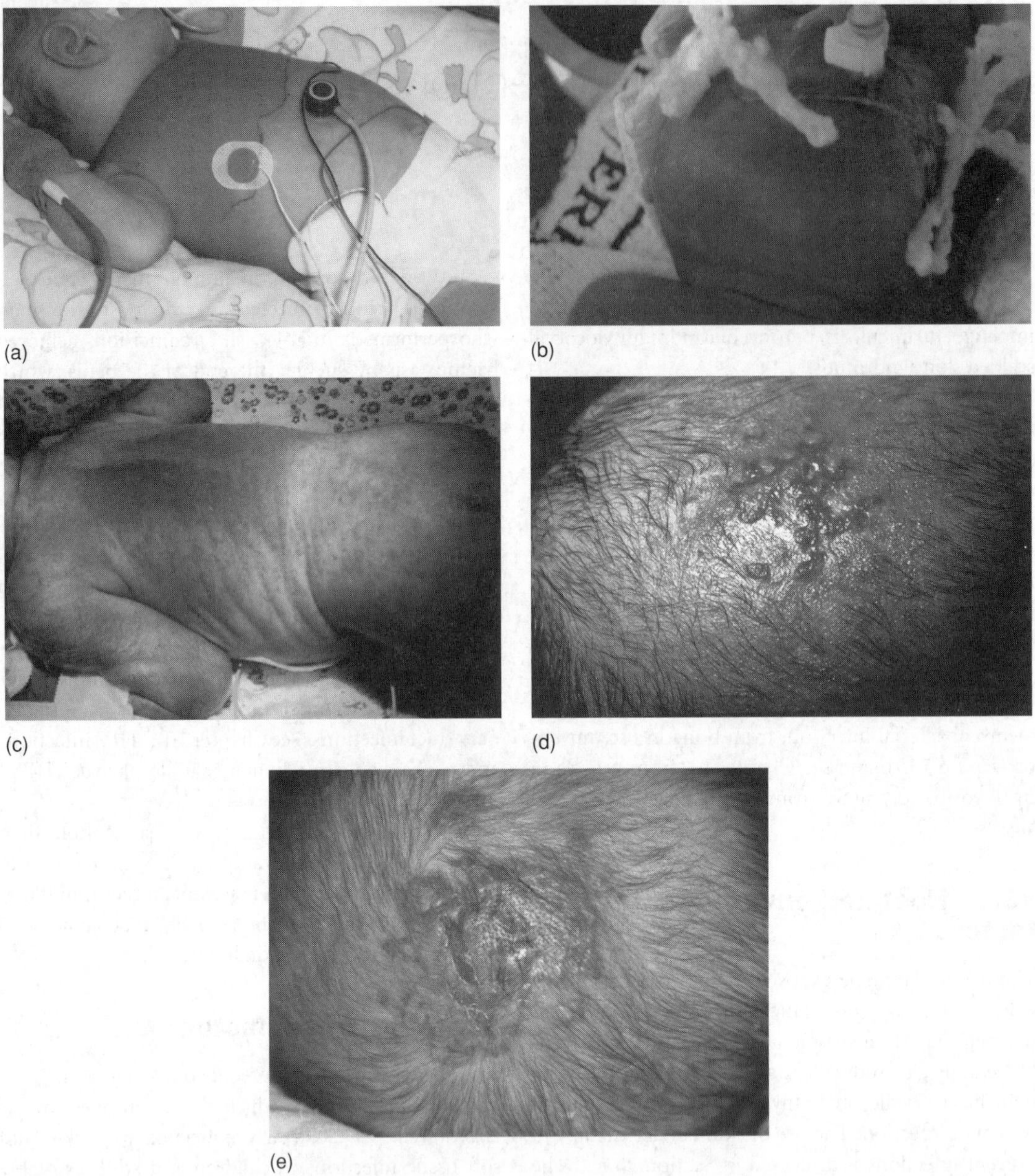

Figure 13.1 (a) Group A streptococcal (GAS) cellulitis and bacteraemia in 4-day-old term baby who made complete recovery. (b) Group B streptococcal (GBS) facial cellulitis-adenitis in a 32-week-gestation infant aged 20 days, showing right mandibular oedema and redness with central clearing. Reprinted from Reference 26 with permission. (c) Cellulitis. Congenital candidiasis in 32-week-gestation twin presenting day 3 with florid pustulo-vesicular, markedly pruritic truncal rash, with diffuse, patchy erythroderma. Reprinted from Reference 32 with permission. (d) Herpes simplex virus (HSV) cellulitis at the site of scalp electrode: discrete punched out lesions starting to coalesce. (e) HSV cellulitis at the site of scalp electrode: lesions have coalesced making diagnosis difficult.

distinguish hospital-acquired from community-acquired MRSA.[14–16] Hospital-acquired MRSA typically caused isolated cases or epidemics of septicaemia in neonatal units associated with respiratory and gastrointestinal colonization without significant skin and soft tissue infections.[18] A report from Texas showed increasing numbers of community-acquired *S. aureus* infections in previously healthy term and near-term neonates, with 61 of 89 infections (68.5%) caused by MRSA and 86.5% involving skin and soft tissue.[19] Almost all the MRSA belonged to the USA 300 clone and were positive for the Panton–Valentine leukocidin (PVL) gene, which has been associated with skin and soft tissue infections and more severe invasive diseases.[19] If PVL-producing MRSA (and MSSA strains which can also carry the PVL gene) become more prevalent in the community, the incidence of skin and soft tissue infections will probably increase.[20]

Other organisms known to be associated with skin and soft tissue infections include GBS, which can cause neonatal cellulitis, and organisms associated with cellulitis in older children and adults but only rarely in neonates such as GAS (Figure 13.1a).

13.3 Epidemiology

Definitions of skin infections lack precision and epidemiologic data on skin infections are not always reported with precision. Furthermore, some infants with skin infections do not present until after discharge from hospital. The rarity of GAS and *Haemophilus influenzae* type b (Hib) skin infections in neonates is presumably due to uncommon exposure, although it is also possible that the host immune response contributes to the cellulitis and that neonates are protected against cellulitis by the relative immaturity of their immune response.

13.4 Clinical manifestations

13.4.1 Cellulitis

Cellulitis is a diffuse, spreading skin infection, and the term should exclude infections associated with underlying suppurative foci, such as cutaneous abscesses, necrotizing fasciitis, septic arthritis and osteomyelitis.[21] Spreading, tender erythema may be associated with one or more of fever, lymphangitis, lymphadenopathy and systemic toxicity. As the rash progresses, blistering may occur.[21] Cellulitis is rarely reported in the neonatal period and the presence of cellulitis should always alert the clinician to the possibility of underlying osteomyelitis or septic arthritis (see Figure 9.5b). Orbital cellulitis can be the presentation of underlying ethmoid osteomyelitis,[22] while maxillary osteomyelitis can mimic orbital cellulitis.[23]

Cellulitis due to GBS is characteristically facial submandibular cellulitis with associated adenitis.[24–26] This is a late-onset manifestation of GBS commonly associated with GBS bacteraemia and presenting at a mean age of onset of five weeks with marked local swelling and erythema (Figure 13.1b), poor feeding and irritability. In one report, four of five infants with facial or submandibular GBS cellulitis had ipsilateral otitis media at the time of admission and the authors postulated that primary otitis media with subsequent lymphatic spread to facial or submandibular areas could be the pathogenesis. GBS can cause cellulitis elsewhere, including the inguinal region.[27]

GAS is an occasional cause of neonatal cellulitis (Figure 13.1a),[28] including facial cellulitis: in one series of streptococcal facial cellulitis, five of six cases were due to GBS and the other due to GAS.[25] Hib can cause a vesicular eruption at birth although not the classical facial cellulitis of older children, which is often buccal or peri-orbital.[29] Gram-negative bacilli are rare causes of cellulitis: one of 14 infants with Serratia infections secondary to contaminated shampoo had cellulitis.[30] Other organisms reported to cause occasional cases of cellulitis are Candida which can cause burn-like truncal erythema (Figure 13.1c)[31, 32] as well as more classic rashes in diaper and intertriginous areas, and anaerobes which can be found in scalp cellulitis secondary to scalp electrodes.[33]

Cellulitis of the scalp secondary to scalp electrodes may be due to HSV, (see Chapter 17) even if there is bacterial secondary infection.[34, 35] HSV cellulitis is characterized by discrete punched out lesions (Figure 13.1d) which may coalesce and become secondarily infected making the diagnosis difficult (Figure 13.1e). The diagnosis is a vital one because of the danger of rapid dissemination of HSV.

Cellulitis of the abdomen should alert the physician to a possible diagnosis of necrotizing fasciitis (Section 13.4.2). Empiric treatment of cellulitis should include both anti-staphylococcal and Gram-negative cover given parenterally until blood culture results are back because of the relatively high rate of associated bacteraemia. US clinicians often suggest aspirating the leading edge of an area of cellulitis after infusing saline subcutaneously.

13.4.2 Necrotizing fasciitis and myonecrosis

Necrotizing skin and soft-tissue infections are deeper than cellulitis and may involve the fascial compartment (necrotizing fasciitis) or the muscle compartment (myonecrosis).[21] They cause major tissue destruction and have a high mortality. Extensive necrosis is called gangrene.[21]

A review of the world literature in 1999 yielded 66 cases of neonatal necrotizing fasciitis.[36] Only 3 infants were pre-term. Underlying conditions that might have contributed to the development of necrotizing fasciitis included omphalitis (47 or 71%), breast abscess (5), balanitis (4), foetal scalp monitoring (2), necrotizing enterocolitis (1), immune deficiency (1) and bullous impetigo (1). The most common site was the abdominal wall (53 or 80%), followed by the thorax (7), back (2), scalp (2) and extremity (2). The initial skin presentation ranged from a minimal rash to erythema, oedema, induration or cellulitis and spread was characteristically rapid. The overlying skin appearance was variously described as violaceous, *peau d'orange*, bullae or necrosis. Crepitus was rare. Pain, which is typical of the disease in older children and adults, was hard to evaluate. Fever and tachycardia were common but not invariable. Most infants had neutrophil leukocytosis and half had thrombocytopenia. Of the 53 wound cultures available for bacteriologic evaluation, 13 had a pure growth of one organism, 39 were polymicrobial and one was sterile. Among the 39 specimens with polymicrobial infections, the predominant aerobic bacteria were *S. aureus*, *Escherichia coli* and enterococci, and the predominant anaerobes were *Clostridium* and *Bacteroides*. *S. aureus* was the most common organism recovered from the wound cultures with one organism. Blood culture was performed in 40 cases and was positive in half, 15 with a single organism, and 5 polymicrobial. There were 13 episodes of bacteraemia caused by organisms identical to those found in the wound cultures. Two blood cultures and one wound culture grew *Candida*. The mortality rate was 59% (39 of 66). Twelve of the 27 survivors needed skin grafting because of poor healing or large post-operative skin defects.[36] A later case was associated with a PVL-producing strain of methicillin-sensitive *S. aureus*.[37]

13.4.3 Omphalitis

S. aureus has caused nursery outbreaks of skin infections (bullous impetigo) and umbilical infection (omphalitis) in the United States[38] and United Kingdom[39] since at least the 1920s. The introduction of skin and umbilical cord care using antiseptics and topical antibiotics to the cord in the 1960s and 1970s was associated with a marked reduction in staphylococcal skin infections and omphalitis. A sequential US study[40] showed that staphylococcal colonization and infection were low when babies had total body bathing with 3% hexachlorophene but increased dramatically (80% colonization, 9.5% infection) when hexachlorophene was discontinued and replaced by Ivory Soap baths. Reinstitution of hexachlorophene reduced colonization and infection, although not to the initial low levels. A second Ivory Soap period (period 4) was associated with a return to high rates of colonization (77%) and infection (11.5%). Subsequently, when daily Ivory Soap baths were continued but topical bacitracin ointment was applied regularly to the umbilicus, colonization fell to 10% and infection to 3%. Colonization with Gram-negative enteric bacilli was highest while using hexachlorophene or Ivory bacitracin, but there was no increase in Gram-negative infections.[40] Triple dye (brilliant green, proflavine hemisulphate, and crystal violet in aqueous solution) once widely used was effective against *S. aureus* but less effective against Gram-negative organisms.[41] A 6 year study of infected umbilical stumps in the 1970s found an infection rate of 0.7% (200 of 27 107 infants) with Gram-negative organisms ($n = 171$) isolated more often than Gram-positive ($n = 118$).[42]

More recently, the need for umbilical cord care in Western countries has been questioned because of concerns about toxicity of topical agents, resistance and improvements in infection control which make nosocomial transmission less likely. Many institutions changed to dry cord care and non-antiseptic whole-body baths although there was no prior strong evidence for or against this change. One institution reported three cases of omphalitis following such a change (Figure 13.2).[43] An RCT compared antiseptic care with dry care.[44] Newborns were randomly allocated to either

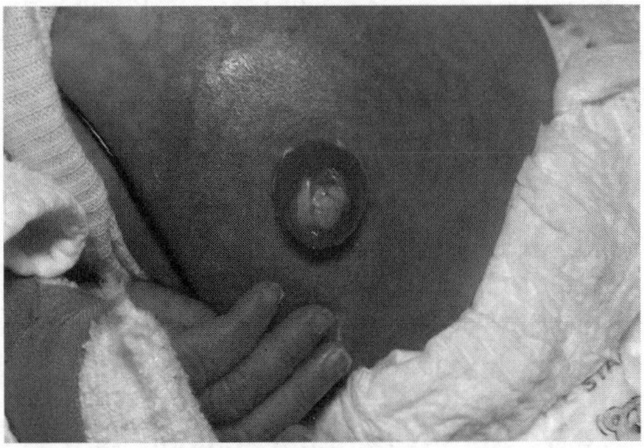

Figure 13.2 Severe omphalitis with abdominal wall cellulitis

two applications of triple dye to the umbilical cord stump on the day of birth plus twice daily alcohol swabbing until the cord fell off ($n = 384$) or to dry care ($n = 382$) which consisted of cleaning the peri-umbilical area with soap and water, wiping it with a dry cotton swab or cloth and allowing it to dry in the air. No infants in the triple dye group and one in the dry care group developed omphalitis. Infants in the dry care group were significantly more likely to be colonized with *S. aureus* (31.3% vs 2.8%) and with *E. coli*, CoNS and GBS. Community health nurses visiting infants at home were significantly more likely to report exudate and foul odour in infants in the dry care group.[44] A Cochrane systematic review of umbilical cord care found 21 studies ($n = 8959$) mostly in high income countries.[45] Antiseptics significantly reduced colonization with *S. aureus* by about half, but there were no systemic infections in any infants and no deaths. Umbilical infection was rare (about 1%) and not reported in most of the studies. Antiseptic cord care compared with dry cord care was associated with a non-significant but almost 50% reduction in umbilical infection (9 of 1431 vs 18 of 1400, RR 0.53, 95% CI 0.25, 1.13).[45]

Omphalitis is a far greater problem in developing countries and there is much stronger evidence that umbilical cord care reduces omphalitis and all-cause mortality[46–48] (see Section 23.3.1). The reported incidence of omphalitis varies hugely with how cases are found and how omphalitis is defined. A hospital-based study from a special care baby unit in Oman reported an incidence of 1.8%,[49] whereas a Pakistani study that used community health workers to diagnose cases found an incidence of 21.7%.[50] In both countries *S. aureus* was the major pathogen, predominantly methicillin sensitive. In Pakistan the next most common pathogens were GAS and GBS, then Pseudomonas, Aeromonas and Klebsiella; in Oman *E. coli* and Klebsiella predominated.[49, 50]

The treatment of omphalitis should be with parenteral antibiotics guided by cultures of the umbilicus and blood. Empiric regimens should include Gram positive including staphylococcal cover and Gram-negative cover. The choice will depend on local prevalence of MRSA and resistance patterns to Gram negatives (see Chapter 5).

13.4.4 Impetigo

Impetigo or *impetigo contagiosa* is a contagious, superficial, bacterial skin infection (Figures 13.3a and 13.3b).[51] Like staphylococcal scalded skin syndrome, impetigo is mediated by exfoliative toxins causing blistering which affects only the superficial epidermis and heals without scarring.[52, 53] Impetigo is often classified as bullous or non-bullous, although these may be matters of degree. Bullous impetigo means the skin eruption is mainly bullae (blisters) which often affect the trunk, although they may occur elsewhere (Figure 13.3a). The bullae contain purulent material with organisms and leukocytes and may rupture leaving red, scaly, circular lesions (Figure 13.3b). Non-bullous impetigo commonly affects the face and limbs and is characterized by thin-walled vesicles which rupture easily leaving superficial erosions covered with yellow or honey-coloured crusts that resolve to leave a red lesion. The term 'impetigo contagiosa' is sometimes used to denote non-bullous impetigo, and at other times it is used to mean all impetigo.[51]

In neonates, impetigo is more commonly due to *S. aureus* than GAS or GBS, whereas in older children Group A streptococci are the commonest cause.[51] Neonatal impetigo needs to be distinguished from other causes of bullous lesions: in a study of 44 neonates with vesico-bullous lesions in India, only 4 had impetigo, 2 with *S. aureus* and 2 with GAS[54] and there was a wide range of other diagnoses including erythema toxicum.

For impetigo in older children and adults, topical antibiotics are as effective as oral antibiotics and more effective than placebo,[51] but there are no data

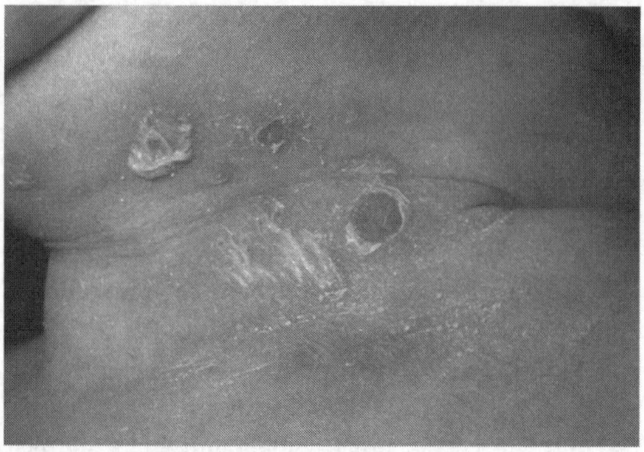

(a)

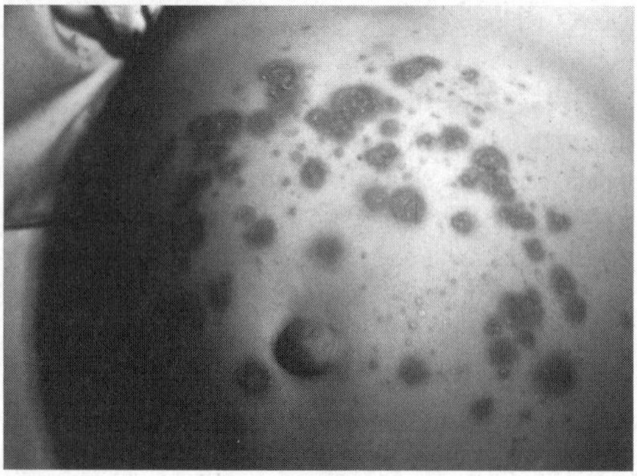

(b)

Figure 13.3 (a) Bullous impetigo due to *Staphylococcus aureus* with blisters filled with yellow purulent fluid. (b) Bullous impetigo due to *Staphylococcus aureus* with burst blisters.

in neonates. However, neonates with skin sepsis are far more likely than older children to develop bacteraemia. A 5-year retrospective US hospital-based study identified 126 cases of community-acquired staphylococcal skin sepsis in term and pre-term neonates, of whom 6 (5%) had bacteraemia.[55] If there is any concern about systemic toxicity, including fever or soft signs of possible sepsis, it is safest to treat with IV antibiotics until blood culture results are back.[55, 56]

Nursery outbreaks of staphylococcal bullous impetigo have been described in association with one or more staff who are nasal carriers.[57, 58] If an apparent nursery outbreak does not respond to enhanced infection control measures and is shown by molecular techniques to be caused by a common strain, it may be necessary to screen staff for nasal carriage and to try to eradicate any carriage, for example with nasal mupirocin.

A double-blind placebo-controlled RCT in Bangladesh tested the hypothesis that maternal zinc deficiency might predispose to impetigo in infancy. Zinc supplementation during pregnancy halved the risk of and the incidence of impetigo in the first 6 months.[59] Zinc was most effective in growth restricted or low birth-weight infants and in those with low socioeconomic status.[59]

13.4.5 Staphylococcal scalded skin syndrome

Neonatal staphylococcal scalded skin syndrome (SSSS) is rare, but can be caused by methicillin-sensitive *S. aureus* and MRSA, can occur in term and pre-term neonates,[60] can cause nursery outbreaks[61, 62] and can be associated with fatal staphylococcal septicaemia.[60] The neonatal form, first described in infants in 1878 by Ritter Van Rittershain, is sometimes called Ritter's disease. SSSS is caused predominantly by phage group 2 staphylococci and like bullous impetigo (Section 13.4.4) is induced by staphylococcal exfoliative toxins. These are serine proteases that cause epidermolysis by interfering with the function of desmogleins, trans-membrane glycoproteins that mediate cell-to-cell adhesion of keratinocytes. The toxins cause blistering restricted to the superficial epidermis that heals without scarring.[52, 53]

Infants characteristically present with no or low-grade fever and with erythematous patches on the face and body which progress rapidly within a day to blister and desquamate. The underlying skin is red and tender and resembles a scald (Figures 13.4a and 13.4b). Nikolsky's sign (gentle rubbing of the skin causes desquamation) is positive. Mucous membranes are not involved. The skin surface is often sterile but *S. aureus* can usually be isolated from nose swab, nasopharyngeal or endotracheal aspirates or from conjunctival swabs, and sometimes from blood.[60]

Treatment is with parenteral anti-staphylococcal antibiotics (see Section 14.1.2.1), pain relief and fluid resuscitation as necessary. There is no evidence that intravenous immunoglobulins help, although their use has sometimes been advocated.[60] Descriptions of the use of special skin dressings[63] are difficult to interpret because of the natural history of healing without scarring.

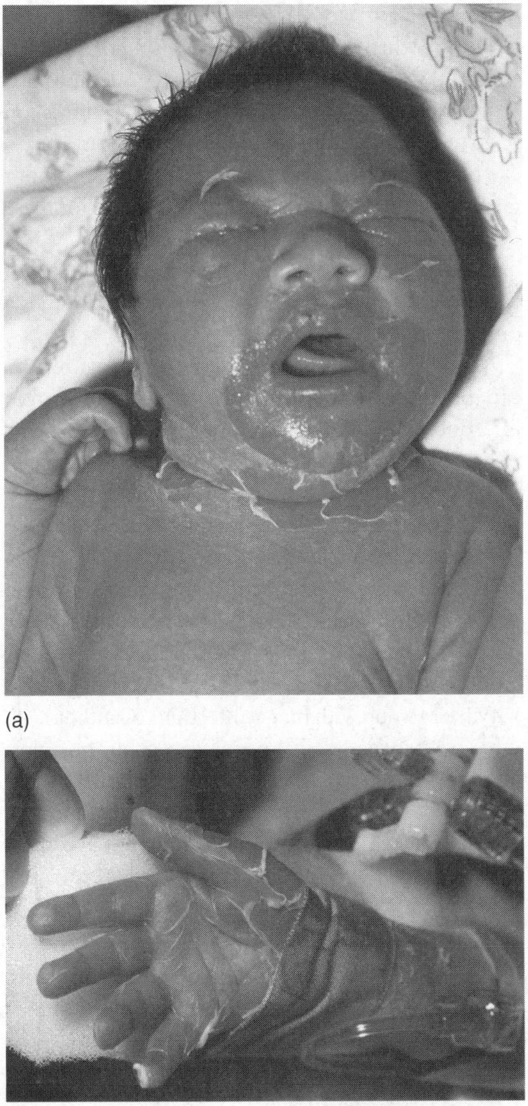

(a)

(b)

Figure 13.4 (a) Staphylococcal scalded skin syndrome: face and neck. (b) Staphylococcal scalded skin syndrome: hand with skin desquamation and underlying erythema.

13.4.6 Toxic shock syndrome

There are anecdotal reports of infants with features consistent with toxic shock syndrome, in association with the production of staphylococcal toxic shock syndrome toxin (TSST). A Japanese group reported 20 neonates with widespread exanthema and thrombocytopenia in association with MRSA strains which produced toxic shock syndrome toxin-1 (TSST-1).[64] Two of the Japanese cohort died.[64] They subsequently gave this syndrome the name neonatal toxic shock syndrome-like erythematous disease (NTED),[65] although the infants appeared to fulfil classic criteria for toxic shock syndrome. A nationwide Japanese survey identified 540 neonates with NTED over a 10-year period.[66] The frequency was decreasing. No term infants developed shock or died but pre-term infants sometimes developed severe symptoms.[66] Surprisingly, there have been no reports from outside Japan, which suggests under-recognition, under-reporting or a surprising restriction of this syndrome to Japan.

13.4.7 Skin abscess

Skin abscesses can be florid abscesses involving the nails (paronychia Figure 13.5), breast (Figure 13.6) or may come in the form of showers of small abscesses (sometimes called pustulosis, Figure 13.7). The general rule is to obtain purulent material for Gram stain and

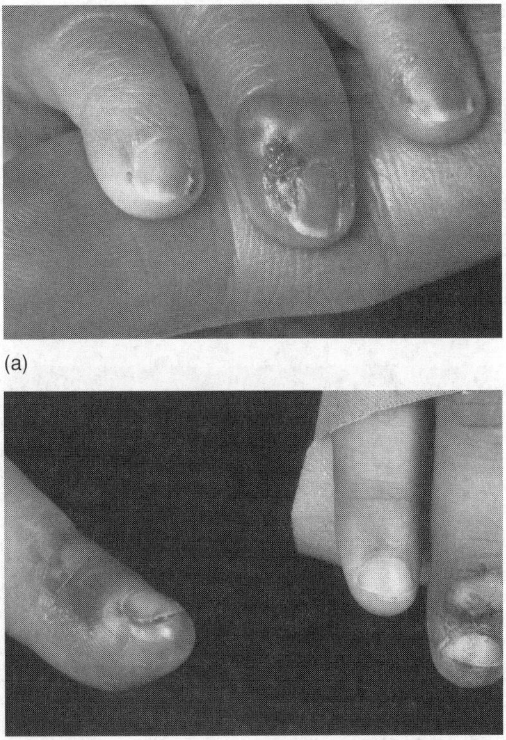

(a)

(b)

Figure 13.5 (a) Paronychia due to *Staphylococcus aureus.* (b) Herpetic whitlow, easily mistaken for paronychia.

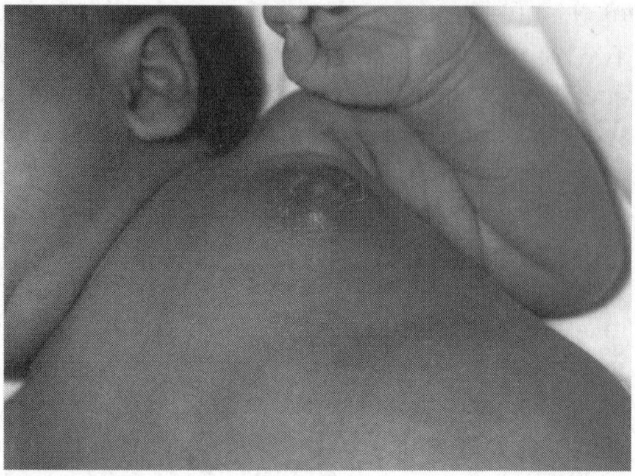

Figure 13.6 Breast abscess due to *Staphylococcus aureus*.

culture because, although *S. aureus* is the commonest organism by far, it is important to distinguish MSSA from MRSA and to diagnose other organisms which occasionally cause skin abscesses.

Paronychia (Figure 13.5a) are usually caused by *S. aureus*, but occasionally by Group A or B streptococci. Herpetic whitlow (Figure 13.5b) caused by HSV, which is more characteristic of older infants and children, can mimic paronychia and can occur in the neonatal period. It is a critical differential diagnosis not to miss because of the risk of disseminated HSV infection if untreated (see Chapter 17).[67] If attempts to obtain pus from a paronychia are unsuccessful, the possibility of herpetic whitlow should be considered.

Breast abscesses are usually caused by *S. aureus*, but occasionally by other organisms including Gram-negative bacilli.[68–71] MRSA breast abscesses occurring in both mother and infant have been reported.[72] The terms mastitis and breast abscess are sometimes used synonymously and sometimes the term mastitis is confined to inflammation without pus formation. The two can be distinguished by ultrasound,[73] which is important when considering incision and drainage for therapeutic and diagnostic purposes.[74] In a US hospital-based case series, 16 of 20 patients with staphylococcal mastitis were managed with oral antibiotics as outpatients.[55]

Neonatal pustulosis due to infection (Figure 13.7) can be difficult to distinguish from benign non-infectious conditions including erythema toxicum, milia and neonatal acne.[75] In a series of 126 children with community-acquired neonatal staphylococcal infections, 43 had pustulosis and none of these had positive blood cultures. However, 31 (72%) of the 43 were treated with empiric intravenous anti-staphylococcal antibiotics.[55] Pustulosis has been described with congenital Listeria infection (usually septicaemic), with herpetic virus infections (HSV, VZV), CMV and with fungal infections (Candida).[75, 76] It has been suggested that neonatal cephalic pustulosis might be caused by one or other species of Malassezia, but case-control studies found Malassezia colonization normally increases with age and as common in controls as cases.[77, 78]

13.4.8 Vasculitic lesions

Vasculitis or inflammation of blood vessels may affect capillaries, small vessels or arteries. It often results in

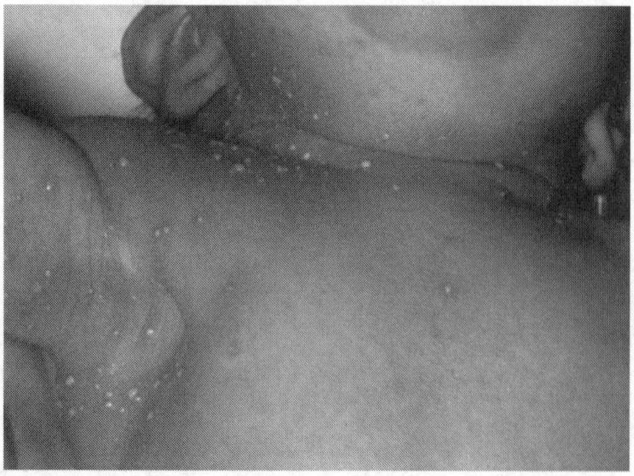

Figure 13.7 Neonatal pustulosis: multiple small micro-abscesses (due to *Staphylococcus aureus* in this case).

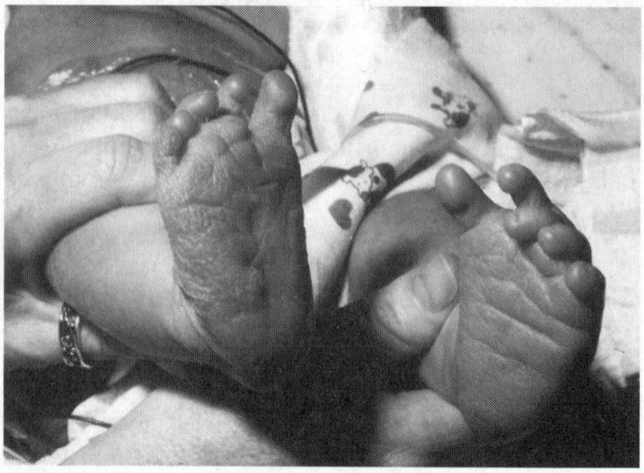

Figure 13.8 Vasculitic necrotic lesions on feet secondary to bacterial endocarditis.

palpable purpura, red, purple or black necrotic haemorrhagic macules, papules and plaques, but a range of morphologies may occur including urticated plaques, nodules and ulcers. Vasculitic lesions are unusual in the neonatal period and usually occur as a result of maternal auto-immune disease.[79–81] However, they can rarely be seen as an embolic feature of bacteraemia, particularly caused by *S. aureus* endovasculitis[82] or infective endocarditis (Figure 13.8).[83]

References

1. Speert H. Neonatal circumcision. *ObstetGynecol* 1953; 2:164–172.
2. Howell AJ, Cummins G, Isaacs D. Inguinal lymph nodes and penile lesions after circumcision. *Pediatr Infect Dis J* 2009; 28:344–347.
3. Aridogan IA, Izol V, Ilkit M. Superficial fungal infections of the male genitalia: a review. *Crit Rev Microbiol* 2011; 37:237–244.
4. Circumcision policy statement. American Academy of Pediatrics. Task Force on Circumcision. *Pediatrics* 1999; 103:686–693.
5. Lerman SE, Liao JC. Neonatal circumcision. *PediatrClin North Am* 2001; 48:1539–1557.
6. Perera CL, Bridgewater FH, Thavaneswaran P, Maddern GJ. Safety and efficacy of nontherapeutic male circumcision: a systematic review. *Ann Fam Med* 2010; 8:64–72.
7. Weiss HA, Thomas SL, Munabi SK, Hayes RJ. Male circumcision and risk of syphilis, chancroid, and genital herpes: a systematic review and meta-analysis. *Sex Transm Infect* 2006; 82:101–109.
8. Singh-Grewal D, Macdessi J, Craig J. Circumcision for the prevention of urinary tract infection in boys: a systematic review of randomised trials and observational studies. *Arch Dis Child* 2005; 90:853–858.
9. Wiysonge CS, Kongnyuy EJ, Shey M, Muula AS, Navti OB, Akl EA, Lo YR. Male circumcision for prevention of homosexual acquisition of HIV in men. *Cochrane Database Syst Rev* 2011, Issue 6. Art. No.: CD007496. doi:10.1002/14651858.CD007496.pub2.
10. Larke N, Thomas SL, Dos Santos Silva I, Weiss HA. Male circumcision and human papillomavirus infection in men: a systematic review and meta-analysis *J Infect Dis* 2011; 204:1375–1390.
11. Albero G, Castellsagué X, Giuliano AR, Bosch FX. Male circumcision and genital human papillomavirus: a systematic review and meta-analysis. *Sex Transm Dis* 2012; 39:104–113.
12. Thompson DJ, Gezon HM, Hatch TF, Rycheck RR, Rogers KD. Sex distribution of *Staphylococcus aureus* colonization and disease in newborn infant. *N Engl J Med* 1963; 269:337–341.
13. Thompson DJ, Gezon HM, Rogers KD, Yee RB, Hatch TF. Excess risk of staphylococcal infection and disease in newborn males. *Am J Epidemiol* 1966; 84:314–328.
14. Chuang YY, Huang YC, Lee CY, Lin TY, Lien R, Chou YH. Methicillin-resistant *Staphylococcus aureus* bacteraemia in neonatal intensive care units: an analysis of 90 episodes. *ActaPaediatr* 2004; 93:786–790.
15. Kuint J, Barzilai A, Regev-Yochay G, Rubinstein E, Keller N, Maayan-Metzger A. Comparison of community-acquired methicillin-resistant *Staphylococcus aureus* bacteremia to other staphylococcal species in a neonatal intensive care unit. *Eur J Pediatr* 2007; 166:319–325.
16. Carey AJ, Duchon J, Della-Latta P, Saiman L. The epidemiology of methicillin-susceptible and methicillin-resistant *Staphylococcus aureus* in a neonatal intensive care unit, 2000-2007. *J Perinatol* 2010; 30:135–139.
17. Carey AJ, Long SS. Staphylococcus aureus: a continuously evolving and formidable pathogen in the neonatal intensive care unit. *ClinPerinatol* 2010; 37:535–546.
18. King MD, Humphrey BJ, Wang YF, Kourbatova EV, Ray SM, Blumberg HM. Emergence of community-acquired methicillin-resistant *Staphylococcus aureus* USA 300 clone as the predominant cause of skin and soft-tissue infections. *Ann Intern Med* 2006; 144:309–317.
19. Fortunov RM, Hulten KG, Hammerman WA, Mason Jr EO, Kaplan SL.Community-acquired *Staphylococcus aureus* infections in term and near-term previously healthy neonates. *Pediatrics* 2006; 118:874–881.
20. Wu D, Wang Q, Yang Y, et al. Epidemiology and molecular characteristics of community-associated methicillin-resistant and methicillin-susceptible Staphylococcus aureus from skin/soft tissue infections in a children's hospital in Beijing, China. *DiagnMicrobiol Infect Dis* 2010; 67: 1–8.
21. Stevens DL, Bisno AL, Chambers HF, et al.; Infectious Diseases Society of America. Practice guidelines for the diagnosis and management of skin and soft-tissue infections. *Clin Infect Dis* 2005; 41:1373–1406.
22. Cruz AA, Mussi-Pinhata MM, Akaishi PM, Cattebeke L, Torrano da Silva J, Elia Jr J. Neonatal orbital abscess. *Ophthalmology* 2001; 108:2316–2320.
23. Loh FC, Ling SY. Acute osteomyelitis of the maxilla in the newborn. *J Laryngol* 1993; 107:627–628.
24. Patamasucon P, Seigel JD, McCracken Jr GH. Streptococcal submandibular cellulitis in young infants. *Pediatrics* 1981; 67:378–380.
25. Baker CJ. Group B streptococcal cellulitis-adenitis in infants. *Am J Dis Child* 1982; 136:631–633.
26. Chakkarapani E, Bill Yoxall C, Morgan C. Facial submandibular cellulitis-adenitis in a preterm infant. *Arch Dis Child Fetal Neonatal Ed* 2007; 92:F153.
27. Doedens RA, Miedema CJ, Oetomo SB, Kimpen JL. Atypical cellulitis due to group B streptococcus. *Scand J Infect Dis* 1995; 27:399–400.
28. Martic J, Mijac V, Jankovic B, Sekulovic LK, Vasiljevic Z, Vuksanovic J. Neonatal cellulitis and sepsis caused by group A streptococcus. *PediatrDermatol* 2010; 27:528–530.
29. Halal F, Delorme L, Brazeau M, Ahronheim G. Congenital vesicular eruption caused by Haemophilusinfluenzae type b. *Pediatrics* 1978; 62:494–496.

30. Madani TA, Alsaedi S, James L, et al. Serratia marcescens-contaminated baby shampoo causing an outbreak among newborns at King Abdulaziz University Hospital, Jeddah, Saudi Arabia. *J Hosp Infect* 2011; 78:16–19.
31. Baley JE, Silverman RA. Systemic candidiasis: cutaneous manifestations in low birth weight infants. *Pediatrics* 1988; 82:211–215.
32. Carmo K, Evans N, Isaacs D. Congenital candidiasis presenting as septic shock without rash. *Arch Dis Child* 2007; 92:627–628.
33. Brook I. Anaerobic infections in children. *AdvExp Med Biol* 2011; 697:117–152.
34. Goldkrand JW. Intrapartum inoculation of herpes simplex virus by fetal scalp electrode. *ObstetGynecol* 1982; 59:263–265.
35. Overall Jr JC. Herpes simplex virus infection of the fetus and newborn. *Pediatr Ann* 1994; 23:131–136.
36. Hsieh WS, Yang PH, Chao HC, Lai JY. Neonatal necrotizing fasciitis: a report of three cases and review of the literature. *Pediatrics* 1999; 103:e53.
37. Dunlop RL, Eadie P. Idiopathic neonatal necrotising fasciitis caused by community-acquired MSSA encoding Panton Valentine Leukocidin genes. *J PlastReconstrAesthetSurg* 2011; 64:1522–1524.
38. Rulison ET. Control of impetigo neonatorum: advisability of a radical departure in obstetrical care. *J Am Med Assoc* 1929; 93:903–904.
39. Poole WH, Whittle CH. Epidemic pemphigus of the newly born. *Lancet* 1935; 225:1323–1327.
40. Johnson J, Malachowski N, Vosti K, Sunshine P. A sequential study of various modes of skin and umbilical care and the incidence of staphylococcal colonization and infection in the neonate. *Pediatrics* 1976;58:354–361.
41. Speck W, Driscoll J, O'Neil J, RosenKranz H. Effect of antiseptic cord care on bacterial colonization in the newborn infant. *Chemotherapy* 1980; 26:372–376.
42. McKenna H, Johnson D. Bacteria in neonatal omphalitis. *Pathology* 1977; 9:111–113.
43. Simon NP, Simon MW. Changes in newborn bathing practices may increase the risk for omphalitis. *ClinPediatr (Phila)* 2004; 43:763–767.
44. Janssen PA, Selwood BL, Dobson SR, Peacock D, Thiessen PN. To dye or not to dye: a randomized, clinical trial of a triple dye/alcohol regime versus dry cord care. *Pediatrics* 2003; 111:15–20.
45. Zupan J, Garner P, Omari AAA. Topical umbilical cord care at birth. *Cochrane Database Syst Rev* 2004, Issue 3. Art. No.: CD001057. doi:10.1002/14651858.CD001057.pub2.
46. Mullany LC, Darmstadt GL, Khatry SK, et al. Topical applications of chlorhexidine to the umbilical cord for prevention of omphalitis and neonatal mortality in southern Nepal: a community-based, cluster-randomised trial. *Lancet* 2006; 367:910–918.
47. Arifeen SE, Mullany LC, Shah R, et al. The effect of cord cleansing with chlorhexidine on neonatal mortality in rural Bangladesh: a community-based, cluster-randomised trial. *Lancet* 2012; 379:1022–1028.
48. Soofi S, Cousens S, Imdad A, Bhutto N, Ali N, Bhutta ZA. Topical application of chlorhexidine to neonatal umbilical cords for prevention of omphalitis and neonatal mortality in a rural district of Pakistan: a community-based, cluster-randomised trial. *Lancet* 2012; 379:1029–1036.
49. Sawardekar KP. Changing spectrum of neonatal omphalitis. *Pediatr Infect Dis J* 2004; 23:22–26.
50. Mir F, Tikmani SS, Shakoor S, et al. Incidence and etiology of omphalitis in Pakistan: a community-based cohort study. *J Infect DevCtries* 2011; 5:828–833.
51. Koning S, van der Sande R, Verhagen AP, et al. Interventions for impetigo. *Cochrane Database Syst Rev* 2012, (Issue 1). Art. No.: CD003261. doi:10.1002/14651858.CD003261.pub3.
52. Hanakawa Y, Schechter NM, Lin C, Garza L, Li H, Yamaguchi T, et al. Molecular mechanisms of blister formation in bullous impetigo and staphylococcal scalded skin syndrome. *J Clin Invest* 2002; 110:53–60.
53. Nishifuji K, Sugai M, Amagai M. Staphylococcal exfoliative toxins: "molecular scissors" of bacteria that attack the cutaneous defense barrier in mammals. *J DermatolSci* 2008; 49:21–31.
54. Tarang G, Anupam V. Incidence of vesicobullous and erosive disorders of neonates. *J Dermatol Case Rep* 2011; 5:58–63.
55. Fortunov RM, Hulten KG, Hammerman WA, Mason Jr EO, Kaplan SL. Evaluation and treatment of community-acquired Staphylococcus aureus infections in term and late-preterm previously healthy neonates. *Pediatrics* 2007; 120:937–945.
56. Johnston GA. Treatment of bullous impetigo and the staphylococcal scalded skin syndrome in infants. *Expert Rev Anti Infect Ther* 2004; 2:439–446.
57. Nakashima AK, Allen JR, Martone WJ, et al. Epidemic bullous impetigo in a nursery due to a nasal carrier of *Staphylococcus aureus*: role of epidemiology and control measures. *Infect Control* 1984; 5:326–331.
58. Belani A, Sherertz RJ, Sullivan ML, Russell BA, Reumen PD. Outbreak of staphylococcal infection in two hospital nurseries traced to a single nasal carrier. *Infect Control* 1986; 7:487–490.
59. Darmstadt GL, Osendarp SJ, Ahmed S, et al. Effect of antenatal zinc supplementation on impetigo in Bangladesh. *Pediatr Infect Dis J* 2012; 31:407–409.
60. Kapoor V, Travadi J, Braye S. Staphylococcal scalded skin syndrome in an extremely premature neonate: a case report with a brief review of literature. *J Paediatr Child Health* 2008; 44:374–376.
61. El Helali N, Carbonne A, Naas T, et al. Nosocomial outbreak of staphylococcal scalded skin syndrome in neonates: epidemiological investigation and control. *J Hosp Infect* 2005; 61:130–138.
62. Neylon O, O'Connell NH, Slevin B, et al. Neonatal staphylococcal scalded skin syndrome: clinical and outbreak containment review. *Eur J Pediatr* 2010; 169:1503–1509.
63. Baartmans MG, Dokter J, den Hollander JC, Kroon AA, Oranje AP. Use of skin substitute dressings in the treatment of staphylococcal scalded skin syndrome in neonates and young infants. *Neonatology* 2011; 100:9–13.

64. Takahashi N, Nishida H, Kato H, Imanishi K, Sakata Y, Uchiyama T.Exanthematous disease induced by toxic shock syndrome toxin 1 in the early neonatal period. *Lancet* 1998; 351:1614–1619.
65. Takahashi N. Neonatal toxic shock syndrome-like exanthematous disease (NTED). *PediatrInt* 2003; 45:233–237.
66. Takahashi N, Uehara R, Nishida H, et al. Clinical features of neonatal toxic shock syndrome-like exanthematous disease emerging in Japan. *J Infect* 2009; 59:194–200.
67. Jordan MB, Abramo TJ. Occurrence of herpetic whitlow in a twelve-day-old infant. *Pediatr Infect Dis J* 1994; 13:832–833.
68. Rudoy RC, Nelson JD. Breast abscess during the neonatal period. A review. *Am J Dis Child* 1975; 129:1031–1034.
69. Efrat M, Mogilner JG, Iujtman M, Eldemberg D, Kunin J, Eldar S. Neonatal mastitis - diagnosis and treatment. *Isr J Med Sci* 1995; 31:558–560.
70. Faden H. Mastitis in children from birth to 17 years. *Pediatr Infect Dis J* 2005; 24:1113.
71. Stricker T, Navratil F, Sennhauser FH. Mastitis in early infancy. *ActaPaediatr* 200; 94:166–169.
72. Montalto M, Lui B. MRSA as a cause of postpartum breast abscess in infant and mother. *J Hum Lact* 2009; 25:448–450.
73. Borders H, Mychaliska G, Gebarski KS. Sonographic features of neonatal mastitis and breast abscess. *PediatrRadiol* 2009; 39:955–958.
74. Turbey WJ, Buntain WL, Dudgeon DL. The surgical management of pediatric breast masses. *Pediatrics* 1975; 56:736–739.
75. Van Praag MC, Van Rooij RW, Folkers E, Spritzer R, Menke HE, Oranje AP. Diagnosis and treatment of pustular disorders in the neonate. *PediatrDermatol* 1997; 14:131–143.
76. Smolinski KN, Shah SS, Honig PJ, Yan AC. Neonatal cutaneous fungal infections. *CurrOpinPediatr* 2005; 17:486–493.
77. Niamba P, Weill FX, Sarlangue J, Labrèze C, Couprie B, Taïeh A. Is common neonatal cephalic pustulosis (neonatal acne) triggered by Malasseziasympodialis?. *Arch Dermatol* 1998; 134:995–998.
78. Ayhan M, Sancak B, Karaduman A, Arikan S, Sahin S. Colonization of neonate skin by Malassezia species: relationship with neonatal cephalic pustulosis. *J Am AcadDermatol* 2007; 57:1012–1018.
79. Neiman AR, Lee LA, Weston WL, Buyon JP. Cutaneous manifestations of neonatal lupus without heart block: characteristics of mothers and children enrolled in a national registry. *J Pediatr* 2000; 137:674–680.
80. Barr KL, O'Connell F, Wesson S, Vincek V. Nonbullous-neutrophilicdermatosis: sweet's syndrome, neonatal lupus erythematosus, or both?. *Mod Rheumatol* 2009; 19:212–215.
81. Gray PE, Bock V, Ziegler DS, Wargon O. Neonatal sweet syndrome: a potential marker of serious systemic illness. *Pediatrics* 2012; 129(5): e1353–e1359.
82. Abramovits W, Stevenson LC. Sweet's syndrome associated with Staphylococcus aureus. *Int J Dermatol.* 2004; 43:938–941.
83. Gould KP, Jones JD, Callen JP. Sweet's syndrome in a patient with enterococcal subacute bacterial endocarditis. *J Am AcadDermatol* 2004; 50:798–799.

CHAPTER 14
Bacterial infections

14.1 Gram-positive cocci

14.1.1 Group B streptococcus

In the nineteenth and early twentieth centuries, GAS were the major cause of puerperal and neonatal sepsis. *Streptococcus agalactiae*, the original name for GBS, was described in cattle as a cause of bovine mastitis and there is continued speculation whether human strains evolved from bovine strains. Rebecca Lancefield published her famous serologic classification of haemolytic streptococci in 1933.[1] The first description of human GBS infection was a 1938 report of three women with fatal puerperal sepsis.[2] Neonatal GBS infection was not reported until the late 1960s,[3] but was a recognized major problem by the early 1970s.[4]

14.1.1.1 Epidemiology of GBS infections

GBS occurs globally, although the incidence of infection varies with maternal colonization rates, organism virulence, low birth-weight incidence and intrapartum antibiotic use. The reported incidence is also affected by the completeness of case ascertainment, including the availability of optimal culture facilities. A systematic review and meta-analysis of global reports on GBS (8718 infants in 36 countries) reported the mean incidence of GBS infections in infants aged 0–89 days globally was 0.53 per 1000 live births and the incidence was almost twice as high in the first week (0.43 per 1000 live births) as subsequently (0.24).[5] The authors acknowledge that the true incidence is underestimated because of ascertainment difficulties. The reported incidence was highest in Africa (1.21 per 1000 live births) and the Americas (0.67), intermediate in Europe (0.57) and the Middle East/Eastern Mediterranean (0.35) and lowest in South-East Asia (0.02) and the Western Pacific (0.15 per 1000). The global mean case fatality was 9.6% and was almost twice as high in the first week (12.1%) as subsequently (6.8%).[5]

Serotype distribution was available for a small proportion of infections, mainly from high income countries. Five serotypes (Ia, Ib, II, III, V) accounted for more than 85% of serotypes and the distribution across WHO regions was largely similar. Serotype III was responsible for 37% of early-onset (<7 days) and 53% of late-onset infection, while the figures for serotype I were 40% and 30%, respectively.[5]

The reported incidence of GBS infection was not significantly different between countries whose gross national income was low or high, although there was a trend towards higher incidence (0.94 per 1000 live births) in the lowest income countries. The only variable strongly predictive of GBS risk was the proportion of infants positive for GBS who were low birth weight.[5] The increasing incidence of both early- and late-onset GBS infection with decreasing gestation and birth weight is well known, and is thought to be due at least in part to lower levels of protective maternal antibodies.

In a US case-control study of 90 infants with early-onset GBS infection (<7 days) and 489 controls, infected infants were more likely to be low birth weight, to have been delivered pre-term, or to have a mother with chorioamnionitis, intrapartum fever or premature rupture of the membranes. Intrauterine foetal monitoring was also associated with more than double the risk of neonatal GBS disease.[6] In a case-control study of 138 infants with GBS infection age <90 days in the United Kingdom, where intrapartum antibiotics were rarely used, 74% of cases presented in the first week of life (defined as early onset) and 89% of these early-onset cases presented on day one.[7] Only 65% of early-onset cases had one or more clinical risk

Evidence-Based Neonatal Infections, First Edition. David Isaacs.

factors (prematurity, prolonged rupture of membranes, known maternal GBS carriage or intrapartum fever). The strongest independent associations with GBS disease were known maternal carriage of GBS, maternal infection in the peripartum period and maximum temperature in labour (the OR increased by 2.2 per °C). Early-onset cases had lower Apgar scores and were more likely than controls to have respiratory distress and convulsions, and to require tube feeding.[7]

A 1999 literature review gave a summary analysis of the OR for risk factors for early-onset GBS infection.[8] The major risk factors were GBS-positive vaginal culture at delivery (OR: 204), GBS-positive recto-vaginal culture at 28 (OR: 9.6) or 36 weeks gestation (OR: 26.7), vaginal GBS rapid test positive at delivery (OR: 15.4), birth weight </= 2500 g (OR: 7.4), gestation <37 weeks (OR: 4.8), gestation <28 weeks (OR: 21.7), prolonged rupture of membranes (PROM) >18 hours (OR: 7.3), intrapartum fever >37.5°C (OR: 4.1), intrapartum fever, PROM, or prematurity (OR: 9.7), intrapartum fever or PROM at term (OR: 11.5) and chorioamnionitis (OR: 6.4). Chorioamnionitis was reported in 88% of cases in which neonatal infection occurred despite intrapartum maternal antibiotic therapy. The ORs could not be estimated for maternal GBS bacteriuria during pregnancy, pre-term premature rupture of membranes, or a sibling or twin with invasive GBS disease, although these findings are apparently associated with a very high risk. Multiple gestation was not an independent risk factor for GBS infection.[8] These findings provide important data, but their relative importance depends on local epidemiologic factors.

Prematurity is the major risk for late-onset GBS infection. In a US case-control study of 122 infants with late-onset GBS infection, 84% of patients were <34 weeks gestation and the risk of infection increased by a factor of 1.34 for each week of decreased gestation.[9]. Additional risk factors were Afro-American status and maternal colonization with GBS.[9] GBS can be acquired post-natally and indeed occasional nosocomial outbreaks of GBS infection have been reported in neonatal nurseries, implying transmission on the hands of staff.[10, 11] Breast milk transmission of GBS was first reported in 1977[12, 13] and there have been a number of subsequent reports of late-onset and recurrent GBS infection thought to be transmitted by infected breast milk, including in twins and even triplets, although proof is lacking that the infected breast milk actually caused the neonatal infection (see Chapter 19).[14, 15] In full-term infants, the most common route of late infection is invasion by GBS colonizing the nasopharynx. This contrasts with meningococcal infection, where carriage is often protective and persons newly acquiring the organism are at greatest risk of invasive infection.

In the United States, 15–40% of pregnant women are colonized with GBS. The risk of maternal GBS colonization is increased with age <20 years, diabetes and African-American race, factors which also increase the risk of pre-term birth.[10,16–18] Heavy maternal colonization with GBS increases the risk of pre-term birth by 50%.[18] About half of all neonates born to colonized mothers themselves become colonized at birth, although the proportion varies from 30% to 85% and is higher with increased intensity of maternal colonization.[10] About 1–2% of colonized infants develop GBS infection.[10, 17] Maternal colonization rates in Western Europe are 11–21%, Eastern Europe 19.7–29.3%, Scandinavia 24.3–36%, and Southern Europe 6.5–32%.[19] Colonization of mucous membranes persists for weeks and is not eradicated by parenteral antibiotics. Intrapartum antibiotics do not reduce the incidence of late-onset GBS infection.[17]

14.1.1.2 Microbiology of GBS

Virulence factors for GBS pathogenicity include its thick polysaccharide (sugar) outer capsule, capsular sialic acid, lipoteichoic acid and various enzymes including neuraminidase and an enzyme that cleaves complement component C5a.[10, 16] Varying strain virulence may be the main explanation for the high rate of neonatal GBS infection in North America compared to Europe before the era of intrapartum antibiotic prophylaxis (IAP) despite very similar rates of maternal colonization.[10] However, other factors such as intensity of colonization and host genetic factors determining immune response are also important.

The capsular polysaccharide is probably the most important virulence factor. There is a correlation between low maternal antibodies to the polysaccharide and neonatal infection,[20] and a correlation between maternal capsular polysaccharide antibodies and protection of the neonate against infection.[21, 22] The major focus of vaccine development has been to develop conjugate vaccines (capsular polysaccharide conjugated to protein) to stimulate capsular polysaccharide antibody production.[23, 24] Conjugate vaccines induce T-cell immunity and memory. One possible reason for problems developing an effective conjugate vaccine is that the sialylated polysaccharides of types Ia, Ib and III GBS are structurally similar to human serum glycoproteins and thus these strains may be able to avoid the immune response by molecular mimicry.[10]

In the United States, the distribution of serotypes differs for early- and late-onset neonatal diseases. In particular, serotype III causes around 30% of early-onset infection, similar to the proportion colonizing pregnant women, but around 65% of late-onset infections and 90% of late-onset meningitis are due to serotype III. This suggests that early-onset sepsis is more dependent on environmental factors than on organism virulence, whereas the increased virulence of serotype III is responsible for it causing an increased proportion of late-onset sepsis, particularly meningitis.

A German study compared invasive and non-invasive strains of serotype III GBS isolated from infants with proven sepsis and from colonized infants without systemic sepsis. Non-invasive strains were far more genetically and phenotypically heterogeneous whereas the invasive strains showed considerable clustering. The authors concluded that GBS strains are subject to selection pressures favouring more virulent strains during invasion.[25]

14.1.1.3 Clinical features of GBS infection

Early- and late-onset GBS neonatal infections are clinically distinct entities.

(i) Early-onset infection is typically caused by ascending infection from the maternal genital tract and most cases (>80%) present within hours of birth with respiratory distress, manifested as grunting, recession, tachypnoea or apnoea.[10] The chest radiographic appearance is often indistinguishable from hyaline membrane disease (Figure 8.4A), but patchy (Figure 8.4B) or lobar pneumonic changes are also described and the chest radiograph may even rarely be normal.[10] Infants who develop respiratory distress after day 2 are unlikely to have GBS pneumonia or hyaline membrane disease. The differential diagnosis of respiratory illness developing after 2 days includes treatable infectious causes such as HSV pneumonitis, which must not be missed because of the danger of disseminated HSV infection, and Chlamydia pneumonitis, and non-infectious causes including congenital heart disease.

Between 25% and 40% of infants with early-onset GBS infection are bacteraemic, often at birth, and will progress to meningitis if untreated. They typically present with non-specific features of sepsis such as poor feeding, lethargy, fever or hypothermia, abdominal distension and even with shock or convulsions. Convulsions are most typically due to meningitis but babies with meningitis only infrequently develop seizures so lumbar puncture (LP) should be performed in suspected GBS sepsis and, if not performed acutely, should certainly be performed if blood cultures are positive to guide duration of therapy and to inform prognosis.

(ii) Late-onset GBS infection is a bacteraemic illness with or without meningitis typically presenting at 2–4 weeks of age, although infants may develop GBS infection up to and rarely beyond 3 months of age, particularly pre-term infants. A history of preceding upper respiratory tract infection is obtained in about a quarter of infants with late-onset GBS meningitis, so invasion may occur when the nasal mucosa is damaged, for example by respiratory viral infection, allowing GBS to invade the bloodstream.

The presentation may be fulminant or indolent, usually with non-specific signs of sepsis, including fever or hypothermia, poor feeding, irritability, lethargy, abdominal distension and sometimes convulsions. Respiratory signs are rare. Other manifestations of late-onset GBS infection are with signs due to osteomyelitis and/or septic arthritis or cellulitis (often facial or submandibular, less commonly neck, scrotum, inguinal or pre-patellar, see Chapter 13). These infants are usually bacteraemic suggesting metastatic spread is the likely pathogenesis. Rare manifestations of neonatal GBS infection include cardiac (endocarditis, myocarditis, pericarditis, mycotic aneurysm of the aorta), gastrointestinal (adrenal abscess, peritonitis), and central nervous system (brain abscess, subdural empyema).[10]

14.1.1.4 Probable early-onset GBS infection

A clinical entity is well described of severe early-onset respiratory disease in relatively mature newborns colonized with GBS but with negative blood cultures.[26, 27] The chest radiograph is usually consistent with hyaline membrane disease or pneumonia,[26] although may be normal.[27] These infants are often categorized as having probable GBS infection. The reported frequency of probable GBS infection is approximately the same as proven, blood-culture-positive, early-onset GBS infection,[26, 27] although is likely to be affected by the extent of intrapartum antibiotic use. It is by no means certain that infants with probable GBS sepsis truly have GBS infection, since the GBS colonization may be coincidental. For example, if the infant was not colonized with GBS, alternate diagnoses considered would include hyaline membrane disease, persistent foetal circulation and idiopathic pneumonia. Nevertheless, the existence of true blood-culture-negative GBS pneumonia/infection cannot be excluded and cannot be ignored. Clinicians are recommended to manage infants with probable GBS sepsis as for true GBS sepsis.

14.1.1.5 Twins and late-onset GBS infection

Multiple gestation is not in itself a risk factor for GBS infection,[8] but there are a number of reports of one twin developing late-onset GBS infection, followed rapidly by the other twin.[28] The reason for these concordant infections is unknown. Possible explanations include simultaneous exposure to an increased load of GBS or simultaneous exposure of colonized infants to a risk factor such as a respiratory viral infection. When one twin develops late-onset GBS sepsis, the other should be examined urgently. If clinically well, the approach will depend on gestation and family circumstances, but in view of the speed and severity with which late-onset GBS infection can present, a cautious approach is to admit the baby, perform a blood culture and treat empirically with IV penicillin G. This does not eradicate carriage,[29] but neither does rifampicin (rifampin).[30] Because treatment does not eradicate carriage, it does not seem indicated to persist with treatment beyond 2–3 days in the well sibling unless blood cultures are positive.

14.1.1.6 Treatment of GBS infection

All strains of GBS are susceptible to penicillin G, the antibiotic of choice for established GBS infection.[10, 19] Ampicillin and cephalosporins, which are often used, have never been shown to be superior to penicillin G for treating GBS infections, including meningitis.[10] Penicillin allergy is vanishingly rare in neonates, but alternatives to β-lactams include vancomycin and linezolid. Up to 20% of GBS strains in Europe are resistant to erythromycin and clindamycin.[19] There is *in vitro* evidence and also *in vivo* evidence from animal studies of synergy between penicillin G and gentamicin against GBS, but no human studies. For this reason, GBS infection is often treated with a combination of penicillin G (or ampicillin) plus gentamicin. Aminoglycosides accumulate in renal tissue and otolymph, so gentamicin should be ceased as soon as the infant is stable and certainly not continued longer than 7 days.

There are no studies on optimal duration of antibiotics for proven GBS infection. It is generally advised to give parenteral penicillin for 7–10 days for bacteraemia without meningitis, for at least 14 days for meningitis, for 3 weeks for septic arthritis, and for 4 weeks for osteomyelitis or endocarditis (Table 14.1). These recommendations are empiric and not based on well-conducted scientific studies. The high doses in Table 14.1 are based on the relatively high minimum inhibitory concentration (MIC) of penicillin G

Table 14.1 Recommended antimicrobial treatment of proven neonatal group B streptococcal infections (all given parenterally).

Infection	Antibiotics	Duration
Bacteraemia (without meningitis)	Penicillin G 200 000 U/Kg IV daily (plus gentamicin 7.5 mg/kg IV daily until resolved)	7–10 days
Meningitis	Penicillin G 500 000 U/Kg IV daily (plus gentamicin 7.5 mg/kg IV daily until resolved)	At least 14 days
Septic arthritis	Penicillin G 200 000 U/Kg IV daily	3 weeks
Osteomyelitis	Penicillin G 200 000 U/Kg IV daily	4 weeks
Endocarditis	Penicillin G 400 000 U/Kg IV daily (plus gentamicin 3 mg/kg IV daily for first 14 days)	4 weeks

for GBS (median 0.04 μg/mL) and the phenomenon of *in vitro* tolerance of about 5% of strains, although neither of these has been shown definitively to be associated with treatment failures. There are anecdotal reports of relapse and recurrence when lower doses or shorter durations are used, but babies occasionally relapse after even the recommended antibiotic course (Section 14.1.1.5). Nevertheless, the severity of the disease mitigates caution.

14.1.1.7 Relapse or recurrence of GBS

Relapse during treatment or recurrence of GBS infection occurs in 0.5–3% of infections.[17] Studies in non-identical twins concordant for disease and recurrence suggest that recurrence is likely to be due to persistent mucosal colonization rather than acquisition of new strains.[31] Studies have shown that neither penicillin nor rifampin (rifampicin) eradicate colonization effectively, although the latter may be tried in addition to penicillin in hope rather than expectation. It is not logical to treat recurrences longer than the normal treatment duration.[10]

14.1.1.8 Prevention of neonatal GBS infection

Question: What is the most effective way to prevent neonatal GBS infection?

There is strong evidence that IAP of colonized mothers during labour prevents most early-onset neonatal GBS infection. A Cochrane systematic review identified three RCTs (852 GBS-colonized women) which evaluated the effects of IAP versus no treatment.[32] The use of IAP reduced the incidence of early-onset neonatal GBS infection by 83% compared to no treatment (95% CI 26–96). In these studies 25 women needed to be treated with antibiotics to prevent one case of early-onset neonatal infection, although the number varies depending on the level of maternal risk. Ampicillin and penicillin are equally effective.[33] IAP does not prevent late-onset GBS infection (Figure 14.1).[17, 32]

There is no effective alternative to IAP. Vaginal chlorhexidine reduced early neonatal GBS colonization by 28%, but did not prevent early-onset neonatal GBS sepsis.[34]

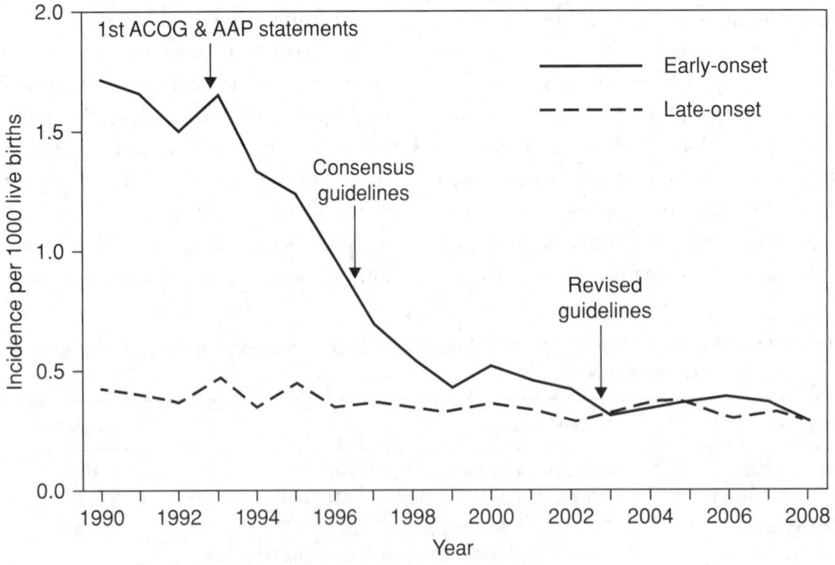

ACOG = American College of Obstetricians and Gynecologists
AAP = American Academy of Pediatrics

Figure 14.1 Decline in early-onset neonatal group B streptococcal infection in the United States. Reproduced with permission from Reference 17).

In modelling studies, a cheap, effective vaccine is the most cost-effective way of preventing GBS infection.[35] Furthermore, an effective vaccine that would also interrupt carriage might be expected to prevent late-onset GBS neonatal infection.

A cheap, effective vaccine is still awaited, although several candidate vaccines are in development.[23] It has been difficult to develop an effective vaccine. Problems will include identifying and accessing the target population (e.g. pregnant women, schoolgirls, all adolescents) and assessing vaccine cost-effectiveness.

Answer: An effective vaccine would be ideal but currently IAP of colonized women is the most effective way to prevent early-onset neonatal GBS infection.

IAP for colonized women prevents early-onset neonatal GBS infection,[32] which raises two important questions:

(1) Should all pregnant women be screened for carriage, and if so at what gestation?

(2) Should all GBS-colonized women be treated with IAP or only those with additional risk factors for having a baby with early infection?

Cost and cost-effectiveness is one issue. There is also a need to achieve the optimal balance between the number of women treated with parenteral antibiotics (which medicalizes women and occasionally hazardous) and the number of cases of GBS prevented.

Question: What is the best way to target intrapartum antibiotic therapy?

A **risk-based approach** involves empiric antibiotic treatment of women with known risk factors for neonatal GBS infection. The major risk factors are prematurity (the risk of sepsis increases with decreasing gestation), spontaneous onset of pre-term labour, prolonged rupture of membranes, maternal fever and colonization with GBS or a previous baby infected with GBS.[36, 37] Post-maturity (gestation >42 weeks) is also a risk factor (Table 14.2). These risks are cumulative, so if more than one is present, the risk is greatly increased.[36, 37]

A **screening-based approach** involves screening pregnant women for GBS carriage. This was originally at 26–28 weeks, but is now recommended at 35–37 weeks in the United States.[17] Either all carriers are treated or only those with risk factors. Maternal colonization can be high or low density and can be chronic, transient or intermittent or transient, so carriers may screen as negative and pregnant women may become colonized after screening.[38, 39] Accurate point-of-care tests for identifying GBS carriage in women in labour would be ideal, but current tests are not sufficiently accurate to be relied upon to exclude GBS carriage.[40, 41]

The incidence of GBS neonatal infection is important: no preventative strategy is indicated if there is no GBS infection, whereas the higher the incidence the greater the need for the most effective approach. Cost is an issue and the approach adopted will differ between high- and low-income countries. A cost-effectiveness study[42] compared four strategies.

(1) Screening cultures at 26–28 weeks; universal intrapartum chemoprophylaxis of all carriers

(2) Screening cultures at 26–28 weeks; selective intrapartum chemoprophylaxis of carriers with risk factors

(3) No screen; intrapartum chemoprophylaxis for women with risk factors

(4) Intrapartum chemoprophylaxis until 37 weeks; screening cultures at 37 weeks; universal intrapartum chemoprophylaxis for all carriers.

Strategy 4, currently recommended by the Centers for Disease Control in the United States, prevents most cases.[17] On the other hand, strategy 3 is the cheapest and was still cost-effective for a country with an incidence of 2 per 1000 live births.[42] A

Table 14.2 Risk factors for early-onset neonatal group B streptococcal (GBS) infection.[6–8]

Prematurity: risk increases with decreasing gestation and birth weight
Spontaneous pre-term onset of labour
Spontaneous pre-term rupture of membranes
Prolonged rupture of membranes (increases with increasing duration >12 hours)
Maternal intrapartum fever >38°C
Maternal clinical chorioamnionitis
Maternal urinary tract infection with GBS
Maternal colonisation with group B streptococcus (GBS)
Previous baby with early-onset GBS infection
Intrauterine foetal monitoring

cost-effectiveness analysis based on US data suggested that a hypothetical vaccine would be the best option, but in its absence a risk-factor-based approach (strategy 3 above) costs less per case prevented than a screening-based approach (strategy 2) but prevents fewer cases.[43] The study found the cost of introducing a risk-based strategy exceeded the calculated cost of GBS infection until the baseline incidence exceeded 0.6 per 1000 live births, although the figures and assumptions are open to challenge.[43] The study did not consider the combined approach now used in the United States.[17] A complex cost-effectiveness analysis for the United Kingdom found that a risk-based approach treating all women with pre-term and other high risk factors was superior to the United Kingdom's current selective approach.[44]

Screening at 26–28 weeks gestation has been dropped in the United States because about 10% of non-colonized women become colonized by delivery.[45] In addition, only 67% of women colonized at 26–28 weeks are still positive at delivery, which could lead to over-treatment.[45]

The United States recommends a combined approach, risk-based until 35–37 weeks of gestation, then universal maternal screening at 35–37 weeks of gestation and the treatment of all carriers with intrapartum antibiotics.[17] In the United States, the incidence of early-onset sepsis fell nationally from 1.7 per 1000 live births in 1990 to 0.4 per 1000 in 2008 (Figure 14.1).[17] Australia has not mandated one particular approach, but all large maternity units surveyed have adopted one or other approach[46, 47] and the combined incidence of early-onset GBS infection in these hospitals fell from 2 cases per 1000 live births in 1991 before widespread chemoprophylaxis[46] to 0.25 per 1000 in 2001,[47] which if valid nationally extrapolates to 4500 cases of early-onset GBS infection prevented over 10 years (Figure 14.2).

Answer: The optimal approach is determined by the incidence of neonatal GBS infection and the affordability. In low-income countries with an incidence >0.6 per 1000 live births a risk-based approach is the cheapest way to prevent cases. In high-income countries, a combined approach using risk-based treatment until 35–37 weeks and screening-based subsequently prevents more cases than other approaches.

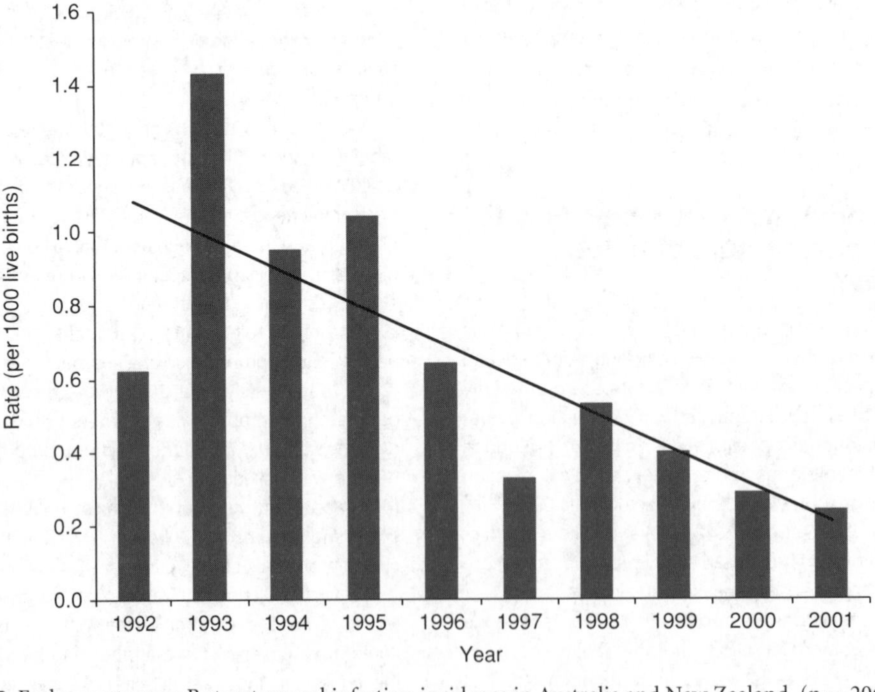

Figure 14.2 Early-onset group B streptococcal infection incidence in Australia and New Zealand, (n = 206, $p < 0.001$)[47].

14.1.1.9 IAP and antibiotic resistance

One concern has been that IAP could select for infection with other organisms resistant to penicillin or ampicillin. Most studies have found the incidence of early-onset sepsis due to other organisms has remained unchanged[48–56] or decreased.[47, 57] Some papers reported an increased incidence of *Escherichia coli* infections in pre-term infants temporally related to antepartum prophylaxis and some studies reported increasing ampicillin resistance in these *E. coli* isolates.[58–63] Claims that these changes were caused by IAP rather than a chance association ignored the fact that increasing ampicillin resistance was occurring simultaneously elsewhere,[64] and that it was biologically implausible that short-term antibiotic prophylaxis would have such a profound effect on resistance.[65] Further studies have not suggested a consistent increase in ampicillin-resistant *E. coli* infections in term or pre-term infants.[65–67]

14.1.1.10 Management of newborns whose mothers received intrapartum antibiotic prophylaxis

The management of newborns born to mothers who received IAP, particularly mothers known to be GBS-colonized, is problematic. The current IAP recommendation is that women receive penicillin G or ampicillin IV 4 hourly until delivery. A Spanish study showed that the neonatal colonization rate fell from 46% if the baby was delivered less than an hour after antibiotics were started to 2.9% at 2–4 hours and 1.2% after 4 hours.[68] While further studies have confirmed that the effectiveness increases after 2 hours,[69] the quality of the data on the duration of maternal antibiotics has been questioned.[70, 71]

The US CDC recommendations[17] on management of all infants, including those born to mothers who received intrapartum antibiotics, are summarized in Figure 14.3. A retrospective Israeli study questioned the need to perform full blood counts and blood cultures on well babies whose GBS-carrier mothers received only one dose of antibiotic before delivery. Full blood counts sent on infants whose mothers received only one dose of intrapartum antibiotics were non-contributory.[72] All 11 infants with proven early-onset GBS sepsis were symptomatic. The authors suggest it is reasonable to observe well, full-term babies whose GBS carrier mothers received only one dose of intrapartum antibiotics without performing haematologic investigations, although cautious clinicians will perform a blood culture.[72]

14.1.2 Coagulase-negative staphylococci

CoNS cause more than half of all late-onset infections in Western neonatal intensive care units, mostly in pre-term infants receiving invasive respiratory support and/or intravenous nutrition.[73] CoNS infections can cause true infection but are also frequent contaminants of blood cultures. Contamination can occur at the time of sampling or in the laboratory. Approximately half of all neonatal blood cultures that grow CoNS are thought to be true infections and the rest are contaminants. The best evidence comes from comparisons of clinical findings with quantitative cultures.[74–76] However, quantitative cultures are too time-consuming and expensive to perform except as a research tool. Although time to growth of a positive culture correlates usefully with quantitative cultures,[74–76] all studies of neonatal CoNS infection need to be read with caution because a significant proportion of reported cases may not be truly infected. In particular, reports of CoNS causing early-onset infection on the first day of life and of causing late-onset meningitis in the absence of predisposing factors (e.g. shunt, surgery) should be treated with scepticism. Of course the epidemiologist can afford a great deal more scepticism than the clinician. Nevertheless, many infants treated with antibiotics for positive blood or CSF CoNS cultures are probably not infected.

14.1.2.1 Epidemiology of coagulase-negative staphylococcal infections

The definition of CoNS sepsis varies and can greatly affect reported incidence. A definition based on positive cultures plus clinical features compatible with sepsis is not very effective at excluding contaminants, because possible sepsis is the usual indication for blood culture. In the United States it is common to take two blood cultures at the time of investigation for possible sepsis and many studies specify that both have to be classified epidemiologically as a true case. In other countries, the definition of CoNS sepsis may require one or more abnormal laboratory tests (e.g. CRP, I:T ratio).

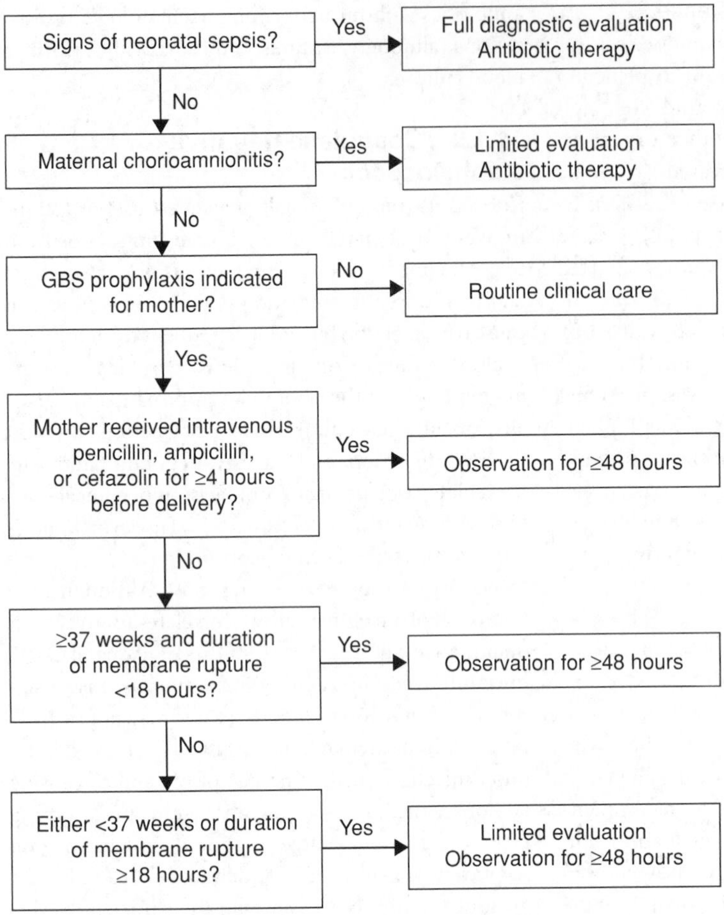

Figure 14.3 CDC algorithm for secondary prevention of early-onset group B streptococcal (GBS) disease among all newborns (Reproduced with permission from Reference 17).

A prospective multi-centre NICU-based study in Australia and New Zealand defined CoNS sepsis as a pure growth of CoNS from blood or CSF plus clinical sepsis plus at least one abnormal haematologic test (I:T ratio, white count or platelet count) or raised serum C-reactive protein.[73] There were 1281 cases of CoNS sepsis in 10 years, comprising 57.1% of all late-onset infections. The incidence of CoNS sepsis was 3.5 episodes per 1000 live births. Most infected babies (71%) were 24–29 weeks of gestation at birth (mode 26 weeks). Half of all babies' positive CoNS culture was in week 2 (mode 10 days, see Figure 14.4). Five cases of meningitis were reported (incidence 0.4% of all CoNS infections). Twenty nine babies (2.3%) had CoNS septicaemia in association with necrotizing enterocolitis. Four babies (0.3%) were assessed as having died from CoNS infection, while CoNS infection was assessed as possibly contributing to the death of an additional 20 babies (1.6%). The mortality of 0.3% directly attributed to CoNS infection was significantly lower than the 13.1% from *Staphylococcus aureus* (relative risk (RR) = 36.1 (95% CI 13–100.2) or 14.2% from Gram-negative bacilli (RR = 45.5, 95% CI 16.8–123.3) in the same cohort.[73]

The incidence of CoNS rises with falling birth weight, as for all late-onset neonatal infections, due to both immaturity and increased length of stay which are major independent risk factors.[77] In one study, the rate of CoNS infection was 44.5 times higher in infants <750 g than in infants >2000 g, but only 5.3 times higher after allowing for length of stay.[77] Risk factors for CoNS include prematurity, intravascular catheters particularly intracardiac catheters and endotracheal intubation. Parenteral nutrition fluids, particularly lipids, are a rich growth medium and are a risk factor for CoNS sepsis in addition to the

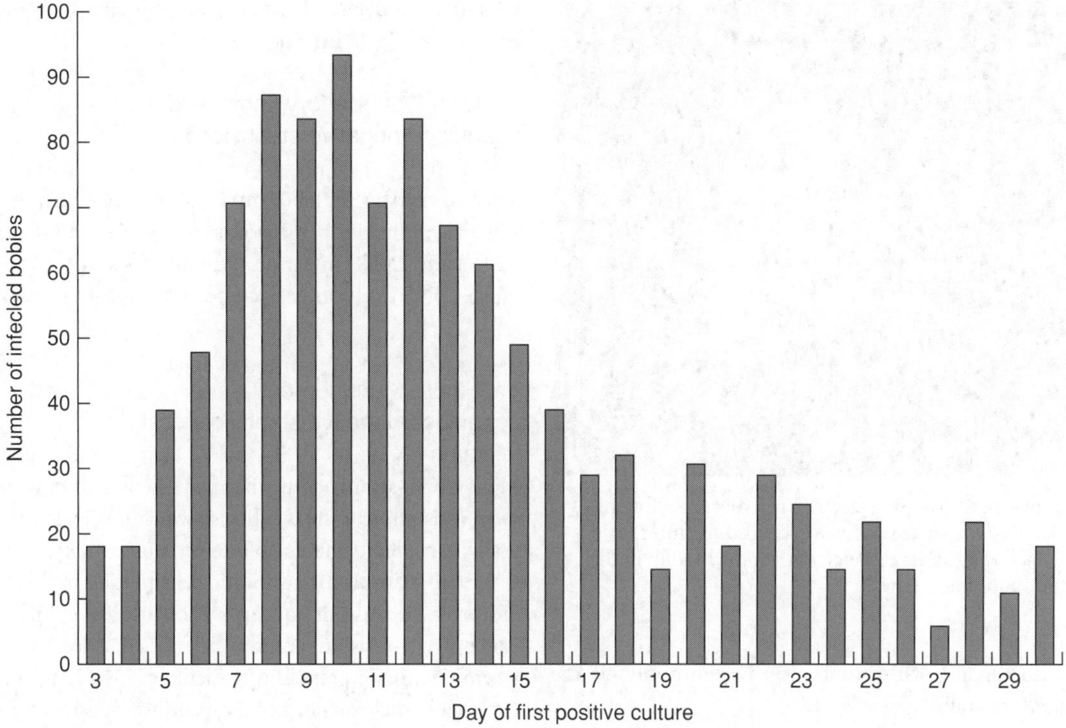

Figure 14.4 Day of first positive culture of coagulase-negative staphylococci from blood or CSF. Infants <3 days old are not included. (Reproduced with permission from Reference 72).

presence of an intravascular catheter.[78] CoNS are the most frequent cause of central line-associated bacteraemias (CLABs).[75, 79]

14.1.2.2 Microbiology of coagulase-negative staphylococci

There are 31 species of CoNS, of which 13 colonize human skin and 7 cause neonatal infections: *S. epidermidis, S. haemolyticus, S. hominis, S. warneri, S. saprophyticus, S. capitis* and *S. cohnii. S. epidermidis* are responsible for 50–80% of colonization and 60–93% of CoNS bloodstream infection.[16] Capsular polysaccharide adhesins help CoNS stick to skin, mucosal surfaces or indwelling intravascular catheters or intracerebral shunts. Some CoNS produce an exopolysaccharide 'slime' layer mainly made of N-acetylglucosamine, which acts as a biofilm and protects the organism from host defences and from antibiotics. Slime production has been linked to virulence and also to persistent CoNS infection.[78] Interestingly, there is *in vitro* evidence that the slime produced by *S. epidermidis* can inhibit the penetration of fluconazole into mixed Candida and *S. epidermidis* biofilms while *Candida albicans* biofilm protects CoNS from vancomycin,[80] which could explain mixed neonatal infections with Candida and *S. epidermidis.* CoNS adhere, but also secrete enzymes that allow colonies to burrow into the surface of silastic catheters (Figure 14.5).

Staphylococcus lugdunensis is more pathogenic than most CoNS strains, sometimes approaching *S. aureus* in virulence. It can cause endocarditis in older children and adults, although not reported in neonates yet. Like other CoNS it is often an asymptomatic commensal that has been reported to cause catheter-associated bacteraemia. Some laboratories report *S. lugdunensis* isolates. Clinicians should only be concerned if they suspect sepsis but should not be more worried about colonization with *S. lugdunensis* than they would by *S. aureus* colonization.

CoNS can rarely be acquired from the maternal genital tract at birth, but most infants become colonized soon after birth with other strains.

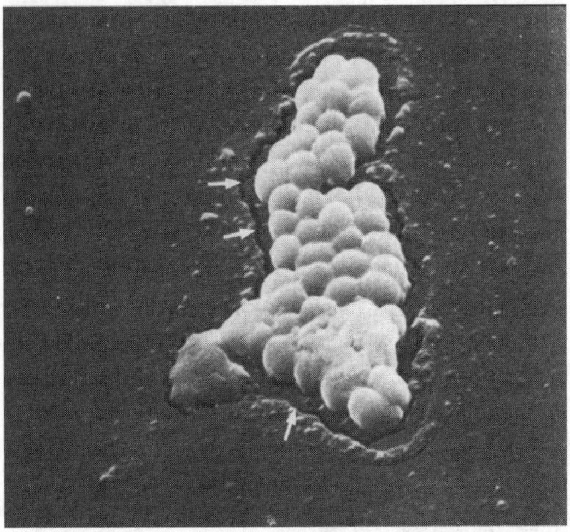

Figure 14.5 Scanning electron micrograph showing coagulase-negative staphylococci eroding into the surface of a silastic catheter, with some biofilm at the bottom of the colony.

Nosocomial CoNS colonization is commonly via the hands of staff.[16]

14.1.2.3 Clinical features of coagulase-negative staphylococcal infection

There are no specific clinical features of CoNS infection, which is usually indolent, presenting with apnea, bradycardia, increased ventilatory requirements, irritability and feeding intolerance. Fever may or may not be present.[81, 82] In a retrospective study, fulminant sepsis, defined as death within 48 hours of a positive blood culture, occurred in 4 of 277 infants >3 days old who grew CoNS in their blood culture.[83]

14.1.2.4 Early-onset coagulase-negative staphylococcal infection

A retrospective study identified 11 infants out of a population of approximately 7800 extremely low birthweight infants <1500 g who were thought on chart review to have true early-onset CoNS sepsis (10 on day 1, 1 on day 2) in association with ventilator-dependent respiratory distress. Three had repeat positive cultures, 4 had pulmonary haemorrhage and 3 died.[84] The retrospective nature of this study, the potential that an extremely pre-term infant would have a similarly severe course without sepsis and the lack of autopsy data makes it debatable whether these infants had true early-onset CoNS infection.

14.1.2.5 Laboratory findings in coagulase-negative staphylococcal infection

There are no specific laboratory features of CoNS infection. Thrombocytopenia occurs in 15–25% of infants with acute CoNS infection, but this does not distinguish CoNS from other bacterial and fungal causes of sepsis.[85, 86]

14.1.2.6 Management of coagulase-negative staphylococcal infection

Most CoNS strains carry the mecA gene and have *in vitro* resistance to cloxacillin, so vancomycin is generally considered the antibiotic of choice for treating CoNS infection until antibiotic sensitivities are back. However, because of concerns about the selection of vancomycin-resistant enterococci, it is common to use a semi-synthetic penicillin (oxacillin, cloxacillin, flucloxacillin, dicloxacillin) plus an aminoglycoside, usually gentamicin, for empiric treatment of suspected late-onset sepsis (see Section 5.1.2). There are no RCTs, but sequential studies comparing empiric vancomycin plus aminoglycoside with empiric oxacillin/cloxacillin plus aminoglycoside for suspected late-onset sepsis showed no difference in outcomes from CoNS infection treated with either regimen.[83, 87, 88] While it is generally recommended to change to vancomycin if CoNS infection with a resistant strain is proven, infants with oxacillin-resistant organisms have often responded to the oxacillin plus aminoglycoside regimen by the time cultures are back.[83,87–89] This may be because aminoglycosides have some activity against CoNS, it may be due to catheter removal, or because the isolates were contaminants. A Dutch study of 163 infants with CoNS bacteraemia reported that 140 had a cefazolin-susceptible strain (86%). The authors reported a good response to cefazolin in most infants with cefazolin-sensitive or cefazolin-resistant strains, although 22% of infants failed cefazolin and the response was better in those whose central venous catheter was removed.[89]

The need for removal of central lines in CoNS bacteraemia is considered in Section 6.10.1. Early central venous catheter removal improves the likelihood of resolution of CoNS but clinicians often want to preserve a precious catheter. About half of all infants can be successfully treated without removing the central line.[79, 90] However, bacteraemia which persists >4 days does not resolve without central venous catheter removal.[90]

The optimal duration of antibiotics for CoNS bacteraemia is unknown. A Dutch group hypothesized that most CoNS infections respond within 3 days and stopped antibiotics after 3 days if infants with CoNS infection had responded clinically, had normal platelets and had no catheter *in situ* (never present or removed). All 80 infants treated with 3 days of antibiotics recovered without relapse.[91]

Question: Should an infant with late-onset coagulase-negative staphylococcal bacteraemia have an LP?

While LP is often recommended in the initial investigation of all infants with suspected late-onset sepsis (see Section 4.1.3), in clinical practice immediate LP is often omitted. If an infant investigated for suspected late-onset sepsis without an LP grows CoNS from the blood culture, should we perform an LP?

If the infant has not been started on antibiotics and is well, blood cultures can be repeated and if negative, LP is unnecessary. Most infants, however, will have been started on empiric antibiotics. What is the likelihood that they have meningitis and what are the risks and benefits of LP?

CoNS is a common cause of intraventricular shunt infection (see Section 7.10), but an extremely rare cause of meningitis in the absence of a shunt and there is some doubt whether CoNS meningitis without a shunt is a true clinical entity. However, the risk of LP is low and the potential risk of under-treatment of CoNS meningitis is life-long morbidity. For this reason, it seems sensible to recommend LP for an infant with CoNS bacteraemia, if only to accumulate more information about whether or not CoNS meningitis in the absence of a shunt is a real entity. We recognize that many clinicians do not perform delayed LP on infants with CoNS bacteraemia.

Recommendation: Because of the potential risk of missing CoNS meningitis it is recommended to LP an infant with CoNS bacteraemia, although this recommendation is not based on classical evidence of harm if LP is omitted.

14.1.2.7 Persistent coagulase-negative staphylococcal infections

CoNS infections have a propensity to persist, with or without fever or other signs of infection, and often in association with thrombocytopenia.[92, 93] Endocarditis should always be considered in any child with persistent bacteraemia. In one study, 5 of 58 infants with persistent CoNS bacteraemia had right-sided endocarditis in association with umbilical catheters in the right atrium.[92] Most cases of persistent CoNS bacteraemia are thought to be due to endovasculitis, to which central venous catheters probably predispose, although persistent CoNS bacteraemia can occur in infants who never had a central venous catheter.

In one study, 31 (18%) of 171 infants with CoNS bacteraemia had persistent infection. The incidence of thrombocytopenia was 84% for persistent CoNS infection compared with 13% for those whose infection resolved.[93]

In a retrospective case-control study, 52 infants with persistent CoNS bacteraemia >48 hours were significantly more likely than controls to have feed intolerance and to need ventilatory support, inotropes, and blood transfusion but mortality was not increased. Risk factors for persistent infection were duration of parenteral nutrition, hydrocortisone, antibiotics, and mechanical ventilation prior to infection.[94] In another study, endotracheal intubation, central venous catheters and biofilm production were significant risk factors for persistent infection.[95] An Israeli study found persistent CoNS bacteraemia resolved quicker in breastfed infants.[96]

A retrospective Dutch study identified 137 infants with CoNS bacteraemia, which persisted in 18 (13%) who had three positive cultures at least 48 hours apart and were treated with vancomycin and rifampicin (rifampin). The authors reported a rapid response to rifampicin, although the retrospective design casts doubt on the validity of this observation.[97]

14.1.2.8 Outcome of coagulase-negative staphylococcal infections

The mortality of CoNS infection is low, 0.3% in the largest prospective study[73] and 1.4% in a retrospective US study.[83] A very large multi-centre study identified 16 629 infants with 17 624 episodes of CoNS infection in 248 NICUs, and classified the CoNS infections as definite (10%), probable (17%) and possible (73%).

Surprisingly, the mortality was significantly lower in infants with CoNS infection than in controls matched for gestational, birth weight and Apgar score for all three categories.[98] It does not seem credible that CoNS infection would prevent deaths, and the retrospective nature of the study makes it likely that the results are confounded.

Other studies have shown that CoNS bacteraemia is associated with prolonged duration of NICU stay, on average 14 days longer than controls, and with significantly increased hospital costs.[99] A follow-up study of over 6000 infants born weighing 401–1000 g assessed at 18–22 months found that infants with CoNS infection were significantly more likely than non-infected infants to have impaired neurodevelopment.[100]

14.1.2.9 Prevention of coagulase-negative staphylococcal infections

Evidence from before and after studies suggests that improved hand hygiene[101–103] and clusters of infection control measures involving care of peripheral and central lines[104] reduce the incidence of CoNS infections.[105] While these measures are probably truly effective, our previous caveat about distinguishing true infections from contaminants is pertinent. The measures might reduce blood culture contaminants rather than true CoNS infections. In one study improved hand hygiene was associated with a significant reduction in CoNS blood culture contaminants, whereas the lesser reduction in 'true' CoNS infections did not reach statistical significance.[106]

There is RCT evidence that early introduction of enteral nutrition can prevent CoNS infections. Infants <1750 g randomized to trophic feeds of 0.5–1 mL/hour plus parenteral nutrition from day 3 until ventilator support finished had significantly fewer infections than those on parenteral nutrition (mean 0.5 vs 1.2 episodes of culture-proven sepsis, mainly CoNS).[107] A retrospective Canadian study found that achieving full enteral feeds was associated with an 85% reduction in CoNS infections.[108]

14.1.3 *Staphylococcus aureus*

S. aureus was a major cause of hospital-acquired neonatal sepsis between the 1950s and the 1970s, causing major nursery outbreaks. These were often associated with skin sepsis and omphalitis (see Chapter 13), while osteomyelitis and septic arthritis (see Chapter 9) were rare, serious complications. *S. aureus* strains produce an enzyme, coagulase, which is detected in the laboratory to distinguish them from CoNS. *S. aureus* has a cell wall with two major components, peptidoglycan and teichoic acid, and an outer capsule. Antibiotic resistance genes are mainly carried on mobile genetic elements which include a so-called resistance island. The organism can also carry gene clusters called pathogenicity islands coding for production of exotoxins like toxic shock syndrome toxin and for enterotoxins. The basis for methicillin resistance of all MRSA isolates is the *mecA* gene, which codes for a penicillin-binding protein with greatly reduced affinity for β-lactam antibiotics. The Panton–Valentine leukocidin (PVL) gene, which is associated with increased virulence, can be carried by strains of MRSA and strains of methicillin-sensitive *S. aureus* (MSSA).[109]

S. aureus can cause both early- and late-onset infections. In Western countries, early-onset *S. aureus* infections are rare,[110, 111] and most empiric antibiotic regimens for early-onset sepsis do not include an anti-staphylococcal antibiotic (see Chapter 5). However, the mortality of early-onset *S. aureus* infection is high: in one study the incidence of early-onset *S. aureus* infection (all MSSA) was 0.08 per 1000 live births but the mortality was 39%.[110] Empiric antibiotic regimens for possible early-onset infection may need to be reviewed if MSSA or community MRSA strains emerge as a common cause of early-onset infection,[112] although currently MRSA are much more likely to cause late-onset infections.[109–113] In most developing countries, in contrast, MSSA is an important early-onset pathogen.[114] *S. aureus* is also an important late-onset pathogen worldwide (see Chapter 2) and it is recommended that all empiric regimens for suspected late-onset sepsis should provide anti-staphylococcal cover (see Chapter 5).

The clinical presentation of *S. aureus* infections will mainly be considered under the relevant chapters. *S. aureus* can cause skin and soft tissue infections including omphalitis, mastitis, staphylococcal scalded skin syndrome and toxic shock syndrome (see Chapter 13), osteomyelitis and septic arthritis (see Chapter 9), pneumonia (see Chapter 8), endocarditis and bacteraemia, including CLAB. *S. aureus* can cause central nervous system shunt infections and are a rare cause of meningitis in the absence of CNS shunts. *S. aureus* meningitis can occur secondary to endocarditis, due to rupture of a mycotic aneurysm, secondary to epidural abscess and rarely in isolation secondary to bacteraemia.[109, 110] Similar to CoNS bacteraemia, although *S. aureus* meningitis is rare, it is recommended to perform an LP for an infant with *S. aureus* bacteraemia who did not have an original LP because of the danger of under-treatment if meningitis is missed.

14.1.3.1 Treatment of infections due to *Staphylococcus aureus*

S. aureus were originally universally susceptible to penicillin, but strains soon emerged that produced β-lactamases (called penicillinases). About 10% of strains of *S. aureus* are sensitive to penicillin and have a much lower MIC for penicillin than for semi-synthetic penicillins such as oxacillin. Penicillin G is the antibiotic of choice for invasive infections due to penicillin-sensitive strains of *S. aureus*.

For methicillin-sensitive penicillin-resistant strains, the treatment of choice is a β-lactamase-resistant semi-synthetic penicillin, e.g. cloxacillin, flucloxacillin, oxacillin or nafcillin. There is no good evidence for adding an aminoglycoside or rifampin (rifampicin) for synergy. First generation cephalosporins such as cefazolin or cephalothin are also active against MSSA.

Methicillin resistance is a problem worldwide. Strains that are resistant to methicillin (MRSA) are also resistant to other semi-synthetic penicillins (oxacillin, cloxacillin, dicloxacillin, flucloxacillin, nafcillin), to all cephalosporins, and may be resistant to other classes of antibiotics. MRSA are not necessarily more virulent than MSSA strains, and both MRSA and MSSA can carry the PVL gene which is a major virulence determinant.

Vancomycin is the treatment of choice for bacteraemic MRSA infections. It is often used in conjunction with an aminoglycoside or rifampin (rifampicin) without good evidence. Most strains (around 90%) of community-acquired MRSA are susceptible to clindamycin, which has activity against toxins and is, therefore, often used against clindamycin-sensitive PVL-producing strains and also in toxic shock syndrome and staphylococcal scalded skin syndrome. Clindamycin is bacteriostatic, so is not recommended as sole treatment for suspected or proven bacteraemic MRSA infection, but may be used in conjunction with another anti-staphylococcal agent, for example vancomycin for clindamycin-sensitive MRSA or with flu/cl/oxacillin for clindamycin-sensitive MSSA. Most MRSA are sensitive to linezolid, which is a possible alternative. They are also usually sensitive to trimethoprim–sulfamethoxazole and quinolones, antibiotics not usually used in neonates because of concerns about toxicity.

Although isolates of vancomycin-intermediate *S. aureus* (VISA) and vancomycin-resistant *S. aureus* (VRSA) have been detected in adults since the 1980s, there are no reports of outbreaks of VISA or VRSA in neonatal units, although failure of an MRSA-infected infant to respond to vancomycin should raise the possibility of VISA. VISA are usually susceptible to linezolid, quinupristin–dalfopristin and trimethoprim–sulfamethoxazole. Alternatives with activity against MRSA include other glycopeptides such as teicoplanin and newer antibiotics such as linezolid, which has been shown to be at least as effective as vancomycin but more expensive and possibly more toxic,[115, 116] and daptomycin, for which there are scanty data.[116]

14.1.3.2 Infection control measures for *Staphylococcus aureus*

Both MRSA and MSSA can cause nursery outbreaks. These will be discussed in detail in Chapter 21.

14.1.4 Enterococci

Enterococci are faecal streptococci. The most common enterococci to be neonatal pathogens are *Enterococcus faecalis* and *E. faecium*. Some but not all enterococci belong to Lancefield group D. *Streptococcus bovis* and *S. mitis* are not enterococci.

Enterococci can cause early- and late-onset neonatal infection,[117, 118] but can also be blood culture contaminants. Enterococci are sometimes isolated in blood cultures with another organism and, while in general polymicrobial blood cultures are often due to contamination (see Section 4.1.1.4), if enterococci are isolated with other enteric organisms, the positive blood cultures could represent true polymicrobial bacteraemia secondary to gut pathology, for example necrotizing enterocolitis. Enterococci can cause early- or late-onset meningitis, so LP should be performed if blood cultures are positive.[118] In one report, early-onset enterococcal sepsis was relatively benign with respiratory distress or diarrhoea whereas late-onset sepsis presented with severe apnea, bradycardia, circulatory collapse and increased ventilatory requirements and was associated with scalp abscess, catheter-related infection, pneumonia and meningitis.[118]

Vancomycin-resistant enterococci (VRE) carry resistance genes, usually *vanA* or *vanB*, which they can pass on to *S. aureus* to confer vancomycin resistance (VRSA). VRE can colonize infants and a proportion may develop nosocomial sepsis. It has been suggested that even a single case of VRE sepsis should prompt screening of other infants on the NICU because asymptomatic colonization is common and because it is important to know which infants are colonized in case they develop sepsis and need targeted antibiotic treatment and for infection control purposes, to prevent other babies becoming colonized.[119, 120]

Most enterococci are sensitive to ampicillin, the treatment of choice for susceptible enterococci, and gentamicin appears to provide synergistic activity, at least *in vitro*. Vancomycin is an alternative except for VRE. Enterococci are inherently resistant to cephalosporins, including cefotaxime, and overzealous use of third generation cephalosporins has been linked to increased colonization and infection with enterococci. Some VRE are susceptible to ampicillin which is then the drug of choice. Linezolid can be used to treat systemic infections with VRE resistant to both ampicillin and vancomycin. Quinupristin/dalfopristin is active against *E. faecium* infections. Teicoplanin is sometimes used to treat *vanB*-producing strains, but teicoplanin resistance can emerge during therapy.

14.1.5 Other streptococci

Group A streptococcus (*Streptococcus pyogenes*), which was the cause of severe neonatal and maternal sepsis a hundred years ago ('puerperal fever') is now a rare cause of early-onset or late-onset neonatal sepsis. It can cause cellulitis (see Chapter 13) and osteoarticular infections (see Chapter 9).[121] There are occasional reports of neonatal infections with groups C and G streptococci.

The pneumococcus (*Streptococcus pneumoniae*) is a rare cause of early-onset neonatal bacteraemia with pneumonia and sometimes meningitis and can cause late-onset infections, including bacteraemia, meningitis, otitis media, pneumonia and osteomyelitis or septic arthritis.[122]

Viridans streptococci (α-haemolytic streptococci) are more likely than not to be contaminants in cultures of blood or CSF, but can cause endocarditis and convincing cases of sepsis and of meningitis with *S. viridans* and *S. mitis* have been reported.[123–125] *S. milleri*, an organism more classically associated with deep abscess formation, has been described as a cause of early-onset neonatal infection, although the validity of the diagnosis of true sepsis in retrospective case series is arguable.[126]

14.2 Gram-negative bacilli

Gram-negative bacilli are a major cause of neonatal sepsis and mortality in resource-rich and resource-poor countries and increasing antibiotic resistance is a major problem. The Enterobacteriaceae (*E. coli*, *Enterobacter*, *Klebsiella*, *Serratia* and *Citrobacter* species) are normal gut commensals that can invade to cause septicaemia and meningitis and are associated with outbreaks of nosocomial neonatal infections. They are encapsulated and have fimbriae for attachment.[16] Other Gram-negative organisms (e.g. *Pseudomonas*, *Acinetobacter*) are often water-loving and may be acquired on the hands of staff and colonize the respiratory tract or the gastro-intestinal tract and invade. All Gram-negative bacilli have endotoxin (also called lipopolysaccharide) as a major component of the cell wall and endotoxinaemia is known to be associated with septic shock.

Combination therapy with two or more classes of antimicrobials, usually a β-lactam and an aminoglycoside, is often used to treat proven Gram-negative bacteraemia. A non-Cochrane systematic review and meta-analysis of 17 studies in all age groups found no mortality benefit with combination therapy for Gram-negative bacteraemia overall (OR 0.96, 95% CI 0.70–1.32).[127] However, combination therapy halved mortality for Pseudomonas (OR 0.50, 95% CI 0.30–0.79).[127] A Cochrane systematic review of 20 studies in all ages which compared β-lactam monotherapy with the same β-lactam combined with an aminoglycoside found no difference in mortality (RR 1.01, 95% CI 0.75–1.35) or clinical failure rate (RR 1.11, 95% CI 0.95–1.21).[128] A meta-analysis of 44 trials which compared monotherapy using a broader-spectrum β-lactam with combination therapy using a different, narrower-spectrum β-lactam and an aminoglycoside favoured monotherapy in terms of mortality (RR 0.85, 95% CI 0.71–1.01) and clinical failure (RR 0.77, 95%

CI 0.69–0.86).[128] There was no significant difference in sub-group analyses of patients with Gram-negative or Pseudomonas infections. Nephrotoxicity was more than 3 times as common with combination therapy as with monotherapy.[128] While *in vitro* studies may suggest synergy, there is little convincing *in vivo* evidence to support combination therapy.[129] It is now believed widely that any demonstrated benefits of combination therapy against Pseudomonas are due to the broader spectrum achieved with two agents, rather than to true synergy between them. Using an aminoglycoside as well as a β-lactam for empiric therapy provides 'insurance' against the possibility that the β-lactam agent will be inactive against the pathogen. Once antibiotic sensitivities are known, β-lactam monotherapy with an active agent is usually appropriate.

Gram-negative bacilli can be spread on the hands of staff and NICU outbreaks of Gram-negative bacillary infection have been attributed to poor hand hygiene. There is molecular evidence that the Gram-negative bacilli causing invasive infections are not always found on the hands of nursing staff or other infants, suggesting that prevention strategies may need to concentrate also on ways of reducing transmission from endogenous neonatal flora or environmental sources.[130, 131]

14.2.1 *Escherichia coli*

E. coli can cause early- or late-onset neonatal infection. In general the mortality of early-onset *E. coli* sepsis is higher than that of late-onset *E. coli* infection. In one longitudinal NICU-based multi-centre study the mortality of early-onset *E. coli* sepsis was 36% (and was 50% for infants <1500 g)[132] while the mortality of late-onset *E. coli* sepsis was 14.6%.[133]

Some strains of *E. coli* cause sepsis more than others. Known virulence factors include possession of the K1 polysaccharide capsule, fimbriae for attachment, haemolysins and clusters of genes called pathogenicity islands.[16] The incidence of *E. coli* sepsis has been reported by some but not others to be increasing. There has been an increase in ampicillin resistance in many countries; in most series $>50\%$ and often 80–90% of strains are ampicillin-resistant.[16,58–67] In developing countries, community strains of *E. coli* are increasingly reported as resistant to ampicillin and often to many other antibiotic classes.

E. coli is the major cause of neonatal urinary tract infections (see Chapter 10) and an extremely important cause of neonatal meningitis (see Chapter 7). Lumbar puncture should always be performed in any infant with *E. coli* bacteraemia, because the duration of treatment of meningitis, often associated with ventriculitis which interferes with antibiotic treatment, is for 3 weeks.

14.2.2 Enterobacter species

Enterobacter are mainly transmitted by the hands of staff, although cases and outbreaks of *Enterobacter sakazakii* septicaemia, meningitis and necrotizing enterocolitis have been associated with contaminated powdered infant formula.[134] *E. sakazakii* is sometimes classified as Cronobacter species.[135] Enterobacter species have also been transmitted in contaminated intravenous fluids, both parenteral nutrition and saline.

Enterobacter usually cause late-onset rather than early-onset sepsis. In a multi-centre study, the mortality of late-onset Enterobacter sepsis was 18.6%.[133] *Enterobacter cloacae* is the most commonly reported Enterobacter species. Both *E. cloacae*[136, 137] and *E. sakazakii*[134, 135] can cause necrotizing meningitis with cerebral abscess formation and a high mortality.

All *E. cloacae* carry the gene for an inducible cephalosporinase which is usually not expressed in wild-type strains but can be de-repressed under antibiotic pressure. Thus, even if strains are apparently sensitive to cephalosporins such as cefotaxime and ceftazidime *in vitro*, relapses due to the emergence of resistance during treatment with these agents is common. For this reason it is better to consider *E. cloacae* as inherently resistant to cephalosporins. In addition, many Enterobacter carry genes for extended spectrum β-lactamases (ESBL).[138]

14.2.3 Klebsiella species

Klebsiella oxytoca and *K. pneumoniae* are the main Klebsiella species causing neonatal infections. They can cause early- and late-onset infections, including pneumonia, urinary tract infections, bacteraemia and meningitis.[139] Multi-drug resistance due to ESBL is an increasing problem throughout the world.[138, 139] The mortality of late-onset Klebsiella infection (13.7% in one study[133]) is comparable to that due to other Enterobacteriaceae.

14.2.4 Serratia species

Serratia marcescens is the species causing most neonatal infections and has a similar propensity to cause neonatal meningitis with brain abscesses and a similar mortality (20.9% in a large study[133]) to other Enterobacteriaceae. A non-Cochrane systematic review of 34 outbreaks of *S. marcescens* infections in NICUs and PICUs recommended that two temporally related cases of systemic *S. marcescens* sepsis should raise the possibility of an outbreak and be an indication for improved hygiene precautions (see Chapter 21).[140]

14.2.5 Acinetobacter species

Acinetobacter are immotile, aerobic, non-fermenting Gram-negative bacilli found in soil and fresh water. A non-Cochrane systematic review of outbreaks of invasive Acinetobacter infections in children found 18 reports of nosocomial outbreaks of which 16 were in neonatal intensive care units.[141] Acinetobacter are increasingly reported to be resistant to a broad range of antimicrobials, including β-lactams and even carbapenems.[142–144]

14.2.6 Citrobacter species

Citrobacter species can cause sporadic cases and outbreaks of neonatal infection. Most cases are late-onset but early-onset cases have rarely been reported.[145] *Citrobacter koseri* (previously named *C. diversus*) is particularly associated with necrotizing meningitis and brain abscesses.[145]

14.2.7 *Pseudomonas aeruginosa*

Pseudomonas aeruginosa can cause early- or late-onset infections, although late-onset infections are more common and both have a very high mortality. There are no specific clinical features although, in neutropenic patients, *P. aeruginosa* can cause necrotic skin lesions called ecthyma gangrenosum (Figure 14.6), while *P. aeruginosa* conjunctivitis can progress to endophthalmitis (see Chapter 12). *P. aeruginosa* can cause meningitis and in a case-control study *P. aeruginosa* infection was significantly associated with necrotizing enterocolitis.[146]

The incidence of late-onset Pseudomonas infection was 0.14 per 1000 live births in a multi-centre Australian study.[133] and was 0.7 per 1000 live births in one US hospital.[147] The combined mortality of late-onset Pseudomonas infection in three Australian and US studies was 53% (77 of 146, range 50–56%).[82, 133, 147] For this reason, if a neonatal unit discovers that just one infant is colonized with Pseudomonas, it is reasonable to isolate that infant and culture other babies to try to prevent nursery spread (see Chapters 21 and 22).

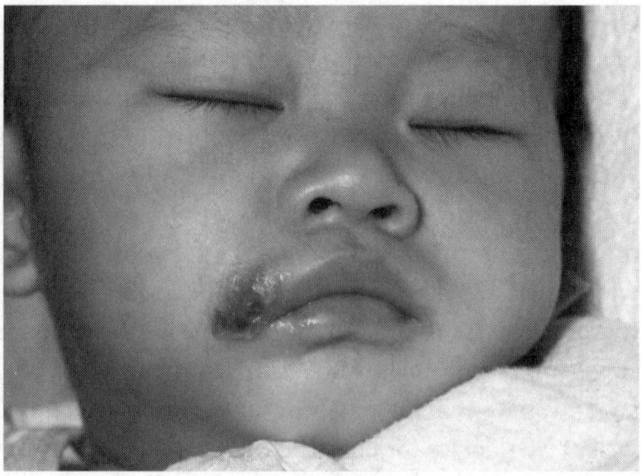

Figure 14.6 Ecthyma gangrenosum-like skin lesion due to *Pseudomonas aeruginosa* in a neutropenic infant.

In a case-control study infants with Pseudomonas bacteraemia or meningitis were more likely than controls to have feeding intolerance and prolonged parenteral hyperalimentation and received intravenous antibiotics for significantly longer than controls.[146] There was an association with prior or concurrent necrotizing enterocolitis.[146]

Pseudomonas species are usually sensitive to aminoglycosides. They are resistant to most third generation cephalosporins, including cefotaxime and ceftriaxone, but are usually sensitive to ceftazidime and to the fourth generation cephalosporin cefepime. Pseudomonas species are usually sensitive to the synthetic penicillins ticarcillin and piperacillin. The use of combination products in which the synthetic penicillin is combined with a β-lactamase inhibitor (ticarcillin–clavulanate or piperacillin–tazobactam) improves activity against staphylococci, anaerobes and ESBL-producing coliforms but does not improve Pseudomonas cover and is not necessary for Pseudomonas strains that are sensitive to ticarcillin and piperacillin. Pseudomonas is also usually sensitive to carbapenems, such as meropenem. Pseudomonas is usually sensitive to quinolones, but quinolones are potentially toxic and should not be used in neonates except as a last resort.

As discussed above (Section 14.2), there are conflicting data on the relative benefits of monotherapy compared with combination therapy using a β-lactam combined with an aminoglycoside: a non-Cochrane systematic review found a survival advantage for combination therapy for Pseudomonas infections[127] whereas a Cochrane review found no advantage in outcome but increased nephrotoxicity with combination therapy.[128] Once sensitivities are back, the data suggest that monotherapy with a β-lactam to which the organism is sensitive is likely to be as effective as combination therapy and less toxic. There are fewer data for an aminoglycoside as monotherapy for Pseudomonas infection and an aminoglycoside should not be used as monotherapy for Pseudomonas meningitis because of relatively poor CSF penetration.

Pseudomonas colonization can become endemic on NICUs. If there is no endemic Pseudomonas colonization on an NICU, it is recommended that finding a single colonized or infected infant should trigger an infection control response with cohorting of the infected infant and screening of other infants for Pseudomonas carriage. Pseudomonas species are water-loving organisms and while they may be found colonizing sinks and humidified incubators, they are most commonly spread on the hands of staff. Management of Pseudomonas outbreaks, including the indications for environmental sampling, will be considered in more detail in Chapter 21.

14.2.8 *Burkholderia cepacia*

Burkholderia cepacia, previously *Pseudomonas cepacia*, is another water-loving organism which can cause neonatal nosocomial outbreaks, usually with a mortality of around 10%,[147, 148] much lower than the 50% or greater mortality of *P. aeruginosa* infection. While some *B. cepacia* outbreaks have been linked to water sources such as infected distilled water[148] or hospital sinks[149] or taps,[150] *B. cepacia* can also contaminate blood culture bottles or blood gas analysers (which can contaminate blood cultures when residents attempt to perform blood gases and blood cultures using the same blood sample) and lead to pseudo-outbreaks of *B. cepacia* infection.[151]

14.2.9 Salmonella

Salmonella are important causes of infant meningitis and septicaemia but are rare causes of neonatal infection. They can cause outbreaks of nosocomial infection, almost always in resource-poor countries, with diarrhoea, fever and sometimes meningitis.[152, 153] Occasional cases of Salmonella meningitis are reported from resource-rich countries.[154, 155] Reptiles and amphibians commonly carry unusual strains of Salmonella and the occurrence of neonatal Salmonella infection in a Western setting should prompt enquiries about maternal exposure to reptiles and amphibians as well as maternal ingestion of eggs or of undercooked chicken.

14.2.10 *Haemophilus influenzae*

Haemophilus influenzae is a vaginal commensal which is a rare cause of early-onset neonatal sepsis with bacteraemia and sometimes meningitis, predominantly occurring in very pre-term infants.[156, 157] Late-onset sepsis is even rarer. There are no specific clinical features of neonatal infection. Infants present with early-onset respiratory distress with pneumonia and the disease has a high mortality particularly in the very low birth-weight infant.[156] Most cases are due to untypeable strains of *H. influenzae* and are not preventable using the type b conjugate vaccines. Occasionally neonatal strains are capsulated. There is some interest in developing vaccines against untypeable strains of *H. influenzae*.[156, 157]

14.3 Gram-positive bacilli

Gram-positive bacilli include Listeria, which is an important neonatal pathogen, and Corynebacteria (diphtheroids) which are common contaminants of neonatal blood cultures and only very rarely pathogenic (Section 14.5).

14.3.1 *Listeria monocytogenes*

Listeria monocytogenes, a Gram-positive bacillus, is an environmental organism found in soil which can infect humans through ingestion of contaminated foods, including undercooked chicken and other meat, unwashed vegetables and unpasteurized dairy products. It can grow at 4°C, so Listeria in undercooked meat can survive and multiply in refrigerators. Listeria is an opportunist intracellular organism which targets cells of the monocyte–macrophage lineage and causes infection almost exclusively in immunocompromised hosts, including pregnant women and newborns.[158–160] *L. monocytogenes* is an important pathogen which can cause early-onset and late-onset neonatal infections, including meningitis, and has a high mortality and morbidity. Most cases are sporadic but community epidemics and nursery outbreaks can occur. However, Listeria infections are responsible for <5% of early-onset infections in most countries and only rare late-onset cases.[158–160]

Maternal *L. monocytogenes* infection can cause miscarriage, stillbirth, pre-term labour, placental infection with granuloma formation and both early- and late-onset neonatal infection. Mothers of infants with early-onset *L. monocytogenes* infection may be asymptomatic around delivery or they may have a bacteraemic febrile influenza-like illness with chills, myalgia and headache. A case series described meconium staining of the liquor in association with pre-term labour in 9 of 13 infants with neonatal listeriosis,[161] but this has been an inconsistent finding and pre-term meconium staining of the liquor also occurs with other organisms and in the absence of infection.[162, 163] Infants with congenital listeriosis may be born with a granulomatous rash (an old name was granulomatosis infantiseptica, see Figure 3.1) indicating haematogenous spread, but infected infants may also have severe respiratory distress with non-specific radiographic changes more suggestive of ascending infection. Early-onset listeriosis may be complicated by meningitis and has a mortality of about 25%.[159–161]

Late-onset infection classically occurs after 7 days and over 90% of infants have meningitis with an acute or sub-acute presentation. There is nothing specific about late-onset Listeria infection. The CSF usually shows a neutrophil predominance although, as the name suggests, *L. monocytogenes* can cause a monocytic pleocytosis in rabbits, and the CSF in human neonates is sometimes predominantly monocytic. A late-onset-like presentation was described at 4–8 days of age in nine infants given a bath soon after birth containing Listeria-contaminated mineral oil.[164] Listeria is a gastro-intestinal organism and one report described transmission from two infants with early-onset *L. monocytogenes* infection to other infants on the nursery, probably through the use of a communal rectal thermometer.[165]

Listeria are inherently resistant to cephalosporins, which is one reason for advising against empiric use of third generation cephalosporins as monotherapy for suspected early-onset neonatal infection or for late-onset meningitis. The treatment of choice is ampicillin plus an aminoglycoside, although clinical reports suggest penicillin G is probably just as effective as ampicillin.

14.4 Gram-negative cocci

14.4.1 *Neisseria meningitidis*

Meningococcus (*Neisseria meningitidis*) is a rare cause of early-onset[166] and late-onset[167, 168] neonatal infections. Fulminant meningococcemia with purpura is described, but many infants have a non-specific presentation of sepsis without rash. Meningococcus can cause conjunctivitis (see Chapter 12).

14.5 Anaerobes

Anaerobes are frequent blood culture contaminants, often in association with other aerobic organisms. Because of this, reports of bacteraemia with anaerobes such as Bacteroides, Clostridium, Peptostreptococcus and Propionibacterium species are difficult to interpret, although some cases are more clinically convincing than others.[169] *Bacteroides fragilis* meningitis is rare, but almost all reported cases have been in neonates.[170] Metronidazole is the treatment of choice for established anaerobic infections.

References

1. Lancefield RC. A serologic differentiation of human and other groups of hemolytic streptococci. *J Exp Med* 1933; 57:591–595.
2. Fry RM. Fatal infections by hemolytic streptococcus group B. *Lancet* 1938; 1:199–201.
3. Jones HE, Howells CH. Neonatal meningitis due to *Streptococcus agalactiae. Postgrad Med J* 1968; 44:549–551.
4. McCracken Jr GH. Group B streptococci: the new challenge in neonatal infections. *J Pediatr* 1973; 82:703–706.
5. Edmond KM, Kortsalioudaki C, Scott S, et al. Group B streptococcal disease in infants aged younger than 3 months: systematic review and meta-analysis. *Lancet* 2012; 379:547–556.
6. Adair CE, Kowalsky L, Quon H, et al. Risk factors for early-onset group B streptococcal disease in neonates: a population-based case-control study. *CMAJ* 2003; 169:198–203.
7. Heath PT, Balfour GF, Tighe H, Verlander NQ, Lamagni TL, Efstratiou A; HPA GBS Working Group. Group B

streptococcal disease in infants: a case control study. *Arch Dis Child* 2009; 94:674–680.
8. Benitz WE, Gould JB, Druzin ML. Risk factors for early-onset group B streptococcal sepsis: estimation of odds ratios by critical literature review. *Pediatrics* 1999; 103:e77.
9. Lin FY, Weisman LE, Troendle J, Adams K. Prematurity is the major risk factor for late-onset group B streptococcus disease. *J Infect Dis* 2003; 188:267–271.
10. Edwards MS, Nizet V. Group B streptococcal infections. In: *Infectious diseases of the fetus and newborn infant*, (eds JS Remington, JO Klein, CB Wilson, V Nizet, Y Maldonado). 7th edn. Philadelphia: Elsevier, 2011. pp 419–469.
11. Noya FJD, Rench MA, Metzger TG, et al. Unusual occurrence of an epidemic of type Ib/c group B streptococcal sepsis in a neonatal intensive care unit. *J Infect Dis* 1987; 155:1135–1144.
12. Kenny JF. Recurrent group B streptococcal disease in an infant associated with the ingestion of infected mother's milk. *J Pediatr* 1977; 91:158–159.
13. Schreiner RL, Coates T, Shackelford PG. Possible breast milk transmission of group B streptococcal infection. *J Pediatr* 1977; 91:159.
14. Olver WJ, Bond DW, Boswell TC, Watkin SL. Neonatal group B streptococcal disease associated with infected breast milk. *Arch Dis Child Fetal Neonatal Ed* 2000; 83:F48–F49.
15. Gagneur A, Héry-Arnaud G, Croly-Labourdette S, et al. Infected breast milk associated with late-onset and recurrent group B streptococcal infection in neonatal twins: a genetic analysis. *Eur J Pediatr* 2009; 168:1155–1158.
16. Kaufman D, Fairchild KD. Clinical microbiology of bacterial and fungal sepsis in very-low-birth-weight infants. *Clin Microbiol Rev* 2004; 17:638–680.
17. Centers for Disease Control and Prevention. Prevention of perinatal Group B streptococcal disease. *MMWR Recommendations and Reports* 2010; 59(RR-10):1–32. Available at: http://www.cdc.gov/mmwr/pdf/rr/rr5910.pdf.
18. Regan JA, Klebanoff MA, Nugent RP, et al. Colonization with group B streptococci in pregnancy and adverse outcome. VIP Study Group. *Am J Obstet Gynecol* 1996; 174:1354–1360.
19. Barcaite E, Bartusevicius A, Tameliene R, Kliucinskas M, Maleckiene L, Nadisauskiene R. Prevalence of maternal group B streptococcal colonisation in European countries. *Acta Obstet Gynecol Scand* 2008; 87:260–271.
20. Baker CJ, Kasper DL. Correlation of maternal antibody deficiency with susceptibility to neonatal group B streptococcal infection. *N Engl J Med* 1976; 294:753–756.
21. Lin FY, Philips 3rd JB, Azimi PH, et al. Level of maternal antibody required to protect neonates against early-onset disease caused by group B streptococcus type Ia: a multicenter, seroepidemiology study. *J Infect Dis* 2001; 184:1022–1028.
22. Lin FY, Weisman LE, Azimi PH, et al. Level of maternal IgG anti-group B streptococcus type III antibody correlated with protection of neonates against early-onset disease caused by this pathogen. *J Infect Dis* 2004; 190:928–934.
23. Heath PT. An update on vaccination against group B streptococcus. *Expert Rev Vaccines* 2011; 10:685–694.
24. Palmeiro JK, De Carvalho NS, Botelho AC, Fracalanzza SE, Madeira HM, Dalla-Costa LM. Maternal group B streptococcal immunization: capsular polysaccharide (CPS)-based vaccines and their implications on prevention. *Vaccine* 2011; 29:3729–3730.
25. Fluegge K, Wons J, Spellereberg B, et al. Geneteic differences between invasive and non-invasive neonatal group B streptococcal isolates. *Pediatr Infect Dis J* 2011; 30:1027–1031.
26. Webber S, Lindsell D, Wilkinson AR, Hope PL, Dobson SRM, Isaacs D. Neonatal pneumonia. *Arch Dis Child* 1990; 65:207–211.
27. Carbonell-Estrany X, Figueras-Aloy J, Salcedo-Abizanda S, de la Rosa-Fraile M; Castrillo Study Group. Probable early-onset group B streptococcal sepsis: a serious clinical condition related to intrauterine infection. *Arch Dis Child Fetal Neonatal Ed* 2008; 93:F85–F89.
28. Edwards MS, Jackson CV, Baker CJ. Increased risk of group B streptococcal disease in twins. *J Am Med Assoc* 1981; 245:2044–2046.
29. Paredes A, Wong P, Yow MD. Failure of penicillin to eradicate the carrier state of group B Streptococcus in infants. *J Pediatr* 1976; 89:191–193.
30. Fernandez M, Rench MA, Albanyan EA, Edwards MS, Baker CJ. Failure of rifampin to eradicate group B streptococcal colonization in infants. *Pediatr Infect Dis J* 2001; 20:371–376.
31. Moylett EH, Fernandez M, Rench MA, Hickman ME, Baker CJ. A 5-year review of recurrent group B streptococcal disease: lessons from twin infants. *Clin Infect Dis* 2000; 30:282–287.
32. Ohlsson A, Shah VS. Intrapartum antibiotics for known maternal Group B streptococcal colonization. Cochrane Database of Systematic Reviews 2009, Issue 3. Art. No.: CD007467. doi: 10.1002/14651858.CD007467.pub2.
33. Edwards RK, Clark P, Sistrom CL, Duff P. Intrapartum antibiotic prophylaxis 1: relative effects of recommended antibiotics on Gram-negative pathogens. *Obstet Gynecol* 2002; 100:534–539.
34. Stade BC, Shah VS, Ohlsson A. Vaginal chlorhexidine during labour to prevent early-onset neonatal group B streptococcal infection. Cochrane Database of Systematic Reviews 2004, Issue 3. Art. No.: CD003520. doi: 10.1002/14651858.CD003520.pub2.
35. Colbourn TE, Asseburg C, Bojke L, et al. Preventive strategies for group B streptococcal and other bacterial infections in early infancy: cost effectiveness and value of information analyses. *BMJ* 2007; 335:655.
36. BBenitz WE, Gould JB, Druzin ML. Risk factors for early-onset group B streptococcal sepsis: estimation of odds ratios by critical literature review. *Pediatrics* 1999; 103:e77.
37. Puopolo KM, Draper D, Wi S, et al. Estimating the probability of neonatal early-onset infection on the basis of maternal risk factors. *Pediatrics* 2011; 128:e1155–e1163; Anthony BF, Okada DM, Hobel CJ. Epidemiology of group B

Streptococcus: longitudinal observations during pregnancy. *J Infect Dis* 1978; 137: 524–530.

38. Yow MD, Leeds LJ, Thompson PK, Mason Jr EO, Clark DJ, Beachler CW. The natural history of group B streptococcal colonization in the pregnant woman and her offspring. I. Colonization studies. *Am J Obstet Gynecol* 1980; 137:34–38.
39. Honest H, Sharma S, Khan KS. Rapid tests for group B Streptococcus colonization in laboring women: a systematic review. *Pediatrics* 2006; 117:1055–1066.
40. Daniels J, Gray J, Pattison H, et al. Rapid testing for group B streptococcus during labour: a test accuracy study with evaluation of acceptability and cost-effectiveness. *Health Technol Assess* 2009; 13:1–154, iii–iv.
41. Gilbert GL, Isaacs D, Burgess MA, et al. Prevention of neonatal group B streptococcal sepsis: is routine antenatal screening appropriate? *Aust NZ J Obstet Gynecol* 1995; 35:120–126.
42. Mohle-Boetani JC, Schuchat A, Plikyatis BD, Smith JD, Broome CV. Comparison of prevention strategies for neonatal group B streptococcal infection. A population-based economic analysis. *J Am Med Assoc* 1993; 270:1442–1448.
43. Colbourn T, Asseburg C, Bojke L, et al. Prenatal screening and treatment strategies to prevent group B streptococcal and other bacterial infections in early infancy: cost-effectiveness and expected value of information analyses. *Health Technol Assess* 2007; 11:1–226, iii.
44. Boetani JC, Schuchat A, Plikyatis BD, Smith JD, Broome CV. Comparison of prevention strategies for neonatal group B streptococcal infection. A population-based economic analysis. *J Am Med Assoc* 1993; 270:1442–1448.
45. Boyer KM, Gadzala CA, Kelly PD, Burd LI, Gotoff SP. Selective intrapartum chemoprophylaxis of neonatal group B streptococcal early-onset disease. II. Predictive value of prenatal cultures. *J Infect Dis* 1983; 148:802–809.
46. Isaacs D, Royle J, Australasian Study Group for Neonatal Infections. Intrapartum antibiotics and early onset neonatal sepsis caused by group B streptococcus and other organisms. *Pediatr Infect Dis J* 1999; 18:354–358.
47. Daley AJ, Isaacs D. Ten year study on the effects of intrapartum antibiotic prophylaxis on early onset group B Streptococcal and *Escherichia coli* neonatal sepsis in Australasia. *Pediatr Infect Dis J* 2004; 23:630–634.
48. Main EK, Slagle T. Prevention of early-onset invasive neonatal group B streptococcal disease in a private hospital setting: the superiority of culture-based protocols. *Am J Obstet Gynecol* 2000; 182:1344–1354.
49. Baltimore RS, Huie SM, Meek JI, Schuchat A, O'Brien KL. Early-onset neonatal sepsis in the era of group B streptococcal prevention. *Pediatrics* 2001; 108:1094–1098.
50. Edwards RK, Jamie WE, Sterner D, Gentry S, Counts K, Duff P. Intrapartum antibiotic prophylaxis and early-onset neonatal sepsis patterns. *Infect Dis Obstet Gynecol* 2003; 11:221–226.
51. Alarcon A, Pena P, Salas S, Sancha M, Omenaca F. Neonatal early onset *Escherichia coli* sepsis: trends in incidence and antimicrobial resistance in the era of intrapartum antimicrobial prophylaxis. *Pediatr Infect Dis J* 2004; 23:295–299.
52. Rentz AC, Samore MH, Stoddard GJ, Faix RG, Byington CL. Risk factors associated with ampicillin-resistant infection in newborns in the era of group B streptococcal prophylaxis. *Arch Pediatr Adolesc Med* 2004; 158:556–560.
53. Sutkin G, Krohn MA, Heine RP, Sweet RL. Antibiotic prophylaxis and non-group B streptococcal neonatal sepsis. *Obstet Gynecol* 2005; 105:581–586.
54. Angstetra D, Ferguson J, Giles WB. Institution of universal screening for group B *Streptococcus* (GBS) from a risk management protocol results in reduction of early-onset GBS disease in a tertiary obstetric unit. *Aust N Z J Obstet Gynaecol* 2007; 47:378–382.
55. Puopolo K, Eichenwald E. No change in the incidence of ampicillin-resistant, neonatal, early-onset sepsis over 18 years. *Pediatrics* 2010; 125:e1031–e1038.
56. Joseph TA, Pyati SP, Jacobs N. Neonatal early-onset *Escherichia coli* disease: the effect of intrapartum ampicillin. *Arch Pediatr Adolesc Med* 1998; 152:35–40.
57. Cordero L, Sananes M, Ayers LW. Bloodstream infections in a neonatal intensive-care unit: 12 years' experience with an antibiotic control program. *Infect Control Hosp Epidemiol* 1999; 20:242–246.
58. Towers CV, Carr MH, Padilla G, Asrat T. Potential consequences of widespread antepartal use of ampicillin. *Am J Obstet Gynecol* 1998; 179:879–883.
59. Levine EM, Ghai V, Barton JJ, Strom CM. Intrapartum antibiotic prophylaxis increases the incidence of gram-negative neonatal sepsis. *Infectious diseases in Obstet Gynecol* 1999; 7:210–213.
60. Bizzarro MJ, Dembry LM, Baltimore RS, Gallagher PG. Changing patterns in neonatal *Escherichia coli* sepsis and ampicillin resistance in the era of intrapartum antibiotic prophylaxis. *Pediatrics* 2008; 121:689–696.
61. Stoll BJ, Hansen N, Fanaroff AA, et al. Changes in pathogens causing early-onset sepsis in very-low-birth-weight infants. *N Engl J Med* 2002; 347:240–247.
62. Hyde TB, Hilger TM, Reingold A, Farley MM, O'Brien KL, Schuchat A. Trends in incidence and antimicrobial resistance of early-onset sepsis: population-based surveillance in San Francisco and Atlanta. *Pediatrics* 2002; 110:690–695.
63. Al-Hasan MN, Lahr BD, Eckel-Passow JE, Baddour LM. Antimicrobial resistance trends of *Escherichia coli* bloodstream isolates: a population-based study, 1998–2007. *J Antimicrob Chemother* 2009; 64:169–174.
64. Moore MR, Schrag SJ, Schuchat A. Effects of intrapartum antimicrobial prophylaxis for prevention of group-B-streptococcal disease on the incidence and ecology of early-onset neonatal sepsis. *Lancet Infect Dis* 2003; 3:201–213.
65. Stoll BJ, Hansen NI, Higgins RD, et al. Very low birth weight preterm infants with early onset neonatal sepsis: the predominance of gram-negative infections continues in the National Institute of Child Health and Human Development Neonatal Research Network, 2002–2003. *Pediatr Infect Dis J* 2005; 24:635–639.

66. Schrag SJ, Hadler JL, Arnold KE, Martell-Cleary P, Reingold A, Schuchat A. Risk factors for invasive, early-onset *Escherichia coli* infections in the era of widespread intrapartum antibiotic use. *Pediatrics* 2006; 118:570–576.
67. de Cueto M, Sanchez MJ, Sampedro A, Miranda JA, Herruzo AJ, Rosa-Fraile M. Timing of intrapartum ampicillin and prevention of vertical transmission of group B *Streptococcus. Obstet Gynecol* 1998; 91:112–114.
68. Lin FY, Brenner RA, Johnson YR, et al. The effectiveness of risk-based intrapartum chemoprophylaxis for the prevention of early-onset neonatal group B streptococcal disease. *Am J Obstet Gynecol* 2001; 184:1204–1210.
69. Illuzzi JL, Bracken MB. Duration of intrapartum prophylaxis for neonatal group B streptococcal disease: a systematic review. *Obstet Gynecol* 2006; 108:1254–1265.
70. Barber EL, Zhao G, Buhimschi IA, Illuzzi JL. Duration of intrapartum prophylaxis and concentration of penicillin G in fetal serum at delivery. *Obstet Gynecol* 2008; 112:265–270.
71. Hashavya S, Benenson S, Ergaz-Shaltiel Z, Bar-Oz B, Averbuch D, Eventov-Friedman S. The use of blood counts and blood cultures to screen neonates born to partially treated group B Streptococcus-carrier mothers for early-onset sepsis: is it justified? *Pediatr Infect Dis J* 2011; 30:840–843.
72. Isaacs D, Australasian Study Group for Neonatal Infections. A ten-year multi-centre study of coagulase negative staphylococcal infections. *Arch Dis Child Fetal Neonatal Ed* 2003; 88:F89–F93.
73. St Geme 3rd JW, Bell LM, Baumgart S, D'Angio CT, Harris MC. Distinguishing sepsis from blood culture contamination in young infants with blood cultures growing coagulase-negative staphylococci. *Pediatrics* 1990; 86:157–162.
74. Mueller-Premru M, Gubina M, Kaufmann ME, Primozic J, Cookson BD. Use of semi-quantitative and quantitative culture methods and typing for studying the epidemiology of central venous catheter-related infections in neonates on parenteral nutrition. *J Med Microbiol* 1999; 48:451–460.
75. Kassis C, Rangaraj G, Jiang Y, Hachem RY, Raad I. Differentiating culture samples representing coagulase-negative staphylococcal bacteremia from those representing contamination by use of time-to-positivity and quantitative blood culture methods. *J Clin Microbiol* 2009; 47:3255–3260.
76. Freeman J, Platt R, Epstein MF, Smith NE, Sidebottom DG, Goldmann DA. Birth weight and length of stay as determinants of nosocomial coagulase-negative staphylococcal bacteremia in neonatal intensive care unit populations: potential for confounding. *Am J Epidemiol* 1990; 132:1130–1140.
77. Freeman J, Goldmann DA, Smith NE, Sidebottom DG, Epstein MF, Platt R. Association of intravenous lipid emulsion and coagulase-negative staphylococcal bacteremia in neonatal intensive care. *N Engl J Med* 1990; 323:301–308.
78. Benjamin Jr DK, Miller W, Garges H, Benjamin DK, McKinney Jr RE, Cotton M, et al. Bacteremia, central catheters, and neonates: when to pull the line. *Pediatrics* 2001; 107:1272–1276.
79. Schulman J, Stricof R, Stevens TP, et al; New York State Regional Perinatal Care Centers. Statewide NICU central-line-associated bloodstream infection rates decline after bundles and checklists. *Pediatrics* 2011; 127:436–444.
80. Maayan-Metzger A, Linder N, Marom D, Vishne T, Ashkenazi S, Sirota L. Clinical and laboratory impact of coagulase-negative staphylococci bacteremia in preterm infants. *Acta Paediatr* 2000; 89:690–693.
81. Healy CM, Palazzi DL, Edwards MS, Campbell JR, Baker CJ. Features of invasive staphylococcal disease in neonates. *Pediatrics* 2004; 114:953–961.
82. Karlowicz MG, Buescher ES, Surka AE. Fulminant late-onset sepsis in a neonatal intensive care unit, 1988-1997, and the impact of avoiding empiric vancomycin therapy. *Pediatrics* 2000; 106:1387–1390.
83. Stoll BJ, Fanaroff A. Early-onset coagulase-negative staphylococcal sepsis in preterm neonate. *Lancet* 1995; 345:1236–1237.
84. Fowlie PW, Schmidt B. Diagnostic tests for bacterial infection from birth to 90 days – a systematic review. *Arch Dis Child Fetal Neonatal Ed* 1998; 78:F92–F98.
85. Manzoni P, Mostert M, Galletto P, et al. Is thrombocytopenia suggestive of organism-specific response in neonatal sepsis? Pediatr Int 2009; 51:206–210.
86. Krediet TG, Jones ME, Gerards LJ, Fleer A. Clinical outcome of cephalothin versus vancomycin therapy in the treatment of coagulase-negative staphylococcal septicemia in neonates: relation to methicillin resistance and mec A gene carriage of blood isolates. *Pediatrics* 1999; 103:E29.
87. Lawrence SL, Roth V, Slinger R, Toye B, Gaboury I, Lemyre B. Cloxacillin versus vancomycin for presumed late-onset sepsis in the Neonatal Intensive Care Unit and the impact upon outcome of coagulase negative staphylococcal bacteremia: a retrospective cohort study. *BMC Pediatr* 2005; 5:49.
88. Blayney MP, Al Madani M. Coagulase-negative staphylococcal infections in a neonatal intensive care unit: In vivo response to cloxacillin. *Paediatr Child Health* 2006; 11:659–663.
89. Hemels MA, van den Hoogen A, Verboon-Maciolek MA, Fleer A, Krediet TG. A seven-year survey of management of coagulase-negative staphylococcal sepsis in the neonatal intensive care unit: vancomycin may not be necessary as empiric therapy. *Neonatology* 2011; 100:180–185.
90. Karlowicz MG, Furigay PJ, Croitoru DP, Buescher ES. Central venous catheter removal versus in situ treatment in neonates with coagulase-negative staphylococcal bacteremia. *Pediatr Infect Dis J* 2002; 21:22–27.
91. Hemels MA, van den Hoogen A, Verboon-Maciolek MA, Fleer A, Krediet TG. Shortening the antibiotic course for the treatment of neonatal coagulase-negative staphylococcal sepsis: fine with three days? *Neonatology* 2012; 101:101–105.
92. Noel GJ, O'Loughlin JE, Edelson PJ. Neonatal *Staphylococcus epidermidis* right-sided endocarditis: description of five catheterized infants. *Pediatrics* 1988; 82:234–239.

93. Khashu M, Osiovich H, Henry D, Al Khotani A, Solimano A, Speert DP. Persistent bacteremia and severe thrombocytopenia caused by coagulase-negative Staphylococcus in a neonatal intensive care unit. *Pediatrics* 2006; 117:340–348.
94. Anderson-Berry A, Brinton B, Lyden E, Faix RG. Risk factors associated with development of persistent coagulase-negative staphylococci bacteremia in the neonate and associated short-term and discharge morbidities. *Neonatology* 2011; 99:23–31.
95. Dimitriou G, Fouzas S, Giormezis N, et al. Clinical and microbiological profile of persistent coagulase-negative staphylococcal bacteraemia in neonates. *Clin Microbiol Infect* 2011; 17:1684–1690.
96. Linder N, Hernandez A, Amit L, Klinger G, Ashkenazi S, Levy I. Persistent coagulase-negative staphylococci bacteremia in very-low-birth-weight infants. *Eur J Pediatr* 2011; 170:989–995.
97. van der Lugt NM, Steggerda SJ, Walther FJ. Use of rifampin in persistent coagulase negative staphylococcal bacteremia in neonates. *BMC Pediatr* 2010; 10:84.
98. Jean-Baptiste N, Benjamin Jr DK, Cohen-Wolkowiez M, et al. Coagulase-negative staphylococcal infections in the neonatal intensive care unit. *Infect Control Hosp Epidemiol* 2011; 32:679–686.
99. Gray JE, Richardson DK, McCormick MC, Goldmann DA. Coagulase-negative staphylococcal bacteremia among very low birth weight infants: relation to admission illness severity, resource use, and outcome. *Pediatrics* 1995; 95:225–230.
100. Stoll BJ, Hansen NI, Adams-Chapman I, et al; National Institute of Child Health and Human Development Neonatal Research Network. Neurodevelopmental and growth impairment among extremely low-birth-weight infants with neonatal infection. *J Am Med Assoc* 2004; 292:2357–2365.
101. Kilbride HW, Wirtschafter DD, Powers RJ, Sheehan MB. Implementation of evidence-based potentially better practices to decrease nosocomial infections. *Pediatrics* 2003; 111:e519–e533.
102. Sharek PJ, Benitz WE, Abel NJ, Freeburn MJ, Mayer ML, Bergman DA. Effect of an evidence-based hand washing policy on hand washing rates and false-positive coagulase negative staphylococcus blood and cerebrospinal fluid culture rates in a level III NICU. *J Perinatol* 2002; 22:137–143.
103. Lam BC, Lee J, Lau YL. Hand hygiene practices in a neonatal intensive care unit: a multimodal intervention and impact on nosocomial infection. *Pediatrics* 2004; 114:e565–e571.
104. Horbar JD, Rogowski J, Plsek PE, Delmore P, Edwards WH, Hocker J, et al. Collaborative quality improvement for neonatal intensive care. NIC/Q Project Investigators of the Vermont Oxford Network. *Pediatrics* 2001; 107:14–22.
105. Kane E, Bretz G. Reduction in coagulase-negative staphylococcus infection rates in the NICU using evidence-based research. *Neonatal Netw* 2011; 30:165–174.
106. Sharek PJ, Benitz WE, Abel NJ, Freeburn MJ, Mayer ML, Bergman DA. Effect of an evidence-based hand washing policy on hand washing rates and false-positive coagulase negative staphylococcus blood and cerebrospinal fluid culture rates in a level III NICU. *J Perinatol* 2002; 22:137–143.
107. McClure RJ, Newell SJ. Randomised controlled trial of clinical outcome following trophic feeding. *Arch Dis Child Fetal Neonatal Ed* 2000; 82:F29–F33.
108. Lavoie PM. Earlier initiation of enteral nutrition is associated with lower risk of late-onset bacteremia only in most mature very low birth weight infants. *J Perinatol* 2009; 29:448–454.
109. Carey AJ, Long SS. *Staphylococcus aureus*: a continuously evolving and formidable pathogen in the neonatal intensive care unit. *Clin Perinatol* 2010; 37:535–546.
110. Isaacs D, Fraser S, Hogg G, Li HY. *Staphylococcus aureus* infections in Australasian neonatal nurseries. *Arch Dis Child Fetal Neonatal Ed* 2004; 89:F331–F335.
111. Vergnano S, Menson E, Smith Z, et al. Characteristics of invasive *Staphylococcus aureus* in United Kingdom neonatal units. *Pediatr Infect Dis J* 2011; 30:850–854.
112. Fortunov RM, Hulten KG, Hammerman WA, Mason Jr EO, Kaplan SL. Community-acquired *Staphylococcus aureus* infections in term and near-term previously healthy neonates. *Pediatrics.* 2006; 118:874–881.
113. Fortunov RM, Hulten KG, Hammerman WA, Mason Jr EO, Kaplan SL. Evaluation and treatment of community-acquired Staphylococcus aureus infections in term and late-preterm previously healthy neonates. *Pediatrics* 2007; 120:937–945.
114. Zaidi AKM, Thaver D, Ali AS, Khan TA. Pathogens associated with sepsis in newborns and young infants in developing countries. *Pediatr Infect Dis J* 2009; 28:S10–S18.
115. Deville JG, Adler S, Azimi PH, et al. Linezolid versus vancomycin in the treatment of known or suspected resistant Gram-positive infections in neonates. *Pediatr Infect Dis J* 2003; 22:S158–S163.
116. Gray JW, Patel M. Management of antibiotic-resistant infection in the newborn. *Arch Dis Child Educ Pract Ed* 2011; 96:122–127.
117. Siegel JD, McCracken Jr GH. Group D streptococcal infections. *J Pediatr* 1978; 93:542–543.
118. Dobson SR, Baker CJ. Enterococcal sepsis in neonates: features by age at onset and occurrence of focal infection. *Pediatrics* 1990; 85:165–171.
119. Duchon J, Graham Iii P, Della-Latta P, et al. Epidemiology of enterococci in a neonatal intensive care unit. *Infect Control Hosp Epidemiol* 2008; 29:374–376.
120. Malik RK, Montecalvo MA, Reale MR, et al. Epidemiology and control of vancomycin-resistant enterococci in a regional neonatal intensive care unit. *Pediatr Infect Dis J* 1999; 18:352–356.
121. Greenberg D, Leibovitz E, Shinnwell ES, Yagupsky P, Dagan R. Neonatal sepsis caused by *Streptococcus pyogenes*: resurgence of an old etiology? *Pediatr Infect Dis J* 1999; 18:479–481.
122. Hoffman JA, Mason EO, Schutze GE, et al. *Streptococcus pneumoniae* infections in the neonate. *Pediatrics* 2003; 112:1095–1102.

123. Freedman RM, Baltimore R. Fatal *Streptococcus viridans* septicemia and meningitis: relationship to fetal scalp electrode monitoring. *J Perinatol* 1990; 10:272–274.
124. Bignardi G, Isaacs D. Neonatal *Streptococcus mitis* meningitis. *Rev Infect Dis* 1989; ii: 86–88.
125. Adams JT, Faix RG. *Streptococcus mitis* infection in newborns. *J Perinatol* 1994; 14:473–478.
126. Raymond J, Bergeret M, Francoual C, Chavinié J, Gendrel D. Neonatal infection with *Streptococcus milleri. Eur J Clin Microbiol Infect Dis* 1995; 14:799–801.
127. Safdar N, Handelsman J, Maki DG. Does combination antimicrobial therapy reduce mortality in Gram-negative bacteraemia? A meta-analysis. *Lancet Infect Dis* 2004; 4:519–527.
128. Paul M, Grozinsky S, Soares-Weiser K, Leibovici L. Beta lactam antibiotic monotherapy versus beta lactam-aminoglycoside antibiotic combination therapy for sepsis. Cochrane Database of Systematic Reviews 2006, Issue 1. Art. No.: CD003344. doi: 10.1002/14651858.CD003344.pub2.
129. Paul M, Leibovici L. Combination antimicrobial treatment versus monotherapy: the contribution of meta-analyses. *Infect Dis Clin North Am* 2009; 23:277–293.
130. Waters V, Larson E, Wu F, et al. Molecular epidemiology of gram-negative bacilli from infected neonates and health care workers' hands in neonatal intensive care units. *Clin Infect Dis* 2004; 38:1682–1687.
131. Larson EL, Cimiotti JP, Haas J, et al. Gram-negative bacilli associated with catheter-associated and non-catheter-associated bloodstream infections and hand carriage by healthcare workers in neonatal intensive care units. *Pediatr Crit Care Med* 2005; 6:457–461.
132. Daley AJ, Isaacs D. Ten year study on the effects of intrapartum antibiotic prophylaxis on early onset group B *Streptococcal* and *Escherichia coli* neonatal sepsis in Australasia. *Pediatr Infect Dis J* 2004; 23:630–634.
133. Gordon A, Isaacs D, Australasian Study Group for Neonatal Infections. Late onset Gram negative bacillary infections in Australia and New Zealand, 1992-2002. *Pediatr Infect Dis J* 2006: 25:25–29.
134. Drudy D, Mullane NR, Quinn T, Wall PG, Fanning S. Enterobacter sakazakii: an emerging pathogen in powdered infant formula. *Clin Infect Dis* 2006; 42:996–1002.
135. Healy B, Cooney S, O'Brien S, et al. Cronobacter (Enterobacter sakazakii): an opportunistic foodborne pathogen. *Foodborne Pathog Dis* 2010; 7:339–350.
136. Dalben M, Varkulja G, Basso M, et al. Investigation of an outbreak of Enterobacter cloacae in a neonatal unit and review of the literature. *J Hosp Infect* 2008; 70:7–14.
137. Chen HN, Lee ML, Yu WK, Lin YW, Tsao LY. Late-onset Enterobacter cloacae sepsis in very-low-birth-weight neonates: experience in a medical center. *Pediatr Neonatol* 2009; 50: 3–7.
138. Paterson DL. Resistance in gram-negative bacteria: enterobacteriaceae. *Am J Med* 2006; 119 (6 Suppl 1): S20–S28.
139. Cordero L, Rau R, Taylor D, Ayers LW. Enteric gram-negative bacilli bloodstream infections: 17 years' experience in a neonatal intensive care unit. *Am J Infect Control* 2004; 32:189–195.
140. Voelz A, Müller A, Gillen J, et al. Outbreaks of Serratia marcescens in neonatal and pediatric intensive care units: clinical aspects, risk factors and management. *Int J Hyg Environ Health* 2010; 213:79–87.
141. Hu J, Robinson JL. Systematic review of invasive Acinetobacter infections in children. *Can J Infect Dis Med Microbiol* 2010; 21:83–88.
142. Afzal-Shah M, Livermore D. Worldwide emergence of carapanem-resistant *Acinetobacter* spp. *J Antimicrob Chemother* 1998; 41:576–577.
143. Coelho J, Woodford N, Turton J, Livermore D. Multiresistant *Acinetobacter* in the UK: How big a threat? *J Hosp Infect* 2004; 58:167–169.
144. Kuo L, Yu C, Lee L, et al. Clinical features of pandrug-resistant *Acinetobacter baumannii* bacteremia at a university hospital in Taiwan. *J Formos Med Assoc* 2003; 102:601–606.
145. Doran TI. The role of Citrobacter in clinical disease of children: review. *Clin Infect Dis* 1999; 28:384–394.
146. Leigh L, Stoll BJ, Rahman M, McGowan J. *Pseudomonas aeruginosa* infection in very low birth weight infants: a case-control study. *Pediatr Infect Dis J* 1995; 14:367–371.
147. Rapkin RH. Pseudomonas cepacia in an intensive care nursery. *Pediatrics* 1976; 57:239–243.
148. Lee JK. Two outbreaks of *Burkholderia cepacia* nosocomial infection in a neonatal intensive care unit. *J Paediatr Child Health* 2008; 44:62–66.
149. Lucero CA, Cohen AL, Trevino I, et al. Outbreak of *Burkholderia cepacia* complex among ventilated pediatric patients linked to hospital sinks. *Am J Infect Control* 2011; 39:775–778.
150. Kotsanas D, Brett J, Kidd TJ, Stuart RL, Korman TM. Disinfection of *Burkholderia cepacia* complex from non-touch taps in a neonatal nursery. *J Perinat Med* 2008; 36:235–239.
151. Manzar S, Nair AK, Pai MG, Al-Khusaiby SM. Pseudo-outbreak of *Burkholderia cepacia* in a neonatal intensive care unit. *J Hosp Infect* 2004; 58:159.
152. Mahajan R, Mathur M, Kumar A, Gupta P, Faridi MM, Talwar V. Nosocomial outbreak of *Salmonella typhimurium* infection in a nursery intensive care unit (NICU) and paediatric ward. *J Commun Dis* 1995; 27:10–14.
153. Newman MJ. Multiple-resistant Salmonella group G outbreak in a neonatal intensive care unit. *West Afr J Med* 1996; 15:165–169.
154. Hansen LN, Eschen C, Bruun B. Neonatal Salmonella meningitis: two case reports. *Acta Paediatr* 1996; 85:629–631.
155. Cooke FJ, Ginwalla S, Hampton MD, et al. Report of neonatal meningitis due to *Salmonella enterica* serotype Agona and review of breast milk-associated neonatal Salmonella infections. *J Clin Microbiol* 2009; 47:3045–3049.
156. Hershckowitz S, Elisha MB, Fleisher-Sheffer V, et al. A cluster of early neonatal sepsis and pneumonia caused by

nontypable *Haemophilus influenzae. Pediatr Infect Dis J* 2004; 23:1061–1062.

157. Gkentzi D, Slack MP, Ladhani SN. The burden of non-encapsulated *Haemophilus influenzae* in children and potential for prevention. *Curr Opin Infect Dis* 2012; 25:266–272.
158. Mylonakis E, Paliou M, Hohmann EL, Calderwood SB, Wing EJ. Listeriosis during pregnancy: a case series and review of 222 cases. *Medicine (Baltimore)* 2002; 81:260–269.
159. Jackson KA, Iwamoto M, Swerdlow D. Pregnancy-associated listeriosis. *Epidemiol Infect* 2010; 138:1503–1509.
160. Lamont RF, Sobel J, Mazaki-Tovi S, et al. Listeriosis in human pregnancy: a systematic review. *J Perinat Med* 2011; 39:227–236.
161. Becroft DM, Farmer K, Seddon RJ, et al. Epidemic listeriosis in the newborn. *Br Med J* 1971; 3:747–751.
162. Siriwachirachai T, Sangkomkamhang US, Lumbiganon P, Laopaiboon M. Antibiotics for meconium-stained amniotic fluid in labour for preventing maternal and neonatal infections. Cochrane Database of Systematic Reviews 2010, Issue 12. Art. No.: CD007772. doi: 10.1002/14651858.CD007772.pub2.
163. Tran SH, Caughey AB, Musci TJ. Meconium-stained amniotic fluid is associated with puerperal infections. *Am J Obstet Gynecol* 2003; 189:746–750.
164. Schuchat A, Lizano C, Broome CV, Swaminathan B, Kim C, Winn K. Outbreak of neonatal listeriosis associated with mineral oil. *Pediatr Infect Dis J* 1991; 10:183–189.
165. Larsson S, Cederberg A, Ivarsson S, Svanberg L, Cronberg S. Listeria monocytogenes causing hospital-acquired enterocolitis and meningitis in newborn infants. *Br Med J* 1978; 2: 473–474.
166. Lo WT, Yuh YS, Wang CC, Chu ML. Early onset neonatal infection with Neisseria meningitidis serogroup C: case report and literature review. *Eur J Pediatr* 2003; 162:785–787.
167. Falcão MC, Andrade SB, Ceccon ME, Costa Vaz FA. Neonatal sepsis and meningitis caused by Neisseria meningitidis: a case report. *Rev Inst Med Trop Sao Paulo* 2007; 49:191–194.
168. Tinsa F, Jallouli M, Ben Lassouad M, et al. Neonatal meningitis by Neisseria meningitidis B. *Tunis Med* 2008; 86:1014–1015.
169. Brook I. Anaerobic infections in children. *Adv Exp Med Biol* 2011; 697:117–152.
170. Feder Jr HM. Bacteroides fragilis meningitis. *Rev Infect Dis* 1987; 9:783–786.

CHAPTER 15
Mycoplasmas

15.1 Microbiology

Mycoplasmas, which include Mycoplasma and Ureaplasma, are the smallest free-living organisms that can live outside cells, distinguishing them from viruses which are obligate intracellular organisms. Mycoplasmas have both DNA and RNA and can grow in cell-free culture media. They are bound by a cell membrane and have no rigid cell wall, which explains their inherent resistance to antibiotics acting by inhibiting cell wall synthesis such as β-lactams. They have small genomes and need exogenous nutrients, obtaining these by colonizing mucosal surfaces of the human respiratory and genitourinary tracts.[1,2]

Mycoplasmas stain poorly with Gram's iodine and can only be cultured using special culture media not routinely available in diagnostic laboratories. Detection in diagnostic laboratories is usually by PCR.[3,4]

15.2 Epidemiology

The most common Mycoplasmas present in the female genital tract, *Mycoplasma hominis*, *Ureaplasma urealyticum* and *Ureaplasma parvum* are also the most common neonatal Mycoplasmas. Maternal colonization with Mycoplasma and Ureaplasma is common (20–80%) and the prevalence is increased in pregnant women of lower socioeconomic status and women with multiple partners.[1,2] *U. parvum* (parvum meaning small) is a tiny Mycoplasma that was not separated into a distinct species until 2002. In future, however, it is important to differentiate *U. parvum* and *U. urealyticum* because of their different pathologic effects on the neonatal lung (Section 15.4).

Mycoplasma pneumoniae, an important respiratory pathogen of infants and older children, is rarely implicated in neonatal infection.[5]

15.3 Chorioamnionitis

Mycoplasmas are detected equally commonly in women with and without clinical chorioamnionitis. However, detection of *U. urealyticum* in the chorioamniotic fluid or chorioamnion is associated with histologic chorioamnionitis, premature rupture of the membranes and pre-term labour,[1,2,6–8] although finding these associations does not prove causality. There are conflicting data regarding the association between *M. hominis* and chorioamnionitis.[1,8] Although infants delivered vaginally are more likely to become colonized with Ureaplasma, colonization can also follow elective Caesarean section.[1,2,6–8]

While some authorities have found associations between maternal and neonatal Ureaplasma colonization or infection, chorioamnionitis and neonatal chronic lung disease, there are many potential confounding factors and the association is not proof of causality. Indeed, in a prospective study of infants <30 weeks of gestation chorioamnionitis with umbilical vasculitis was associated with a reduced risk of chronic lung disease.[9] A meta-analysis of 59 studies found a significant association between chorioamnionitis and bronchopulmonary dysplasia (BPD) (OR 1.89, 95% CI 1.56–2.30) and infants exposed to chorioamnionitis were significantly lighter and less mature at birth. However, there was significant heterogeneity and the authors suspected publication bias and concluded that chorioamnionitis cannot be definitively considered a risk factor for BPD.[10]

A systematic review of the association between chorioamnionitis and neonatal neurodevelopment found conflicting data regarding the benefits and risks of chorioamnionitis on the pre-term infant brain. The authors postulated that inflammation might enhance brain maturation of the pre-term infant and have

Evidence-Based Neonatal Infections, First Edition. David Isaacs.

protective effects balancing its potential harmful effects.[11]

15.4 Ureaplasmas and respiratory distress syndrome

Although there is a well-recognized association between Ureaplasma neonatal infection and chronic lung disease, most studies find no association between Ureaplasma and respiratory distress syndrome (RDS).[1,8] An Australian study reported that maternal and infant colonization with *U. urealyticum* was associated with a 64% decrease in the risk of RDS but a threefold increase in chronic lung disease.[12] Similarly, a British study reported that infants <30 weeks of gestation colonized with *U. urealyticum* had a milder initial course of RDS clinically and radiographically than non-colonized infants of the same gestation, but were subsequently more likely to develop chronic lung disease with pulmonary interstitial emphysema (Figure 15.1).[13] In contrast, an Italian study found colonization with Ureaplasma, particularly *U. parvum*, was significantly more common in infants with RDS than infants without RDS.[14] Possibly the earlier study was unable to distinguish *U. parvum* from *U. urealyticum* infections and the two Ureaplasma species differ with respect to their effect on RDS. However, if Ureaplasma colonization does indeed protect against RDS, this urges caution in planning intervention studies which attempt to reduce chronic lung disease using antibiotic treatment of pregnant women or pre-term newborns.

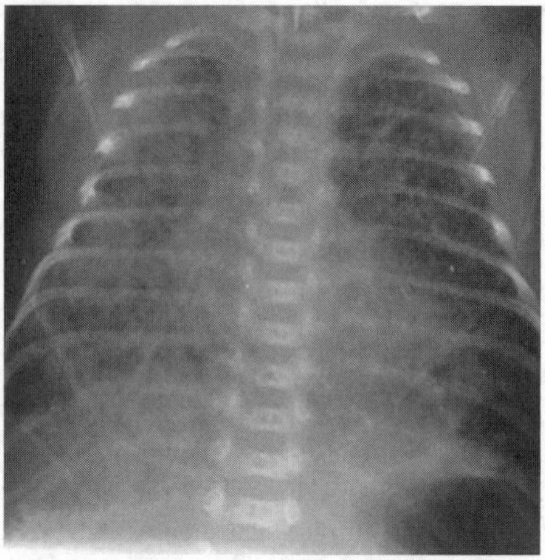

(a)

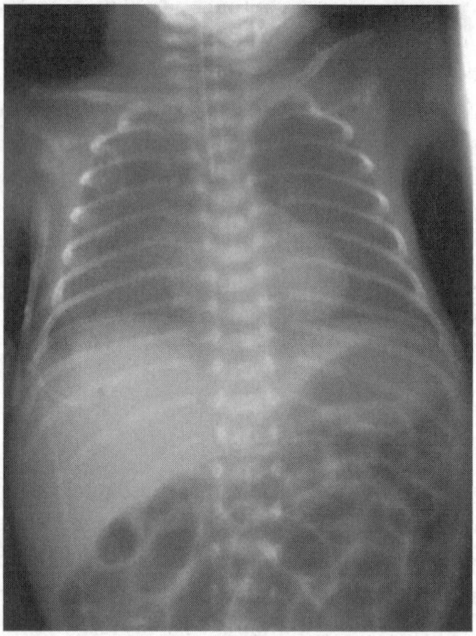

(b)

Figure 15.1 Chest radiographs of infants aged 10 days with *Ureaplasma urealyticum* infection and chronic lung disease with pulmonary interstitial emphysema (a) and Ureaplasma-negative infant (b). Reproduced from Reference 13 with permission.

15.5 Ureaplasmas, Mycoplasmas and neonatal pneumonia

There have been reports of congenital and neonatal pneumonia, including fatal cases, in which either *U. urealyticum* or *M. hominis* was the only pathogen isolated from the respiratory tract.[1] Neonates with Ureaplasma pneumonia have had concurrent bloodstream isolation of Ureaplasmas occasionally.[1] While most infants were pre-term, a case report describes a term infant with fatal congenital pneumonia, presumably acquired intrauterine, from which *U. parvum* was the sole organism cultured.[15] While it has been argued that "the ability of Ureaplasma species and *M. hominis* to cause pneumonia, bacteraemia and meningitis in newborns can no longer be questioned,"[1] Mycoplasmas and Ureaplasmas may be cleared spontaneously without specific antibiotic treatment from the respiratory tract, bloodstream or CSF and it has been problematic to demonstrate that antibiotics make any difference to the clinical course of neonatal Ureaplasma or Mycoplasma infection.

15.6 Ureaplasmas and chronic lung disease of prematurity

The association between neonatal *U. urealyticum* respiratory tract colonization and chronic lung disease of prematurity or BPD has been described in a number of case-control studies.[6, 12,16–26] There are some reservations, however, regarding the strength of the association and causality. A 1993 critical appraisal of four studies found that the association between *U. urealyticum* colonization and chronic lung disease was not observed in infants <1250 g, while uncolonized infants <750 g had such a high risk (82%) of chronic lung disease that no association with colonization could be demonstrated.[27] A more recent critical appraisal of 23 studies (2216 infants) found a significant association between *U. urealyticum* colonization and BPD at age 28 days or at 36 weeks post-menstrual age, but found substantial heterogeneity with the greatest contribution to the effect from small studies enrolling fewer than 100 infants each, suggesting possible publication bias.[28]

A Cochrane systematic review[29] found only two RCTs of macrolides and BPD in patients colonized with *U. urealyticum*.[30, 31] In one study colonized neonates <30 weeks of gestation who were intubated received erythromycin (40 mg/kg/day) or placebo for 10 days, started at a mean age of 7 days: erythromycin did not reduce rates of BPD.[30] Only 28 patients in this study had *U. urealyticum* colonization, of whom 5 had positive nasopharyngeal but negative endotracheal cultures; 14 of the 28 were treated with erythromycin; repeat cultures were negative in 12 of these 14 whereas untreated patients remained culture positive.[30] However, there was no clinical improvement. In the other study, infants <30 weeks of gestation (irrespective of Ureaplasma status) were randomized to prophylactic erythromycin or placebo. There was no reduction in the rate of BPD, but the study was seriously underpowered.[31]

A subsequent study found that neither 5 nor 10 days of intravenous erythromycin eradicated *U. urealyticum* colonization in infants <1500 g,[32] a result discordant with the previously described study,[30] despite using similar doses and duration of erythromycin.

Two more recent RCTs of macrolides reported slightly more promising results. A trial of 6 weeks of azithromycin prophylaxis of infants <1250 g demonstrated no significant reduction in death or BPD.[33] However, the incidence of BPD in infants colonized with Ureaplasma was 73% with azithromycin versus 94% with placebo ($p = 0.03$). Sub-analysis demonstrated a decrease in BPD or death in the azithromycin group (estimated OR 0.026, 95% CI 0.001–0.618).[33] As the benefit of azithromycin was confined to infants colonized with Ureaplasma, azithromycin was presumably acting through an antimicrobial rather than an anti-inflammatory mechanism.

In a single centre, unblinded study from Turkey, infants 750–1250 g colonized with *U. urealyticum* received 10 days of intravenous clarithromycin or placebo.[34] One of 35 (2.9%) treated with clarithromycin developed BPD compared with 12 of 33 (36.4%) placebo recipients ($p < 0.001$), although *U. urealyticum* was eradicated in only 68.5% of patients treated with clarithromycin.[34] The results are surprisingly different from other macrolide studies. The authors suggest clarithromycin may have better *in vitro* activity than erythromycin against *U. urealyticum* and better penetration into bronchial mucosa and secretions. There was no difference in duration of mechanical ventilation or in mortality, so the clinical significance is uncertain.[34]

Safety may be a concern. There is an association between erythromycin and pyloric stenosis,[35, 36] and pyloric stenosis was also described in two of three triplets given azithromycin,[37] which suggests a possible class effect of macrolides.

15.7 *Mycoplasma hominis*, Ureaplasma and central nervous system infection

There are around 30 reports of *M. hominis* meningitis and/or brain abscess in neonates.[1, 35, 36, 38] Meningitis may be associated with intraventricular haemorrhage and hydrocephalus, is often diagnosed late and the outcome is usually poor. Most infants are pre-term although cases occur in full-term infants.[1] *U. urealyticum* and *U. parvum* have also been isolated as the sole organism from the CSF of preterm and full-term infants with proven or suspected meningitis.[1, 39, 40] Both *M. hominis* and a Ureaplasma species were isolated from one infant with a brain abscess.[41] The organism may also be isolated from the bloodstream.[1] These cases are clinically convincing, but the response to antibiotics is often poor.

However, the interpretation of finding *M. hominis* or Ureaplasma in CSF is complicated. Symptoms can vary from none (asymptomatic) to severe neurologic impairment, sometimes fatal. The CSF cell count and chemistry is often normal and the organisms may persist with or without treatment.[1,42,43] *U. urealyticum* infection and CSF pleocytosis sometimes resolve spontaneously without antibiotics.[44]

For these reasons the decision to treat an infant for *M. hominis* or Ureaplasma CNS infection needs to be made on an individual basis.

15.8 Treatment of Mycoplasma or Ureaplasma

Treatment decisions are complicated by uncertainty about the organism's contribution to the illness, about the effectiveness of treatment and concern about potential toxicity.

Macrolides, erythromycin and more recently azithromycin and clarithromycin, are the usual mainstays of treatment of Ureaplasma infections not involving the central nervous system. Lincosamide clindamycin is active against Ureaplasma but has limited CNS penetration.[45] Alternatives with improved CSF penetration are doxycycline, which can be used for short periods without staining teeth and affecting bone, and quinolones, including moxifloxacin and gatifloxacin.[45] In recent reports doxycycline is often used in conjunction with moxifloxacin or gatifloxacin to treat severe Ureaplasma infection, particularly if the CNS is involved.[1]

Macrolides have limited efficacy in *M. pneumoniae* lower respiratory tract infections in older children and have poor CNS penetration.[5] Doxycycline is the usual drug of choice for *M. hominis*, which is resistant to macrolides, although doxycycline resistance has been reported. *M. hominis* is sensitive to quinolones *in vitro*, and moxifloxacin or gatifloxacin is often used in conjunction with doxycycline to treat severe *M. hominis* infection, particularly if the CNS is involved.[46]

15.9 Prevention

Prophylactic antibiotics do not prevent neonatal chronic lung disease convincingly in pre-term infants colonized with Ureaplasma (Section 15.6) and might even exacerbate respiratory distress (Section 15.4).

Antibiotic treatment of Ureaplasma-colonized pregnant women might prevent pre-term birth. A Cochrane review[47] identified one trial in which colonized women of 22–32 weeks of gestation were randomized to antibiotic (erythromycin estolate, $n = 174$; erythromycin stearate, $n = 224$; or clindamycin hydrochloride, $n = 246$) or placebo ($n = 427$). The incidence of low birth weight <2500 g was only evaluated for the two erythromycin groups combined compared to placebo and was not statistically significant different (RR 0.70, 95% CI 0.46–1.07).[47]

References

1. Waites KB, Schelonka RL, Xiao L, Grigsby PL, Novy MJ. Congenital and opportunistic infections: Ureaplasma species and *Mycoplasma hominis*. *Semin Fetal Neonatal Med* 2009; 14:190–199.
2. Viscardi RM. Ureaplasma species: role in diseases of prematurity. *Clin Perinatol* 2010; 37:393–409.
3. Diaz N, Dessì D, Dessole S, Fiori PL, Rappelli P. Rapid detection of coinfections by *Trichomonas vaginalis*, *Mycoplasma hominis*, and *Ureaplasma urealyticum* by a new multiplex polymerase chain reaction. *Diagn Microbiol Infect Dis* 2010; 67:30–36.
4. Enomoto M, Morioka I, Morisawa T, Yokoyama N, Matsuo M. A novel diagnostic tool for detecting neonatal infections using multiplex polymerase chain reaction. *Neonatology* 2009; 96:102–108.
5. Mulholland S, Gavranich JB, Gillies MB, Chang AB. Antibiotics for community-acquired lower respiratory tract infections secondary to *Mycoplasma pneumoniae* in children. Cochrane Database of Systematic Reviews 2012, Issue 9. Art. No.: CD004875. doi: 10.1002/14651858.CD004875.pub4.
6. Honma Y, Yada Y, Takahashi N, Momoi MY, Nakamura Y. Certain type of chronic lung disease of newborns is associated with *Ureaplasma urealyticum* infection in utero. *Pediatr Int* 2007; 49:479–484.
7. Kirchner L, Helmer H, Heinze G, et al. Amnionitis with *Ureaplasma urealyticum* or other microbes leads to increased morbidity and prolonged hospitalization in very low birth weight infants. *Eur J Obstet Gynecol Reprod Biol* 2007; 134:44–50.
8. Goldenberg RL, Andrews WW, Goepfert AR, et al. The Alabama Preterm Birth Study: umbilical cord blood *Ureaplasma urealyticum* and *Mycoplasma hominis* cultures in very preterm newborn infants. *Am J Obstet Gynecol* 2008; 198:43.e1–43.e5.
9. Lahra MM, Beeby PJ, Jeffery HE. Intrauterine inflammation, neonatal sepsis, and chronic lung disease: a 13-year hospital cohort study. *Pediatrics* 2009; 123:1314–1319.

10. Hartling L, Liang Y, Lacaze-Masmonteil T. Chorioamnionitis as a risk factor for bronchopulmonary dysplasia: a systematic review and meta-analysis. *Arch Dis Child Fetal Neonatal Ed* 2012; 97:F8–F17.
11. Ylijoki M, Ekholm E, Haataja L, Lehtonen L. PIPARI study group. Is chorioamnionitis harmful for the brain of preterm infants? A clinical overview. *Acta Obstet Gynecol Scand* 2012; 91:403–419.
12. Hannaford K, Todd DA, Jeffery H, John E, Blyth K, Gilbert GL. Role of *Ureaplasma urealyticum* in lung disease of prematurity. *Arch Dis Child Fetal Neonatal Ed* 1999; 81:F162–F167.
13. Theilen U, Lyon AJ, Fitzgerald T, Hendry GM, Keeling JW. Infection with *Ureaplasma urealyticum*: is there a specific clinical and radiological course in the preterm infant? *Arch Dis Child Fetal Neonatal Ed* 2004; 89:F163–F167.
14. Cultrera R, Seraceni S, Germani R, Contini C. Molecular evidence of *Ureaplasma urealyticum* and *Ureaplasma parvum* colonization in preterm infants during respiratory distress syndrome. *BMC Infect Dis* 2006; 6:166.
15. Morioka I, Fujibayashi H, Enoki E, Yokoyama N, Yokozaki H, Matsuo M. Congenital pneumonia with sepsis caused by intrauterine infection of *Ureaplasma parvum* in a term newborn: a first case report. *J Perinatol* 2010; 30:359–362.
16. Cassell GH, Waites KB, Crouse DT, et al. Association of *Ureaplasma urealyticum* infection of the lower respiratory tract with chronic lung disease and death in very-low-birth-weight infants. *Lancet* 1988; 2:240–245.
17. Sánchez PJ, Regan JA. *Ureaplasma urealyticum* colonization and chronic lung disease in low birth weight infants. *Pediatr Infect Dis J* 1988; 7:542–546.
18. Wang EE, Frayha H, Watts J, et al. Role of *Ureaplasma urealyticum* and other pathogens in the development of chronic lung disease of prematurity. *Pediatr Infect Dis J* 1988; 7:547–551.
19. Payne NR, Steinberg SS, Ackerman P, et al. New prospective studies of the association of *Ureaplasma urealyticum* colonization and chronic lung disease. *Clin Infect Dis* 1993; 17 (Suppl. 1):S117–S121.
20. Pacifico L, Panero A, Roggini M, Rossi N, Bucci G, Chiesa C. *Ureaplasma urealyticum* and pulmonary outcome in a neonatal intensive care population. *Pediatr Infect Dis J* 1997; 16:579–586.
21. Abele-Horn M, Genzel-Boroviczény O, Uhlig T, Zimmermann A, Peters J, Scholz M. *Ureaplasma urealyticum* colonization and bronchopulmonary dysplasia: a comparative prospective multicentre study. *Eur J Pediatr* 1998; 157:1004–1011.
22. Perzigian RW, Adams JT, Weiner GM, et al. *Ureaplasma urealyticum* and chronic lung disease in very low birth weight infants during the exogenous surfactant era. *Pediatr Infect Dis J* 1998; 17:620–625.
23. Agarwal P, Rajadurai VS, Pradeepkumar VK, Tan KW. *Ureaplasma urealyticum* and its association with chronic lung disease in Asian neonates. *J Paediatr Child Health* 2000; 36:487–490.
24. Colaizy TT, Morris CD, Lapidus J, Sklar RS, Pillers DA. Detection of ureaplasma DNA in endotracheal samples is associated with bronchopulmonary dysplasia after adjustment for multiple risk factors. *Pediatr Res* 2007; 61:578–583.
25. Kasper DC, Mechtler TP, Böhm J, et al. In utero exposure to Ureaplasma spp. is associated with increased rate of bronchopulmonary dysplasia and intraventricular hemorrhage in preterm infants. *J Perinat Med* 2011; 39:331–336.
26. Inatomi T, Oue S, Ogihara T, et al. Antenatal exposure to Ureaplasma species exacerbates bronchopulmonary dysplasia synergistically with subsequent prolonged mechanical ventilation in preterm infants. *Pediatr Res* 2012; 71:267–273.
27. Wang EE, Cassell GH, Sánchez PJ, Regan JA, Payne NR, Liu PP. *Ureaplasma urealyticum* and chronic lung disease of prematurity: critical appraisal of the literature on causation. *Clin Infect Dis* 1993; 17(Suppl. 1):S112–S116.
28. Schelonka RL, Katz B, Waites KB, Benjamin Jr DK. Critical appraisal of the role of Ureaplasma in the development of bronchopulmonary dysplasia with meta-analytic techniques. *Pediatr Infect Dis J* 2005; 24:1033–1039.
29. Mabanta CG, Pryhuber GS, Weinberg GA, Phelps D. Erythromycin for the prevention of chronic lung disease in intubated preterm infants at risk for, or colonized or infected with Ureaplasma urealyticum. Cochrane Database of Systematic Reviews 2003, Issue 4. Art. No.: CD003744. doi: 10.1002/14651858.CD003744.
30. Jónsson B, Rylander M, Faxelius G. *Ureaplasma urealyticum*, erythromycin and respiratory morbidity in high-risk preterm neonates. *Acta Paediatr* 1998; 87:1079–1084.
31. Lyon AJ, McColm J, Middlemist L, Fergusson S, McIntosh N, Ross PW. Randomised trial of erythromycin on the development of chronic lung disease in preterm infants. *Arch Dis Child Fetal Neonatal Ed* 1998; 78:F10–F14.
32. Baier RJ, Loggins J, Kruger TE. Failure of erythromycin to eliminate airway colonization with ureaplasma urealyticum in very low birth weight infants. *BMC Pediatr* 2003; 3:10.
33. Ballard HO, Shook LA, Bernard P, et al. Use of azithromycin for the prevention of bronchopulmonary dysplasia in preterm infants: a randomized, double-blind, placebo controlled trial. *Pediatr Pulmonol* 2011; 46:111–118.
34. Ozdemir R, Erdeve O, Dizdar EA, et al. Clarithromycin in preventing bronchopulmonary dysplasia in *Ureaplasma urealyticum*-positive preterm infants. *Pediatrics* 2011; 128:e1496–e1501.
35. Hauben M, Amsden GW. The association of erythromycin and infantile hypertrophic pyloric stenosis: causal or coincidental? *Drug Saf* 2002; 25:929–942.
36. Maheshwai N. Are young infants treated with erythromycin at risk for developing hypertrophic pyloric stenosis? *Arch Dis Child* 2007; 92:271–273.
37. Morrison W. Infantile hypertrophic pyloric stenosis in infants treated with azithromycin. *Pediatr Infect Dis J* 2007; 26:186–188.
38. Hata A, Honda Y, Asada K, Sasaki Y, Kenri T, Hata D. *Mycoplasma hominis* meningitis in a neonate: case report and review. *J Infect* 2008; 57:338–343.
39. Watt KM, Massaro MM, Smith B, Cohen-Wolkowiez M, Benjamin Jr DK, Laughon MM. Pharmacokinetics of

moxifloxacin in an infant with *Mycoplasma hominis* meningitis. *Pediatr Infect Dis J* 2012; 31:197–199.
40. Clifford V, Tebruegge M, Everest N, Curtis N. Ureaplasma: pathogen or passenger in neonatal meningitis? *Pediatr Infect Dis J* 2010; 29:60–64.
41. Biran V, Dumitrescu AM, Doit C, et al. Ureaplasma parvum meningitis in a full-term newborn. *Pediatr Infect Dis J* 2010; 29:1154.
42. Rao RP, Ghanayem NS, Kaufman BA, Kehl KS, Gregg DC, Chusid MJ. *Mycoplasma hominis* and Ureaplasma species brain abscess in a neonate. *Pediatr Infect Dis J* 2002; 21:1083–1085.
43. Waites KB, Rudd PT, Crouse DT, et al. Chronic *Ureaplasma urealyticum* and *Mycoplasma hominis* infections of central nervous system in preterm infants. *Lancet* 1988; 1: 17–21.
44. Waites KB, Duffy LB, Crouse DT, et al. Mycoplasmal infections of cerebrospinal fluid in newborn infants from a community hospital population. *Pediatr Infect Dis J* 1990; 9:241–245.
45. Neal TJ, Roe MF, Shaw NJ. Spontaneously resolving *Ureaplasma urealyticum* meningitis. *Eur J Pediatr* 1994; 153:342–343.
46. Krausse R, Schubert S. 'In-vitro activities of tetracyclines, macrolides, fluoroquinolones and clindamycin against Mycoplasma hominis and Ureaplasma ssp. isolated in Germany over 20 years. *Clin Microbiol Infect* 2012; 16:1649–1655.
47. Raynes-Greenow CH, Roberts CL, Bell JC, Peat B, Gilbert GL, Parker S. Antibiotics for ureaplasma in the vagina in pregnancy. Cochrane Database of Systematic Reviews 2011, Issue 9. Art. No.: CD003767. doi: 10.1002/14651858.CD003767.pub3.

CHAPTER 16

Fungal infections

16.1 Epidemiology

Neonatal systemic fungal infection can be defined as the identification (by culture, nucleic acid amplification or histology) of fungi from a normally sterile body site. Colonization is defined as the identification of fungi from skin and mucosal surfaces without invasion. The distinction is straightforward for blood and/or meninges, but urine cultures are easily contaminated with fungus on the infant's skin or genitalia. Other fungi and yeasts such as Malassezia and moulds such as zygomycetes can infect neonates, but the great majority of neonatal fungal infections are caused by Candida species.

16.1.1 Risk factors for invasive fungal infection

Neonates are at significantly increased risk of invasive fungal infection (IFI) compared with older age groups.[1] Extreme prematurity is the single greatest risk factor for IFI: the risk increases with decreasing gestation and is highest in infants <1000 g.[2–8] Any epidemiologic study of risk factors therefore needs to control for birth weight. For example, case-control studies should match cases and controls for birth weight and gestation, when several risk factors emerge as significant (Table 16.1).[2–14] Of these, the most potentially preventable are prolonged antibiotic therapy,[3–5,9,10] use of broad-spectrum antibiotics, particularly third generation cephalosporins,[9,10,12] prolonged parenteral nutrition with lipid emulsions,[5,6,12,13] prolonged presence of central venous catheters, prolonged endotracheal intubation and acid suppression using histamine H2-receptor blockers (Table 16.1). Prior fungal colonization is a risk factor for IFI unsurprisingly, and the risk increases with density of colonization.[7,8]

A case-control study in which controls were matched for birth weight found duration of antibiotics was the single variable most associated with candidaemia.[3] In a large multi-centre US study, infants <1000 g treated with a third generation cephalosporin had more than double the risk of developing invasive Candida infection, RR = 2.2 (95% CI 1.4–3.3).[9] In this study the incidence of candidiasis varied from 2.4% to 20.4% in different centres and correlated with broad-spectrum antibiotic use in different centres.[9] A large multi-centre cohort study found the incidence of invasive candidiasis in infants <1500 g receiving third generation cephalosporins on day 3 of life was 15.3%, compared with 5.6% for infants <1500 g on other antibiotics and 0.9% on no antibiotics.[12]

Prolonged use of parenteral nutrition is a risk factor for invasive candidiasis, particularly intravenous fat emulsions which favour fungal growth.[3,5,6,8] Infants <1500 g who started enteral feeds by day 3 had just over half the incidence of invasive candidiasis of infants <1500 g who did not.[12]

In an Israeli study comparing infants with bacterial and fungal sepsis corticosteroids given for bronchopulmonary dysplasia were a risk factor for systemic Candida infection,[13] but a US case-control study did not find any association between corticosteroid use and IFI.[6]

More than 90% of invasive candidiasis occurs in infants <1500 g.[5,15] Invasive candidiasis is unusual in full-term infants, but in a population-based surveillance study, infants who had abdominal surgery were more than 10 times as likely as controls to have IFI (adjusted OR 10.9, 95% CI 1.9–62).[7] We do not know what proportion of neonates who have abdominal surgery develop IFI and, therefore, the likely risks and benefits of antifungal prophylaxis.

Evidence-Based Neonatal Infections, First Edition. David Isaacs.

Table 16.1 Risk factors for neonatal systemic candidiasis.

Birth weight (incidence increases with decreasing birth weight)[2–10]
Prolonged antibiotic therapy[3–5,9,10]
Broad-spectrum antibiotics,[3,5,11] e.g. third generation cephalosporins[9,10,12]
Antenatal antibiotics[12]
Vaginal delivery[7]
Prolonged parenteral nutrition, including lipid formulations[3,5,6,8,12,13]
Presence of central venous catheter[6,12,13]
Prolonged endotracheal intubation[4–6,10,12,13]
Use of histamine H2-receptor blockers[6]
Colonization, particularly heavy colonization, with fungi[6,11,13]
Abdominal surgery[7]

16.1.2 Incidence of invasive fungal infection

The reported incidence of neonatal fungal infection varies enormously with geographic location, definitions and means of reporting infections.

Infants <1000 g:

The largest US multi-centre cohort studies reported an incidence of invasive candidiasis in infants <1000 g of 7% when the definition was restricted to infants with candidaemia or meningitis[8] and 9% in a study which also included infants with renal candidiasis.[12] In the latter study, the incidence in different centres ranged widely from 2% to 28%.[12] In a US RCT of prophylactic antifungals for infants <1000 g, the incidence of invasive Candida infection in the control arm was 26% (13 of 50).[16] In a Turkish trial, the incidence in control infants <1000 g was 31.1%.[17] In a UK trial using an active prospective surveillance mechanism the reported incidence of IFI including renal candidiasis in infants <1000 g was 2.1% (95% CI 1.7–2.6).[18] In Australia and New Zealand, the incidence of IFI excluding renal candidiasis was 2.7% (2–3.4%) in units using no antifungal prophylaxis, 1.2% (0.9–1.5%) for babies <1000 g in units using nystatin prophylaxis and 1.8% overall (95% CI 1.4–2.1).[15]

Infants <1500 g:

The incidence of IFI in infants <1500 g was 36.2% in a study from Turkey,[17] 25% from India,[19] and 13.2%[20] and 16.7%[21] in two studies from Italy. It was only 1.0% (95% CI 0.8–1.2) using surveillance to identify infected UK infants <1500 g.[18] In Australia and New Zealand it was 0.8% (0.7%–0.9%) overall, but 1.2% (0.8–1.6%) in units using no prophylaxis and 0.5% (0.4%–0.7%) in units using selective or universal nystatin prophylaxis.[15]

It has not been possible to ascertain the reasons for the large differences in incidence between and within countries, although it has been postulated that in the United States it may be due mainly to prolonged use of broad-spectrum antibiotics in some but not other neonatal units.[9]

Infants >1500 g:

There is an increased incidence of IFI in infants who have had gastrointestinal surgery[7] and also an association with major congenital malformations (Section 16.3.4) although it is not clear how much of this increased risk is due to the use of parenteral nutrition and how much due to translocation of fungi across the intestinal wall or entry at other sites.

16.2 Microbiology

The name Candida means glowing white in Latin, so *Candida albicans* could be translated loosely as 'white on white' or 'a whiter shade of pale'. Candida are ubiquitous yeasts which reproduce by budding. Most Candida can produce filamentous pseudo-hyphae (Figure 16.1). There are over 150 different species of Candida, mostly environmental saprophytes, and only a few invade humans (Table 16.2). Candida have various adhesion molecules. They are primarily colonizers of the mucosa of the gastrointestinal, genital and respiratory tracts and only invade very immunocompromised hosts, hosts with major gastrointestinal breaches (e.g. surgery, NEC) or hosts whose normal mucocutaneous integrity is breached (such as by catheters or mucositis). Their pathogenicity is thought to be related to hyphae formation and also biofilm production, a property of *C. albicans*, *C. parapsilosis* and *C. glabrata*. Biofilm formation may aid survival of Candida adherent to catheters and be a factor in central catheter-associated Candida infections.

Malassezia species are lipophilic yeasts and can cause catheter-related bloodstream infection in association with lipid emulsions.[22,23] They require lipid supplementation in culture media and can be difficult to

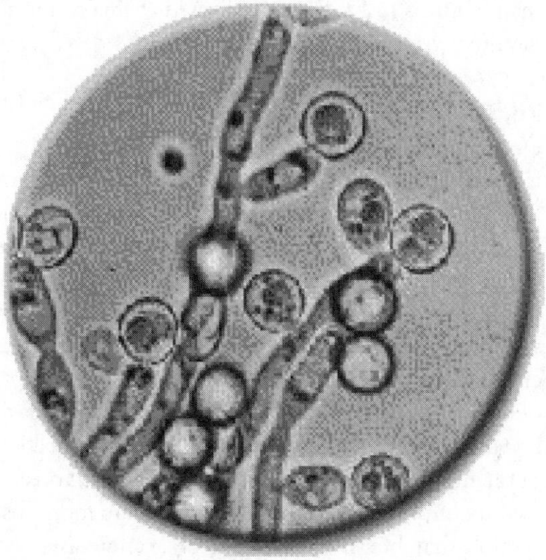

Figure 16.1 *Candida albicans*: budding yeast cells and pseudo-hyphae.

grow in the laboratory. Infections with the ubiquitous moulds Mucor, Rhizopus and Absidia (confusingly collectively termed zygomycosis or mucormycosis) are rare, but mortality is high. Most cases occur in pre-term infants and have a gastrointestinal or skin focus, unlike the sinopulmonary and rhinocerebral presentation seen in older immunocompromised hosts.[24–26]

16.3 Clinical features of Candida infections

The vast majority of IFIs are nosocomial, but infants can rarely present at or soon after birth with congenital candidiasis.

16.3.1 Congenital candidiasis

Most infants with congenital candidiasis are symptomatic at birth or soon afterwards, and infection is thought to come from maternal intrauterine infection or high-level vaginal colonization. The usual presentation is with a generalized eruption of erythematous macules, papules, and/or pustules that sometimes evolve to include vesicles and bullae (see Figure 13.1C).[27] Extremely low birth-weight infants <1000 g often present with a widespread desquamating and/or erosive dermatitis and often have had systemic candidiasis with a 40% mortality.[27] Presence of an intrauterine foreign body, including a cervical stitch, is a predisposing factor for congenital cutaneous candidiasis in pre-term infants.[27]

Some infants with congenital cutaneous candidiasis also have respiratory distress and hepatosplenomegaly, suggesting ascending infection and possible haematogenous spread.[28, 29] Infants may rarely have fulminant disease without rash. In one report a 32-week gestation twin was well although neutropenic at birth but developed septic shock and died at 22 hours. The other twin did not develop a typical

Table 16.2 Usual sensitivities of fungal species to antifungals.

Organism	Amphotericin B	Fluconazole	Flucytosine[a]
Candida albicans	99% sensitive	95–98% sensitive	90% sensitive
Candida parapsilosis	Sometimes resistant	Usually sensitive	Usually sensitive
Candida guilliermondii	Usually sensitive	Usually sensitive	Usually sensitive
Candida glabrata	Usually sensitive	Reduced susceptibility	Usually sensitive
Candida krusei	Usually sensitive	Intrinsically resistant	Usually resistant
Candida tropicalis	Usually sensitive	Up to 20% resistant	Usually sensitive
Candida lusitaniae	Often resistant or resistance develops during therapy	Usually sensitive	Usually sensitive
Candida dubliniensis	Usually sensitive	Usually sensitive	Usually sensitive
Aspergillus	Sensitive	Resistant	Resistant
Zygomycetes	Sensitive	Resistant	Resistant

[a]Flucytosine should not be used on its own because resistance rapidly develops.

Candida rash (see Figure 13.1C) until day 3 of age.[30] A form of congenital candidiasis affecting only the nails has been described.[31]

16.3.2 Candida dermatitis

Most Candida dermatitis occurs in term infants and is benign. It particularly affects the diaper (napkin or nappy) region and is often associated with oral thrush and gastrointestinal colonization. However, damp and soiling are more common causes of diaper dermatitis and require barrier creams or topical steroids rather than antifungals.[32, 33] Candida classically causes a red, confluent, pruritic (itchy) rash with satellite lesions (Figure 16.2).

Candida dermatitis is more sinister in infants <1500 g. In a prospective study 9 (32%) of 28 infants <1500 g with mucocutaneous candidiasis developed invasive candidiasis despite topical antifungals.[34] Candida skin lesions in infants <1000 g are often more severe, with erythema, erosion, desquamation and draining wounds which crust and can bleed, sometimes called invasive fungal dermatitis, and associated with a high incidence of invasive infection.[35, 36] In a case-control study, affected infants were more likely than controls to have been delivered vaginally and to have received post-natal corticosteroids.[35]

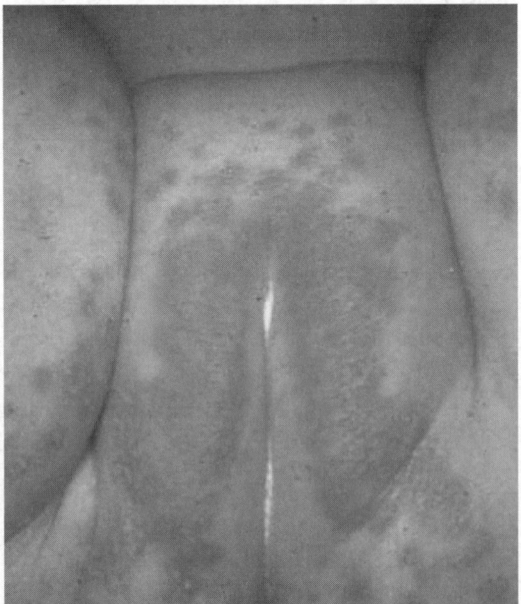

Figure 16.2 Candida diaper (napkin) dermatitis showing erythema and satellite lesions.

16.3.3 Oral candidiasis

Oral candidiasis (thrush) is extremely common. There is a well-recognized association with antibiotics, particularly broad-spectrum antibiotics, but oral candidiasis is also common in infants who have not received antibiotics.[37, 38] Mild oral candidiasis causes white plaques on the tongue and buccal mucosa with few symptoms. Severe disease can cause painful mucosal erythema which may interfere with feeding. Infants of breastfeeding mothers can develop oral candidiasis and the mother may develop painful Candida infection of the nipple, both of which can interfere with breastfeeding until treated. Bottle-fed infants are more susceptible than breastfed infants to oral candidiasis.[37, 38]

16.3.4 Systemic fungal infection

Candidaemic infants generally present with non-specific features indistinguishable from bacterial sepsis, including lethargy, feed intolerance, apnoea, increased need for respiratory support, abdominal distension, hyperglycaemia, temperature instability and hypotension.[1,39–42] Infections can be fulminant with circulatory failure and shock.[39–42] End-organ involvement is common, causing one or more of meningitis, chorioretinitis (see Figure 12.5) or endophthalmitis, renal abscesses (Figure 16.3), brain abscesses (Figure 16.4), endocarditis and hepatosplenomegaly.[1, 39]

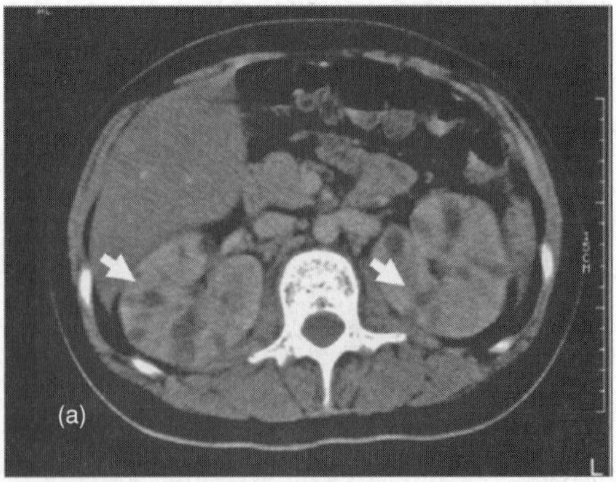

Figure 16.3 Renal candidiasis: computerized tomographic (CT) scan showing filling deposits (arrows) in both kidneys due to renal lesions (fungal balls).

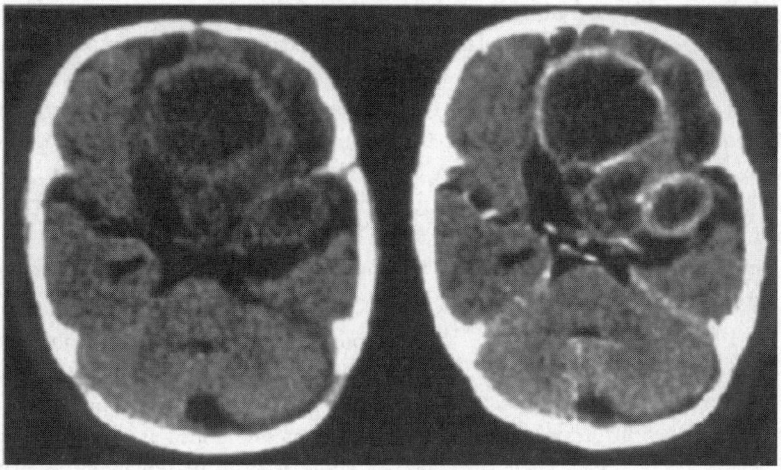

Figure 16.4 Cerebral candidiasis: CT scan unenhanced (a) and after iodine contrast (b). Shows rounded lesions with low-density centres and a ring-like periphery which enhances with contrast in the frontal and temporal regions of the left hemisphere. There is midline shift to the right.

The clinical examination should include specialist eye examination with retinoscopy. Urine microscopy and CSF examination may reveal yeasts. Meningitis occurs in around 10–15% of all infants with Candida sepsis[14, 39,40] and the blood culture is negative in 50–60% of them.[8, 43] This shows that Candida can be difficult to grow from blood and that Candida meningitis will be missed in half of all infants if LP is not performed immediately.

The clinician would like to know whether a baby with suspected sepsis has IFI. Infants at increased risk of IFI (<1500 g and infants who have had gastrointestinal surgery and major congenital malformations) are at even greater risk of bacterial infection. A maternal history of severe vaginal candidiasis or intrauterine foreign body is helpful but rare (Section 16.3.1). The most common age of presentation of invasive candidiasis is between 10 and 20 days when bacterial infection is also common but the range is from birth to over 100 days of age.[8, 36,44] A history of current or prolonged broad-spectrum antibiotic use may help. In one case series, 38% of infants with either *C. albicans* or *C. parapsilosis* infection and 67% with *C. glabrata* infection were on broad-spectrum antibiotics at the time of infection.[44] In another series, infants with *C. albicans* or *C. parapsilosis* bloodstream infection, were more likely than infants with or CoNS bacteraemia to have been exposed to broad-spectrum antibiotics, systemic steroids and catecholamines, and 29 of 32 infants (90%) treated with third generation cephalosporins developed fungaemia compared with 5 of 19 (26%) not treated with third generation cephalosporins.[45] Candida can cause central venous catheter-associated infections, but in an Israeli case series of infants <1500 g with candidaemia, there was a strong association with hyperalimentation and lipid emulsions, but alimentation was delivered by peripheral venous catheters for all but one infant.[5] This suggests that hyperalimentation fluids and lipids may be a more important risk factor than the type of catheter used.

Thrombocytopenia is common in both invasive fungal and bacterial infections (see Section 4.3.2). In an Italian study of septic infants <1500 g, thrombocytopenia $<80 \times 10^9$/L occurred in 16% of infants with Gram-negative, 18% with Gram-positive (16% of CoNS) and 20% with fungal infections.[46] In a US study, Gram-positive bacteria predominated as the cause of sepsis,[47] whereas in India, Gram-negative sepsis predominated.[48] Although most infants with fungal infections were thrombocytopenic in both sites, a clinically septic thrombocytopenic infant was far more likely to have bacterial sepsis.[47, 48]

Benjamin et al. used a large database of 6172 infants <1250 g to develop a clinical predictive model and generate a 'candidaemia score'.[49] In multivariate modelling, thrombocytopenia ($<150 \times 10^9$/L) and use of a third generation cephalosporin or carbapenem in the 7 days before the blood culture were the major risk factors for candidaemia in addition to the risk increasing with decreasing gestation. A candidaemia score of 2 or greater had a sensitivity of 85% and a specificity of 47% for predicting invasive candidiasis. The authors concluded that clinicians should consider empiric fungal therapy for thrombocytopenic infants <25 weeks of gestation with suspected late-onset sepsis.[49] However, the strength of this recommendation depends on the frequency of fungal infection compared with bacterial infection and the risks and benefits of antifungal therapy. It is less valid when the incidence of fungal infection is low.

16.3.5 Urinary tract Candida infection (renal candidiasis)

Candida grown from urine obtained by a freshly inserted catheter or suprapubic aspiration is considered diagnostic of a Candida urinary tract infection.[50–53] There is a distinct syndrome of renal parenchymal candidiasis, presumed to arise by haematogenous seeding, which often coexists with hepatic and/or splenic Candida lesions ('chronic disseminated' or 'hepatosplenic' candidiasis).

In a study of 57 NICU infants with 60 urinary tract infections, 25 (42%) were caused by Candida, 13 of whom (52%) also had candidaemia, while renal pelvis fungal balls were present in 7 of 20 who had renal ultrasound scans.[50] Renal fungus balls or renal fungal abscess were found in 13 of 41 infants with candiduria in another single-centre study, and the abnormality developed more than a week after the initial positive culture in 6 infants.[51] Only 10 of 30 Canadian NICU infants with candiduria were <30 weeks of gestation, while 10 had congenital heart disease. Fifteen of 26 tested had abnormal renal ultrasound scans and 4 infants developed disseminated candidiasis.[53] Mortality and morbidity in infants <1000 g with isolated candiduria is not significantly different from infants <1000 g with candidaemia (Section 16.5),[54] so confirmed candiduria in an infant <1000 g should prompt full evaluation with cultures of blood and CSF and a renal ultrasound scan.[54]

About 5% of all infants with candidaemia have an abnormal renal ultrasound consistent with renal candidiasis.[38] The investigation of an infant with proven candidaemia should, therefore, always include renal imaging, ideally with a renal ultrasound scan, although computerized tomography (CT) (Figure 16.4) may sometimes be necessary. In the above studies 12% and 20% of infants, respectively, with proven candiduria did not have any renal imaging performed.[51, 53]

16.3.6 Candida eye infections

A meta-analysis of papers published from 1979 to 1992 found that Candida endophthalmitis occurred in 3% of infants with candidaemia.[39] Candida chorioretinitis causes white or cream-coloured fluffy raised exudates, sometimes described as 'snowballs' (see Figure 12.6). Candidiasis can be unilateral or bilateral, can occur in the posterior fundus or the vitreous, rarely infects the lens and is often clinically silent. For this reason fundoscopy should be performed on all infants with possible IFI, and a formal ophthalmologic consultation is recommended for any infant with candidaemia, Candida meningitis or renal candidiasis. All Candida strains in Table 16.2 can cause Candida eye infections.

16.3.7 Intestinal candidiasis

Spontaneous intestinal perforation not due to NEC is an entity that often presents acutely with bluish discoloration of the abdominal wall.[55–58] Invasive Candida infection of the intestinal wall is an important cause of spontaneous intestinal perforation. It often affects infants <1000 g and has a high mortality.[59] It is not clinically distinguishable from other forms of perforation and may be mistaken clinically for NEC.[60] It is potentially treatable with antifungals and is an important diagnosis not to miss.

16.3.8 Candida meningitis and brain abscess

Candida meningitis occurs in 10–15% of all infants with candidaemia[12, 39,40] and brain abscess (Figure 16.4) or ventriculitis in 4% of candidaemic infants.[39] Early fungal abscesses can be microscopic and not detected by ultrasound or CT, and LP may be normal.[40, 61,62]

Most infants with Candida meningitis are <1000 g and <28 weeks of gestation. The median age of onset was 8 days in one study.[63] The clinical manifestations of central nervous system Candida infections include bulging fontanelle, increased head circumference, seizures or focal neurologic signs but presentation may be non-specific.[61–63] The CSF Gram stain is usually negative and there may be no white cells, while the CSF glucose is typically but not always low.[39, 40,61–63] Blood culture is negative in around 50% of infants with Candida meningitis,[8, 43] emphasizing the importance of LP in the diagnostic work-up of an infant with suspected late-onset infection and certainly one with proven candidaemia.

16.3.9 Candida endocarditis

Endocarditis is diagnosed in 5% of infants with candidaemia.[39] Candida is the most common organism causing neonatal endocarditis after *S. aureus*.[64] Most neonatal Candida endocarditis occurs in infants without congenital heart disease,[65] and while there is a reported association with central venous catheters, such catheters are almost universal in extremely preterm infants and many infants who develop endocarditis do not have a catheter in the right atrium at the time of diagnosis.[65] Infants with Candida endocarditis often have persistently positive blood cultures.[66] In a review of 30 reported cases of Candida endocarditis the mortality was 27%.[65]

16.4 Diagnosis

The diagnosis of fungal infections is based on clinical suspicion and supported by culture and sometimes radiology. A blood or CSF culture that grows Candida, even if it also grows a likely skin contaminant such as CoNS, should never be dismissed as a contaminant. Rapid tests such as PCR for fungal DNA[67] and rapid tests to identify fungal mannan proteins in serum[68] can potentially identify up to 90% of infants with candidaemia at the time of presentation, allowing timely empiric antifungal therapy. However, the relatively low sensitivity of these tests and the relatively low incidence of neonatal systemic fungal infection mean that routine use of the tests in suspected sepsis will result in large numbers of uninfected infants being treated with empiric antifungals. These tests are also expensive and not widely available, and PCR in particular is not well-standardized and relies on assays developed and validated locally, so inter-laboratory performance comparisons are generally lacking.

16.5 Treatment

Some authorities have argued that empiric antifungal therapy should be started or at least strongly considered for those infants with suspected late-onset sepsis who are at greatest risk of IFI.[49, 69] One proposal is to consider starting empiric antifungals for thrombocytopenic infants <25 weeks of gestation with suspected late-onset sepsis.[49] Another proposal is to use prophylactic antifungals for infants <1000 g and consider empiric antifungal therapy for thrombocytopenic infants 1000–1500 g with negative blood cultures who are not responding to anti-bacterial antibiotics after 48 hours.[69] Finally, empiric antifungal treatment could be initiated in infants who have a positive fungal PCR[67] or positive mannan test[68] (Section 16.4). None of these approaches has been formally evaluated and, while they may appear attractive initially, it is important to know how many infants will receive empiric fungal infection for every one with true fungal infection. Furthermore, unless cultures subsequently become positive, it may be difficult to know when to stop antifungal therapy once started.

16.5.1 Antifungal treatment of invasive fungal infection

The agents most commonly used and most studied in neonatal fungal infections are amphotericin B and fluconazole.

Amphotericin B is a polyene macrolide antifungal which increases cell membrane permeability by binding to ergosterols in the fungal membrane leading to cell death. Amphotericin B is active against Candida species except *C. lusitaniae* (Table 16.2) and is active against Aspergillus and the zygomycetes.[70] While nephrotoxicity and systemic reactions are major problems when using conventional amphotericin B in cancer patients, conventional amphotericin B is surprisingly well-tolerated in neonates[71–73] and although nephrotoxicity can occur, it rarely limits treatment. In older children and adults, liposomal amphotericin is often used to decrease toxicity and improve tissue penetration, notably to the CSF. However, CSF penetration of conventional amphotericin is much higher in pre-term neonates (40–90% vs. 2–4% of blood levels).[71] A retrospective review of invasive Candida infections in US neonatal units from 1997 to 2003 found an overall mortality of 19%, but the mortality was considerably higher in infants receiving liposomal amphotericin (29%) than in those receiving conventional amphotericin (18%) (OR 2.0, 95% CI 1.2–3.3) or fluconazole (16%) (OR 2.4, 95% CI 1.2–4.8).[74] Although this was a retrospective study, not an RCT, the data suggest extreme caution in the use of liposomal amphotericin, which incidentally is far costlier than conventional amphotericin. Liposomal amphotericin should not be used to treat neonates unless RCT evidence becomes available showing it is superior to conventional amphotericin B or fluconazole. A small test dose of amphotericin B used to be recommended for neonates in case of allergic reactions, as is recommended for adults, but since allergic reactions have not been described in neonates, test doses are no longer recommended. The dose of conventional amphotericin B is 0.5–1 mg/kg/day IV once daily.[71–73]

Fluconazole is a triazole antifungal which inhibits a fungal cytochrome P_{450} enzyme involved in ergosterol synthesis by the cell membrane. Fluconazole has excellent CSF penetration, is less nephrotoxic than amphotericin B although hepatotoxicity has been described,[75] and resistance can develop with prolonged or extensive use.[76, 77] While most studies of fluconazole prophylaxis have not shown selection of azole-resistant fungi, in one study from India[77] fluconazole prophylaxis for 6 years was associated with a predominance of non-albicans Candida species, predominantly *C. glabrata*, which is often resistant to fluconazole (Table 16.2). The treatment dose of fluconazole in neonatal fungal infection is 12 mg/kg/day IV or oral once daily, and a loading dose of 25 mg/kg has been recommended on pharmacokinetic grounds.[78, 79] In a small study of 10 infants an initial loading dose of 25 mg/kg IV was safe and achieved therapeutic levels within 24 hours, quicker than without a loading dose.[80]

There is a dearth of RCTs of antifungals in neonatal systemic fungal infections.[81] A small RCT from South Africa compared conventional amphotericin B and fluconazole for 23 infants with disseminated fungal sepsis, 21 with Candida species and 2 with *Rhodotorula rubra*.[82] The case fatality was high: 4 of 12 (33%) for fluconazole and 5 of 11 (45%) for amphotericin B, ($p > 0.05$). The fluconazole group did not need central lines, whereas three babies on amphotericin B did, and intravenous therapy was given for significantly shorter time to the fluconazole group. The safety profiles were similar. It has been argued that if fluconazole is being used for prophylaxis, amphotericin B should be used for empiric antifungal treatment.[69]

The echinocandins (micafungin, caspofungin and anidulafungin) inhibit fungal β-(1,3)-D-glucan synthase, interfering with cell wall biosynthesis. The echinocandins are active against Candida and Aspergillus (although fungistatic against Aspergillus) but inactive against zygomycetes.[69, 83] All three echinocandins have been used in neonates,[83] particularly micafungin[84] but also anidulafungin[85] and caspofungin.[86] A small RCT from Egypt which compared caspofungin and amphotericin B reported no significant difference in mortality, although caspofungin was superior in terms of a poorly defined endpoint of a 'favourable response'.[87] In the absence of adequate efficacy and safety data, echinocandins should not be used as first-line antifungal therapy, although salvage therapy use is understandable.[83]

Flucytosine (5-flucytosine, fluorocytosine) is a fluorine analogue of cytosine which inhibits DNA synthesis when converted to 5-fluorouracil. It is active against all Candida species except *C. krusei*, but resistance develops rapidly if it is used as monotherapy (Table 16.2). It has excellent CSF penetration and is well absorbed orally and excreted through the kidneys, so has been used in combination therapy of renal candidiasis and of Candida meningitis. However, there is no objective evidence that its use improves outcome compared to monotherapy with amphotericin B or fluconazole. There is considerable individual variation in serum concentrations and clearance after oral doses.[71] The recommended dose is 25–100 mg/kg/day orally once daily, and the dose should be modified based on drug levels.[71]

16.5.2 Duration of antifungal treatment

There are no RCTs on duration of antifungal treatment, but fungi are slow-growing organisms that are difficult to eradicate and prolonged treatment is necessary. On the basis of limited evidence from case series, most authorities recommend systemic therapy for 14–21 days after negative cultures. Amphotericin B has traditionally been given for 3–4 weeks. Candida meningitis may relapse and prolonged therapy for 4–6 weeks is advised. For susceptible Candida species initial IV therapy can be changed to oral fluconazole when the infant is improving and oral feeds are tolerated. Six weeks of parenteral therapy is recommended for endocarditis. Isolated renal candidiasis can be treated with 7 days of therapy but infants with fungal balls or undrainable abscesses should be treated until there is ultrasonographic or radiographic resolution.

16.5.3 Central venous catheter removal in invasive fungal infection

Observational studies report a much worse outcome in infants with candidaemia whose central venous catheters are left in place compared with infants whose catheters are removed immediately (see Section 6.10.5).[88, 89] It is possible that catheters are left in place in infants with difficult vascular access, who are likely to be much sicker. Nevertheless, the data are strong enough to recommend immediate central venous catheter removal unless vascular access is an insurmountable problem.

16.5.4 Ethanol lock therapy for catheter fungal infections

Ethanol has activity against biofilms and ethanol locks have been proposed for treatment of catheter-related infections.[90] Successful treatment of persistent catheter Candida infections using ethanol locks has been described in two 8-month-old infants and a 50-year-old.[91] There are no studies in neonates.

16.5.5 Treatment of oral candidiasis

In immunocompetent full-term infants with oral candidiasis, miconazole gel is more effective than nystatin gel[92] or nystatin suspension.[93] Fluconazole suspension 3 mg/kg daily for 7 days is more effective than nystatin suspension.[94] The cure rate for nystatin was low in all three studies: in the largest study it was 38% by day 8 and 54% by day 12.[93]

16.6 Outcome

Infants who develop IFI are often already at risk of poor outcome. Only controlled comparisons can differentiate morbidity and mortality due to fungal infection from that due to prematurity. A Canadian paper compared 25 infants <1250 g with candidaemia or Candia meningitis (8 had meningitis) with 25 controls matched closely for birth weight and gestation.[95] Eleven infants (44%) with invasive candidiasis died (3 with meningitis) compared with 4 (16%) of the controls, while 4 (29%) of the 14 surviving Candida infants had major neurodevelopmental disability compared with 3 (14%) of the 21 surviving controls. Overall 60% of the infants with invasive candidiasis died or had major neurodevelopmental disability compared with 28% of the controls ($p < 0.05$).[95]

The outcome of infants with isolated renal candidiasis might be expected to be better than for infants with bloodstream or meningeal candidiasis. However, in a large US study the immediate mortality for candiduria was 26% (9 of 34) and 50% had died or had major neurodevelopmental disability at 18 months, not significantly different from the mortality of 28% (19 of 69) and the 18 month outcome of 61% died or with major neurodevelopmental disability for infants with candidaemia.[54]

In two population-based studies the mortality for US infants of any gestation (mean 27 weeks and mean birth weight 1035 g) was 19%,[74] and for infants <1500 g in Australia and New Zealand mortality was 16.5%.[15]

The prognosis is particularly poor for infants <1000 g. In a US cohort of infants <1000 g born from 1993 to 2001, the mortality of IFI was 30%[96] and 57% of the survivors had neurodevelopmental impairment.[97] In a separate multi-centre US cohort from 1998 to 2001, mortality of infants <1000 g with candidiasis was 32% and major neurodevelopmental impairment occurred in 57% of survivors with candidaemia, 53% with Candida meningitis and 36% of infants <1000 g without Candida infection ($p < 0.001$).[8] Overall, death or disability occurred in 73% of infants <1000 g who developed candidiasis,[8] important data when counselling families about decisions on whether or not to continue intensive care for an infected infant.

16.7 Prevention

There are several possible approaches to prevention (Table 16.3). Some involve modification of clinical practice which is cost neutral or even reduces costs. Arguably antifungal prophylaxis should not be used unless prior attempts have been made to correct for bad clinical practices.

16.7.1 Antifungal prophylaxis

If antifungal prophylaxis is used, it is logical to target infants at high risk. Birth weight is the single most important determinant of risk and most studies of

Table 16.3 Strategies to reduce incidence and severity of invasive fungal infection.

Caesarean section delivery of very-low-birth-weight infants
Minimum duration of endotracheal intubation
Minimum duration of antibiotics
Reduce use of broad-spectrum antibiotics
Minimum duration of parenteral nutrition; early enteral feeds
Minimum duration of central venous catheters
Avoid use of histamine H2 blockers
Avoid use of post-natal corticosteroids if possible
Use prophylactic antifungals
Consider empiric antifungal at the time of investigation of an infant <1500 g for late-onset sepsis

prophylaxis have been restricted to infants <1500 g or <1000 g, although some clinicians have included infants on broad-spectrum antibiotics.

Question: Should we use antifungal prophylaxis and what is the best agent?

A Cochrane systematic review and meta-analysis of prophylactic systemic antifungal agents[98] found five eligible trials, all comparing **fluconazole** with placebo.[77,99–102] The methodologic quality of these studies was generally high.[103] The incidence of IFI in infants <1500 g treated with prophylactic fluconazole was 6.1% compared to 16.6% in infants who received placebo, (RR 0.36, 95% CI 0.15–0.89). The mortality was 9.5% of babies receiving fluconazole compared with 14.0% with placebo (RR 0.68, 95% CI 0.47–0.99).[98] No significant toxicity from fluconazole was reported and no babies were withdrawn from the studies because of adverse events.

In one single-centre study from India, prophylactic fluconazole prophylaxis was ineffective.[77] This study was unique in reporting that non-albicans Candida caused 96.8% of cases of IFI (*C. glabrata* 71%, *C. parapsilosis* 14.7% and *C. tropicalis* 9.6%).[77] In all other studies, *C. albicans* predominated, and much lower rates of colonization and IFI with non-albicans species were documented.[99–102] The Indian NICU had been using prophylactic fluconazole for the previous 6 years which may have selected for Candida species with resistance or reduced susceptibility to fluconazole (e.g. *C. glabrata, C. krusei*).[77] They observed reduced colonization by fluconazole-sensitive Candida species (*C. albicans, C. parapsilosis, C. tropicalis*) in infants randomized to receive antifungal prophylaxis and no difference in *C. glabrata* and *C. krusei* colonization rates between infants receiving fluconazole and placebo.[77] If the Indian study is excluded from the Cochrane meta-analysis, the effect of fluconazole is stronger (RR 0.23, 95% CI 0.11–0.46), and for the populations studied nine infants need to be treated (number needed to treat (NNT)) with fluconazole to prevent one invasive infection (95% CI 6, 17).[103] However, in the United Kingdom 125 infants <1500 g need to be treated with fluconazole to prevent one baby developing IFI,[104] and in Australia and New Zealand[15] the NNT is 116. The NNT for fluconazole for babies <1000 g is 45 in the United Kingdom[101] and 69 in Australia and New Zealand.[15]

Fluconazole is usually given from birth for 30 days to babies <1500 g, or 45 days for babies <1000 g and the dose is 3–6 mg/kg IV or oral given every 3 days or twice a week, although regimens vary.[97–102] Some centres have reported selective use of fluconazole prophylaxis. In one study, IV fluconazole was given to all infants <1500 g or <32 weeks of gestation, but only during periods when they received broad-spectrum antibiotics for >3 days.[105] A more targeted approach has been to give selective fluconazole prophylaxis only to infants <1500 g with additional risk factors for fungal infection. A Belfast study targeted infants <1500 g who were receiving treatment with a third generation cephalosporin; or had received treatment for more than 10 consecutive days with a systemic broad-spectrum antibiotic; or had fungal colonization from surface sites and a central venous catheter, and 30% of babies <1500 g were eligible for prophylaxis. The policy was associated with a reduction in fungal sepsis compared to an historic control period.[106]

A Cochrane systematic review of prophylactic oral or topical non-absorbed antifungal agents,[107] included two RCTs comparing oral nystatin with placebo[108,109] and one study comparing miconazole with placebo.[110] The methodologic quality was moderate.[107] Miconazole reduced Candida colonization but not IFI, although the incidence was low.[110] In the meta-analysis, the incidence of IFI in babies <1500 g treated with prophylactic oral nystatin was 5.3% compared to 32.9% in babies receiving placebo (RR 0.16, 95% CI 0.11–0.23). Mortality was 6.4% (39 of 602) with nystatin and 7.5% (45 of 598) with placebo (RR 0.70, 95% CI 0.47–1.06).[107] There was no significant toxicity reported from oral mycostatin or nystatin in the studies reviewed and no babies were withdrawn because of adverse events.[106–109]

Two RCTs compared fluconazole with nystatin.[111, 112] The methodologic quality was moderate.[107] When the two studies were combined, there was no significant difference in incidence of IFI between fluconazole and nystatin (RR 0.54, 95% CI 0.19–1.56). Mortality was 6.1% (8 of 131) with fluconazole and 10.3% (14 of 136) with nystatin (RR 0.96, 95% CI 0.89–1.03).[107]

In a survey of US neonatologists, 21% of those who used antifungal prophylaxis reported using amphotericin B or liposomal amphotericin although there is no formal evidence of efficacy or safety.[113] One small pilot study showed once-weekly liposomal amphotericin prophylaxis was tolerated by 12 infants <1500 g but the study was underpowered.[114]

In summary, there is strong evidence that either fluconazole or nystatin reduces the incidence of IFI and fluconazole reduces mortality. The clinical trial evidence for efficacy of fluconazole is stronger. Fluconazole can cause reversible hepatotoxicity and can select for non-albicans Candida. Oral nystatin is cheap and has no apparent toxicity.

Recommendation: It is recommended that high-risk pre-term infants <1500 g receive antifungal prophylaxis with intravenous or oral fluconazole or with oral nystatin. Fluconazole is indicated when the incidence of IFIs is high. Nystatin may be preferred when the incidence of IFIs is low or if resources are severely limited.

Although IFIs can occur in infants who have undergone gastrointestinal surgery[7] and in infants with major congenital malformations,[115] the incidence of IFIs in these populations is unknown. This makes it impossible to know the relative risks and benefits for antifungal prophylaxis in these populations and to give authoritative advice.

16.7.2 Changes in clinical practice

The incidence of IFI in infants <1500 g increases with use of broad-spectrum antibiotics and with duration of antibiotic use. Although the corollary that avoiding broad-spectrum antibiotics and reducing the duration of antibiotics reduces the incidence of IFI has not been studied, such a change in practice seems a worthwhile goal if it can be achieved safely.

Similarly, early introduction of enteral feeds allows earlier cessation of parenteral nutrition and earlier removal of central venous catheters, the duration of both of which are known to correlate with the incidence of IFIs.

Table 16.3 summarizes other approaches which might be undertaken to reduce the risk or severity of IFIs. The risks and benefits of each recommendation should be considered.

16.7.3 Lactoferrin

Lactoferrin is a naturally occurring glycoprotein in mammalian milk that plays an important part in innate immunity (see Section 23.4.4). An RCT compared supplementation of infants <1500 g with bovine lactoferrin alone, bovine lactoferrin plus the probiotic *Lactobacillus rhamnosus* GG or placebo. IFI incidence was significantly lower with bovine lactoferrin alone (0.7%) or plus *Lactobacillus rhamnosus* GG (2.0%) than with placebo (7.7%).[116] This is the only study of lactoferrin that has reported rates of fungal infection and it is hoped that it will stimulate further studies.

16.7.4 Probiotics

There are contrasting data on the effect of bacterial probiotics on Candida colonization. In the lactoferrin study infants in the lactoferrin plus Lactobacillus arm did not have reduced colonization compared with controls and the addition of Lactobacillus did not reduce the incidence of IFI compared with lactoferrin alone.[116] In contrast, in one study supplementation with either *Lactobacillus rhamnosus* or *Lactobacillus reuteri* reduced Candida stool colonization compared with controls and probiotic-supplemented infants had a better neurologic outcome.[117]

The ability of yeast-based probiotics such as Saccharomyces to protect against IFIs is being studied.

16.8 Malassezia

Malassezia are yeasts which can infect humans and animals and are mostly obligatorily lipophilic.[118, 119] Skin colonization of adults with Malassezia species is extremely common. *M. furfur* can cause the adult skin infection tinea versicolor. *M. globus* and *M. sympodiales* can cause neonatal pustulosis or neonatal acne.[120] *M. pachydermatis* infects dogs and a neonatal unit outbreak involving eight infants with bloodstream infection and one meningitis was thought to have been caused by *M. pachydermatis* carried on the hands of a health-care worker with a pet dog.[121]

Neonatal skin colonization with Malassezia species is extremely common,[122] but invasive infection is rare. Bloodstream infection occurs almost exclusively in association with parenteral nutrition with lipid emulsions, often in infants <1000 g or with severe gastrointestinal disease or congenital heart disease.[120] The clinical presentation of bloodstream infection, especially if catheter-associated, is indistinguishable from other bacterial and fungal infections. Fever and thrombocytopenia each occur in about half of all cases.[118, 119] Fungaemia often persists but disseminated fungal infection is very rare, although meningitis, urinary tract infection, and liver abscess have been described[118, 119, 121]

Malassezia are only moderately sensitive to amphotericin B *in vitro*. The mainstay of treatment is to remove central venous catheters and stop parenteral nutrition and particularly lipid emulsions. The outlook of bloodstream infection is generally good, although occasional deaths have been reported.[118, 119]

16.9 Pichia

Pichia anomala (previously called *Hansenula anomala*) are Saccharomycetes, budding yeasts found in soil and pigeon droppings, which can cause single cases or outbreaks of bloodstream infection, usually in extremely pre-term infants in association with central venous catheters and lipid-containing parenteral nutrition.[123, 124] Treatment is with amphotericin B and catheter removal.

16.10 Zygomycosis

The zygomycetes, Rhizopus, Mucor and Absidia, are found in soil, animal manure and on fruits. They can cause infections in immunocompromised hosts including neonates and have caused NICU outbreaks, including skin and systemic Rhizopus infection associated with the use of wooden tongue depressors as armboards for drips.[24–26,125] A systematic review found 59 neonatal cases of zygomycosis published up to 2007, 77% born pre-term.[26] The commonest sites were gastrointestinal (54%) and cutaneous (36%), a different pattern from the typical sinopulmonary and rhinocerebral zygomycosis in older children.[126] Most cases (57%) were diagnosed by histology only and 44% by histology and culture. Rhizopus species were isolated from 18 of 25 cases (72%). The mortality was high (64%). Over a third of patients did not receive antifungal therapy. The survival was 70% for neonates treated with amphotericin B and surgery compared with 5% for those who received no therapy. A combination of amphotericin B and surgery was a common management strategy and associated with improved survival.[26]

References

1. Blyth CC, Chen SC, Slavin MA et al. Not just little adults: candidemia epidemiology, molecular characterization, and antifungal susceptibility in neonatal and pediatric patients. *Pediatrics* 2009; 123:1360–1368.
2. Baley JE, Kliegman RM, Fanaroff AA. Disseminated fungal infections in very low birth-weight infants: clinical manifestations and epidemiology. *Pediatrics* 1984; 73:144–152.
3. Weese-Mayer DE, Fondriest DW, Brouilette RT, Shulman ST. Risk factors associated with candidemia in the neonatal intensive care unit: a case-control study. *Pediatr Infect Dis J* 1987; 6:190–196.
4. Faix RG, Kovarik SM, Shaw TR, Johnson RV. Mucocutaneous and invasive candidiasis among very low birth weight (<1500 grams) infants in intensive care nurseries: a prospective study. *Pediatrics* 1989; 83:101–107.
5. Leibovitz E, Iuster-Reicher A, Amitai M, Mogilner B. Systemic candida infections associated with use of peripheral venous catheters in neonates: a 9-year experience. *Clin Infect Dis* 1992; 14:485–491.
6. Saiman L, Ludington E, Pfaller M, et al. Risk factors for candidemia in neonatal intensive care unit patients: the National Epidemiology of Mycosis Survey Study Group. *Pediatr Infect Dis J* 2000; 19:319–324.
7. Shetty SS, Harrison LH, Hajjeh RA, et al. Determining risk factors for candidemia among newborn infants from population-based surveillance: Baltimore, Maryland, 1998–2000. *Pediatr Infect Dis J* 2005; 24:601–604.
8. Benjamin DK Jr, Stoll BJ, Fanaroff AA, et al. Neonatal candidiasis among extremely low birth weight infants: risk factors, mortality rates, and neurodevelopmental outcomes at 18 to 22 months. *Pediatrics* 2006; 117:84–92.
9. Cotten CM, McDonald S, Stoll B, et al. The association of third-generation cephalosporin use and invasive candidiasis in extremely low birth-weight infants. *Pediatrics* 2006; 118:717–722.
10. Manzoni P, Farina D, Leonessa M, d'Oulx EA, Galletto P, Mostert M, Miniero R, Gomirato G. Risk factors for progression to invasive fungal infection in preterm neonates with fungal colonization. *Pediatrics* 2006; 118:2359–2364.
11. Manzoni P, Farina D, Galletto P, et al. Type and number of sites colonized by fungi and risk of progression to invasive

fungal infection in preterm neonates in neonatal intensive care unit. *J Perinat Med* 2007; 35:220–226.
12. Benjamin DK, Stoll BJ, Gantz MG, et al. Neonatal candidiasis: epidemiology, risk factors, and clinical judgment. *Pediatrics* 2010; 126:e865–e873.
13. Farmaki E, Evdoridou J, Pouliou T, et al. Fungal colonization in the neonatal intensive care unit: risk factors, drug susceptibility, and association with invasive fungal infections. *Am J Perinatol* 2007; 24:127–135.
14. Makhoul IR, Bental Y, Weisbrod M, Sujov P, Lusky A, Reichman B. Candidal versus bacterial late-onset sepsis in very low birthweight infants in Israel: a national survey. *J Hosp Infect* 2007; 65:237–243.
15. Howell A, Isaacs D, Halliday R. Oral nystatin prophylaxis and neonatal fungal infections. *Arch Dis Child Fetal Neonatal Ed* 2009; 94:F429–F433.
16. Kaufman D, Boyle R, Hazen KC, Patrie JT, Robinson M, Donowitz LG. Fluconazole prophylaxis against fungal colonization and infection in preterm infants. *N Engl J Med* 2001; 345:1660–1666.
17. Ozturk MA, Gunes T, Kokiu E, Cetin N, Koc N. Oral nystatin prophylaxis to prevent invasive candidiasis in Neonatal Intensive Care Unit. *Mycoses* 2006; 49:484–492.
18. Clerihew L, Lamagni TL, Brocklehurst P, McGuire W. Invasive fungal infection in very low birthweight infants: national prospective surveillance study. *Arch Dis Child Fetal Neonatal Ed* 2006; 91:F188–F192.
19. Parikh TB, Nanavati RN, Patankar CV, et al. Fluconazole prophylaxis against fungal colonization and invasive fungal infection in very low birth weight infants. *Indian Pediatr* 2007; 44:830–837.
20. Manzoni P, Stolfi I, Pugni L, et al. A multicenter, randomized trial of prophylactic fluconazole in preterm neonates. *N Engl J Med* 2007; 356:2483–2495.
21. Manzoni P, Arisio R, Mostert M, et al. Prophylactic fluconazole is effective in preventing fungal colonization and fungal systemic infections in preterm neonates: a single-center, 6-year, retrospective cohort study. *Pediatrics* 2006; 117:e22–e32.
22. Dankner WM, Spector SA, Fierer J, Davis CE. Malassezia fungemia in neonates and adults: complication of hyperalimentation. *Rev Infect Dis* 1987; 9:743–753.
23. Oliveri S, Trovato L, Betta P, Romeo MG, Nicoletti G. Malassezia furfur fungaemia in a neonatal patient detected by lysis-centrifugation blood culture method: first case reported in Italy. *Mycoses.* 2011; 54:e638–e640.
24. Antoniadou A. Outbreaks of zygomycosis in hospitals. *Clin Microbiol Infect* 2009; 15(Suppl 5):55–59.
25. Roilides E, Zaoutis TE, Walsh TJ. Invasive zygomycosis in neonates and children. *Clin Microbiol Infect* 2009; 15(Suppl 5):50–54.
26. Roilides E, Zaoutis TE, Katragkou A, Benjamin DK Jr, Walsh TJ. Zygomycosis in neonates: an uncommon but life-threatening infection. *Am J Perinatol* 2009; 26:565–573.
27. Darmstadt GL, Dinulos JG, Miller Z. Congenital cutaneous candidiasis: clinical presentation, pathogenesis, and management guidelines. *Pediatrics* 2000; 105:438–444.
28. Almeida Santos L, Beceiro J, Hernandez R, et al. Congenital cutaneous candidiasis: report of four cases and review of the literature. *Eur J Pediatr* 1991; 150:336–338.
29. Cosgrove BF, Reeves K, Mullins D, Ford MJ, Ramos-Caro FA. Congenital cutaneous candidiasis associated with respiratory distress and elevation of liver function tests: a case report and review of the literature. *J Am Acad Dermatol.* 1997; 37:817–823.
30. Carmo K, Evans N, Isaacs D. Congenital candidiasis presenting as septic shock without rash. *Arch Dis Child* 2007; 92:627–628.
31. Sánchez-Schmidt JM, Vicente-Villa MA, Viñas-Arenas M, Gené-Giralt A, González-Enseñat MA. Isolated congenital nail candidiasis: report of 6 cases. *Pediatr Infect Dis J* 2010; 29:974–976.
32. Scheinfeld N. Diaper dermatitis: a review and brief survey of eruptions of the diaper area. *Am J Clin Dermatol* 2005; 6:273–281.
33. Adalat S, Wall D, Goodyear H. Diaper dermatitis-frequency and contributory factors in hospital attending children. *Pediatr Dermatol* 2007; 24:483–488.
34. Faix RG, Kovarik SM, Shaw TR, Johnson RV. Mucocutaneous and invasive candidiasis among very low birth weight (less than 1,500 grams) infants in intensive care nurseries: a prospective study. *Pediatrics* 1989; 83:101–107.
35. Rowen JL, Atkins JT, Levy ML, Baer SC, Baker CJ. Invasive fungal dermatitis in the ≤1000-gram neonate. *Pediatrics* 1995; 95:682–687.
36. Brenuchon C, Lebas D, Rakza T, Piette F, Storme L, Catteau B. [Invasive fungal dermatitis in extremely premature newborns: a specific clinical form of systemic candidiasis]. *Ann Dermatol Venereol* 2006; 133:341–346.
37. Hoppe JE. Treatment of oropharyngeal candidiasis and candidal diaper dermatitis in neonates and infants: review and reappraisal. *Pediatr Infect Dis J* 1997; 16:885–894.
38. Pankhurst CL. Candidiasis (oropharyngeal). *Clin Evid (Online).* 2012; 2012 pii:1304.
39. Benjamin DK Jr, Poole C, Steinbach WJ, Rowen JL, Walsh TJ. Neonatal candidemia and end-organ damage: a critical appraisal of the literature using meta-analytic techniques. *Pediatrics* 2003; 112:634–640.
40. Kaufman D, Fairchild KD. Clinical microbiology of bacterial and fungal sepsis in very-low-birth-weight infants. *Clin Microbiol Rev* 2004; 17:638–680.
41. Clerihew L, Lamagni TL, Brocklehurst P, McGuire W. *Candida parapsilosis* infection in very low birthweight infants. *Arch Dis Child Fetal Neonatal Ed* 2007; 92:F127–F129.
42. Kaufman DA. Neonatal candidiasis: clinical manifestations, management, and prevention strategies. *J Pediatr* 2010; 156(Suppl 2): S53–S67.
43. Cohen-Wolkowiez M, Smith PB, Mangum B, et al. Neonatal Candida meningitis: significance of cerebrospinal fluid parameters and blood cultures. *J Perinatol* 2007; 27:97–100.
44. Fairchild KD, Tomkoria S, Sharp EC, Mena FV. Neonatal *Candida glabrata* sepsis: clinical and laboratory features compared with other Candida species. *Pediatr Infect Dis J* 2002; 21:39–43.

45. Benjamin DK Jr, Ross K, McKinney RE Jr, Benjamin DK, Auten R, Fisher RG. When to suspect fungal infection in neonates: A clinical comparison of *Candida albicans* and *Candida parapsilosis* fungemia with coagulase-negative staphylococcal bacteremia. *Pediatrics* 2000; 106:712–718.
46. Manzoni P, Mostert M, Galletto P, et al. Is thrombocytopenia suggestive of organism-specific response in neonatal sepsis? *Pediatr Int* 2009; 51:206–210.
47. Guida JD, Kunig AM, Leef KH, McKenzie SE, Paul DA. Platelet count and sepsis in very low birth weight neonates: is there an organism-specific response?. *Pediatrics* 2003; 111:1411–1415.
48. Bhat MA, Bhat JI, Kawoosa MS, Ahmad SM, Ali SW. Organism-specific platelet response and factors affecting survival in thrombocytopenic very low birth weight babies with sepsis. *J Perinatol* 2009; 29:702–708.
49. Benjamin DK Jr, DeLong ER, Steinbach WJ, Cotton CM, Walsh TJ, Clark RH. Empirical therapy for neonatal candidemia in very low birth weight infants. *Pediatrics* 2003; 112:543–547.
50. Phillips JR, Karlowicz MG. Prevalence of Candida species in hospital-acquired urinary tract infections in a neonatal intensive care unit. *Pediatr Infect Dis J* 1997; 16:190–194.
51. Bryant K, Maxfield C, Rabalais G. Renal candidiasis in neonates with candiduria. *Pediatr Infect Dis J* 1999; 18:959–963.
52. Karlowicz MG. Candidal renal and urinary tract infection in neonates. *Semin Perinatol* 2003; 27:393–400.
53. Robinson JL, Davies HD, Barton M, et al. Characteristics and outcome of infants with candiduria in neonatal intensive care - a Paediatric Investigators Collaborative Network on Infections in Canada (PICNIC) study. *BMC Infect Dis* 2009; 9:183.
54. Wynn JL, Tan S, Gantz MG, et al. Outcomes following candiduria in extremely low birth weight infants. *Clin Infect Dis* 2012; 54:331–339.
55. Meyer CL, Payne NR, Roback SA. Spontaneous, isolated intestinal perforations in neonates with birth weight less than 1,000 g not associated with necrotizing enterocolitis. *J Pediatr Surg* 1991; 26:714–717.
56. Mintz AC, Applebaum H. Focal gastrointestinal perforations not associated with necrotizing enterocolitis in very low birth weight neonates. *J Pediatr Surg* 1993; 28:857–860.
57. Adderson EE, Pappin A, Pavia AT. Spontaneous intestinal perforation in premature infants: a distinct clinical entity associated with systemic candidiasis. *J Pediatr Surg* 1998; 33:1463–1467.
58. Pumberger W, Mayr M, Kohlhauser C, Weninger M. Spontaneous localized intestinal perforation in very-low-birth-weight infants: a distinct clinical entity different from necrotizing enterocolitis. *J Am Coll Surg* 2002; 195:796–803.
59. Bond S, Stewart DL, Bendon RW. Invasive Candida enteritis of the newborn. *J Pediatr Surg* 2000; 35:1496–1498.
60. Robertson NJ, Kuna J, Cox PM, Lakhoo K. Spontaneous intestinal perforation and Candida peritonitis presenting as extensive necrotizing enterocolitis. *Acta Paediatr* 2003; 92:258–261.
61. Faix RG, Chapman RL. Central nervous system candidiasis in the high-risk neonate. *Semin Perinatol* 2003; 27:384–392.
62. Moylett EH. Neonatal Candida meningitis. *Semin Pediatr Infect Dis* 2003; 14:115–122.
63. Fernandez M, Moylett EH, Noyola DE, Baker CJ. Candidal meningitis in neonates: a 10-year review. *Clin Infect Dis* 2000; 31:458–463.
64. Daher AH, Berkowitz FE. Infective endocarditis in neonates. *Clin Pediatr (Phila)* 1995; 34:198–206.
65. Levy I, Shalit I, Birk E, et al. Candida endocarditis in neonates: report of five cases and review of the literature. *Mycoses* 2006; 49:43–48.
66. Chapman RL, Faix RG. Persistently positive cultures and outcome in invasive neonatal candidiasis. *Pediatr Infect Dis J* 2000; 19:822–827.
67. Trovato L, Betta P, Romeo MG, Oliveri S. Detection of fungal DNA in lysis-centrifugation blood culture for the diagnosis of invasive candidiasis in neonatal patients. *Clin Microbiol Infect* 2012; 18:E63–E65.
68. Oliveri S, Trovato L, Betta P, Romeo MG, Nicoletti G. Experience with the Platelia Candida ELISA for the diagnosis of invasive candidosis in neonatal patients. *Clin Microbiol Infect* 2008; 14:391–393.
69. Kaufman DA. Challenging issues in neonatal candidiasis. *Curr Med Res Opin* 2010; 26:1769–1778.
70. Cohen-Wolkowiez M, Moran C, Benjamin DK Jr, Smith PB. Pediatric antifungal agents. *Curr Opin Infect Dis* 2009; 22:553–558.
71. Baley JE, Meyers C, Kliegman RM, et al. Pharmacokinetics, outcome of treatment, and toxic effects of amphotericin B and 5-fluorocytosine in neonates. *J Pediatr* 1990; 116:791–797.
72. Holler B, Omar SA, Farid MD, et al. Effects of fluid and electrolyte management on amphotericin B-induced nephrotoxicity among extremely low birth weight infants. *Pediatrics* 2004; 113:e608–e616.
73. Turkova A, Roilides E, Sharland M. Amphotericin B in neonates: deoxycholate or lipid formulation as first-line therapy - is there a 'right' choice?. *Curr Opin Infect Dis* 2011; 24:163–171.
74. Ascher SB, Smith PB, Watt K, et al. Antifungal therapy and outcomes in infants with invasive Candida infections. *Pediatr Infect Dis J* 2012; 31:439–443.
75. Aghai ZH, Mudduluru M, Nakhla TA, et al. Fluconazole prophylaxis in extremely low birth weight infants: association with cholestasis. *J Perinatol* 2006; 26:550–555.
76. Brion LP, Uko SE, Goldman DL. Risk of resistance associated with fluconazole prophylaxis: systematic review. *J Infect* 2007; 54:521–529.
77. Parikh TB, Nanavati RN, Patankar CV, et al. Fluconazole prophylaxis against fungal colonization and invasive fungal infection in very low birth weight infants. *Indian Pediatr* 2007; 44:830–837.
78. Wade KC, Wu D, Kaufman DA, et al. Population pharmacokinetics of fluconazole in young infants. *Antimicrob Agents Chemother* 2008; 52:4043–4049.

79. Wade KC, Benjamin DK Jr, Kaufman DA, et al. Fluconazole dosing for the prevention or treatment of invasive candidiasis in young infants. *Pediatr Infect Dis J* 2009; 28:717–723.
80. Piper L, Smith PB, Hornik CP, et al. Fluconazole loading dose pharmacokinetics and safety in infants. *Pediatr Infect Dis J* 2011; 30:375–378.
81. Clerihew L, McGuire W. Systemic antifungal drugs for invasive fungal infection in preterm infants. *Cochrane Database of Systematic Reviews* 2004, (Issue. 1). Art. No.: CD003953. doi:10.1002/14651858.CD003953.pub2.
82. Driessen M, Ellis JB, Cooper PA, et al. Fluconazole versus amphotericin B for the treatment of neonatal fungal septicemia: a prospective randomized trial. *Pediatr Infect Dis J* 1996; 15:1107–1112.
83. Caudle KE, Inger AG, Butler DR, Rogers PD. Echinocandin use in the neonatal intensive care unit. *Ann Pharmacother* 2012; 46:108–116.
84. Manzoni P, Benjamin DK, Hope W, et al. The management of Candida infections in preterm neonates and the role of micafungin. *J Matern Fetal Neonatal Med* 2011; 24(Suppl. 2):24–27.
85. Cohen-Wolkowiez M, Benjamin DK Jr, Piper L, et al. Safety and pharmacokinetics of multiple-dose anidulafungin in infants and neonates. *Clin Pharmacol Ther* 2011; 89:702–707.
86. Somer A, Törün SH, Salman N. Caspofungin therapy in immunocompromised children and neonates. *Expert Rev Anti Infect Ther* 2011; 9:347–355.
87. Mohamed WA, Ismail M. A randomized, double-blind, prospective study of caspofungin vs. amphotericin B for the treatment of invasive candidiasis in newborn infants. *J Trop Pediatr* 2012; 58:25–30.
88. Eppes SC, Troutman JL, Gutman LT. Outcome of treatment of candidemia in children whose central catheters were removed or retained. *Pediatr Infect Disease J* 1989; 8:99–104.
89. Karlowicz MG, Hashimoto LN, Kelly RE Jr, Buescher ES. Should central venous catheters be removed as soon as candidemia is detected in neonates? *Pediatrics* 2000; 106:E63.
90. Qu Y, Istivan TS, Daley AJ, Rouch DA, Deighton MA. Comparison of various antimicrobial agents as catheter lock solutions: preference for ethanol in eradication of coagulase-negative staphylococcal biofilms. *J Med Microbiol.* 2009; 58:442–450.
91. Blackwood RA, Klein KC, Micel LN, et al. Ethanol locks therapy for resolution of fungal catheter infections. *Pediatr Infect Dis J* 2011; 30:1105–1107.
92. Hoppe JE, Hahn H. Randomized comparison of two nystatin oral gels with miconazole oral gel for treatment of oral thrush in infants. *Antimycotics Study Group. Infection* 1996; 24:136–139.
93. Hoppe JE. Treatment of oropharyngeal candidiasis in immunocompetent infants: a randomized multicenter study of miconazole gel vs. nystatin suspension. The Antifungals Study Group. *Pediatr Infect Dis J* 1997; 16:288–293.
94. Goins RA, Ascher D, Waecker N, Arnold J, Moorefield E. Comparison of fluconazole and nystatin oral suspensions for treatment of oral candidiasis in infants. *Pediatr Infect Dis J* 2002; 21:1165–1167.
95. Lee BE, Cheung PY, Robinson JL, Evanochko C, Robertson CM. Comparative study of mortality and morbidity in premature infants (birth weight, <1,250 g) with candidemia or candidal meningitis. *Clin Infect Dis* 1998; 27:559–565.
96. Stoll B, Hansen N, Fanaroff AA, et al. Late onset sepsis in very low birth weight neonates: The experience of the NICHD Neonatal Research Network. *Pediatrics* 2002; 110:285–291.
97. Stoll BJ, Hansen NI, Adams-Chapman I, et al; Neurodevelopmental and growth impairment among extremely low-birth-weight infants with neonatal infection. *J Am Med Assoc* 2004; 292:2357–2365.
98. Clerihew L, Austin N, McGuire W. Prophylactic systemic antifungal agents to prevent mortality and morbidity in very low birth weight infants. *Cochrane Database of Systematic Reviews* 2007, (Issue. 4). Art. No.: CD003850. doi: 10.1002/14651858.CD003850.pub3.
99. Kaufman D, Boyle R, Hazen KC, Patrie JT, Robinson M, Donowitz LG. Fluconazole prophylaxis against fungal colonization and infection in preterm infants. *N Engl J Med* 2001; 345:1660–1666.
100. Kicklighter SD, Springer SC, Cox T, Hulsey TC, Turner RB. Fluconazole for prophylaxis against candidal rectal colonization in the very low birth weight infant. *Pediatrics* 2001; 107:293–298.
101. Cabrera C, Frank M, Carter D, Bhatia J. Fluconazole prophylaxis against systemic candidiasis after colonization: a randomized, double-blinded study. *J Perinatol* 2002; 22:604.
102. Manzoni P, Stolfi I, Pugni L, et al. A multicenter, randomized trial of prophylactic fluconazole in preterm neonates. *N Engl J Med* 2007; 356:2483–2495.
103. Blyth CC, Barzi F, Hale K, Isaacs D. Chemoprophylaxis of neonatal fungal infections in very low birth weight infants: efficacy and safety of fluconazole and nystatin. *J Paed Child Health* 2012; 48(9):846–851.
104. Clerihew L, Lamagni TL, Brocklehurst P, McGuire W. Invasive fungal infection in very low birthweight infants: national prospective surveillance study. *Arch Dis Child Fetal Neonatal Ed* 2006; 901:F188–F192.
105. Uko S, Soghier LM, Vega M, et al. Targeted short-term fluconazole prophylaxis among very low birth weight and extremely low birth weight infants. *Pediatrics* 2006; 117:1243–1252.
106. McCrossan BA, McHenry E, O'Neill F, Ong G, Sweet DG. Selective fluconazole prophylaxis in high-risk babies to reduce invasive fungal infection. *Arch Dis Child Fetal Neonatal Ed* 2007; 92:F454–F458.
107. Austin N, Darlow BA, McGuire W. Prophylactic oral/topical non-absorbed antifungal agents to prevent invasive fungal infection in very low birth weight infants. *Cochrane Database of Syst Rev* 2009, (Issue. 4). Art. No.: CD003478. doi:10.1002/14651858.CD003478.pub3.

108. Sims ME, Yoo Y, You H, Salminen C, Walther FJ. Prophylactic oral nystatin and fungal infections in very-low-birthweight infants. *Am J Perinatol* 1988; 5:33–36.
109. Ozturk MA, Gunes T, Kokiu E, Cetin N, Koc N. Oral nystatin prophylaxis to prevent invasive candidiasis in Neonatal Intensive Care Unit. *Mycoses* 2006; 49:484–492.
110. Wainer S, Cooper PA, Funk E, Bental RY, Sandler DA, Patel J. Prophylactic miconazole oral gel for the prevention of neonatal fungal rectal colonization and systemic infection. *Pediatr Infect Dis J* 1992; 11:713–716.
111. Aydemir C, Oguz SS, Dizdar EA, et al. Randomised controlled trial of prophylactic fluconazole versus nystatin for the prevention of fungal colonisation and invasive fungal infection in very low birth weight infants. *Arch Dis Child Fetal Neonatal Ed* 2011; 96:F164–F168.
112. Violaris K, Carbone D, Bateman D, Olawepo O, Doraiswamy B, LaCorte M. Comparison of fluconazole and nystatin oral suspensions for prophylaxis of systemic fungal infection in very low birth weight infants. *Am J Perinatol* 2010; 27:73–78.
113. Burwell LA, Kaufman D, Blakely J, Stoll BJ, Fridkin SK. Antifungal prophylaxis to prevent neonatal candidiasis: a survey of perinatal physician practices. *Pediatrics* 2006; 118:e1019–e1026.
114. Arrieta AC, Shea K, Dhar V, et al. Once-weekly liposomal amphotericin B as Candida prophylaxis in very low birth weight premature infants: a prospective, randomized, open-label, placebo-controlled pilot study. *Clin Ther* 2010; 32:265–271.
115. Rabalais GP, Samiec TD, Bryant KK, Lewis JJ. Invasive candidiasis in infants weighing more than 2500 grams at birth admitted to a neonatal intensive care unit. *Pediatr Infect Dis J* 1996; 15:348–352.
116. Manzoni P, Stolfi I, Messner H, et al. Bovine lactoferrin prevents invasive fungal infections in very low birth weight infants: a randomized controlled trial. *Pediatrics* 2012; 129:116–123.
117. Romeo MG, Romeo DM, Trovato L, et al. Role of probiotics in the prevention of the enteric colonization by Candida in preterm newborns: incidence of late-onset sepsis and neurological outcome. *J Perinatol* 2011; 31:63–69.
118. Stuart SM, Lane AT. Candida and Malassezia as nursery pathogens. *Semin Dermatol* 1992; 11:19–23.
119. Devlin RK. Invasive fungal infections caused by Candida and Malassezia species in the neonatal intensive care unit. *Adv Neonatal Care* 2006; 6:68–79.
120. Bernier V, Weill FX, Hirigoyen V, et al. Skin colonization by Malassezia species in neonates: a prospective study and relationship with neonatal cephalic pustulosis. *Arch Dermatol* 2002; 138:215–218.
121. Chang HJ, Miller HL, Watkins N, et al. An epidemic of *Malassezia pachydermatis* in an intensive care nursery associated with colonization of health care workers' pet dogs. *N Engl J Med* 1998; 338:706–711.
122. Nagata R, Nagano H, Ogishima D, Nakamura Y, Hiruma M, Sugita T. Transmission of the major skin microbiota, Malassezia, from mother to neonate. *Pediatr Int* 2012; 54(3):350–355.
123. Aragão PA, Oshiro IC, Manrique EI, et al. Pichia anomala outbreak in a nursery: exogenous source? *Pediatr Infect Dis J* 2001; 20:843–848.
124. Paula CR, Krebs VL, Auler ME, et al. Nosocomial infection in newborns by Pichia anomala in a Brazilian intensive care unit. *Med Mycol* 2006; 44:479–484.
125. Smolinski KN, Shah SS, Honig PJ, Yan AC. Neonatal cutaneous fungal infections. *Curr Opin Pediatr* 2005; 17:486–493.
126. Zaoutis TE, Roilides E, Chiou CC, et al. Zygomycosis in children: a systematic review and analysis of reported cases. *Pediatr Infect Dis J* 2007; 26:723–727.

CHAPTER 17
Viral infections

17.1 Cytomegalovirus

17.1.1 Virology of cytomegalovirus

Cytomegalovirus (CMV) is a herpesvirus and shares the characteristics of all herpesviruses including the ability to cause latent (hidden) infection and to reactivate with intermittent viral shedding. CMV can cause latent infection of macrophages but may also cause chronic, low-level infection rather than true latency. CMV is the largest herpesvirus and the most structurally complex. Genomic variation among human cytomegalovirus (HCMV) wild-type strains is well documented and the differences between strains are sufficient that CMV-seropositive individuals can be reinfected with new strains.[1] CMV can infect many different cell types. As the name implies (*cyto* = cell and *megalo* = large), infection results in large cells with inclusions likened to an owl's eye appearance. An old name for CMV infection was cytomegalic inclusion disease.

17.1.2 Epidemiology of cytomegalovirus

CMV is the commonest congenital infection in Western countries.[2] Congenital CMV infection can follow either primary maternal CMV infection or CMV reactivation or possibly reinfection in a seropositive mother. In populations with very high maternal CMV seroprevalence most cases of congenital CMV are caused by reactivation, whereas primary maternal CMV is an important mode of transmission in Western countries. Infants with congenital CMV infection can be symptomatic or asymptomatic at birth. The relative severity of congenital CMV acquired through primary or reactivated maternal infection is an important epidemiologic question.

Humans are thought to be the only reservoir for CMV, which is an advantage for vaccine development. The virus is ubiquitous. CMV is acquired at an earlier age in developing countries, and in sub-Saharan Africa, South America and the Pacific almost all school children (>95%) are seropositive. A literature review found that CMV seroprevalence in women of reproductive age ranged from 45% to 100%, being highest in South America, Africa and Asia and lowest in Western Europe and United States.[2] CMV seroprevalence also varied substantially within the United States, differing by as much as 30 percentage points between states. The seroprevalence was higher by an average 20–30% points globally in non-whites than whites and increased with lower socioeconomic status. In Western populations up to 55% of women of child-bearing age are CMV seronegative and at risk of primary CMV infection during pregnancy.[2]

Modes of transmission of CMV are poorly understood. CMV is shed intermittently and can be found in nasopharyngeal secretions, urine, tears, breast milk and genital secretions and can spread transplacentally to cause congenital infection. Evidence for breast milk transmission is not conclusive[3] (see Section 19.4.1.3). A review of studies of CMV shedding in body fluids, detected by culture or PCR, found the highest prevalence (median 80%) and duration of shedding in children with congenital CMV infection, declining steeply by 5 years of age.[4] Healthy children attending day care shed twice as frequently (median 23%) as healthy children not attending day care (median 12%) and more often in urine than in saliva. Peak shedding occurred at 1–2 years of age. Adults with risk factors, for example attendance at a sexual health clinic, were three times more likely to shed than adults without risk factors. The prevalence of CMV shedding in

Evidence-Based Neonatal Infections, First Edition. David Isaacs.

pregnant women increased with gestation. In children with congenital CMV infection, higher viral load at birth correlated strongly with being symptomatic at birth and an increased risk of sensorineural hearing loss.[4]

A systematic review and meta-analysis of studies of systematic CMV screening of foetuses and/or live-born infants found the overall birth prevalence of congenital CMV infection was 0.64%, with considerable variation among different study populations.[5] About 11% of live-born infants with congenital CMV infection were symptomatic, although different definitions of 'symptomatic' limited interpretation. The main risk factors for congenital CMV infection were non-white race and low socioeconomic status. Congenitally infected infants were more likely to be born pre-term and to be admitted to NICUs. Birth prevalence increased with maternal CMV seroprevalence. The rate of intrauterine transmission to infants was 32% with primary maternal CMV infection and 1.4% with recurrent infection.[5]

The incidence of congenital CMV infection is 1–5% in developing countries, mostly due to reactivation or reinfection, although the data are not always reliable.[6] The incidence in the United States is around 1% (varying from 0.2% to 2.2%).[2] Sequelae such as hearing loss can follow congenital CMV infection from both primary and post-primary maternal CMV and congenital CMV is the commonest cause of acquired sensorineural hearing loss (Section 17.1.3). Symptomatic congenital CMV resulting in severe neurodevelopmental sequelae is more common following primary maternal CMV infection. An Australian study found the seroprevalence in pregnant women was 57% (53–60%) and the rate of CMV seropositivity increased markedly with lower SES ($p < 0.001$).[7] However, more congenital CMV cases were reported in the highest socioeconomic groups (55%) than in the lowest (9%) ($p < 0.001$), implying that symptomatic congenital CMV is more likely to follow primary maternal infection.[7]

The timing in pregnancy of primary maternal CMV infection is also an important determinant of neonatal outcome. In one study first trimester primary maternal infection was more likely to result in sensorineural hearing loss than later maternal infection (24% vs. 2.5%) and more likely to be associated with CNS sequelae such as hearing loss, mental retardation, cerebral palsy, seizures or chorioretinitis (32% vs. 15%).[8] Unlike congenital rubella, which causes foetal malformations only with first trimester infection, late pregnancy CMV can also cause CNS sequelae, suggesting deformation.

17.1.3 Clinical manifestations of congenital cytomegalovirus infection

About 10–11% of infants with congenital CMV infections are symptomatic at birth. The rest are asymptomatic and not detected unless by screening.[5]

17.1.3.1 Clinical signs

The most common clinical findings at or soon after birth in symptomatic infants are a petechial or less commonly purpuric rash, jaundice and hepatosplenomegaly (Figure 17.1). About half of all symptomatic babies have intrauterine growth retardation and about half have microcephaly. Microcephaly, often defined as a head circumference below the fifth or third percentile, may be proportionate to generalized growth retardation and resolve with catch-up growth or may be out of proportion and persist. Microcephaly is a particularly sinister sign in terms of predicting death or poor neurologic outcome if it is associated with intracranial calcification, which is classically periventricular (Figure 17.2).[9] Chorioretinitis occurs in an estimated 14% of symptomatic infants[10] and may resemble toxoplasma retinitis (see Figure 18.5). A delayed presentation of congenital CMV with strabismus sometimes occurs, as with congenital toxoplasmosis.

Hepatitis and pneumonitis are rare in congenital infection and suggest CMV infection acquired post-natally (Section 17.1.4). They rarely occur concurrently.

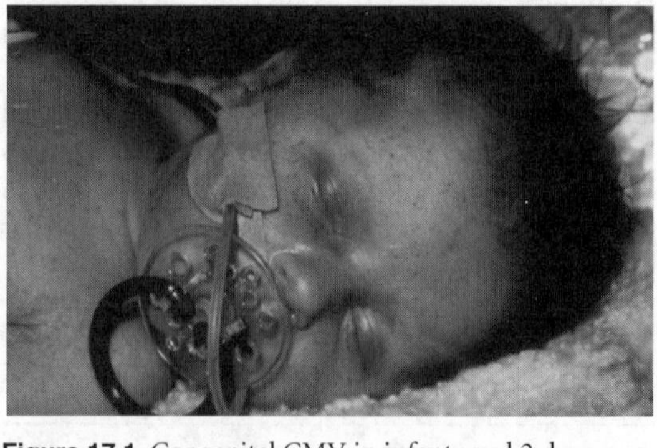

Figure 17.1 Congenital CMV in infant aged 2 days. Petechial rash and jaundice.

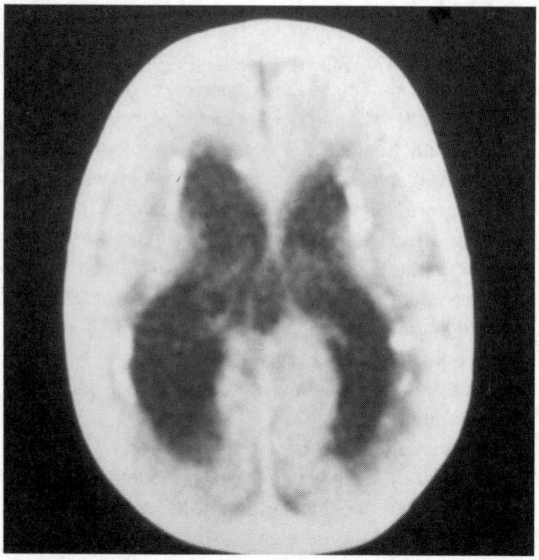

Figure 17.2 Congenital CMV. CT scan: periventricular calcification and ventricular dilatation (due to cerebral atrophy, not hydrocephalus).

17.1.3.2 Sensorineural hearing loss

Sensorineural hearing loss is commonest in symptomatic children, but asymptomatic infected infants can develop progressive sensorineural hearing loss. Severity is variable: unilateral or bilateral, mild to profound. Severity correlates with CMV DNA viral load.[11] The mechanism of hearing loss is poorly understood.

A systematic review found approximately 14% of children with congenital CMV infection develop sensorineural hearing loss, which is bilateral moderate-to-profound in 3–5%.[12] An estimated 15–20% of all cases of bilateral moderate-to-profound sensorineural hearing loss are caused by congenital CMV infection.[12] In a large study from Brazil, a population with almost 100% CMV seroprevalence in pregnancy, the infection rate in newborns screened for congenital CMV infection was 10 per 1000 (1%) and 10% were symptomatic at birth.[13] At 12 months, 9.8% had sensorineural hearing loss. Symptomatic infection at birth increased the risk of sensorineural hearing loss many fold (OR 38.1, 95% CI 1.6–916.7). In this population, only 4 of 10 infants with sensorineural hearing loss were born to mothers with primary CMV infection.[13] Thus, congenital CMV infection is a major cause of sensorineural hearing loss in children worldwide, even in countries where most mothers are seropositive.

There is an ongoing debate whether or not to screen newborn infants and, if so, whether to screen them for hearing loss or congenital CMV infection.[14] Onset of hearing loss is late in approximately 50% of congenital CMV and will not be detected by newborn hearing screening. Screening is unlikely to be worthwhile unless hearing loss is preventable (Section 17.1.5).

17.1.4 Clinical manifestations of post-natal cytomegalovirus infection

Post-natal CMV infection can result from maternal genital tract secretions at the time of birth, infected breast milk, blood products and respiratory exposure. It is usually asymptomatic although persistent infection with intermittent excretion is common. The level and route of virus exposure compared to intrauterine exposure may explain why post-natal CMV is less severe than congenital CMV infection. Infants born to CMV-seropositive mothers may also be relatively protected by transplacentally acquired CMV IgG. Manifestations include hepatitis, pneumonitis, sepsis, neutropoenia and thrombocytopaenia.[15]

17.1.4.1 Cytomegalovirus hepatitis

Hepatitis is unusual with congenital CMV infection but has been described, but is more characteristic of post-natally acquired CMV infection, particularly pre-term infants.[16, 17] In an observational study, signs and symptoms improved in seven infants treated with IV ganciclovir for 21 days but not in five untreated infants.[16]

17.1.4.2 Cytomegalovirus pneumonitis

CMV pneumonitis is characteristically afebrile and clinically and radiologically indistinguishable from Chlamydia pneumonitis (see Figure 8.2). Symptoms include increased oxygen requirement, tachypnoea and/or apnoea, cough, respiratory distress and increased respiratory secretions.[10] There are no RCTs or even case series of ganciclovir in CMV pneumonitis.

17.1.4.3 Sepsis syndrome

In 1979, 16 (31%) of 51 infants <1500 g screened for post-natal CMV excretion began excreting CMV in urine or nasopharynx after >28 days, and 14 of the 16 had a sepsis-like syndrome characterized by grey pallor, hepatosplenomegaly, respiratory deterioration and atypical lymphocytosis.[18] The syndrome was thought to be caused by blood transfusion. In later studies, acquired CMV infection could be prevented by using CMV-seronegative blood donors[19] or by filtering blood to remove white cells.[20]

17.1.4.4 Haematologic

Acquired CMV infection can result in persistent neutropoenia, thrombocytopaenia and lymphocytosis.[21]

17.1.5 Treatment of congenital cytomegalovirus infection

Studies of antiviral treatment for this condition are extremely difficult to perform. Treatment is prolonged, parenteral and toxic.

Question: Does antiviral treatment compared with no antiviral treatment improve outcome in infants with congenital CMV infection?

We found no systematic reviews, one set of 'evidence-based' guidelines[22] and one RCT.[23] The RCT, a multicentre US study, randomly assigned 100 infants with symptomatic congenital CMV infection to 6 weeks of IV ganciclovir or no treatment. The study was unblinded with no placebo arm. Only 42 of 100 patients achieved the primary end-point of both a baseline and 6-month follow-up brain stem-evoked response (BSER) audiometric examination. The results approached statistical significance: 21 (84%) of 25 infants given ganciclovir had improved hearing or maintained normal hearing compared with 10 (59%) of 17 controls ($p = 0.06$). Hearing deteriorated in 7 (41%) of 17 controls but none of 25 ganciclovir recipients ($p < 0.01$). Significant neutropoenia developed in 63% of ganciclovir patients and 21% of controls ($p < 0.01$).[23] The long-term rate of hearing loss is not known yet.

Some study infants were assessed at 1 year using Denver developmental tests, which developmental paediatricians consider of uncertain validity for predicting neurodevelopmental outcome.[24] The study used a non-validated approach of comparing mean number of 'delays' (milestones not met) in ganciclovir-treated infants and controls. Although they found significant differences at 6 and 12 months, the high drop-out rate and weak study design render the study far from conclusive.

The length of intravenous therapy (6 weeks) and its toxicity are significant constraints on ganciclovir use in clinical practice. Studies are underway of oral valganciclovir, usually following IV ganciclovir. An observational Israeli study treated 23 infants with symptomatic congenital CMV infection using ganciclovir for 6 weeks followed by oral valganciclovir to age 12 months. The main adverse effect was transient neutropoenia. At a year of age or greater, hearing was normal in 76% of affected ears compared to 54% at baseline, supposedly better results than historical infants treated for 6 weeks only. Even if these results are valid, it is unknown whether antiviral treatment merely postpones rather than prevents hearing loss.[25]

Short periods of IV ganciclovir followed by oral valganciclovir or even valganciclovir monotherapy are probably more acceptable to families, but their effectiveness awaits further studies. The role of viral load monitoring is also unclear.

Recommendation: Antivirals may be beneficial in terms of audiologic and neurodevelopmental outcome for infants with symptomatic congenital CMV infection, but the extent and duration of benefit is uncertain and antivirals are associated with significant toxicity. Treatment decisions should be made individually.

The recommended doses of antivirals based on pharmacokinetic data[26] are

Ganciclovir 6 mg/kg/dose IV 12 hourly.
Valganciclovir 16 mg/kg/dose orally 12 hourly.

17.1.6 Prevention of congenital infection

A Cochrane systematic review[27] of RCTs and quasi-RCTs found six studies of antenatal interventions for preventing the transmission of CMV from the mother to foetus during pregnancy including one using hyperimmune globulin,[28] one using a candidate recombinant CMV envelope glycoprotein vaccine[29] and one using parental education,[30] but none met the study entry criteria.

17.1.7 Prevention of acquired cytomegalovirus infection

The rate of transfusion-acquired post-natal CMV infection can be reduced considerably by using

CMV-seronegative blood donors[19] or by filtering blood to remove white cells.[20]

17.1.8 Risk to staff

Pregnant nursing, medical and paramedical staff are often concerned about working with infants with congenital CMV infection but evidence shows health-care workers (HCW) are not at increased risk. In a longitudinal study the annual rate of seroconversion of seronegative medical students (0.6%), house staff (2.7%) and nurses (3.3%) was not significantly higher than young women in the community (2.5% during pregnancy and 5.5% between pregnancies).[31] In a review of similar serologic studies the annual seroconversion rate ranged from 1% to 7% of pregnant women (summary annual rate 2.3%) and was also 2.3% in HCWs, including those caring for infants and children.[32] Most parents exposed to a CMV-shedding child do not become infected. However, seroconversion rates were higher in **day-care** providers (range 0–12.5%, summary annual rate 8.5%),[32] perhaps because exposure is greater and/or hand hygiene is poorer in day care.

We recommend **not** evaluating CMV serostatus routinely in pregnant HCWs, because their risk is no higher than the general population. Congenital CMV can follow primary or post-primary maternal infection, so serologic interpretation is complex. However, serology for CMV IgM may be indicated if a pregnant HCW develops a glandular fever-like illness.

17.2 Herpes simplex virus

Herpes (Greek) means both 'creeping like a snake' and 'latent'. Spreading skin lesions may appear to creep. The ancient Greeks knew of herpes infections and Herodotus used the term *herpes febrilis* to describe the association between oral herpes and fever.

Neonatal herpes simplex virus (HSV) infection was first described in the 1930s. HSV can cause blistering skin lesions, conjunctivitis, mouth blisters and ulceration, isolated pneumonitis or a sepsis-like syndrome with thrombocytopaenia. Suspicion needs to be high because, unless treated early, localized infections usually disseminate and mortality is high.

17.2.1 Virology

HSV, like all herpesviruses, can cause latent (hidden) infection and reactivate with intermittent viral shedding. It was recognized in the mid-1960s that there were two antigenic types of HSV (HSV-1 and HSV-2) and that infection with one provided at best partial protection against infection with the other type.[33]

HSV is neurotropic: the site of latency is sensory neurones. Primary infection is followed by productive replication in mucosal epithelial cells. HSV enters the sensory neurones through nerve terminals, is transported to neuronal cell bodies and establishes latency. HSV can reactivate intermittently resulting in new virus progeny that are transported axonally back to the periphery. The ability to establish lifelong latency and reactivate periodically to facilitate dissemination is central to the virus' survival strategy. The molecular mechanisms are only partially understood.[34]

17.2.2 Epidemiology

HSV needs to be in contact with mucosa or broken skin to initiate infection, generally requiring person-to-person contact. HSV spreads readily among infants and toddlers in day care through infected secretions or respiratory droplets.

HSV can cause classic transplacental congenital HSV infection but neonatal HSV infection is far more commonly acquired perinatally. True congenital HSV infection due to transplacental infection is responsible for around 3–5% of neonatal HSV infections; the remaining 95–97% are post-natally acquired.[35]

Neonatal HSV infection can occur following maternal primary infection or reactivation. In a study from Sweden and the United States, HSV-1 was far more readily transmissible to the neonate than HSV-2 during reactivation (adjusted pooled OR 19.2; 95% CI 5.8–63.6), and the authors expressed concern in view of the rising frequency of genital HSV-1 infection.[33]

Maternal IgG antibody is relatively but not absolutely protective against neonatal HSV infection. In a prospective study, HSV was isolated from 56 (0.35%) of 15 923 genital viral cultures performed on women in early labour with no symptoms or signs of genital HSV infection.[36] There was serologic evidence of subclinical primary genital HSV infection in 18 (35%) of the 56, while 34 (65%) had HSV reactivation. Six of 18 infants (33%) of women with primary genital HSV developed neonatal HSV compared with 1 of 34 infants (3%) of women with HSV reactivation ($p < 0.01$). The risk of neonatal HSV was increased in association with proven viral shedding from the cervix and with use of foetal scalp electrodes.[36]

In another large prospective US study, HSV was isolated from 202 women (5 per 1000) at the time of labour and 10 (5%) of them had neonates with HSV infection.[37] Risk factors for neonatal HSV included first-episode infection (OR 33.1; 95% CI 6.5–168), HSV isolation from the cervix (OR 32.6; 95% CI 4.1–260), HSV-1 versus HSV-2 isolation at the time of labour (OR 16.5; 95% CI 4.1–65), invasive monitoring (OR, 6.8; 95% CI, 1.4–32), delivery before 38 weeks (OR 4.4; 95% CI 1.2–16) and maternal age <21 years (OR 4.1; 95% CI 1.1–15). Neonatal HSV infection rates per 100 000 live births were 54 (95% CI 19.8–118) among HSV-seronegative women, 26 (95% CI 9.3–56) among women who were HSV-1 seropositive only and 22 (95% CI 4.4–64) among all HSV-2-seropositive women. The HSV transmission rate was 1 of 85 (1.2%) delivered by caesarean section and 9 of 117 (7.7%) delivered vaginally (OR 0.14; 95% CI 0.02–1.08).[37]

The incidence of neonatal HSV infection was 9.6 per 100 000 live births in 2006 in the United States[38] and 5.9 per 100 000 in Canada from 2000 to 2003.[39] The incidence of HSV-1 infection is rising in many countries in adults, and so is the proportion of neonatal HSV infections due to HSV-1.[40]

17.2.3 Clinical presentation

17.2.3.1 Congenital herpes simplex virus infection

The classic triad of congenital HSV infection presenting at birth is involvement of the skin (vesicular or bullous skin lesions), eye (chorioretinitis and/or keratoconjunctivitis) and CNS (microcephaly). A literature review yielded only 64 published cases of intrauterine HSV infection, of which less than one-third fit the typical triad.[35] Almost half (44%) of the infants with skin manifestations had lesions other than vesicles or bullae. Diagnosis was delayed >3 days after birth in 15 infants (23%) with the median age 10 days. HSV was often not considered in the differential diagnosis of infants with birth skin lesions that were not vesicles or bullae. New vesicles appeared in a number of infants.

A rare but important manifestation of congenital and neonatal HSV infection is with hepatomegaly and cytopaenia of two or more cell lines due to hemophagocytic lymphohistiocytosis or HLH (see Section 18.6).[41] If HSV is recognized early as the cause of HLH, acyclovir treatment is often curative.

17.2.3.2 Neonatal herpes simplex virus infection

Neonatal HSV infection is usually characterized as localized skin, eye or mouth (SEM) disease; encephalitis; or disseminated infection. HSV can also present in week 1 ('5-day pneumonitis') or 2 as isolated respiratory distress. Encephalitis and disseminated infection have a very poor prognosis. Localized disease including pneumonitis progresses to disseminated disease if not recognized and treated early.

17.2.3.2.1 Skin, eye and mouth infections

The hallmark of HSV skin lesions is the tendency to form individual punched-out vesicles about 0.5 cm in diameter which often rupture and coalesce (see Figures 13.1d, 13.1e and 17.3). Lesions can be anywhere on the infant's skin (Figure 17.3). The scalp is a common site (see Figures 13.1d and 13.1e). It is important to have a high index of suspicion and a low threshold for investigation of neonatal skin lesions. Lesions around the eye are suspicious, particularly if there is associated conjunctivitis (see Figures 12.3a, 12.3b and 17.4). Dendritic ulcers are a late manifestation of HSV eye infection (see Figure 12.4). Oral ulceration due to HSV in neonates is much less commonly reported than skin and eye lesions, because it is truly rare, atypical or

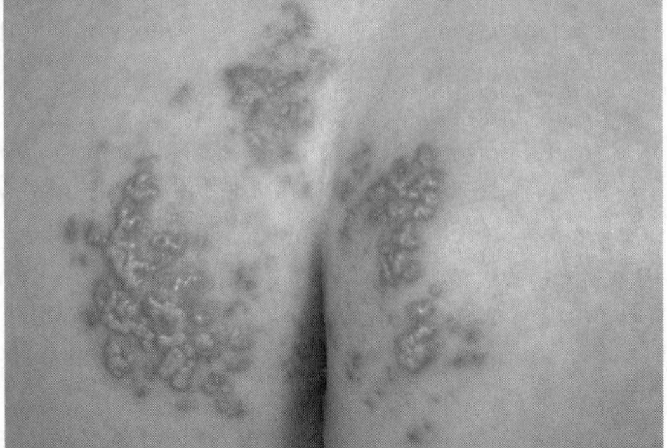

Figure 17.3 HSV infection with vesicles which have mostly coalesced on buttocks.

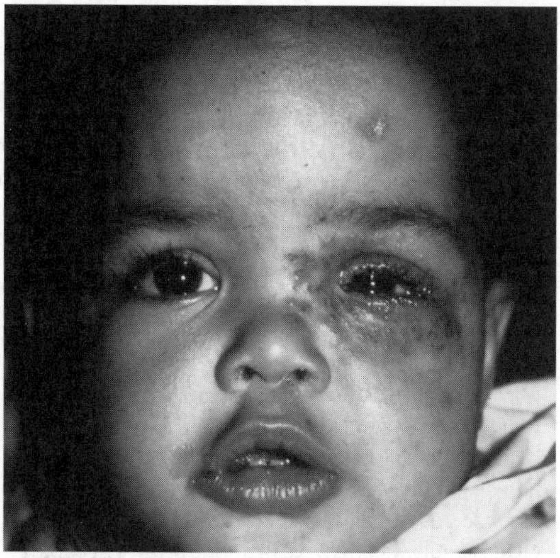

Figure 17.4 HSV infection of eye and skin. Left eyelid swollen and inflamed. Periorbital herpetic skin lesions have coalesced. Skin lesions also present on forehead and lips.

oral examination is performed badly. Rapid diagnosis is essential (Section 17.2.4).

Finding localized disease does not guarantee a good outcome. In a case series around 10% of infants with SEM disease have had long-term neurologic impairment, sometimes severe. The reason is uncertain: undiagnosed acute CNS infection and progressive CNS disease due to chronic or recurrent HSV infection are possible mechanisms.

17.2.3.2.2 Herpes simplex virus pneumonitis

Isolated HSV pneumonitis presents with respiratory distress 3–14 days after birth and is often misdiagnosed as bacterial pneumonia, even when this is clinically unlikely, or as chlamydial or viral pneumonia. The classic chest radiograph shows hilar and central interstitial infiltrate (see Figure 8.3), but HSV pneumonitis is not distinguishable radiologically from other pneumonitides.[42] Rapid viral diagnosis should be performed on respiratory secretions (nasopharyngeal or endotracheal secretions) using immunofluorescence, ELISA or PCR. If the test is positive for HSV, or rapid tests are not available or even if there is a negative test but high clinical suspicion, empiric acyclovir therapy should be started pending further investigation.

17.2.3.2.3 Herpes simplex virus encephalitis

Encephalitis is the sole manifestation of about a third of neonatal HSV infections or can occur with disseminated infection. Infants with neonatal encephalitis usually present in the second week of life, occasionally in the first week or >14 days with seizures, fever, lethargy, poor feeding, irritability, jitteriness and rigidity. The presentation of HSV-2 encephalitis is more fulminant than HSV-1 and the outcome poorer.[43–45]

LP usually shows a mononuclear cell pleocytosis although acellular CSF has rarely been reported from infants with HSV on brain biopsy (in the days before brain biopsy was replaced by PCR). HSV encephalitis is often haemorrhagic, resulting in micro- or macroscopic blood in the CSF. CSF glucose may be low and protein may be normal initially but rise with illness progression. Although false positives do rarely occur, a positive CSF PCR is an absolute indication for acyclovir therapy. CSF PCR is positive in at least 70% of infants with HSV encephalitis, but may be negative early in the course; as a negative PCR does not exclude HSV encephalitis acyclovir treatment may be necessary until a repeat LP can be performed.[45, 46]

Brain imaging may show temporal, parietal, frontal or sub-cortical parenchymal damage. Although temporal changes are common in HSV encephalitis, there are no specific radiologic changes that distinguish HSV reliably from other causes of encephalitis.

17.2.3.2.4 Disseminated herpes simplex virus infection

The clinical features of disseminated HSV infection overlap with severe bacterial sepsis. Infants with disseminated HSV infection often have hepatitis and features of disseminated intravascular coagulopathy such as thrombocytopaenia and a bleeding tendency. Other clinical features such as jaundice, irritability, seizures and shock may not be specific enough to alert the clinician to the diagnosis. Rash is rarely present initially although it may develop. HSV may be detected by PCR or cultured from peripheral blood: a high index of suspicion is the clue to diagnosis.

17.2.3.2.5 Hemophagocytic lymphohistiocytosis

Neonatal HSV infection can occasionally cause hemophagocytic lymphohistiocytosis (HLH) presenting clinically with hepatomegaly and/or splenomegaly and possibly fever, lymphadenopathy, respiratory failure or seizures.[41] Affected infants have cytopaenia of two or more cell lines and greatly elevated serum ferritin levels. Hemophagocytosis is often difficult to prove, but biopsies of bone marrow, lymph nodes (see Figure 18.10) or spleen may be characteristic. If HSV infection is the cause, diagnosis is critical to initiate acyclovir treatment (see Section 18.6).

17.2.4 Diagnosis

Rapid virologic techniques (e.g. nucleic acid amplification by PCR; antigen detection by ELISA; immunofluorescence) have revolutionized the diagnosis of neonatal HSV infection. HSV culture is rarely performed in many centres, because although sensitive it is not timely. PCR can be performed on most body fluids including blood and CSF.

17.2.5 Treatment

A Cochrane systematic review of antivirals for neonatal HSV infection[47] found two RCTs (273 infants). One study compared vidarabine with placebo in 63 infants.[48] There was no significant reduction in mortality overall, but mortality was significantly reduced in infants with either CNS or disseminated disease. There was no difference in the rate of neurologic abnormalities in survivors at 1 year when analysed as an entire group or by disease category.[48]

An RCT comparing acyclovir and vidarabine in 210 infected infants found no difference in mortality, disease progression, incidence of neurologic abnormality at 1 year or incidence of drug-induced renal or bone marrow toxicity. In infants with SEM disease, there was no significant difference in neurologic outcome.[49] Despite the similar outcomes, acyclovir is the only agent used nowadays because of the prohibitive volume of administration of vidarabine.

Current guidelines, based on pharmacokinetic data, recommend treatment with intravenous acyclovir (20 mg/kg/dose 8 hourly). Localized disease is treated for 14 days, provided that investigations include CSF examination to exclude CNS involvement. Disseminated disease and encephalitis should be treated for 21 days. It is recommended to monitor the neutrophil count and, if the absolute neutrophil count falls below 500/mm^3, decreasing the acyclovir dose or giving granulocyte colony stimulating factor (G-CSF) should be considered.

Question: Should infants with neonatal herpes simplex virus infection receive long-term suppressive therapy?

A multi-centre study reported the results of placebo-controlled RCTs of 6 months of suppressive acyclovir therapy (300 mg/m^2/dose 8 hourly orally) for 45 infants with neonatal HSV encephalitis and for 29 i6nfants with SEM disease.[50] Infants with CNS involvement who received acyclovir suppression compared with placebo had significantly higher mean Bayley mental development scores at 12 months (88.2 vs. 68.1, $p = 0.046$). Of the infants with CNS disease who received suppressive acyclovir, 69% had normal neurologic outcomes, 6% had mild impairment, 6% had moderate impairment and 19% had severe impairment; the corresponding proportions among subjects assigned to placebo were 33%, 8%, 25%, and 33%. There was no significant difference in Bayley mental development scores in infants with SEM disease, although numbers were small, and no difference in local skin recurrences. There was a trend to increased neutropoenia with acyclovir.

Recommendation: Infants with CNS involvement should be on long-term suppressive therapy with acyclovir for at least 6 months. For infants with neonatal HSV localized to skin, eye or mouth, suppressive therapy is not recommended because the risk of neutropoenia outweighs the benefits.

17.2.6 Prognosis

Despite concern that antivirals might increase survival at the cost of increased neurologic morbidity, one RCT[48] and observational studies have suggested this is not the case.[51]

Prior to antiviral therapy, the 12-month mortality of disseminated HSV disease was 85% and of HSV encephalitis was 50%. Since high-dose acyclovir has been used, the 12-month mortality for disseminated neonatal HSV has fallen to 29% and for HSV encephalitis to 4%.[51, 52] Morbidity has improved compared to historic data, but remains high. Most survivors of disseminated HSV disease (83%) but only 31% of survivors of HSV encephalitis are assessed as having normal neurodevelopment.[53] The morbidity of SEM disease has improved and <2% of survivors have impaired neurodevelopment.[53]

17.2.7 Prevention of neonatal herpes simplex virus infection

Unfortunately there is no effective vaccine commercially available yet. A trial of a herpes simplex virus type 2 (HSV-2) subunit vaccine containing glycoprotein D in women aged 18–30 years seronegative for HSV-1 and HSV-2 surprisingly showed that although the vaccine did not protect against HSV-2, HSV-1 genital disease was reduced by 58% (95% CI 12–80) and HSV-1 infection (with or without disease) by 35% (95% CI 13–52).[54]

A Cochrane systematic review of antenatal antiviral prophylaxis for recurrent genital herpes found seven eligible RCTs (1249 participants) which compared acyclovir to placebo or no treatment (five trials) and valaciclovir to placebo (two trials).[55] There were no cases of symptomatic neonatal herpes in either treatment or placebo groups. Women who received antiviral prophylaxis were less likely to have a recurrence of genital herpes at delivery and less likely to have a caesarean delivery for genital herpes.[55]

If an asymptomatic mother is shedding HSV, transmission can be reduced several fold by caesarean delivery (Section 17.2.2). If the mother has symptomatic genital HSV infection, caesarean section is certainly recommended for primary infection. However, even if a history of prior genital herpes proves the mother's symptoms are due to reactivation, caesarean is recommended because symptomatic infection is associated with a high viral load which may swamp any passively acquired maternal antibody.[37] Neonatal transmission can be reduced by limiting the use of invasive monitors among women shedding HSV at the time of labour.[37]

17.3 Varicella zoster virus

Varicella zoster virus (VZV) shares the ability of all herpesviruses to cause acute infection but also lie dormant in peripheral nerves and reactivate intermittently. Acute infection is called varicella or more colloquially chickenpox; reactivation disease is called zoster or herpes zoster. Varicella and zoster are caused by the same virus, hence varicella zoster virus. VZV is important in perinatology for three reasons:

- Maternal VZV primary infection in pregnancy can be life-threatening.
- Maternal VZV primary infection can cause congenital varicella syndrome.
- Neonatal VZV infection can be life-threatening.

Varicella zoster immunoglobulin (VZIG or ZIG) is an immunoglobulin preparation derived from blood donors with high VZV antibody titres. In 1969 VZIG was shown to protect healthy children against chickenpox.[56] It has been shown since then that VZIG does not always prevent chickenpox but reduces its severity. Passive protection is particularly important for unimmunized hosts with impaired T-cell function at risk of severe VZV infection. Both pregnant women and their newborns have relatively poor T-cell function.

17.3.1 Maternal primary varicella zoster virus infection in pregnancy

Primary VZV infection in pregnancy is relatively rare. The incidence of chickenpox in pregnant women in the United Kingdom has been estimated to be at least 1 per 2000 pregnancies.[57] The true incidence depends on local epidemiology, including whether or not countries have routine infant VZV immunization programmes, and if not whether most of the population are infected in childhood.[58–60] Primary VZV in adolescence or adulthood can be complicated by life-threatening pneumonitis and the immunosuppressive nature of pregnancy may predispose to severe primary infection. In a case series of adults without severe immunodeficiency managed in a high dependency unit for chickenpox pneumonitis, 30% were pregnant women.[61] However, there are no definitive studies showing chickenpox is more severe in pregnancy than in non-pregnant adults.

An evidence-based systematic review of prevention and treatment of VZV in pregnancy from Canada[62] recommended varicella immunization for all non-immune women as part of pre-pregnancy and postpartum care. VZV is a live attenuated vaccine and so, although vaccination within 2–3 days of exposure is protective,[63] immunization in pregnancy is not recommended. However, the vaccine is probably not teratogenic and termination of pregnancy should not be advised because of inadvertent vaccination during pregnancy.

A pregnant woman with unknown VZV serostatus exposed to VZV should have serologic testing. If the mother is seronegative or the serum result is unavailable within 96 hours from exposure, varicella zoster immunoglobulin (ZIG or VZIG) should be administered,[62] because VZIG reduces the risk both of the pregnant woman developing pneumonitis[62] and of congenital varicella (Section 17.3.2).[64] Prophylactic acyclovir is not recommended for maternal VZV exposure due to safety concerns, although it should be effective if VZIG is unavailable. Normal human immunoglobulin and intravenous immunoglobulin are other alternatives to VZIG.

Women who develop varicella infection in pregnancy should be counselled of the potential adverse maternal and foetal sequelae, the risk of transmission to the foetus and the options available for prenatal diagnosis. It is recommended that all women who develop varicella in pregnancy have serial ultrasounds to screen for congenital varicella infection.[59] Women with significant varicella infection in pregnancy should be treated with acyclovir; pneumonitis is usually an indication for hospital admission and IV acyclovir.[62]

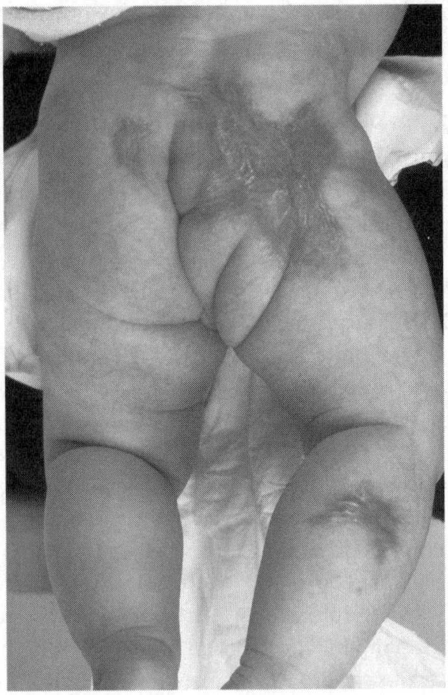

Figure 17.5 Cicatricial skin lesion of congenital varicella syndrome (possibly due to in utero zoster).

17.3.2 Congenital varicella syndrome

Congenital varicella syndrome is characterized by cicatricial (scarring) skin lesions and/or hypoplasia of a limb and severe CNS (microcephaly, cortical atrophy, seizures, developmental delay) and ocular abnormalities (chorioretinitis, microphthalmia).[65, 66] The cicatricial limb lesions may represent scarring from intrauterine zoster (Figure 17.5).

Diagnosis of congenital varicella syndrome is primarily clinical. VZV-specific IgM antibody was detected at birth in 4 (25%) of 16 infants with clinical congenital varicella syndrome and persistent specific IgG antibody in 5 of 7 infants tested.[11] The viral load in congenitally infected infants is much lower than in congenital rubella or CMV and PCR for VZV is diagnostically unreliable.

The strongest evidence on the risk of congenital varicella syndrome following maternal chickenpox or zoster comes from a large prospective study in Germany and the United Kingdom.[67] Nine babies with congenital varicella syndrome were all exposed to maternal varicella in the first 20 weeks of gestation. The highest risk was observed between 13 and 20 weeks of gestation, with 7 of 351 affected pregnancies resulting in congenital varicella (risk 2%, 95% CI 0.8–4.1). Two of 472 infections <13 weeks resulted in congenital varicella (risk 0.4%, 95% CI 0.05–1.5). A smaller US study (106 women with clinical varicella) reported the risk of varicella embryopathy following maternal varicella <20 weeks was 1.2% (95% CI 0–2.4).[68]

None of 366 infants born to women with herpes zoster in pregnancy developed congenital varicella (risk 0; 95% CI 0–1).[67] Congenital varicella syndrome has never been described following maternal zoster, so mothers can be counselled that the risk from maternal zoster is almost negligible.

A non-Cochrane systematic review[64] of the efficacy of maternal VZIG in preventing congenital varicella syndrome found three studies.[65, 69, 70] Congenital varicella syndrome developed in 14 (2.8%) of 498 infants whose mothers were not given VZIG but in no foetus or infant born to 142 mothers who received VZIG ($p < 0.01$ by Fisher exact test).[64]

This supports the recommendation to give VZIG to non-immune pregnant women exposed to VZV in the first 20 weeks of gestation to protect the foetus (Section 17.3.1) as well as the mother.

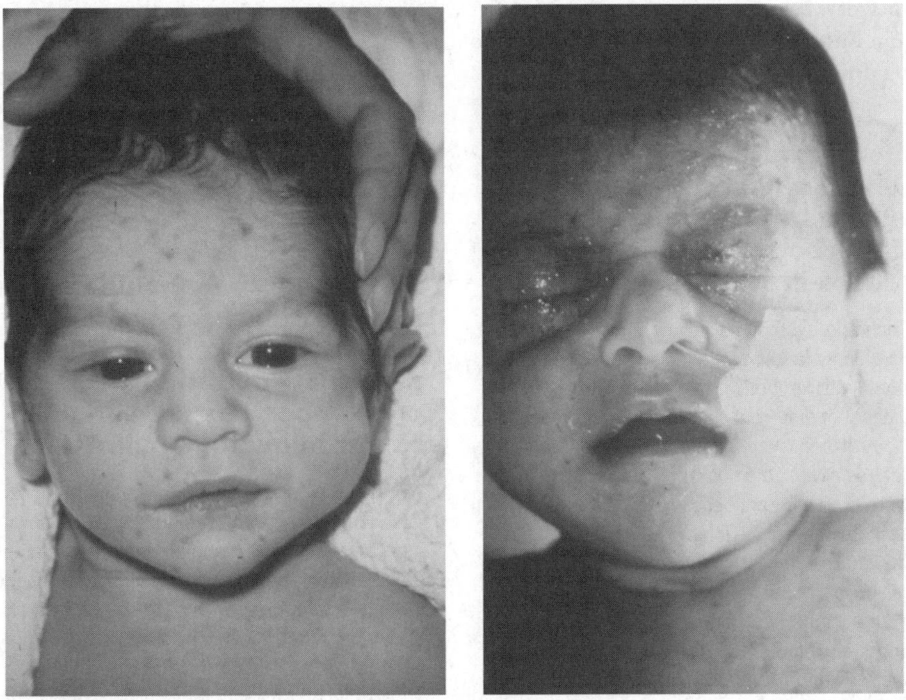

(a) (b)

Figure 17.6 Neonatal chickenpox. (a) Mother had chickenpox 10 days before delivery, baby born with spots but well. (b) Mother had chickenpox 4 days before delivery, baby born well but developed severe chickenpox and pneumonitis age 7 days (see Figure 17.7).

17.3.3 Neonatal varicella

Some infants whose mothers have perinatal chickenpox develop pneumonitis with a high mortality (Figures 17.6a and 17.7) while others are only mildly infected (Figure 17.6b). The critical determinants of severity are the viral load and the amount of protective maternal IgG antibody which has crossed the placenta. These correlate with the timing of maternal chickenpox. Historically, newborns of mothers who develop chickenpox from 4 days prior to delivery until 2 days after delivery were at greatest risk, with an estimated mortality rate of approximately 20–30%.[71, 72]

VZIG is recommended as soon as possible after birth for babies exposed to maternal VZV. The US *Red Book* recommends VZIG for neonates born to mothers with onset of chickenpox from 5 days before delivery to 2 days after delivery.[73] If VZIG is unavailable they recommend 400 mg/kg of intravenous immunoglobulin (IVIG).[73] Canada makes the same recommendation.[62] The recommendation in the United Kingdom is for

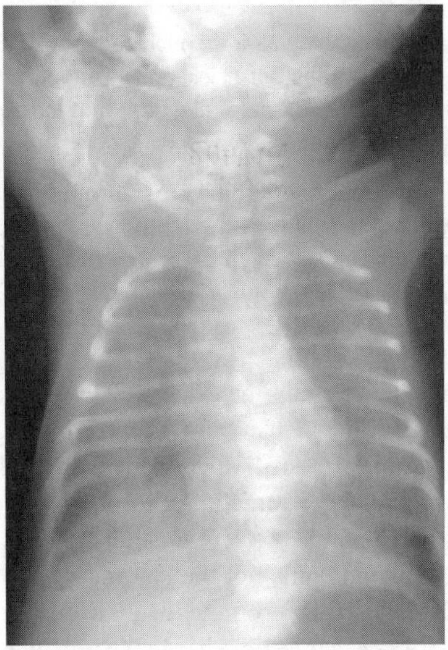

Figure 17.7 Severe VZV pneumonitis in baby whose mother developed chickenpox 4 days before delivery.

VZIG from 7 days before delivery to 7 days after delivery[74] and in Australia from 7 days before delivery to 2 days after delivery.[75]

Question: What is the evidence base about efficacy and timing of varicella zoster immunoglobulin for infants born to mothers with chickenpox around delivery?

A non-Cochrane systematic review[76] found only one prospective study, a UK study including 281 mothers with perinatal chickenpox.[77] All babies born >7 days after the onset of maternal chickenpox had detectable IgG antibody at birth. When maternal rash onset was 3–7 days before delivery, the nearer the delivery the fewer infants were born with antibody. When rash appeared <3 days before delivery, no infant had antibody at birth.

Infants were given 100 or 250 mg of VZIG shortly after birth or the onset of post-natal maternal chickenpox.[77] One infant died from an unrelated cause. Of the 280 surviving infants, 169 (60%) were infected, 134 (48%) with chickenpox and 35 (13%) subclinically. The clinical attack rate was highest (60%) in infants whose mothers had chickenpox between 7 days before and 7 days after delivery. Chickenpox was severe in 19 infants, 16 of whom were exposed to maternal chickenpox between 4 days before and 2 days after delivery. Perinatal maternal herpes zoster did not cause neonatal infection.

The authors of the review concluded that VZIG prevents clinically apparent chickenpox in approximately half of neonates born to mothers with chickenpox around the time of delivery.[76]

Recommendation: The data most strongly support giving VZIG to infants whose mothers have chickenpox with onset 7 days before and up to 2 days after delivery.

Infants may sometimes develop severe varicella despite receiving VZIG.[76,77] One possible reason is delayed administration, which may be due to human error or ignorance. Sometimes hospital staff do not know where to find VZIG (in Australian hospitals it is usually in Blood Bank, not the Pharmacy). If VZIG is unavailable, IVIG is recommended if available. Other reasons for severe infection despite ZIG include a large viral load and/or an inadequate dose of VZIG. There is no point in giving fractions of a vial when the rest will be discarded, so in Australia the whole 2 mL (200 mg) vial is given. In the United States the recommended dose is 125 units (one vial).[78] The difference between units and milligram is confusing. There is no direct relationship because the number of units depends on the titre of VZV antibodies: 125 units is equivalent to 60–200 mg.

Question: What should be done for a newborn exposed to maternal chickenpox around delivery who develops chickenpox despite varicella zoster immunoglobulin?

An infant who develops severe chickenpox despite VZIG needs urgent treatment with acyclovir 20 mg/kg/dose 8 hourly intravenously. A case report documented two infants with severe VZV despite VZIG; the authors reported a 3-day delay between the onset of symptoms and initiation of acyclovir.[79] It is unclear what to do if an infant develops mild varicella despite early VZIG prophylaxis. Most mild disease remains mild but some becomes severe. There is no formal evidence other than case reports.

Recommendation: A cautious approach is to admit and treat with IV acyclovir all neonates who develop chickenpox despite VZIG. An alternative approach is to only admit infants with respiratory symptoms and/or feeding difficulties. Because varicella pneumonitis can be fulminant and fatal, the more cautious approach is recommended.

17.4 Rubella

Rubella, literally 'a little red' in Latin, was first described in the eighteenth century in Germany, which explains its alternative name of German measles. In 1941, an Australian ophthalmologist Norman Gregg noted a sudden increase in the number of infants with congenital cataracts and overheard two mothers in his waiting room saying they both had rubella in early pregnancy. He started asking other mothers of affected infants about rash in pregnancy and performed serologic studies which confirmed recent rubella infection in many mothers and infants.[80] Gregg's observations predated thalidomide and his was the first description of toxic foetal embryopathy. His observation also accelerated the development of effective live attenuated rubella vaccines, first licensed in 1969.

17.4.1 Virology

Rubella is a so-called togavirus (toga = cloak). Man is the only natural host, although other mammals can be infected in the laboratory. There is relatively little antigenic variation which has aided vaccine development. The virus can be grown in cell culture.

17.4.2 Epidemiology

In non-immunized populations rubella causes epidemics every 3–4 years. Between epidemics there are too few susceptible hosts to transmit the virus efficiently, but the number of susceptibles builds until an epidemic can occur. The attack rate is highest in non-immune school-age children aged 5–14 years. When immunization levels are high the incidence of congenital rubella falls. However, the introduction of infant measles, mumps, rubella (MMR) vaccine in Greece without the infrastructure to attain high vaccination coverage and without immunization of adolescents and young women caused a paradoxical outbreak of congenital rubella syndrome. MMR vaccine coverage remained low (<50%) for years. The proportion of seronegative pregnant women increased resulting in an epidemic of rubella in young Greek adults and 25 infants developed congenital rubella syndrome (24.6 per 100 000 live births).[81]

The incidence of congenital rubella syndrome remains unacceptably high in countries which are unable to afford rubella or MMR vaccine.[82–84]

17.4.3 Foetal rubella infection

Rubella embryopathy is a malformation of the developing foetus.

Maternal rubella infection is transmitted to 90% of foetuses <11 weeks, 67% at 11–12 weeks, 54% at 13–14 weeks and 39% in the second trimester.[85] Severe defects, principally congenital heart disease and deafness, occurred in all infants infected before 11 weeks. Infants infected at 13–16 weeks had a 35% incidence of deafness alone. No congenital defects attributable to rubella were found in the 63 children infected later than 16 weeks.[85]

In a subsequent prospective study of women with confirmed pregnancy rubella, foetal infection only occurred when maternal rash appeared 12 days or more after the last menstrual period (LMP). Intrauterine infection did not occur when rash appeared before, or within 11 days after, the LMP.[86] All 10 pregnancies in which the rash appeared 3–6 weeks after the LMP resulted in foetal infection: the four infants delivered at term were all severely damaged.[86]

17.4.4 Clinical features

Rubella virus can infect almost all tissues causing a wide range of congenital defects affecting almost any organ (Figure 17.8). The most consistent are severe sensorineural deafness, eye defects including cataract (Figure 17.9) and 'salt-and-pepper' retinopathy (Figure 17.10) and intrauterine growth retardation. The combination of being blind and deaf is a sinister one, making communication extremely difficult; if both are severe the infant can be completely 'locked in'. Microcephaly is associated with neurodevelopmental delay. The commonest congenital heart defects are pulmonary artery hypoplasia and persistent ductus arteriosus.[87]

Late clinical features include diabetes mellitus, autoimmune disease, dental problems, neuropsychiatric problems including autism and a rare progressive

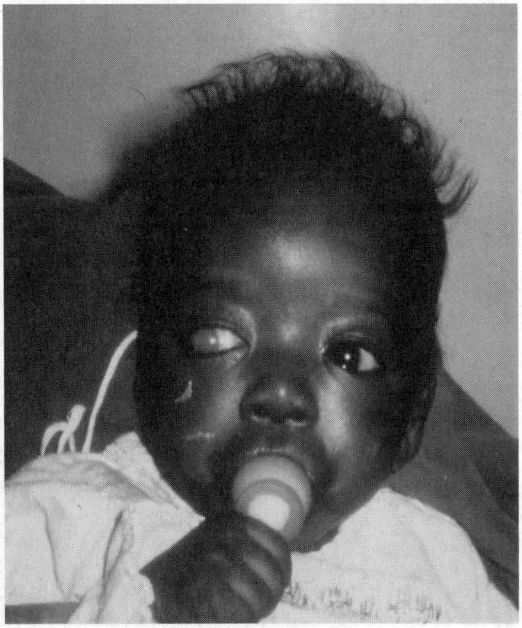

Figure 17.8 Congenital rubella syndrome. Buphthalmos of the right eye with cloudy cornea.

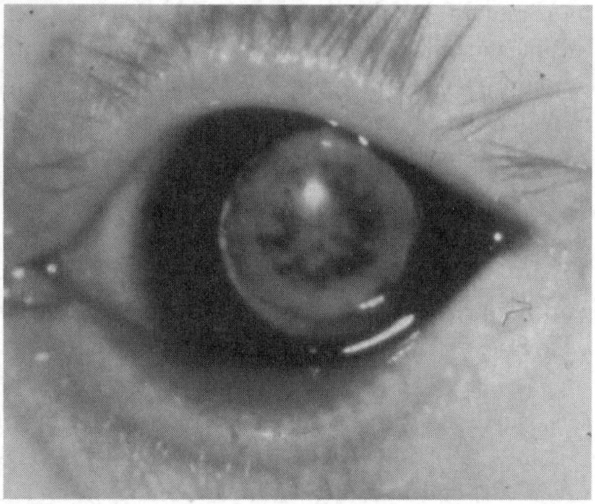

Figure 17.9 Congenital rubella syndrome: stellate cataract.

panencephalitis similar to sub-acute sclerosing panencephalitis of measles.[87]

17.4.5 Diagnosis

Diagnostic confirmation of congenital rubella is almost exclusively serologic by detecting rubella-specific IgM in the infant's serum. Rubella viral culture and PCR are virtually never used. The diagnosis of maternal infection in pregnancy is also exclusively serologic. In Western countries, pregnant women are screened for IgG antibodies and designated immune if IgG is detected. The test is not quantitative, so very occasionally a woman with asymptomatic or mild first trimester primary rubella infection is wrongly assumed to be immune. If there is any clinical doubt, the mother should be tested for IgM antibodies.

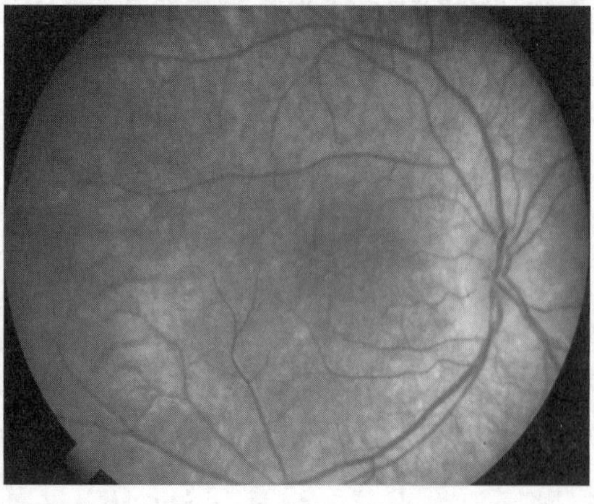

Figure 17.10 Congenital rubella syndrome. Salt-and-pepper retinopathy.

17.4.6 Prevention

Universal infant rubella immunization is the most effective prevention strategy. The United Kingdom and Australia started with a policy of selective immunization of schoolgirls and women who were seronegative postpartum.[88] Although the incidence of congenital rubella syndrome fell, cases continued to occur because rubella circulated among boys and seronegative women were at risk of exposure when pregnant. Both countries changed to routine infant immunization, using one and now two doses of MMR vaccine to boost immunity and 'mop up' any infants who fail to seroconvert after one dose. Universal infant immunization is highly effective: congenital rubella syndrome is extraordinarily rare in countries with an effective infant immunization programme.

Rubella immunization (usually as MMR vaccine nowadays) should still be given to seronegative women postpartum. Immunization is contraindicated in pregnancy, because rubella vaccine is a live attenuated vaccine. However, none of over 300 pregnant women immunized inadvertently who elected to continue the pregnancy had an infant with congenital rubella.[88] The estimated maximum theoretical risk of congenital rubella following maternal immunization is 1.2%, although the true risk may be zero.[88] Women immunized inadvertently with rubella vaccine in pregnancy should be counselled accordingly.

17.5 Enteroviruses

The enteroviruses (gut viruses) include echoviruses, Coxsackieviruses, polioviruses and miscellaneous enteroviruses including enterovirus 71. The parechoviruses, previously called echoviruses, cause very similar clinical features to echoviruses.[89] The enteroviruses are small RNA viruses classified as picornaviruses (from *pico* = small + RNA).

Apart from poliovirus, the enteroviruses do not apparently cause clinically significant transplacental infection and infections are thought to be acquired post-natally.[90] There is an important distinction between 'vertical' mother-to-infant transmission and 'horizontal' transmission, for example, from another infant or a sibling.[91–93] If maternal infection occurs close to delivery, specific IgG antibodies may not cross the placenta and the infant lacks passive protection. This is particularly important for echoviruses: vertical is far more severe than horizontal echovirus infection. Horizontal Coxsackievirus infection, in contrast, which can cause life-threatening myocarditis is apparently as severe as vertical Coxsackievirus infection.[94]

In clinical practice, enterovirus infection may be confirmed by PCR, but this does not distinguish initially between the different enteroviruses. It is often impossible to confirm until much later (from a positive culture or sequencing the PCR product) whether a suspected enterovirus infection is caused by an echovirus, parechovirus or Coxsackievirus.

17.5.1 Clinical features of enterovirus infection

Enterovirus infections may be asymptomatic or symptomatic infection, severity varying from mild to fulminant. The major features are myocarditis (primarily due to Coxsackie B virus but can occur with echoviruses, see Section 17.5.2), hepatitis (severe hepatitis is usually due to vertical echovirus infection but can occur with Coxsackieviruses, see Section 17.5.3), meningitis (either virus) or a sepsis-like picture mimicking bacterial sepsis (any enterovirus).

Around two-thirds of all mothers of infants with vertical infection report respiratory or gastrointestinal symptoms around delivery. Mothers may present with abdominal pain severe enough to be misdiagnosed as abruption.[91]

17.5.2 Enterovirus myocarditis

Coxsackievirus myocarditis is usually more severe than echovirus myocarditis. Both are reported mainly in full-term infants. A case series reported 7 neonates with Coxsackie B virus myocarditis presenting with heart failure and reviewed 28 previously published cases of enterovirus myocarditis.[95] All seven neonates had severe left ventricular dysfunction with dilatation and six had mitral regurgitation. The electrocardiogram resembled myocardial infarction in six infants. Two infants died. The survivors all had long-term cardiac sequelae including delayed left ventricular wall aneurysms, required long-term medication and one is awaiting heart transplantation. The 28 other cases in the review were all either Coxsackie myocarditis or had enterovirus detected by PCR without further testing. The overall mortality was 31% (11 of 35).[95] Sixteen of 24 survivors (66%) had severe cardiac damage and only 8 infants (23% of 35) recovered completely.[95] Because of selective reporting, the true prognosis of enterovirus myocarditis may be considerably better than the published data.

Echovirus myocarditis is rarely fulminant and may manifest only as tachycardia with mild echocardiographic and/or electrocardiogram changes which often resolves without inotropes or other cardiac therapy.

17.5.3 Enterovirus hepatitis

Echovirus hepatitis had a reported mortality >80% in 1986.[91] Most cases present between the third and fifth day after birth.[91] A more recent review of 16 neonates with enterovirus hepatitis and coagulopathy did not distinguish between echovirus and Coxsackie virus hepatitis.[96] The mean onset of symptoms was 3.8 days (range 1–7 days). Frequent clinical and laboratory findings included jaundice, lethargy, anorexia, hepatomegaly, thrombocytopaenia, prolonged clotting, raised liver enzymes and decreased fibrinogen and albumin. Five patients also had myocarditis and four had encephalitis. Ten patients had haemorrhagic complications including five with intracranial haemorrhage. The mortality was 31%; death was associated with myocarditis (5 of 5 vs. 0 of 11, $p < 0.001$), encephalitis (3 of 5 vs. 1 of 11, $p = 0.06$), prothrombin time >30 seconds (4 of 5 vs. 1 of 9, $p = 0.02$) and intracranial haemorrhage (4 of 5 vs. 1 of 8, $p = 0.03$). All survivors recovered completely.[96]

17.5.4 Enterovirus meningitis or encephalitis

Meningitis or encephalitis has been associated with infections caused by Coxsackieviruses, echoviruses and parechoviruses. There are no specific clinical features,[92] although a distinctive palmar-plantar erythematous rash was reported in Japanese infants with parechovirus infection.[89, 90]

The CSF in enterovirus meningitis often has a pleocytosis >1000 cells/mm^3 and a neutrophil predominance, mimicking bacterial meningitis.[92] In a South Korean report, neonates with positive enteroviral CSF PCR often had no white cells. The authors interpreted this as acellular meningitis although false-positive PCR is a possible alternative explanation.[97]

17.5.5 Enterovirus sepsis-like presentation

A sepsis-like presentation with fever, lethargy or irritability, poor feeding, abdominal distension, apnoea and increased oxygen or ventilatory requirement has been described with all the enteroviruses.[92]

17.5.6 Enteroviral rash

Exanthem is common in enterovirus infection and is usually non-specific, although hand-foot-and-mouth distribution has been described with several enteroviruses including enterovirus 71 and palmar-plantar erythematous rash with parechovirus infection.[89, 90]

17.5.7 Diagnosis of enterovirus infections

Viral culture has been replaced in many laboratories by molecular techniques, particularly PCR. The advantage of PCR is speed of diagnosis. The major drawback of PCR is that identification of the specific virus may not be possible or may take a long time. PCR tests are more susceptible than culture to false positives due to contamination. Serology is of no value in diagnosing neonatal enterovirus infections.

17.5.8 Treatment of enterovirus infections

The antiviral pleconaril is no longer commercially available after clinical trials showed disappointing efficacy, and with no specific treatment available, management is supportive. The improved prognosis in echovirus hepatitis is a result of improved neonatal intensive care.

17.5.9 Prevention of enterovirus infections

Enteroviruses spread by the faecal–oral route. Although there have been anecdotal reports of using prophylactic normal human immunoglobulin to interrupt nursery transmission of echoviruses, it is also possible to interrupt transmission through enhanced infection control measures.[98, 99]

Poliovirus immunization is considered briefly in Chapter 23 (see Section 23.5.2.2).

17.6 HIV

At the end of 2011, an estimated 3.4 million children <15 years globally were living with HIV/AIDS.[1] Almost all live in resource-poor countries, an estimated 91% in sub-Saharan Africa, and acquired HIV as a result of mother-to-child transmission (MTCT) during pregnancy, labour or breast feeding.[100]

17.6.1 Prevention of mother-to-child transmission of HIV

Prevention of MTCT of HIV is paramount. Effective strategies reduce the risk of transmission from a historic risk of 15–45% to <1%.[101] The most effective prevention strategies are identification and antiretroviral treatment of HIV-positive pregnant women, prophylactic antiretrovirals given to the infant, caesarean section and interventions surrounding breast feeding (see Section 19.4.1.1).[101] The most important of these is the first. Maternal HIV viral load during pregnancy and particularly at delivery is the single most important determinant of the risk of MTCT. The need for other interventions to prevent HIV depends heavily on whether or not the maternal viral load was undetectable in pregnancy and at delivery.

17.6.1.1 Antiretroviral treatment

In Western countries, most women with HIV are identified in pregnancy and treated effectively with highly active antiretroviral treatment (HAART) which reduces their viral load to undetectable levels. However, this is not always possible for various reasons, including lack of maternal screening for HIV, late maternal acquisition of HIV, late diagnosis and poor maternal adherence to antiretrovirals.

Antiretroviral drugs can be grouped into the following classes:

- Nucleoside analogue reverse transcriptase inhibitors: including zidovudine (ZDV, previously called azidothymidine or AZT), lamivudine (3TC), didanosine (ddI), stavudine (d4T) and abacavir (ABC).
- Non-nucleoside analogue reverse transcriptase inhibitors: including nevirapine (NVP), delavirdine and efavirenz.
- Protease inhibitors: including indinavir, ritonavir, nelfinavir and saquinavir.

- CCR5 receptor antagonists: maraviroc.
- Integrase strand transfer inhibitors: raltegravir and elvitegravir.

A Cochrane systematic review of antiretrovirals for reducing the risk of MTCT found 25 trials (18 901 participants).[102] Most trials (22) randomized mothers (18 prenatally, 4 in labour) but 3 trials randomized infants. The first trial, begun in 1991, compared zidovudine (ZDV/AZT) with placebo. In subsequent trials the type, dosage and duration of drugs have evolved, depending in part on cost, feasibility and setting. The Cochrane review presented the results stratified by regimen and type of feeding.[102]

The results are complex, but should inform national policy when resources are limited. They are presented in the following formats:

- Antiretrovirals versus placebo in breast-feeding populations.
- Antiretrovirals versus placebo in non-breast-feeding populations.
- Duration: longer versus shorter regimens.
- TRIPLE regimens versus other regimens.
- Comparison of different TRIPLE regimens.[102]

The Cochrane review recommended that, if short-course antiretrovirals are required, the current most effective regimen is probably: ZDV to mothers antenatally, followed by ZDV + 3TC intrapartum and postpartum for 1 week, and single-dose NVP to infants within 72 hours of delivery. For infants born to HIV-infected women who present late for delivery, post-exposure prophylaxis of the infant is recommended with a single dose of NVP immediately after birth plus ZDV + 3TC for 6 weeks.[102]

An important message from the Cochrane review is that optimal suppression of maternal HIV in pregnancy using triple therapy plus no breast feeding and post-natal antiretrovirals reduces the rate of MTCT to $<1\%$.[102]

- Adverse effects

The incidence of serious or life-threatening events was not significantly different with any of the different regimens in the Cochrane review.[102] There is no evidence of an increased risk of congenital malformations associated with in utero exposure to zidovudine or other commonly used antiretroviral drugs compared with the general population.

Prophylactic zidovudine is associated with mild, reversible, anaemia in infants and small but persistent reductions in neutrophil, platelet and lymphocyte levels of doubtful clinical significance in children up to 8 years of age.[103] To date, there is no evidence that in utero or neonatal exposure to antiretroviral drugs is associated with an increased risk of childhood cancer, but potential carcinogenic effects cannot be excluded.

Clinically evident mitochondrial disease in children exposed to nucleoside analogue-related antiretrovirals has only been described in Europe,[103, 104] with an estimated 18-month incidence of 'established' mitochondrial dysfunction of 0.26% among exposed children.[103–105] Whether or not these data are generalizable is unclear and so is their clinical significance.

There is some evidence that antiretroviral treatment can result in selection of resistant HIV mutations, although clearly if the infant is uninfected this can only be a problem for the mother.[102]

- Conclusions

Maternal regimens combining triple antiretrovirals are the most effective for preventing transmission of HIV from mothers to babies. The short-term risk of adverse events to both mother and baby appears acceptably low. Studies of the optimal antiretroviral combination and duration to balance optimal prevention against minimal toxicity continue.

One currently recommended Australian neonatal regimen shown in Table 17.1 based on evidence plus UK and US guidelines attempts to balance efficacy and risk. Prophylactic trimethoprim–sulfamethoxazole is no longer recommended because of the low risk of pneumocystis. The regularly updated US NIH guideline[106] available on http://aidsinfo.nih.gov/guidelines/html/3/perinatal-guidelines/187/ currently recommends 6 weeks of zidovudine even in low-risk settings, whereas others recommend 4 weeks when risk is low. UK BHIVA Guidelines are available at http://www.bhiva.org/.[107]

17.6.1.2 Labour ward-based initiation of antiretrovirals

A Cochrane systematic review of studies integrating prevention of MTCT programmes with other HIV health services in developing countries[108] found only one eligible study. A cluster-randomized trial in Zambia (12 clusters, $n = 7664$) compared mother–infant nevirapine coverage in the labour ward between intervention clinics implementing rapid HIV testing with

Table 17.1 Current recommended regimen for prophylactic antiretrovirals (Western setting).

Low risk (no detectable maternal virus load at delivery):
• Zidovudine (AZT) syrup 4 mg/kg/dose orally, 12 hourly × 4 weeks
High risk (maternal virus detectable at delivery):
• Nevirapine syrup 2 mg/kg single dose orally at 48–72 hours old and
• Lamivudine (3TC) syrup 2 mg/kg/dose orally, 12 hourly × 6 weeks and
• Zidovudine (AZT) syrup 4 mg/kg/dose orally, 12 hourly × 6 weeks
Pre-term babies (if can tolerate oral):
>30 weeks of gestation at birth:
• Zidovudine (AZT) syrup: 2 mg/kg/dose orally, 12 hourly
Increase to 2 mg/kg/dose orally, 8 hourly at 2 weeks of age and continue until 4–6 weeks of age
<30 weeks of gestation at birth:
• Zidovudine (AZT) syrup: 2 mg/kg/dose orally, 12 hourly
Increase to 2 mg/kg/dose orally, 8 hourly at 4 weeks of age and continue until 6 weeks of age
There is no dose adjustment of lamivudine (3TC) or nevirapine for pre-term infants
Intravenous therapy (if baby unable to take orally):
Zidovudine (ZDV) is the only IV antiretroviral available. Change to the oral dosage as soon as can tolerate oral feeds
>34 weeks of gestation at birth:
• Zidovudine (ZDV) IV: 1.5 mg/kg/dose IV, 6 hourly
30–34 weeks of gestation at birth:
• Zidovudine (ZDV) IV: 1.5 mg/kg/dose IV, 12 hourly
Increase to 1.5 mg/kg/dose IV, 8 hourly at 2 weeks of age
<30 weeks of gestation at birth:
• Zidovudine (ZDV) IV: 1.5 mg/kg/dose IV, 12 hourly
Increase to 1.5 mg/kg/dose IV, 8 hourly at 4 weeks of age

structured nevirapine assessment and control clinics.[109] Mother–infant nevirapine coverage increased by 10% in the intervention sites and declined by 10% in the control sites, a statistically significant difference.[109]

17.6.1.3 Mobile texting to improve adherence

A Cochrane systematic review of mobile phone text messages, short or long, and adherence found two RCTs, both in Kenya.[110] Meta-analysis found that any weekly text messaging, whether short or long messages, was associated with a lower risk of non-adherence to antiretroviral therapy at 48–52 weeks (RR 0.78, 95% CI 0.68–0.89).

17.6.1.4 Caesarean section

A Cochrane systematic review of caesarean section in MTCT identified 26 potentially relevant studies.[111] Only one RCT compared MTCT according to mode of delivery (caesarean vs. vaginal).[112] Seven (3.4%) of 203 infants delivered by caesarean section were infected compared with 15 (10.2%) of 167 born vaginally ($p = 0.009$).[112] Zidovudine prophylaxis was given to a minority of women in both arms; none received HAART. Caesarean section reduced transmission for women who did not receive zidovudine by 80% (OR 0.2, 95% CI 0–0.8). For women who received zidovudine in pregnancy, the point estimate of efficacy was the same but the reduction was not statistically significant (OR 0.2, 95% CI 0–1.7).[112] For a woman with undetectable viral load it is debatable whether the risks of caesarean section outweigh the benefits.[111, 112]

17.6.1.5 Vaginal disinfection

A Cochrane systematic review of vaginal disinfection to prevent MTCT found two eligible trials (708 patients).

The meta-analysis showed no significant effect of vaginal disinfection on the risk of MTCT, neonatal death or post-neonatal death.[113]

17.6.1.6 Male circumcision

A Cochrane systematic review of male circumcision to prevent heterosexual acquisition of HIV found three RCTS, all in Africa (South Africa, Kenya and Uganda), involving over 10 000 males.[114] All three trials were stopped early because of positive interim analyses. A meta-analysis showed the risk of acquiring HIV in this setting was halved by circumcision (incidence RR 0.5, 95% CI 0.34–0.72 at 12 months and 0.46, 95% CI 0.34–0.62 at 24 months). The risks and benefits of circumcision need to be considered in different settings and the relative merits of other interventions such as promoting condom use.

17.6.2 Diagnosis of HIV infection

Nucleic acid amplification tests using PCR to detect HIV DNA or RNA are the diagnostic modality of choice with a high sensitivity and specificity.[115, 116] The sensitivity is <100% at birth, but by 3 months of age either DNA or RNA PCR has 100% sensitivity and specificity, that is all cases are diagnosed without any false positives.[116]

PCR tests are comparatively expensive and complex tests. In a non-Cochrane review, HIV p24 antigen detection had a sensitivity of 98.8% and specificity of 100% at 6 weeks of age.[117] This test may be useful in resource-poor settings if PCR is unavailable.

17.7 Parvovirus B19

Parvovirus B19 causes a common viral illness associated with rash and fever and sometimes arthralgia or arthritis, which has been given the names slapped cheek disease, fifth disease (it was one of six exanthems described in the nineteenth century) or the uninspiring erythema infectiosum. The importance in neonatology is that acute parvovirus B19 infection causes temporary suppression of erythropoiesis. While this causes the haemoglobin of a normal host to drop by only about 1 g/dL (10 g/L) the neonate has a red cell life span of 40 days compared with 120 days for an adult. Maternal parvovirus B19 infection in pregnancy can infect the foetus, causing severe anaemia and non-immune hydrops. In a Danish study 66% of pregnant women were parvovirus B19 IgG seropositive at screening and the rate of primary maternal infection in pregnancy was 1% between epidemics and 13.5% during an epidemic.[118] Parvovirus B19 IgM seropositivity was associated with an increased risk of late spontaneous abortions and stillbirths (crude OR 9.9; 95% CI 3.3–29.4).[118] However, a Norwegian study found none of 281 foetal deaths were due to parvovirus B19 infection.[119]

If maternal infection is diagnosed early and the foetus is diagnosed as hydropic by ultrasound, intrauterine transfusion is an option, although not without risk. Three (11%) of 28 children who received intrauterine transfusion for this indication developed severe developmental delay; one also had cerebral palsy.[120]

Some reports suggest parvovirus intrauterine B19 infection might result in birth defects. Diverse CNS abnormalities have been described but no consistent syndrome and true embryopathy is unlikely.[121]

17.8 Respiratory viral infections

Neonatal respiratory viral infections can cause significant morbidity.[122] Most infections are community acquired. Nursery infections can be acquired from family or staff. Neonatal infections with influenza, rhinovirus and respiratory syncytial virus (RSV) are clinically indistinguishable. Common symptoms and signs include apnoea or tachypnoea, respiratory distress, feeding difficulties and increased oxygen and/or ventilatory requirements.

Prevention is through improved infection control and hygiene. A Cochrane systematic review of interventions to reduce spread of respiratory virus infections included 67 studies of variable quality.[123] The highest quality cluster-RCTs suggest respiratory virus spread can be prevented by hygienic measures such as hand-washing.

17.8.1 Respiratory syncytial virus infection

A Cochrane systematic review of 12 RCTs found that nebulized ribavirin offers only marginal benefits compared with placebo.[124] Three small trials on ventilated patients suggest ribavirin may reduce duration of ventilation by 1.8 days but does not reduce mortality significantly.[124] These benefits need to be weighed against concerns about teratogenicity in pregnant staff.[125] There have been no new RCTs since this analysis and the Cochrane systematic review has been withdrawn.

The monoclonal antibody palivizumab has been widely promoted as prophylaxis against RSV infection in neonates with chronic lung disease and congenital heart disease. Palivizumab reduces the incidence of hospital admission due to RSV by around 50%. However, the incidence of hospital admission is low, even for high-risk infants. Prophylactic palivizumab has to be given IM monthly for 5 months to 17 pre-term children to prevent one hospital admission with RSV and to 59 children to prevent one intensive care admission.[126] It is expensive and high-quality cost-effectiveness analyses have consistently failed to show palivizumab is cost-effective for any subgroup with sufficient confidence to recommend public funding.[126] Money spent on palivizumab is an opportunity cost which could be spent better on more cost-effective health-care interventions.[126]

17.8.2 Influenza

Influenza virus infection is usually relatively mild in the neonatal period. A fatal case of neonatal influenza infection was reported in 1973,[127] but none since. In nursery outbreaks most infants are only mildly affected. Some neonates were infected with pandemic H1N1 influenza virus in 2009–2010. Fever and cough were common and some pre-term infants required supplemental oxygen or extra ventilatory support, but none died.[128, 129] The risks and benefits of oseltamivir, used in one unit to treat 4 infected infants and 13 neonatal contacts, are unknown.[128]

Influenza should be prevented whenever possible by infection control measures, by immunizing staff and by maternal influenza immunization (see Section 23.5.1.1).

Useful Websites

HIV:

http://aidsinfo.nih.gov/ NIH AIDS information
http://www.bhiva.org/ British HIV Association
http://www.who.int/hiv/topics/paediatric (World Health Organization)

References

1. Pignatelli S, Dal Monte P. Epidemiology of human cytomegalovirus strains through comparison of methodological approaches to explore gN variants. *New Microbiol* 2009; 32:1–10.
2. Cannon MJ, Schmid DS, Hyde TB. Review of cytomegalovirus seroprevalence and demographic characteristics associated with infection. *Rev Med Virol* 2010; 20:202–213.
3. Kurath S, Halwachs-Baumann G, Müller W, Resch B. Transmission of cytomegalovirus via breast milk to the prematurely born infant: a systematic review. *Clin Microbiol Infect* 2010; 16:1172–1178.
4. Cannon MJ, Hyde TB, Schmid DS. Review of cytomegalovirus shedding in bodily fluids and relevance to congenital cytomegalovirus infection. *Rev Med Virol* 2011; 21:240–255.
5. Hyde TB, Schmid DS, Cannon MJ. Cytomegalovirus seroconversion rates and risk factors: implications for congenital CMV. *Rev Med Virol* 2010; 20:311–326.
6. Manicklal S, Emery VC, Lazzarotto T, Boppana SB, Gupta RK. The "silent" global burden of congenital cytomegalovirus. *Clin Microbiol Rev* 2013; 26:86–102.
7. Iwasenko J, Basha J, Robertson P, Craig M, Rawlinson WD. CMV seropositivity is associated with socioeconomic status in pregnant women but not in children in Australia. *J Paediatr Child Health* 2013; 49:In press.
8. Pass RF, Fowler KB, Boppana SB, Britt WJ, Stagno S. Congenital cytomegalovirus infection following first trimester maternal infection: symptoms at birth and outcome. *J Clin Virol* 2006; 35:216–220.
9. Jones CA, Isaacs D. Predicting the outcome of symptomatic congenital cytomegalovirus infection. *J Paediatr Child Health* 1995; 31:70–71.
10. Britt W. Cytomegalovirus. In: *Infectious Diseases of the Fetus and Newborn Infant*, 7th edn (eds JS Remington, JO Klein, CB Wilson, V Nizet, Y Maldonado). Philadelphia: Elsevier, 2011. pp. 706–755.
11. Walter S, Atkinson C, Sharland M, et al. Congenital cytomegalovirus: association between dried blood spot viral load and hearing loss. *Arch Dis Child Fetal Neonatal Ed* 2008; 93:F280–F285.
12. Grosse SD, Ross DS, Dollard SC. Congenital cytomegalovirus (CMV) infection as a cause of permanent bilateral hearing loss: a quantitative assessment. *J Clin Virol* 2008; 41:57–62.
13. Yamamoto AY, Mussi-Pinhata MM, Isaac M de L, et al. Congenital cytomegalovirus infection as a cause of sensorineural hearing loss in a highly immune population. *Pediatr Infect Dis J* 2011; 30:1043–1046.
14. de Vries JJ, Vossen AC, Kroes AC, van der Zeijst BA. Implementing neonatal screening for congenital cytomegalovirus: addressing the deafness of policy makers. *Rev Med Virol* 2011; 21:54–61.
15. Alarcón Allen A, Baquero-Artigao F; Grupo de estudio de la infección por citomegalovirus de la Sociedad

Española de Infectología Pediátrica. [Review and guidelines on the prevention, diagnosis and treatment of postnatal cytomegalovirus infection]. [Article in Spanish]. *An Pediatr (Barc)* 2011; 74:52.e1–52.e13.
16. Ozkan TB, Mistik R, Dikici B, Nazlioglu HO. Antiviral therapy in neonatal cholestatic cytomegalovirus hepatitis. *BMC Gastroenterol* 2007; 7:9.
17. Hasosah MY, Kutbi SY, Al-Amri AW, et al. Perinatal cytomegalovirus hepatitis in Saudi infants: a case series. *Saudi J Gastroenterol* 2012; 18:208–213.
18. Ballard RA, Drew WL, Hufnagle KG, Riedel PA. Acquired cytomegalovirus infection in preterm infants. *Am J Dis Child* 1979; 133:482–485.
19. Yeager AS, Grumet FC, Hafleigh EB, Arvin AM, Bradley JS, Prober CG. Prevention of transfusion-acquired cytomegalovirus infections in newborn infants. *J Pediatr* 1981; 98:281–287.
20. Gilbert GL, Hayes K, Hudson IL, James J. Prevention of transfusion-acquired cytomegalovirus infection in infants by blood filtration to remove leucocytes. Neonatal Cytomegalovirus Infection Study Group. *Lancet* 1989; 1:1228–1231.
21. Yeager AS, Palumbo PE, Malachowski N, Ariagno RL, Stevenson DK. Sequelae of maternally derived cytomegalovirus infections in premature infants. *J Pediatr* 1983; 102:918–922.
22. Kadambari S, Williams EJ, Luck S, Griffiths PD, Sharland M. Evidence based management guidelines for the detection and treatment of congenital CMV. *Early Hum Dev* 2011; 87:723–728.
23. Kimberlin DW, Lin CY, Sánchez PJ, et al.; National Institute of Allergy and Infectious Diseases Collaborative Antiviral Study Group. Effect of ganciclovir therapy on hearing in symptomatic congenital cytomegalovirus disease involving the central nervous system: a randomized, controlled trial. *J Pediatr* 2003; 143:16–25.
24. Oliver SE, Cloud GA, Sánchez PJ, et al.; National Institute of Allergy, Infectious Diseases Collaborative Antiviral Study Group. Neurodevelopmental outcomes following ganciclovir therapy in symptomatic congenital cytomegalovirus infections involving the central nervous system. *J Clin Virol* 2009; 46(Suppl 4):S22–S26.
25. Amir J, Wolf DG, Levy I. Treatment of symptomatic congenital cytomegalovirus infection with intravenous ganciclovir followed by long-term oral valganciclovir. *Eur J Pediatr* 2010; 169:1061–1067.
26. Marshall BC, Koch WC. Antivirals for cytomegalovirus infection in neonates and infants: focus on pharmacokinetics, formulations, dosing, and adverse events. *Paediatr Drugs* 2009; 11:309–321.
27. McCarthy FP, Giles ML, Rowlands S, Purcell KJ, Jones CA. Antenatal interventions for preventing the transmission of cytomegalovirus (CMV) from the mother to fetus during pregnancy and adverse outcomes in the congenitally infected infant. *Cochrane Database Syst Rev* 2011; Issue 3. Art. No.: CD008371. doi: 10.1002/14651858.CD008371.pub2
28. Nigro G, Adler SP, La Torre R, Best AM; Congenital Cytomegalovirus Collaborating Group. Passive immunization during pregnancy for congenital cytomegalovirus infection. *N Engl J Med* 2005; 29:1350–1362.
29. Pass RF, Zhang C, Evans A, et al. Vaccine prevention of maternal cytomegalovirus infection. *N Engl J Med* 2009; 360:1191–1199.
30. Picone O, Vauloup-Fellous C, Cordier AG, et al. A 2-year study on cytomegalovirus infection during pregnancy in a French hospital. *Br J Obstet Gynaecol* 2009; 116:818–823.
31. Dworsky ME, Welch K, Cassady G, Stagno S. Occupational risk for primary cytomegalovirus infection among pediatric health-care workers. *N Engl J Med* 1983; 309:950–953.
32. Hyde TB, Schmid DS, Cannon MJ. Cytomegalovirus seroconversion rates and risk factors: implications for congenital CMV. *Rev Med Virol* 2010; 20:311–326.
33. Brown EL, Gardella C, Malm G, et al. Effect of maternal herpes simplex virus (HSV) serostatus and HSV type on risk of neonatal herpes. *Acta Obstet Gynecol Scand* 2007; 86:523–529.
34. Nicoll MP, Proença JT, Efstathiou S. The molecular basis of herpes simplex virus latency. *FEMS Microbiology Rev* 2012; 36:684–705.
35. Marquez L, Levy ML, Munoz FM, Palazzi DL. A report of three cases and review of intrauterine herpes simplex virus infection. *Pediatr Infect Dis J* 2011; 30:153–157.
36. Brown ZA, Benedetti J, Ashley R, et al. Neonatal herpes simplex virus infection in relation to asymptomatic maternal infection at the time of labor. *N Engl J Med* 1991; 324:1247–1252.
37. Brown ZA, Wald A, Morrow RA, Selke S, Zeh J, Corey L. Effect of serologic status and cesarean delivery on transmission rates of herpes simplex virus from mother to infant. *JAMA* 2003; 289:203–209.
38. Flagg EW, Weinstock H. Incidence of neonatal herpes simplex virus infections in the United States, 2006. *Pediatrics* 2011; 127:e1–e8.
39. Kropp RY, Wong T, Cormier L, et al. Neonatal herpes simplex virus infections in Canada: results of a 3-year national prospective study. *Pediatrics* 2006; 117:1955–1962.
40. Roberts S. Herpes simplex virus: incidence of neonatal herpes simplex virus, maternal screening, management during pregnancy, and HIV. *Curr Opin Obstet Gynecol* 2009; 21:124–130.
41. Janka GE. Familial and acquired hemophagocytic lymphohistiocytosis. *Annu Rev Med* 2012; 63:233–246.
42. Hubbell C, Dominguez R, Kohl S. Neonatal herpes simplex pneumonitis. *Rev Infect Dis* 1988; 10:431–438.
43. Corey L, Whitley RJ, Stone EF, Mohan K. Difference between herpes simplex virus type 1 and type 2 neonatal encephalitis in neurological outcome. *Lancet* 1988; 1:1–4.
44. Toth C, Harder S, Yager J. Neonatal herpes encephalitis: a case series and review of clinical presentation. *Can J Neurol Sci* 2003; 30:36–40.
45. Kimberlin DW, Lakeman FD, Arvin AM, et al.; National Institute of Allergy and Infectious Diseases Collaborative

Antiviral Study Group. Application of the polymerase chain reaction to the diagnosis and management of neonatal herpes simplex virus disease. *J Infect Dis* 1996; 174:1162–1167.
46. Kimberlin D. Herpes simplex virus, meningitis and encephalitis in neonates. *Herpes* 2004; 11(Suppl 2):65A–76A.
47. Jones CA, Walker KS, Badawi N. Antiviral agents for treatment of herpes simplex virus infection in neonates. *Cochrane Database Syst Rev* 2009; Issue 3. Art. No.: CD004206. doi: 10.1002/14651858.CD004206.pub2
48. Whitley RJ, Nahmias MD, Soong S, Galasso GG, Fleming CL, Alford CA. Vidarabine therapy of neonatal herpes simplex virus infection. *Pediatrics* 1980; 66:495–501.
49. Whitley R, Arvin A, Prober C, et al. A controlled trial comparing vidarabine with acyclovir in neonatal herpes simplex virus Infection. *N Engl J Med* 1991; 324:444–449.
50. Kimberlin DW, Whitley RJ, Wan W, et al. Oral acyclovir suppression and neurodevelopment after neonatal herpes. *N Engl J Med* 2011; 365:1284–1292.
51. Thompson C, Whitley R. Neonatal herpes simplex virus infections: where are we now? *Adv Exp Med Biol* 2011; 697:221–230.
52. Kimberlin DW, Lin CY, Jacobs RF, et al. Safety and efficacy of high-dose intravenous acyclovir in the management of neonatal herpes simplex virus infections. *Pediatrics* 2001; 108:230–238.
53. Kimberlin DW, Lin C-Y, Jacobs RF, et al. Natural history of neonatal herpes simplex virus infections in the acyclovir era. *Pediatrics* 2001; 108:223–229.
54. Belshe RB, Leone PA, Bernstein DI, et al.; Herpevac Trial for Women. Efficacy results of a trial of a herpes simplex vaccine. *N Engl J Med* 2012; 366:34–43.
55. Hollier LM, Wendel GD. Third trimester antiviral prophylaxis for preventing maternal genital herpes simplex virus (HSV) recurrences and neonatal infection. *Cochrane Database Syst Rev* 2008; Issue 1. Art. No.: CD004946. doi: 10.1002/14651858.CD004946.pub2
56. Brunell PA, Ross A, Miller LH, et al. Prevention of varicella by zoster immune globulin. *N Engl J Med* 1969; 280:1191–1194.
57. Tebruegge M, Pantazidou A, Curtis N. Towards evidence based medicine for paediatricians. How effective is varicella-zoster immunoglobulin (VZIG) in preventing chickenpox in neonates following perinatal exposure? *Arch Dis Child* 2009; 94:559–561.
58. Fairley CK, Miller E. Varicella-zoster virus epidemiology – a changing scene? *J Infect Dis* 1996; 174(Suppl 3):S314–S319.
59. Lee BW. Review of varicella zoster seroepidemiology in India and Southeast Asia. *Trop Med Int Health* 1998; 3:886–890.
60. Lolekha S, Tanthiphabha W, Sornchai P, et al. Effect of climatic factors and population density on varicella zoster virus epidemiology within a tropical country. *Am J Trop Med Hyg* 2001; 64:131–136.
61. Jones AM, Thomas N, Wilkins EG. Outcome of varicella pneumonitis in immunocompetent adults requiring treatment in a high dependency unit. *J Infect* 2001; 43:135–139.
62. Shrim A, Koren G, Yudin MH, Farine D; Maternal Fetal Medicine Committee. Management of varicella infection (chickenpox) in pregnancy. *J Obstet Gynaecol Can* 2012; 34:287–292.
63. Macartney K, McIntyre P. Vaccines for post-exposure prophylaxis against varicella (chickenpox) in children and adults. *Cochrane Database Syst Rev* 2008; Issue 3. Art. No.: CD001833. doi: 10.1002/14651858.CD001833.pub2
64. Cohen A, Moschopoulos P, Stiehm RE, Koren G. Congenital varicella syndrome: the evidence for secondary prevention with varicella-zoster immune globulin. *CMAJ* 2011; 183:204–208.
65. Paryani SG, Arvin AM. Intrauterine infection with varicella-zoster virus after maternal varicella. *N Engl J Med* 1986; 314:1542–1546.
66. Alkalay AL, Pomerance JJ, Rimoin DL. Fetal varicella syndrome. *J Pediatr* 1987; 111:320–323.
67. Enders G, Miller E, Cradock-Watson J, Bolley I, Ridehalgh M. Consequences of varicella and herpes zoster in pregnancy: prospective study of 1739 cases. *Lancet* 1994; 343:1548–1551.
68. Pastuszak AL, Levy M, Schick B, et al. Outcome after maternal varicella infection in the first 20 weeks of pregnancy. *N Engl J Med* 1994; 330:901–905.
69. Enders G, Miller E. Varicella and herpes zoster in pregnancy and the newborn. In: *Varicella-Zoster Virus: Virology and Clinical Management*, (eds AM Arvin, AA Gershon). Cambridge: Cambridge University Press, 2000. pp. 317–347.
70. Mouly F, Mirlesse V, Meritet J, et al. Prenatal diagnosis of fetal varicella-zoster virus infection with polymerase chain reaction of amniotic fluid in 107 cases. *Am J Obstet Gynecol* 1997; 177:894–898.
71. Meyers JD. Congenital varicella in term infants: risk reconsidered. *J Infect Dis* 1974; 129:215–217.
72. DeNicola LK, Hanshaw JB. Congenital and neonatal varicella. *J Pediatr* 1979; 94:175–176.
73. American Academy of Pediatrics. *The Red Book: 2009 Report of the Committee on Infectious Diseases*, 28th edn. Elk Grove Village, IL: American Academy of Pediatrics, 2009. pp 714–727.
74. Salisbury D, Ramsay M, Noakes K (eds). *Immunisation against Infectious Diseases.* London: Department of Health, 2006. pp. 421–422.
75. NHMRC. *The Australian Immunisation Handbook*, 9th edn. Canberra: Australian Government, 2009. pp. 319–321.
76. Tebruegge M, Pantazidou A, Curtis N. How effective is varicella-zoster immunoglobulin (VZIG) in preventing chickenpox in neonates following perinatal exposure? *Arch Dis Child* 2009; 94:559–561.
77. Miller E, Cradock-Watson JE, Ridehalgh MK. Outcome in newborn babies given anti-varicella-zoster immunoglobulin after perinatal maternal infection with varicella-zoster virus. *Lancet* 1989; 2:371–373.
78. Centers for Disease Control. Managing persons at risk for severe risk varicella. Varicella zoster immune globulin. CDC, 2011. Available at: http://www.cdc.gov/chickenpox/

hcp/persons-risk.html#immune (accessed 2 February 2013).

79. Reynolds L, Struik S, Nadel S. Neonatal varicella: varicella zoster immunoglobulin (VZIG) does not prevent disease. *Arch Dis Child Fetal Neonatal Ed* 1999; 81:F69–F70.
80. Gregg NM. Congenital cataract following German measles in the mother. *Trans Ophthalmol Soc Aust* 1941; 3:35–46 (reproduced as Gregg NM. Congenital cataract following German measles in the mother. *Aust N Z J Ophthalmol* 1991; 19:267–276.)
81. Panagiotopoulos T, Antoniadou I, Valassi-Adam E. Increase in congenital rubella occurrence after immunisation in Greece: retrospective survey and systematic review. *Br Med J* 1999; 319:1462.
82. Lanzieri TM, Parise MS, Siqueira MM, Fortaleza BM, Segatto TC, Prevots DR. Incidence, clinical features and estimated costs of congenital rubella syndrome after a large rubella outbreak in Recife, Brazil, 1999–2000. *Pediatr Infect Dis J* 2004; 23:1116–1122.
83. Jiménez G, Avila-Aguero ML, Morice A, et al. Estimating the burden of congenital rubella syndrome in Costa Rica, 1996–2001. *Pediatr Infect Dis J* 2007; 26:382–386.
84. Dewan P, Gupta P. Burden of congenital rubella syndrome (CRS) in India: a systematic review. *Indian Pediatr* 2012; 49:377–399.
85. Miller E, Cradock-Watson JE, Pollock TM. Consequences of confirmed maternal rubella at successive stages of pregnancy. *Lancet* 1982; 2:781–784.
86. Enders G, Nickerl-Pacher U, Miller E, Cradock-Watson JE. Outcome of confirmed periconceptional maternal rubella. *Lancet* 1988; 1:1445–1447.
87. Plotkin SA, Reef SE, Cooper LZ, Alford Jr CA. Rubella. In: *Infectious Diseases of the Fetus and Newborn Infant*, 7th edn (eds JS Remington, JO Klein, CB Wilson, V Nizet, Y Maldonado). Philadelphia: Elsevier, 2011. pp. 861–898.
88. Miller CL, Miller E, Sequeira PJ, Cradock-Watson JE, Longson M, Wiseberg EC. Effect of selective vaccination on rubella susceptibility and infection in pregnancy. *Br Med J (Clin Res Ed)* 1985; 291:1398–1401.
89. Verboon-Maciolek MA, Krediet TG, Gerards LJ, de Vries LS, Groenendaal F, van Loon AM. Severe neonatal parechovirus infection and similarity with enterovirus infection. *Pediatr Infect Dis J* 2008; 27:241–245.
90. Shoji K, Komuro H, Miyata I, Miyairi I, Saitoh A. Dermatologic manifestations of human parechovirus type 3 infection in neonates and infants. *Pediatr Infect Dis J* 2013; 32:233–236.
91. Modlin JF. Perinatal echovirus infection: insights from a literature review of 61 cases of serious infection and 16 outbreaks in nurseries. *Rev Infect Dis* 1986; 8:918–926.
92. Cherry JD, Krogstad P. Enterovirus and parechovirus infections. In: *Infectious Diseases of the Fetus and Newborn Infant*, 7th edn (eds JS Remington, JO Klein, CB Wilson, V Nizet, Y Maldonado). Philadelphia: Elsevier, 2011. pp. 756–799.
93. Abzug MJ, Levin MJ, Rotbart HA. Profile of enterovirus disease in the first two weeks of life. *Pediatr Infect Dis J* 1993; 12:820–824.
94. Modlin JF. Perinatal echovirus and group B coxsackievirus infections. *Clin Perinatol* 1988; 15:233–246.
95. Freund MW, Kleinveld G, Krediet TG, van Loon AM, Verboon-Maciolek MA. Prognosis for neonates with enterovirus myocarditis. *Arch Dis Child Fetal Neonatal Ed* 2010; 95:F206–F212.
96. Abzug MJ. Prognosis for neonates with enterovirus hepatitis and coagulopathy. *Pediatr Infect Dis J* 2001; 20:758–763.
97. Yun KW, Choi EH, Cheon DS, et al. Enteroviral meningitis without pleocytosis in children. *Arch Dis Child* 2012; 97:874–878.
98. Isaacs D, Dobson SRM, Wilkinson AR, Hope PL, Eglin R, Moxon ER. Conservative management of an echovirus 11 outbreak on a neonatal unit. *Lancet* 1989; 1:543–545.
99. Isaacs D, Wilkinson A, Hope P, Moxon R, Dobson S. Handling echovirus 11 outbreaks. *Lancet* 1989; 1:1337.
100. WHO. Treatment of children living with HIV. Available at: http://www.who.int/hiv/topics/paediatric/en/index.html (accessed 2 February 2013).
101. Brocklehurst P. Interventions for reducing the risk of mother-to-child transmission of HIV infection. *Cochrane Database Syst Rev* 2002; Issue 1. Art. No.: CD000102. doi: 10.1002/14651858.CD000102
102. Siegfried N, van der Merwe L, Brocklehurst P, Sint TT. Antiretrovirals for reducing the risk of mother-to-child transmission of HIV infection. *Cochrane Database Syst Rev* 2011; Issue 7. Art. No.: CD003510. doi: 10.1002/14651858.CD003510.pub3
103. Poirier MC, Divi RL, Al-Harthi L, et al. Long-term mitochondrial toxicity in HIV-uninfected infants born to HIV-infected mothers. *Acquir Immune Defic Syndr* 2003; 33:175–183.
104. Thorne C, Newell ML. Safety of agents used to prevent mother-to-child transmission of HIV: is there any cause for concern? *Drug Saf* 2007; 30:203–213.
105. Hernàndez S, Morén C, López M, et al. Perinatal outcomes, mitochondrial toxicity and apoptosis in HIV-treated pregnant women and in-utero-exposed newborn. *AIDS* 2012; 26:419–428.
106. AIDSinfo. Recommendations for use of antiretroviral drugs in pregnant HIV-1-infected women for maternal health and interventions to reduce perinatal HIV transmission in the United States. Available at: http://aidsinfo.nih.gov/guidelines/html/3/perinatal-guidelines/187/ (accessed 2 February 2013).
107. BHIVA. Guidelines for the management of HIV infection in pregnant women 2012. British HIV Association. Available at: http://www.bhiva.org/PregnantWomen2012.aspx (accessed 2 February 2013).
108. Tudor Car L, van-Velthoven MHMMT, Brusamento S, et al. Integrating prevention of mother-to-child HIV transmission (PMTCT) programmes with other health services for preventing HIV infection and improving HIV outcomes in developing countries. *Cochrane Database Syst Rev* 2011; Issue 6. Art. No.: CD008741. doi: 10.1002/14651858.CD008741.pub2

109. Megazzini K. A cluster-randomised trial of enhanced labor ward-based PMTCT services to increase nevirapine coverage in Lusaka, Zambia. *AIDS* 2010; 24:447–455.
110. Horvath T, Azman H, Kennedy GE, Rutherford GW. Mobile phone text messaging for promoting adherence to antiretroviral therapy in patients with HIV infection. *Cochrane Database Syst Rev* 2012; Issue 3. Art. No.: CD009756. doi: 10.1002/14651858.CD009756
111. Read JS, Newell ML. Efficacy and safety of cesarean delivery for prevention of mother-to-child transmission of HIV-1. *Cochrane Database Syst Rev* 2005; Issue 4. Art. No.: CD005479. doi: 10.1002/14651858.CD005479
112. The European Mode of Delivery Collaboration. Elective caesarean-section versus vaginal delivery in prevention of vertical transmission: a randomised clinical trial. *Lancet* 1999; 353:1035–1039.
113. Wiysonge CS, Shey M, Shang J, Sterne JAC, Brocklehurst P. Vaginal disinfection for preventing mother-to-child transmission of HIV infection. *Cochrane Database Syst Rev* 2005; Issue 4. Art. No.: CD003651. doi: 10.1002/14651858.CD003651.pub2
114. Siegfried N, Muller M, Deeks JJ, Volmink J. Male circumcision for prevention of heterosexual acquisition of HIV in men. *Cochrane Database Syst Rev* 2009; Issue 2. Art. No.: CD003362. doi: 10.1002/14651858.CD003362.pub2
115. Owens DK, Holodniy M, McDonald TW, Scott J, Sonnad S. A meta-analytic evaluation of the polymerase chain reaction for the diagnosis of HIV infection in infants. *JAMA* 1996; 275:1342–1348.
116. Burgard M, Blanche S, Jasseron C, et al. Performance of HIV-1 DNA or HIV-1 RNA tests for early diagnosis of perinatal HIV-1 infection during anti-retroviral prophylaxis. *J Pediatr* 2012; 160:60–66.
117. Wessman MJ, Theilgaard Z, Katzenstein TL. Determination of HIV status of infants born to HIV-infected mothers: a review of the diagnostic methods with special focus on the applicability of p24 antigen testing in developing countries. *Scand J Infect Dis* 2012; 44:209–215.
118. Jensen IP, Thorsen P, Jeune B, Møller BR, Vestergaard BF. An epidemic of parvovirus B19 in a population of 3,596 pregnant women: a study of sociodemographic and medical risk factors. *BJOG* 2000; 107:637–643.
119. Sarfraz AA, Samuelsen SO, Bruu AL, Jenum PA, Eskild A. Maternal human parvovirus B19 infection and the risk of fetal death and low birthweight: a case-control study within 35 940 pregnant women. *BJOG* 2009; 116:1492–1498.
120. De Jong EP, Lindenburg IT, van Klink JM, et al. Intrauterine transfusion for parvovirus B19 infection: long-term neurodevelopmental outcome. *Am J Obstet Gynecol* 2012; 206:204.e1–204.e5.
121. Adler SP, Koch WC. Human parvoviruses. In: *Infectious Diseases of the Fetus and Newborn Infant*, 7th edn (eds JS Remington, JO Klein, CB Wilson, V Nizet, Y Maldonado). Philadelphia: Elsevier, 2011. pp. 834–860.
122. Gunville CF, Sontag MK, Stratton KA, Ranade DJ, Abman SH, Mourani PM. Scope and impact of early and late preterm infants admitted to the PICU with respiratory illness. *J Pediatr* 2010; 157:209–214.e1.
123. Jefferson T, Del Mar CB, Dooley L, et al. Physical interventions to interrupt or reduce the spread of respiratory viruses. *Cochrane Database Syst Rev* 2011; Issue 7. Art. No.: CD006207. doi: 10.1002/14651858.CD006207.pub4
124. Ventre K, Randolph A. Ribavirin for respiratory syncytial virus infection of the lower respiratory tract in infants and young children. *Cochrane Database Syst Rev* 2010; Issue 5. Art. No.: CD000181. doi: 10.1002/14651858.CD000181.pub4
125. Isaacs D. Should respiratory care in preterm infants include prophylaxis against respiratory syncytial virus? *Paediatr Respir Rev* 2013; 14:128–129.
126. Isaacs D. *Evidence-Based Pediatric Infectious Diseases.* Oxford: BMJ Books, 2007. pp. 182–185.
127. Joshi VV, Escobar MR, Stewart L, Bates RD. Fatal influenza A2 viral pneumonia in a newborn infant. *Am J Dis Child* 1973; 126:839–840.
128. Leick-Courtois C, Haÿs S, Perpoint T, et al. Influenza A H1N1 in neonatal intensive care unit: analysis and lessons. *Arch Pediatr* 2011; 18:1069–1075.
129. Zenciroglu A, Kundak AA, Aydin M, et al. Swine influenza A (H1N1) virus infection in infants. *Eur J Pediatr* 2011; 170:333–338.

CHAPTER 18

Other congenital infections

18.1 Tuberculosis

18.1.1 Epidemiology of tuberculosis

Tuberculosis (TB) is one of the most ancient and commonest infections in the world. Egyptian mummies over 5000 years old have had Pott's disease of the spine (spinal TB). Over 2 billion people in the world are estimated to have been infected with TB although infection is latent in the vast majority. This illustrates the important difference between **TB infection**, in which the organism is latent or hidden, and symptomatic **TB disease**. In 2010, TB disease affected an estimated 8.8 million people globally and caused 1.4 million deaths, of which 500 000 were women and at least 64 000 children.[1, 2] TB causes 6–15% of all maternal deaths worldwide and results in nearly 10 million cumulative orphans due to parental deaths.[1] TB is predominantly a developing country disease with the highest rates of disease reported in Africa and South East Asia.[2] Childhood and neonatal TB are under-reported but it is estimated that children <15 years old are responsible for about 10% of new TB cases annually.[2]

Neonatal *Mycobacterium tuberculosis* infection generally occurs in areas of high TB prevalence where TB remains the most common non-obstetric cause of death in women of child-bearing age.[3] In settings such as sub-Saharan Africa, HIV co-infection is common.[4, 5]

In Western countries TB incidence rates are generally low and neonatal TB is uncommon, but it remains an important consideration in communities with increased TB exposure.

18.1.2 Microbiology and immunity

Human TB is caused by *M. tuberculosis*, a very slow-growing bacterium both in the laboratory and in humans. The high lipid content of the cell wall explains mycobacteria being resistant to acid and alkali degradation (hence 'acid-fast bacilli' or AFB), but also difficult to kill with antibiotics and resistant to antibodies. Successful organism containment following *M. tuberculosis* infection is primarily through cell-mediated immunity. People at highest risk for severe TB are those with impaired T-cell immunity, such as neonates, infants, HIV-infected persons and those with congenital immune deficiency (e.g. severe combined immune deficiency) or acquired due to immunosuppressive therapy including corticosteroids and cytotoxics.

18.1.3 Clinical

Neonates exposed to an infectious TB source case are at high risk of developing disease, which may be difficult to diagnose and is frequently fatal if diagnosis is delayed or missed. There are two forms of TB in the perinatal period, congenital and neonatal TB.

Congenital TB is already present at birth (congenital means 'from birth'). Congenital TB results from haematogenous transplacental spread, due to disseminated (miliary) disease in the mother or occult dissemination following recent primary infection, often evidenced by a pleural effusion. Maternal disease can also be confined to the endometrium (tuberculous endometritis) with local spread to the foetus or with aspiration of infected secretions during delivery.

Neonatal TB results from post-natal exposure of a neonate to an infectious source case, usually an adult with 'open/cavitary' TB who coughs tubercle bacilli into the air. The most common source is the infant's mother, but can be a grandparent, the father, other babies' mothers, visitors to the nursery[6] or a member of the nursery staff.

Evidence-Based Neonatal Infections, First Edition. David Isaacs.

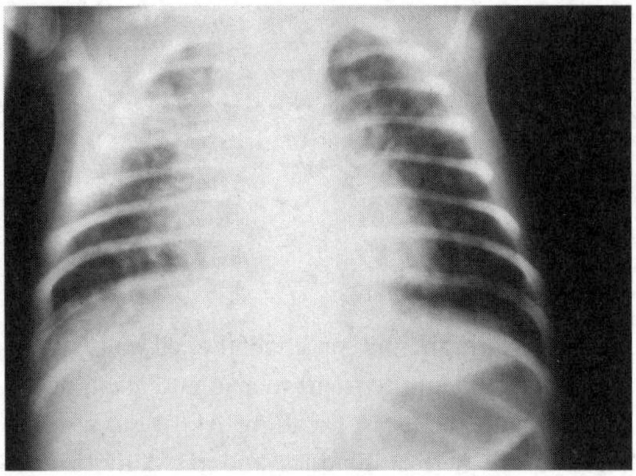

Figure 18.1 Chest radiograph of 3-week-old full-term baby with cough but no fever. Mother had miliary TB. Congenital TB confirmed by gastric aspirate culture.

The clinical manifestations of congenital and neonatal TB are similar, relatively non-specific and include in order of frequency hepatomegaly and/or splenomegaly, respiratory distress, fever, lymphadenopathy, abdominal distension, lethargy or irritability, poor feeding and ear discharge.[7–9] Infants with true congenital TB are usually low birth weight, although symptoms may only present after 1–2 weeks. Those with postpartum exposure may present months later.[10] The chest radiograph is usually abnormal with a miliary or nodular pattern or with hilar lymphadenopathy (Figures 18.1 and 18.2).[7–9]

Unless the mother has overt TB, the diagnosis of perinatal TB is difficult and often delayed. The diagnosis of maternal TB has often been missed during the pregnancy and is only made when the infant presents unwell or if the mother deteriorates after delivery. Infants with signs and symptoms due to TB at birth are usually thought clinically to have a congenital TORCH (toxoplasmosis, rubella, cytomegalovirus, herpes and other) infection (see Chapter 17), congenital syphilis (Section 18.3) or possibly hemophagocytic lymphohistiocytoysis (HLH)[11] (Section 18.4). Infants presenting in the second or third week of life are usually suspected initially as having late-onset bacterial infection.

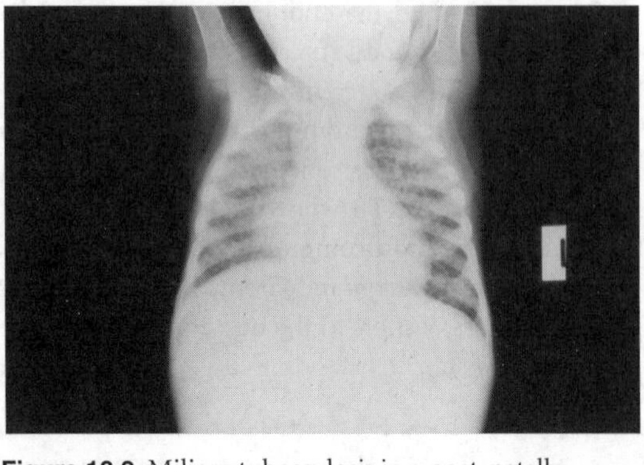

Figure 18.2 Miliary tuberculosis in a post-natally exposed infant.

Neonatal TB meningitis is mercifully rare, except in neonates with disseminated disease, but usually devastating. Lumbar puncture should be performed in newborns with proven or suspected disseminated TB disease.

18.1.4 Diagnosis

The diagnosis of perinatal tuberculosis is usually based on clinical grounds supported by chest radiology. It should be confirmed if possible by accredited laboratory tests including histopathology and/or microbiology testing. A chest radiograph should be performed in all infants with possible TB. Tuberculin skin testing and interferon-gamma release assays may be performed after an interval, but are often negative in neonatal infection, so are only helpful if positive. Respiratory secretions and gastric aspirates should be cultured for *M. tuberculosis* and tested by a polymerase chain reaction (PCR) test (such as Gene X-pert) if available. TB cultures and PCR can also be performed on CSF, pleural or ascitic fluid and blood. The placenta should be examined histopathologically and culture and PCR for *M. tuberculosis* performed. The CSF appearance of TB meningitis is of a lymphocytic pleocytosis with a high CSF protein, often >1 g/L (10 g/dL).[12] The main differential diagnosis of this CSF finding is congenital toxoplasmosis (Section 18.2).

Accredited laboratory tests do not include antibody tests. Serologic antibody testing for *M. tuberculosis* is widely practiced in the private sector in India, at an estimated cost of US $15 million annually, despite strong evidence that serologic tests are unreliable[13] and despite strong recommendations that they should not be used for diagnosis.[14]

18.1.5 Treatment

Treatment often needs to be started empirically prior to laboratory confirmation if there is a strong history of exposure to an infectious source and a typical clinical picture.

Infants from areas with a low prevalence of isoniazid resistance can be treated with three drugs (rifampin also called rifampicin in Europe, isoniazid and pyrazinamide) for 2 months, followed by rifampin/rifampicin plus isoniazid for a further 4 months if there is a good clinical response and/or the source or infant's organism is fully drug susceptible.[15, 16] Infants with extensive infection and infants from areas with a high prevalence of isoniazid resistance should receive a fourth drug (ethambutol) during the 2-month intensive phase of treatment.[9, 10] Despite past concerns about retinal toxicity, the WHO advises that ethambutol is safe in children of all ages.[15, 16]

The recommended doses[16] are as follows:

Isoniazid	10 mg/kg once daily orally (range 7–15 mg/kg)
Rifampin (rifampicin)	15 mg/kg once daily orally (range 10–20 mg/kg)
Pyrazinamide	35 mg/kg once daily orally (range 30–40 mg/kg)
Ethambutol	20 mg/kg once daily orally (range 15–25 mg/kg)

The recommendations for treatment of multiresistant TB are highly specialized, depending on sensitivities and available medications.[17–20]

The treatment of TB meningitis requires specialized advice, if available. It is usual to use the above four drugs if the organism is unlikely to be multiresistant. Corticosteroids, either dexamethasone or prednisone, have been shown to reduce morbidity and mortality in older children and adults with tuberculous meningitis.[21]

18.1.6 Isolation

Recommendations on isolation of the infant and/or mother and separation of an infected mother from her infant need to be based on the risks and benefits. In contrast to adults or adolescents with open or cavitary pulmonary TB, children with primary TB are not usually infectious because the organism load is so much lower. However, infants with congenital TB often have extensive pulmonary involvement with large numbers of AFB.[22] Transmission from infants with congenital TB to health-care workers has only ever been described once[23] and never to other infants.[23–39] Despite this low risk, it is recommended to isolate an infant with suspected congenital TB until it is known whether or not the infant is positive for AFB and also to isolate the mother and screen all relatives or visitors for signs and symptoms suggestive of TB. Infection control precautions and screening of exposed infants and staff should be reviewed in the light of whether or not infectious cases are identified (Section 18.1.7).

There is no evidence that a mother with suspected pulmonary TB needs separating from her infant, and it seems illogical if the mother is on adequate antituberculous treatment and the baby is also receiving preventive therapy or treatment. Nevertheless such separation is sometimes recommended.[22] Continued breastfeeding and development of the important mother–infant relationship should take priority in a situation where the neonate is under close scrutiny and receiving appropriate treatment.

18.1.7 Nursery exposure

If a member of staff on a neonatal nursery or a parent is diagnosed with sputum smear-positive cavitary pulmonary TB (sometimes loosely called 'open TB'), there is understandable concern about exposure of vulnerable neonates and of other parents and staff. Such nursery exposures almost inevitably provoke a vigorous public health response with widespread tracing and testing of contacts, some of whom will have been exposed weeks or months earlier.[23–39] Extensive epidemiologic investigations are usually recommended.[22, 36] The financial and emotional cost of these investigations is high and should be carefully weighed against the risk of potentially devastating disease. The infectiousness of the source case, the duration and the setting of exposure and the evidence from screening other contacts at higher risk may influence the assessment of risk.[32] Important determinants of transmission risk in neonatal units include ventilation, room size, proximity to the index case, infectiousness of the index case and duration of contact.[39] The key determinant influencing transmission is the duration of time spent in a room with the infectious source case.[40]

Exposed infants are recommended to have a clinical examination, a chest radiograph and consideration of prophylactic isoniazid and BCG vaccine. A tuberculin skin test (TST) is not usually performed immediately because of the delay in TST conversion following primary *M. tuberculosis* infection. It is, therefore, delayed until the infant is 3–4 months old. If the TST is negative at this point and the infant is clinically well and thriving, *M. tuberculosis* infection can be ruled out with a fair amount of certainty, chemoprophylaxis can be stopped and BCG vaccination considered.

Investigations of TB outbreaks are extremely time-consuming and costly and generate great anxiety. Prevention is ideal and screening of all staff for tuberculosis is an essential aspect of such prevention.

18.1.8 BCG immunization

Neonatal BCG vaccine will be considered in Section 23.5.1.

18.2 Toxoplasmosis

Congenital toxoplasmosis is a potentially devastating condition that arguably is preventable and the outcome can be improved if diagnosed and treated early.

18.2.1 Epidemiology

Toxoplasmosis is a zoonosis and the cat is the definitive host. The worldwide incidence of toxoplasmosis and congenital toxoplasmosis varies enormously and is an important determinant of the most appropriate detection, prevention and treatment strategies.[41] Factors affecting the incidence of toxoplasmosis include exposure to cats and particularly cat faeces, undercooked meat and climatic conditions, which affect oocyst maturation in soil.[41]

18.2.2 Microbiology

Toxoplasma gondii is a coccidian parasite. Its main host is the cat where it lives in the intestine. Outside the cat intestine it can exist as an oocyst, in which sporozoites form, as a trophozoite (also called an endozoite or tachyzoite) and as a tissue cyst. It is related to *Cryptosporidium* and *Plasmodium*.

Congenital toxoplasmosis follows primary maternal infection. Women infected with *T. gondii* in the first trimester have a relatively low risk (14%) of congenital toxoplasmosis; 6% of their infants are severely affected and 5% are perinatal deaths or stillbirths. In the second and third trimesters, the risk of congenital toxoplasmosis rises (to 29% and 59%, respectively), but the risk of severe disease falls. In the second trimester 2% of infants are severely affected and 2% are perinatal deaths or stillbirths, while babies infected in the third trimester are usually unaffected or sub-clinically infected and only 6% are mildly affected.[41]

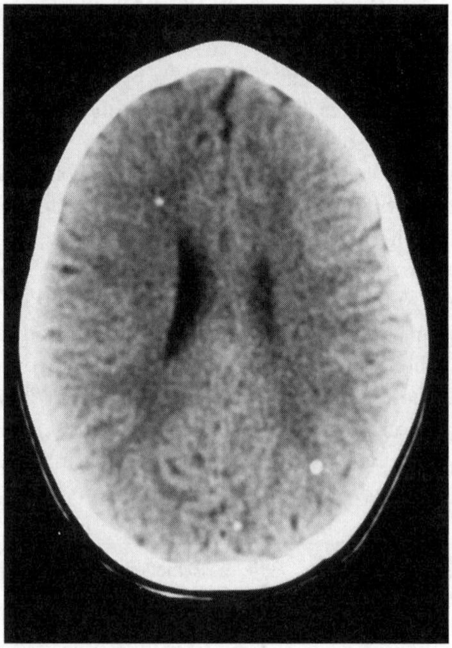

Figure 18.3 Cerebral CT scan showing characteristic punctate calcification of toxoplasmosis and mild ventricular dilatation.

18.2.3 Clinical

The classic triad of congenital toxoplasmosis is hydrocephalus (Figure 18.3), chorioretinitis (Figure 18.4) and brain calcification (Figure 18.3). In a US series of 164 infants with serologically confirmed congenital toxoplasmosis whose mothers had not been treated for the parasite during gestation, from 1991 to 2005, one or more severe clinical manifestations of congenital toxoplasmosis were reported in 84% of the infants. The commonest was eye disease (92.2%), followed by brain calcifications (79.6%) and hydrocephalus (67.7%). In 61.6% of the infants, eye disease, brain calcifications and hydrocephalus were present concurrently.[42] The authors commented that their results contrasted markedly with European investigators who rarely report severe clinical signs in infants with congenital toxoplasmosis.[42]

Other clinical signs and symptoms present in a minority of babies include a blueberry muffin rash

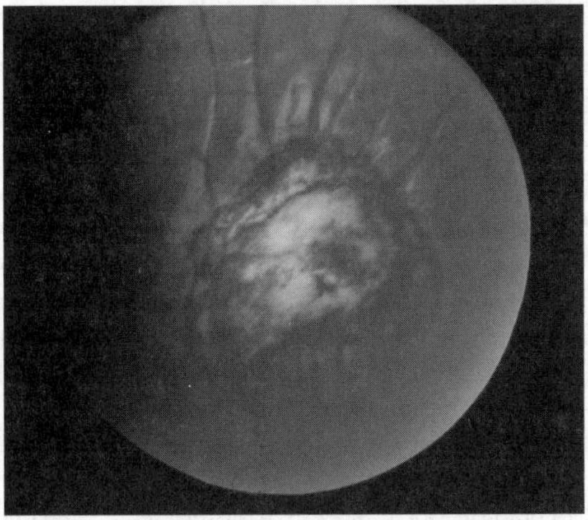

Figure 18.4 Toxoplasma choroidoretinitis showing typical white central area with surrounding pigmentation.

present at birth due to extramedullary haemopoiesis in the skin (Figure 18.5), hepatosplenomegaly and jaundice, all of which may be seen with congenital rubella or congenital CMV infection. Indeed, there have been several case reports of congenital co-infection with *T. gondii* and CMV.[41]

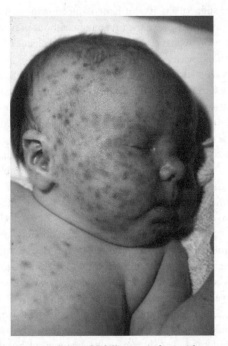

Figure 18.5 One-day-old full-term infant with 'blueberry muffin' appearance, subsequently shown to have congenital toxoplasmosis.

Babies with congenital infection can be asymptomatic at birth. Other presentations include erythroblastosis and hydrops fetalis. Non-specific signs include fever, lymphadenopathy, vomiting, diarrhoea and pneumonitis. Although hydrocephalus is classical, microcephaly is described. The chorioretinitis is a focal necrotizing retinitis, with solitary or multiple yellow or white patches in the fundus with surrounding pigmentation (Figure 18.5). These may be seen at birth if there are other signs or suspicions that lead to a fundoscopic examination. However, it is not uncommon for presentation to be delayed until a few months of age when an infant develops visual signs such as strabismus (Figure 18.4). Rarer eye signs include glaucoma, optic atrophy and microphthalmia.[41, 42]

In addition to the sites already mentioned, toxoplasma can occasionally disseminate and be found in almost any tissue in the body, including ears (deafness), heart (myocarditis), kidney (glomerulonephritis, nephrotic syndrome), adrenals, pancreas and thyroid (patchy necrosis) and skeletal muscle (myositis).[41, 42]

18.2.4 Diagnosis

Clinical examination of the baby with suspected toxoplasmosis should include a full neurologic examination including fundoscopy. Investigations should include lumbar puncture. While CT scan is the radiologic investigation of choice, the radiation exposure has led some clinicians to be more conservative and restrict investigation to skull radiograph and cerebral ultrasound scan.

The definitive laboratory diagnosis of congenital toxoplasmosis is primarily serologic although nucleic acid amplification by PCR on CSF can add valuable confirmatory information. In the large US case series, *T. gondii*-specific IgM, IgA and IgE antibodies were demonstrated in 86.6%, 77.4% and 40.2% of the infants, respectively. Combined testing for both IgM and IgA antibodies increased the diagnostic sensitivity to 93% compared with testing for either IgM or IgA alone. IgM and IgA antibodies were still present in 44% of infants diagnosed between 1 and 6 months of life.[42]

The CSF is abnormal in most infants with congenital toxoplasmosis, classically showing xanthochromia, mononuclear cell pleocytosis and raised CSF protein which, though non-specific, may alert the clinician to request toxoplasma PCR. The CSF protein is often >2 g/L (20 g/dL), higher than in other infections except congenital TB. PCR can also be used to test amniotic fluid for antenatal diagnosis.[35, 37]

18.2.5 Treatment

Authorities recommend 1 year of treatment with anti-parasitic drugs for symptomatic infants with congenital toxoplasmosis. There are no RCTs of duration of treatment of infants with congenital toxoplasmosis.

Remington[41] recommends the following regimen, based on pharmacokinetic data:

- Pyrimethamine: Loading dose of 1 mg/kg 12 hourly for 2 days. From day 3, 1 mg/kg daily for 2–6 months, then 1 mg/kg three times a week to total 1 year.
- Sulfadiazine: 50 mg/kg 12 hourly for 1 year.

Remington also recommends folinic acid 10 mg three times weekly.[41]

There are no data on the adjunctive use of corticosteroids, but prednisone 0.5 mg/kg 12 hourly is sometimes prescribed for infants with CSF protein >10 g/L (1 g/dL) or with vision-threatening chorioretinitis.[41]

Remington[41] recommends treating asymptomatic infants with congenital toxoplasmosis but the risks and benefits of such treatment are unknown.

18.2.6 Prevention

18.2.6.1 Primary prevention: education

Primary prevention consists of educating pregnant women to avoid risk activities such as changing the cat litter and eating undercooked meat.[44] A Cochrane systematic review of RCTs and quasi- RCTs of all types of prenatal education on toxoplasmosis infection during pregnancy[44] found one cluster-RCT (432 women) of poor methodological quality.

18.2.6.2 Secondary prevention: maternal screening and treatment

Maternal toxoplasmosis may be diagnosed if the mother presents with a 'flu-like' illness or by maternal screening. The major problem with the serologic diagnosis of toxoplasmosis is that IgM antibodies can persist for months or even years. For this reason, a single serum sample positive for toxoplasma IgM is difficult to interpret without prior serology. Amniocentesis to perform PCR on amniotic fluid and to test for IgM or IgA antibodies in foetal blood provides a more definitive diagnosis, but is associated with a small but not insignificant risk (up to 1%) of foetal loss.[45]

The rationale for maternal screening for toxoplasmosis is to offer the mother either termination of pregnancy or treatment. In countries where toxoplasmosis is common, maternal screening is often practiced. France began screening for congenital toxoplasmosis in 1978; from 1980 to 1995 the seroconversion rate in non-immune women during pregnancy was 4–5 per 1000.[46] However, there is a significant psychological toll from screening[45] and many women will terminate their pregnancy on the basis of a serologic result of uncertain significance.

Four non-Cochrane systematic reviews[47–50] and one study of case series[51] compared anti-parasitic treatment (spiramycin, pyrimethamine–sulphonamides or both) with no treatment. All four systematic reviews concluded that there are no satisfactory RCTs. The most recent GRADE review concluded that it is not certain whether treating infected pregnant women with spiramycin, pyrimethamine–sulphonamides or both reduces the risk of foetal infection, as the few trials they found produced conflicting results.[47] The authors even suggested that treatment of infection in pregnancy might possibly save the pregnancy without preventing infection, which could increase the prevalence of congenital disease.[47]

A cost-effectiveness analysis based on US data found that screening and treatment of pregnant women was cost-saving for rates of congenital infection above 1 per 10 000 live births, if the parameters in the model were correct.[52] However, since the best evidence cannot confirm that maternal treatment is beneficial, the assumptions in the model are highly questionable, to say the least.

In 2013, Canada made the following recommendations[53]:

(1) Routine universal screening should not be performed for pregnant women at low risk. Serologic screening should be offered only to pregnant women considered to be at risk for primary *T. gondii* infection. (Level of evidence II-3E)

(2) Suspected recent infection in a pregnant woman should be confirmed before intervention by having samples tested at a toxoplasmosis reference laboratory, using tests that are as accurate as possible and correctly interpreted. (II-2B)

(3) If acute infection is suspected, repeat testing should be performed within 2–3 weeks and consideration given to starting therapy with spiramycin immediately, without waiting for the repeat test results. (II-2B)
(4) Amniocentesis should be offered to identify *T. gondii* in the amniotic fluid by PCR (a) if maternal primary infection is diagnosed, (b) if serologic testing cannot confirm or exclude acute infection or (c) in the presence of abnormal ultrasound findings (intracranial calcification, microcephaly, hydrocephalus, ascites, hepatosplenomegaly or severe intrauterine growth restriction). (II-2B)
(5) Amniocentesis should not be offered for the identification of *T. gondii* infection <18 weeks of gestation and should be offered no less than 4 weeks after suspected acute maternal infection to lower the occurrence of false-negative results. (II-2D)
(6) *T. gondii* infection should be suspected and screening should be offered to pregnant women with ultrasound findings consistent with possible TORCH (toxoplasmosis, rubella, cytomegalovirus, herpes and other) infection, including but not limited to intracranial calcification, microcephaly, hydrocephalus, ascites, hepatosplenomegaly or severe intrauterine growth restriction. (II-2B)
(7) Each case involving a pregnant woman suspected of having an acute *T. gondii* infection acquired during gestation should be discussed with an expert in the management of toxoplasmosis. (III-B)
(8) If maternal infection has been confirmed but the foetus is not yet known to be infected, spiramycin should be offered for foetal prophylaxis (to prevent spread of organisms across the placenta from mother to foetus). (I-B)
(9) A combination of pyrimethamine, sulfadiazine and folinic acid should be offered as treatment for women in whom foetal infection has been confirmed or is highly suspected (usually by a positive amniotic fluid PCR). (I-B)
(10) Anti-toxoplasma treatment in immunocompetent pregnant women with previous infection with *T. gondii* should not be necessary. (I-E)
(11) Women who are immunosuppressed or HIV positive should be offered screening because of the risk of reactivation and toxoplasmosis encephalitis. (I-A)
(12) A non-pregnant woman who has been diagnosed with an acute *T. gondii* infection should be counselled to wait 6 months before attempting to become pregnant. Each case should be considered separately in consultation with an expert.

18.2.6.3 Tertiary prevention: infant screening

Tertiary prevention involves serologic screening of all infants for congenital toxoplasmosis. In the absence of high-quality evidence that treatment of any congenital toxoplasmosis is effective, let alone the treatment of asymptomatic congenitally infected infants, it is difficult to justify such a policy. Clearly, we are urgently in need of RCTs to clarify the degree of benefit from treatment, but we may have missed the opportunity. It is unlikely that clinicians and ethics committees would consider it ethical to randomize infants to a placebo arm, although it might be possible to compare two therapies.

18.3 Syphilis

The disease syphilis was first described in the fifteenth century and gets its name from a 1530 poem by Hieronymus Fracastorius about a shepherd called Syphilus.[54] The causative spirochaete organism is called *Treponema pallidum* which resembles a pale, twisted thread. Congenital syphilis was recognized almost as soon as the disease was described.

18.3.1 Epidemiology

Syphilis occurs throughout the world. The widespread introduction of maternal pregnancy screening and treatment led to a marked decline in Western countries. Congenital syphilis increased in the United States in the late 1980s and early 1990s, mainly in urban blacks and Hispanics in association with illicit drug use, particularly crack cocaine.

Syphilis affects the placenta causing a focal villositis and is an important cause of stillbirth and neonatal death globally. A systematic analysis estimated that in 2010, congenital syphilis caused 60 000 deaths in the world (2.1% of the 2 840 157 estimated total neonatal deaths).[55]

18.3.2 Clinical

Congenital syphilis can cause prematurity and intrauterine growth retardation, although infected babies may be born at term of normal weight.

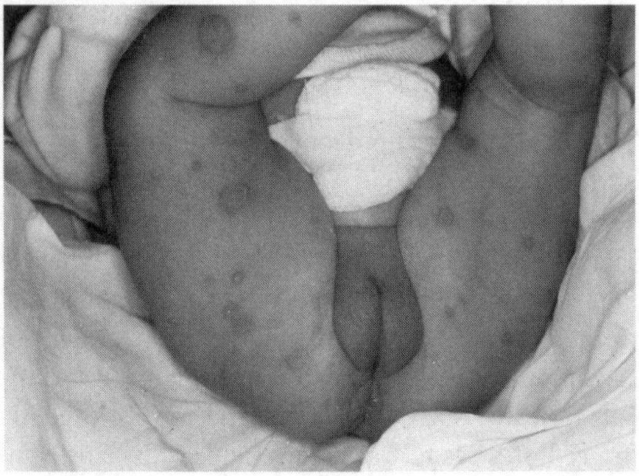

Figure 18.6 Congenital syphilis: vesiculobullous lesions.

The classic rash of congenital syphilis is a macular eruption consisting of pink or copper-coloured oval skin lesions characteristically on the buttocks and trunk (Figure 18.6) and redness of the soles and palms which characteristically desquamates (Figure 18.7). The skin lesions often develop into vesicobullous lesions, often involving the palms and soles, and called pemphigus syphiliticus. The cloudy or blood-stained fluid is full of treponemes, but the bullae readily burst leaving denuded skin that may crust over.[54]

Hepatosplenomegaly is common and often associated with ascites (anasarca). Severely affected infants are often wasted with a pot belly and withered skin and said to resemble little old men.[54]

Generalized painless lymphadenopathy occurs in about half of all babies, usually in association with hepatosplenomegaly. Lymphadenopathy is unusual in the neonatal period, so its presence should raise suspicion of congenital syphilis. Epitrochlear lymphadenopathy is said to be particularly characteristic.[54]

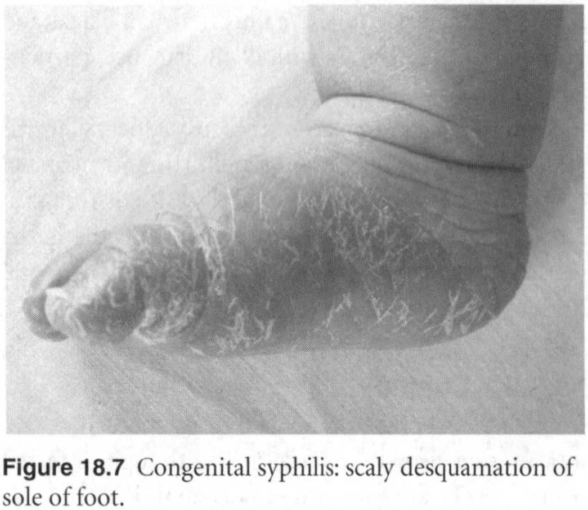

Figure 18.7 Congenital syphilis: scaly desquamation of sole of foot.

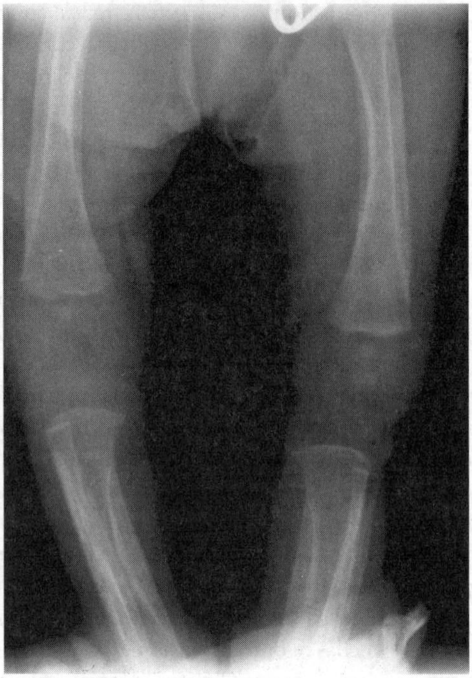

Figure 18.8 Congenital syphilis: extensive bilateral periostitis.

Rhinitis ('snuffles') may develop as early as the second week of life, although usually later, if at all. The mucous discharge is highly infectious. There may be associated laryngitis and a hoarse cry. Mucous patches may be seen in the mouth. Nasal mucosal ulceration can destroy the nasal cartilage and cause a 'saddle nose' deformity.[54]

Bone lesions are common. Osteitis may be present radiologically but will be asymptomatic (Figure 18.8). The osteitis later becomes painful and an infant may refuse to move one limb, a condition called pseudoparalysis of Parrot. The arm is a more common site than the leg and pathological fractures can occur.

Eye involvement is rare but can include a salt-and-pepper retinitis similar to congenital rubella (see Figure 17.10), cataract and glaucoma.[54]

Nephrotic syndrome does not usually present until 2–3 months of age.

Neurosyphilis with leptomeningitis develops in the post-neonatal period and can result in severe neurologic impairment. For this reason it is important to exclude CSF involvement in infants with suspected congenital syphilis.

Babies with congenital syphilis can be asymptomatic at birth, which complicates the frequent clinical situation of a mother treated for syphilis who gives birth to a normal looking baby. One potential problem is that the mother might have been reinfected since being treated.

18.3.3 Diagnosis

The diagnosis of congenital syphilis is not easy. We will consider serology, nucleic acid amplification (PCR) and microscopy.

Maternal IgG antibodies cross the placenta and pass to the infant. The commonly used screening serologic tests, the VDRL (Venereal Disease Research Laboratory) and the RPR (Rapid Plasma Reagin), both measure IgG antibodies and they both detect antibody to cardiolipin. Cardiolipin (previously called reagin, hence Rapid Plasma Reagin) is a membrane lipid and the antibody response in syphilis is non-specific, that is they are non-treponemal antibody tests. False positives can occur in autoimmune conditions such as SLE.

There are a number of confirmatory serologic tests that are specific for *T. pallidum* infection. Most have *Treponema* or *T. pallidum* in the name (e.g. fluorescent treponemal antibody or FTA test; *T. pallidum* particle agglutination or TP-PA). There are also ELISA tests that can detect specific *T. pallidum* IgG and IgM antibodies. Unfortunately IgM tests have shown a low sensitivity of 60–80%, meaning many cases will be missed if IgM is relied upon in isolation, and there are frequent false-positive results, perhaps due to rheumatoid factor which cross-reacts.[54]

When relying on IgG tests, the infant's serologic titre is compared with the mother's. If the infant's titre is substantially higher than the mother's ($\geq$ 4 times), the infant is deemed to be infected. It should be emphasized that the infant's and mother's recent serum need to be tested in parallel, that is on the same laboratory 'run', for this to be a valid approach.

A systematic review of PCR shows a high specificity >95%, but a sensitivity for detecting congenital syphilis of 83% (95% CI 55–95) when used on neonatal blood and of 78% on genital or anal chancres.[56] Therefore, a positive PCR is likely to reflect true infection but a negative PCR does not exclude it.

Dark-field microscopy can confirm congenital syphilis if suitable specimens can be obtained, such as fluid from bullae or nasal discharge, but this is rare.

Because neurosyphilis causes such catastrophic but preventable neurologic impairment it is always recommended to perform a lumbar puncture in the assessment of an infant with possible congenital syphilis. The CSF should be tested by VDRL as well as routine microscopy and chemistry. Some laboratories also test CSF for FTA antibodies which are highly sensitive but less specific, so if negative is useful to rule out CNS involvement. The CSF is often abnormal in infants with symptomatic congenital syphilis (CSF pleocytosis, raised protein, positive CSF VDRL) but rarely abnormal in asymptomatic infants.

In practice, it is often difficult to confirm or exclude the diagnosis of congenital syphilis. The presence of clinical signs when the mother is seropositive is highly suggestive.

18.3.4 Treatment

Infants with proven or probable congenital syphilis should be treated with

- penicillin G 50 000 units/kg IV 12-hourly in the first week of life, 8-hourly thereafter for 10 days.

Procaine penicillin (50 000 units/kg IM once daily) is a painful alternative if IV is not possible for some reason, but the IV regimen is preferable.

If it is uncertain whether or not the infant is infected, we recommend treating the infant empirically if the parents cannot be relied upon to bring the infant for follow-up, which is a common concern. This cautious approach ensures that latent neurologic involvement will not be left untreated. If the infant is asymptomatic and has a titre compatible with transplacental transfer of maternal antibodies (<4 times the maternal titre) and compliance with follow-up is certain, the infant can be followed in clinic. We recommend the full 10-day regimen described above because this treats neurosyphilis effectively. However, the CDC recommends that asymptomatic infants with a normal initial CSF can be treated with a single dose of benzathine penicillin G 50 000 units/kg/dose IM because the risk of neurosyphilis is low.[57]

18.3.5 Prevention: maternal screening in pregnancy

A non-Cochrane systematic review of studies on screening for syphilis in pregnancy[58] found one before and after Chinese study of a universal syphilis screening programme for pregnant women which found a 60% reduction in the rate of congenital syphilis from 54 to 22 cases per 100 000 pregnant women.[59] Two studies on the accuracy of screening for syphilis reported false-positive rates <1%. One study reported an incidence of anaphylaxis after oral penicillin of 1 in 100 000.[58]

Since maternal screening is cheap, safe and effective, the next question is how to improve rates of maternal screening. A non-Cochrane systematic review of different strategies found 10 studies, including two randomized trials, but the effects were variable and could not be combined statistically.[60] However, study interventions were associated with a >50% reduction in perinatal deaths and stillbirths and reduced incidence of congenital syphilis.[60]

Prevention of one case of congenital syphilis costs less than US $1.50 per woman screened.[61]

18.4 Tetanus

Tetanus is caused by a neurotoxin produced by the bacillus *Clostridium tetani. C. tetani* is a spore-forming anaerobic bacillus and is a normal inhabitant of animal intestines and found in soil. Neonatal tetanus results from the contamination of the umbilical cord at delivery, often related to the culturally based applications of substances contaminated with tetanus spores, such as mud or ghee.

The commonest clinical presentation is in the first few days after birth with difficulty feeding and recurrent apnoea.[62, 63] The disease is often called no suck disease because infants are unable to suck due to muscular spasm and they may appear to be smiling (the risus sardonicus), see Figure 18.9. Later the infant has tetanic spasms, often precipitated by sudden loud noises like a door banging and resembling seizures.

Neonatal tetanus is almost completely preventable through tetanus immunization of women of child-bearing age, and tetanus vaccine can be given safely and effectively in pregnancy (see Section 23.5.1.4). Furthermore, even in the absence of maternal tetanus immunization, there is evidence that improved hand-washing around birth can reduce the incidence of neonatal tetanus.[64, 65] However, an estimated 60 000 infants still die each year due to neonatal tetanus.[64] It is unconscionable that we are not able to ensure the equity of health care needed to prevent these horrible and unnecessary deaths.

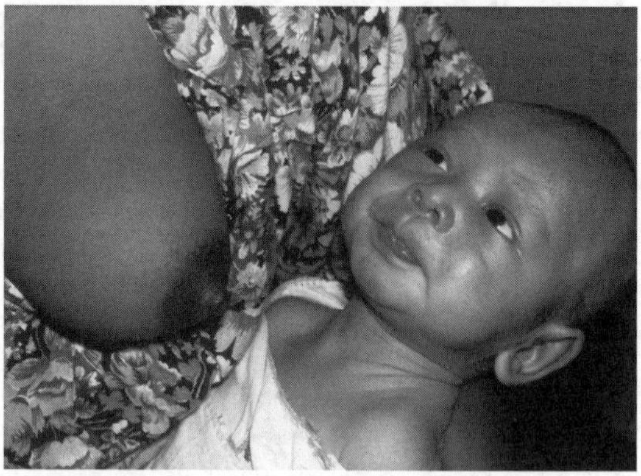

Figure 18.9 Neonatal tetanus ('no suck disease'): 5-day-old infant with risus sardonicus.

18.5 Malaria

There are four species of malarial parasite which affect humans, *Plasmodium falciparum, P. vivax, P. malariae* and *P. ovale. P. falciparum* is the most virulent and predominates in the tropics and throughout Africa. Malaria can be transmitted to the neonate transplacentally, by being bitten by an infected mosquito or by exposure to blood products by blood transfusion. Maternal intravenous drug users may contract malaria from needle-sharing. Placental involvement is common in endemic countries. Intervention studies have shown that strategies to prevent or treat malaria in pregnant women reduce the incidence of low birth weight and reduce neonatal mortality,[66] showing that maternal malaria has a profound effect on foetal growth and survival.

18.5.1 Congenital malaria

Congenital malaria is variably defined as the detection of parasites in the infant's peripheral blood on the first day of life or <7 days of age. Reports of its incidence vary. In a 20-year review of studies from sub-Saharan Africa, five reported that congenital malaria was rare, with prevalence ranging from 0% to 0.7% despite high rates of maternal malaria parasitaemia rates (25–50%).[66] In contrast, nine studies reported a higher prevalence up to 37% and also reported peripheral parasitaemia in 4.0–46.7% of neonates.[66] Babies whose mothers are parasitaemic, particularly if febrile, should be investigated for congenital malaria.[66]

In the United States, 81 cases of congenital malaria were reported over 40 years and 81% were due to *P. vivax*.[67] Most mothers (96%) were born overseas, and 85% were exposed 1 year or less before delivery. Primaquine phosphate was commonly given unnecessarily to infants with congenital *P. vivax* infection.[67] Cases of congenital malaria have also been reported in immigrant mothers in many countries in Europe and Asia, sometimes in association with maternal HIV infection. Usually the mother had had one or more attacks of malaria in pregnancy, although mothers with malaria exposure months or years earlier were occasionally asymptomatic during pregnancy.[68, 69]

Infants with congenital malaria usually present with fever and have anaemia, thrombocytopaenia and splenomegaly.[67–71] Jaundice and hepatomegaly are found in around a third of cases. Infants may have non-specific symptoms including poor feeding, vomiting and diarrhoea. They are sometimes treated empirically for bacterial sepsis and blood films not sent for malaria parasites.[67–71]

Treatment depends on the malarial species. There is scanty safety and efficacy data for any antimalarials in newborns. Chloroquine is the traditional drug of choice for chloroquine-sensitive species infecting babies who can tolerate oral treatment (10 mg/kg of chloroquine base, followed by 5 mg/kg after 6, 24 and 48 hours) and appears safe and effective.[71] For intravenous treatment, quinidine is recommended in the United States (quinidine gluconate 10 mg/kg in normal saline over 1–2 hours, then 0.02 mg/kg/hour infusion until oral therapy tolerated)[71] and quinine in Australia (quinine HCl 20 mg/kg over 4 hours, then starting 4 hours later, 10 mg/kg over 4 hours every 8 hours until oral therapy tolerated).[72] Artemether–lumefantrine was at least as effective as oral quinine and caused fewer adverse events in a randomized trial in pregnant women with *P. falciparum* malaria in Uganda.[73] The current WHO recommendation, to treat uncomplicated falciparum malaria with quinine plus clindamycin in early pregnancy (first trimester) and artemether-based combination therapy in later pregnancy (second and third trimesters), was supported by a systematic review of artemether–lumefantrine in pregnancy.[74] We could find no data on the use of artemether-containing compounds in newborns.

18.5.2 Prevention of malaria in pregnancy

The main interventions to prevent malaria in pregnant women are intermittent antimalarial therapy in pregnancy and insecticide-treated bed nets. A meta-analysis of 32 African national datasets found that full malaria prevention of women in their first or second pregnancy with either of these interventions was associated with an 18% decreased risk of neonatal mortality (95% CI 4–30), compared with newborn babies of mothers with no protection.[6] Malaria prevention in pregnancy also reduced low birth weight by 21% (95% CI 14–27).[66]

18.5.2.1 Antimalarials

A Cochrane systematic review of 16 trials of prophylactic antimalarials (12 638 participants) found that when antimalarials were given to all pregnant women to prevent malaria they reduced antenatal parasitaemia and placental malaria but not perinatal deaths.[75] In women in their first or second pregnancy, antimalarial drugs reduced severe antenatal anaemia and antenatal parasitaemia and reduced perinatal deaths by 27% (RR 0.73, 95% CI 0.53–0.99) and low birth weight by 43% (RR 0.57, 95% CI 0.46–0.72).[75]

A Cochrane systematic review of trials for treating pregnant women with malaria found 10 trials (1805 participants).[76] In general, artemether-containing regimens were less likely to fail.[76]

18.5.2.2 Insecticide-treated bed nets

A Cochrane systematic review of trials of insecticide-treated bed nets identified five eligible RCTs, four from sub-Saharan Africa and one from Asia. In Africa, insecticide-treated bed nets compared with no nets reduced placental malaria in all pregnancies by 21% (RR 0.79, 95% CI 0.63–0.98).[77] They also reduced low birth weight (RR 0.77, 95% CI 0.61–0.98) and foetal loss in the first to fourth pregnancy by 33% (RR 0.67, 95% CI 0.47–0.97), although not in women who had more than four previous pregnancies. One trial in Thailand which randomized individuals to insecticide-treated or untreated nets showed a significant reduction in anaemia and foetal loss in all pregnancies but not for clinical malaria or low birth weight.[77]

18.6 Hemophagocytic lymphohistiocytosis

Hemophagocytic lymphohistiocytosis (HLH) is a disorder of mononuclear cells/phagocytes in which apparently morphologically benign histiocytes proliferate resulting in raised cytokine levels in the blood and uncontrolled T-cell activation. It is rare in neonates, although well described.[78, 79] HLH can be a primary familial genetic condition or can be acquired secondary to infection or other inflammatory conditions such as malignancies and rheumatic diseases.[78, 79]

HLH is a heterogeneous condition. The postulated mechanisms of activation and dysregulation of macrophages and T cells include natural killer cell dysfunction (particularly in association with herpes virus infections) and defects in perforin (which lyses infected cells) and cytotoxic granule exocytosis.[79] There is an animal model of perforin-deficient mice which mimics HLH.

Primary HLH is inherited as an autosomal recessive condition and has an incidence of around 1 in 50 000. Four gene mutations are known to be associated with familial HLH and these gene mutations occur either in the perforin gene or in genes important for the exocytosis of cytotoxic granules. Cytotoxic granules contain perforin and granzymes, which induce apoptosis upon entering (infected) target cells. Additionally, perforin is important for the downregulation of the immune response.[79]

The characteristic clinical presentation of neonatal HLH is with fever, hepatomegaly and/or splenomegaly and cytopoenia of at least two cell lines. Both primary and secondary HLH can present in the neonatal period. In a 10-year Japanese case series of 20 cases, half of them female, hepatomegaly was more common than splenomegaly and fever occurred in 1 of 8 pre-term but 10 of 12 term infants.[79] The overall survival was 40%. Seven of the cases were familial (one associated with severe combined immunodeficiency or SCID) of whom two survived. The rest were secondary to proven or assumed infections, of which the largest number (six) was HSV infection (Chapter 17).

The serum ferritin is characteristically markedly elevated. Hemophagocytosis is often difficult to prove but may be seen in biopsies of bone marrow, lymph nodes (Figure 18.10) or spleen.

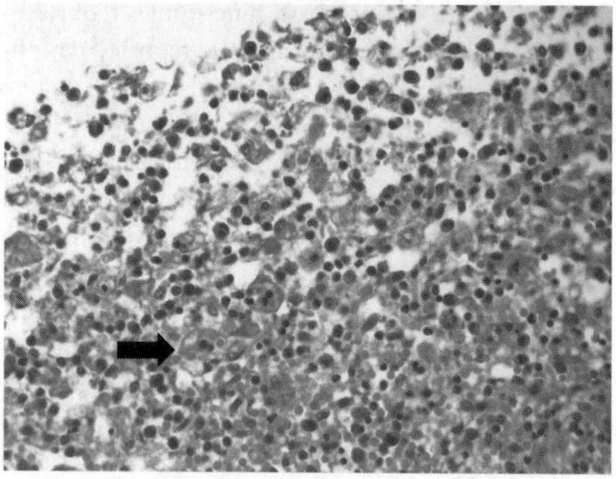

Figure 18.10 Lymph node stained with H&E, showing hemophagocytosis (see arrow).

Some children with HLH and congenital HSV infection respond rapidly to treatment with acyclovir and their HLH resolves without further therapy. More commonly, the HLH needs to be 'switched off' using immunosuppressive or immunomodulatory agents. In the Japanese case series these interventions included corticosteroids, intravenous immunoglobulin, cyclosporine, etoposide and exchange transfusion.[79]

Useful Websites

WHO on tuberculosis http://www.who.int/topics/tuberculosis/en/

References

1. Getahun H, Sculier D, Sismanidis C, Grzemska M, Raviglione M. Prevention, diagnosis, and treatment of tuberculosis in children and mothers: evidence for action for maternal, neonatal, and child health services. *J Infect Dis* 2012; 205 (Suppl 2):S216–S227.
2. Perez-Velez CM, Marais BJ. Tuberculosis in children. *N Engl J Med* 2012; 367:348–361.
3. Marais BJ, Gupta A, Starke JR, El-Sony A. Tuberculosis in women and children. *Lancet* 2010; 375:2057–2059.
4. Mnyani CN, McIntyre JA. Tuberculosis in pregnancy. *BJOG* 2011; 118: 226–231.
5. Bekker A, Du Preez K, Schaaf HS, Cotton MF, Hesseling AC. High tuberculosis exposure among neonates in a high tuberculosis and human immunodeficiency virus burden setting. *Int J Tuberc Lung Dis* 2012; 16:1040–1046.

6. Muñoz FM, Ong LT, Seavy D, Medina D, Correa A, Starke JR. Tuberculosis among adult visitors of children with suspected tuberculosis and employees at a children's hospital. *Infect Control Hosp Epidemiol* 2002; 23:568–572.
7. Cantwell MF, Shehab ZM, Costello AM, et al. Congenital tuberculosis. *N Engl J Med* 1994; 330:1051–1054.
8. Smith KC. Congenital tuberculosis: a rare manifestation of a common infection. *Curr Opin Infect Dis* 2002; 15:269–274.
9. Whittaker E, Kampmann B. Perinatal tuberculosis: new challenges in the diagnosis and treatment of tuberculosis in infants and the newborn. *Early Hum Dev* 2008; 84:795–799.
10. Heyns L, Gie RP, Goussard P, et al. Nosocomial transmission of *M. tuberculosis* in kangaroo mother care units: a risk in tuberculosis endemic areas. *Acta Paediatr* 2006; 95:535–539.
11. Suzuki N, Morimoto A, Ohga S, Kudo K, Ishida Y, Ishii E; HLH/LCH Committee of the Japanese Society of Pediatric Hematology. Characteristics of hemophagocytic lymphohistiocytosis in neonates: a nationwide survey in Japan. *J Pediatr* 2009; 155:235–238.
12. Marais S, Thwaites G, Schoeman J, et al. Tuberculosis meningitis: defining a uniform case definition for use in clinical research. *Lancet Infect Dis* 2010; 10:803–812.
13. Steingart KR, Henry M, Laal S, et al. A systematic review of commercial serological antibody tests for the diagnosis of pulmonary tuberculosis. *Thorax* 2007;62: 911–918.
14. Tuberculosis Coalition for Technical Assistance. *International Standards for Tuberculosis Care (ISTC)*, 2nd edn. The Hague: Tuberculosis Coalition for Technical Assistance, 2009. Available at: http://www.istcweb.org/documents/ISTC_Report_2ndEd_Nov2009.pdf (accessed 2 February 2013).
15. WHO. *Rapid Advice — Treatment of Tuberculosis in Children.* Geneva: World Health Organization, 2010 (WHO/HTM/TB/2010.13).
16. World Health Organization. Essential Medicines for Children. *Tuberculosis Treatment in Children.* Available at: http://www.who.int/topics/tuberculosis/en/ (accessed 2 February 2013).
17. Schaaf HS, Marais BJ. Management of multidrug-resistant tuberculosis in children: a survival guide for paediatricians. *Paediatr Respir Rev* 2011; 12:31–38.
18. Seddon JA, Furin JJ, Gale M, et al; Sentinel Project on Pediatric Drug-Resistant Tuberculosis. Caring for children with drug-resistant tuberculosis: practice-based recommendations. *Am J Respir Crit Care Med* 2012; 186:953–964.
19. Centers for Disease Control and Prevention (CDC). Plan to combat extensively drug-resistant tuberculosis: recommendations of the Federal Tuberculosis Task Force. *MMWR Recomm Rep* 2009; 58(RR-3):1–43.
20. Migliori GB, D'Arcy Richardson M, Sotgiu G, Lange C. Multidrug-resistant and extensively drug-resistant tuberculosis in the West. Europe and United States: epidemiology, surveillance, and control. *Clin Chest Med* 2009; 30:637–665.
21. Prasad K, Singh MB. Corticosteroids for managing tuberculous meningitis. *Cochrane Database Syst Rev* 2008; Issue 1. Art. No.: CD002244. doi:10.1002/14651858.CD002244.pub3
22. American Academy of Pediatrics. Tuberculosis. In: *Red Book: 2009 Report of the Committee on Infectious Diseases*, 28th edn. Elk Grove Village, IL: American Academy of Pediatrics, 2009.
23. Rabalais G, Adams G, Stover B. PPD skin test conversion in health-care workers after exposure to *Mycobacterium tuberculosis* infection in infants. *Lancet* 1991; 338:826.
24. Steiner P, Rao M, Victoria MS, Rudolph N, Buynoski G. Miliary tuberculosis in two infants after nursery exposure: epidemiologic, clinical and laboratory findings. *Am Rev Respir Dis* 1976; 113:267–271.
25. Burk JR, Bahar D, Wolf FS, Greene J, Bailey WC. Nursery exposure of 528 newborns to a nurse with pulmonary tuberculosis. *South Med J* 1978; 71:7–10.
26. Kim KI, Lee JW, Park JH et al. Pulmonary tuberculosis in five young infants with nursery exposure: clinical, radiographic and CT findings. *Pediatr Radiol* 1998; 28: 836–840.
27. Lee LH, Le Vea CM, Graman PS. Congenital tuberculosis in a neonatal intensive care unit: case report, epidemiological investigation, and management of exposures. *Clin Infect Dis* 1998; 27: 474–477.
28. Nivin B, Nicholas P, Gayer M, Frieden TR, Fujiwara PI. A continuing outbreak of multidrug-resistant tuberculosis with transmission in a hospital nursery. *Clin Infect Dis* 1998; 26:303–307.
29. Sen M, Gregson D, Lewis J. Neonatal exposure to active pulmonary tuberculosis in a health care professional. *Can Med Assoc J* 2005; 172:1453–1455.
30. Isaacs D, Jones CA, Dalton D, et al. Exposure to open tuberculosis on a neonatal unit. *J Paediatr Child Health* 2006; 42: 557–559.
31. Light IJ, Saidleman M, Sutherland JM. Management of newborns after nursery exposure to tuberculosis. *Am Rev Respir Med* 1974; 109:415–419.
32. Nania JJ, Skinner J, Wilkerson K, et al. Exposure to pulmonary tuberculosis in a neonatal intensive care unit: unique aspects of contact investigation and management of hospitalized neonates. *Infect Control Hosp Epidemiol* 2007; 28:661–665.
33. Ohno H, Ikegami Y, Kishida K, et al. A contact investigation of the transmission of *Mycobacterium tuberculosis* from a nurse working in a newborn nursery and maternity ward. *J Infect Chemother* 2008; 14:66–71.
34. Millership SE, Anderson C, Cummins AJ, Bracebridge S, Abubakar I. The risk to infants from nosocomial exposure to tuberculosis. *Paediatr Infect Dis J* 2009; 28:915–916.
35. Borgia P, Cambieri A, Chini F, et al. Suspected transmission of tuberculosis in a maternity ward from a smear-positive nurse: preliminary results of clinical evaluations and testing of neonates potentially exposed, Rome, Italy, 1 January to 28 July 2011. *Euro Surveill* 2011; 16(40) pii:19984.
36. Jensen PA, Lambert LA, Iademarco MF, Ridzon R; CDC. Guidelines for preventing the transmission of *Mycobacterium tuberculosis* in health-care settings, 2005. *MMWR Recomm Rep 2005*; 54(RR-17):1–141.
37. Richeldi L, Ewer K, Losi M, et al. T cell-based tracking of multidrug resistant tuberculosis infection after brief exposure. *Am J Respir Crit Care Med* 2004; 170:288–295.

38. Peng W, Yang J, Liu E. Analysis of 170 cases of congenital TB reported in the literature between 1946 and 2009. *Pediatr Pulmonol* 2011; 46: 1215–1224.
39. Fisher K, Guaran R, Stack J, et al. Nosocomial pulmonary tuberculosis contact investigation in a neonatal intensive care unit. *Infect Control Hosp Epidemiol* 2013; 34:754–756.
40. Richeldi L, Ewer K, Losi M, et al. T cell-based tracking of multidrug resistant tuberculosis infection after brief exposure. *Am J Respir Crit Care Med* 2004; 170:288–295.
41. Remington JS, McLeod R, Wilson CB, Desmonts G. Toxoplasmosis. In: *Infectious Diseases of the Fetus and Newborn Infant,* 7th edn (eds JS Remington, JO Klein, CB Wilson, V Nizet, Y Maldonado). Philadelphia: Elsevier, 2011. pp. 918–1041.
42. Olariu TR, Remington JS, McLeod R, Alam A, Montoya JG. Severe congenital toxoplasmosis in the United States: clinical and serologic findings in untreated infants. *Pediatr Infect Dis J* 2011; 30:1056–1061.
43. Gilbert RE, Harden M, Stanford M. Antibiotics versus control for toxoplasma retinochoroiditis. *Cochrane Database Syst Rev* 2002; Issue 1. Art. No.: CD002218. doi:10.1002/14651858.CD002218
44. Di Mario S, Basevi V, Gagliotti C, et al. Prenatal education for congenital toxoplasmosis. *Cochrane Database Syst Rev* 2009; Issue 1. Art. No.: CD006171. doi:10.1002/14651858.CD006171.pub2
45. Khoshnood B, De Vigan C, Goffinet F, Leroy V. Prenatal screening and diagnosis of congenital toxoplasmosis: a review of safety issues and psychological consequences for women who undergo screening. *Prenat Diagn* 2007; 27:395–403.
46. Carme B, Tirard-Fleury V. Toxoplasmosis among pregnant women in France: seroprevalence, seroconversion and knowledge levels. Trends 1965–1995. *Med Malad Infect* 1996; 26:431–436 [in French].
47. Kravetz J. Congenital toxoplasmosis. *Clin Evid (Online).* 2010 Jun 28; 2010. pii: 0906.
48. Wallon M, Liou C, Garner P, et al. Congenital toxoplasmosis: systematic review of evidence of efficacy of treatment in pregnancy. *Br Med Assoc* 1999; 318:1511–1514.
49. Peyron F, Wallon M, Liou C, et al. Treatments for toxoplasmosis in pregnancy. In: *The Cochrane Library,* Issue 1. Chichester, UK: John Wiley & Sons, Ltd, 2010. Available at: http://mrw.interscience.wiley.com/cochrane/clsysrev/articles/CD001684/frame.html (accessed 14 August 2013)
50. SYROCOT (Systematic Review on Congenital Toxoplasmosis) Study Group: Thiebaut R, Leproust S, Chene G, et al. Effectiveness of prenatal treatment for congenital toxoplasmosis: a meta-analysis of individual patients' data. *Lancet* 2007; 369:115–122.
51. Vergani P, Ghidini A, Ceruti P, et al. Congenital toxoplasmosis: efficacy of maternal treatment with spiramycin alone. *Am J Reprod Immunol* 1998; 39:335–340.
52. Stillwaggon E, Carrier CS, Sautter M, McLeod R. Maternal serologic screening to prevent congenital toxoplasmosis: a decision-analytic economic model. *PLoS Negl Trop Dis* 2011; 5:e1333.
53. Paquet C, Yudin MH. Toxoplasmosis in pregnancy: prevention, screening, and treatment. *J Obstet Gynaecol Can* 2013; 35:78–79.
54. Kellmann TR, Dobson S. Syphilis. In: *Infectious Diseases of the Fetus and Newborn Infant,* 7th edn (eds JS Remington, JO Klein, CB Wilson, V Nizet, Y Maldonado). Philadelphia: Elsevier, 2011. pp. 524–563.
55. Lozano R, Naghavi M, Foreman K, et al. Global and regional mortality from 235 causes of death for 20 age groups in 1990 and 2010: a systematic analysis for the Global Burden of Disease Study 2010. *Lancet* 2013; 380:2095–2128.
56. Gayet-Ageron A, Lautenschlager S, Ninet B, Perneger TV, Combescure C. Sensitivity, specificity and likelihood ratios of PCR in the diagnosis of syphilis: a systematic review and meta-analysis. *Sex Transm Infect* 2013; 89:251–256.
57. Workowski KA, Berman S; Centers for Disease Control and Prevention (CDC). Sexually transmitted diseases treatment guidelines, 2010. *MMWR Recomm Rep* 2010; 59(RR-12):1–110. Available at: http://www.cdc.gov/mmwr/preview/mmwrhtml/rr5912a1.htm (accessed 2 February 2013).
58. Wolff T, Shelton E, Sessions C, Miller T. Screening for syphilis infection in pregnant women: evidence for the U.S. Preventive Services Task Force reaffirmation recommendation statement. *Ann Intern Med* 2009; 150:710–716.
59. Cheng JQ, Zhou H, Hong FC, et al. Syphilis screening and intervention in 500,000 pregnant women in Shenzhen, the People's Republic of China. *Sex Transm Infect* 2007; 83:347–350.
60. Hawkes S, Matin N, Broutet N, Low N. Effectiveness of interventions to improve screening for syphilis in pregnancy: a systematic review and meta-analysis. *Lancet Infect Dis* 2011; 11:684–691.
61. Chen XS, Peeling RW, Yin YP, Mabey D. Improving antenatal care to prevent adverse pregnancy outcomes caused by syphilis. *Future Microbiol* 2011; 6:1131–1134.
62. Omoigberale AI, Abiodun PO. Upsurge in neonatal tetanus in Benin City, Nigeria. *East Afr Med J* 2005; 82:98–102.
63. Adeniyi OF, Mabogunje CA, Okoromah CN, Renner JK. Neonatal tetanus: the Massey Street Children's Hospital experience. *Nig Q J Hosp Med* 2010; 20:147–152.
64. Blencowe H, Cousens S, Mullany LC, et al. Clean birth and postnatal care practices to reduce neonatal deaths from sepsis and tetanus: a systematic review and Delphi estimation of mortality effect. *BMC Public Health* 2011; 11 (Suppl. 3):S11. doi:10.1186/1471-2458-11-S3-S11
65. Lassi ZS, Haider BA, Bhutta ZA. Community-based intervention packages for reducing maternal and neonatal morbidity and mortality and improving neonatal outcomes. *Cochrane Database Syst Rev* 2010; Issue 11. Art. No.: CD007754. doi:10.1002/14651858.CD007754.pub2
66. Eisele TP, Larsen DA, Anglewicz PA, et al. Malaria prevention in pregnancy, birthweight, and neonatal mortality: a meta-analysis of 32 national cross-sectional datasets in Africa. *Lancet Infect Dis* 2012; 12:942–949.
67. Uneke CJ. Congenital *Plasmodium falciparum* malaria in sub-Saharan Africa: a rarity or frequent occurrence? *Parasitol Res* 2007; 101:835–842.

68. Lesko CR, Arguin PM, Newman RD. Congenital malaria in the United States: a review of cases from 1966 to 2005. *Arch Pediatr Adolesc Med* 2007; 161:1062–1067.
69. Hagmann S, Khanna K, Niazi M, Purswani M, Robins EB. Congenital malaria, an important differential diagnosis to consider when evaluating febrile infants of immigrant mothers. *Pediatr Emerg Care* 2007; 23:326–329.
70. Vottier G, Arsac M, Farnoux C, Mariani-Kurkdjian P, Baud O, Aujard Y. Congenital malaria in neonates: two case reports and review of the literature. *Acta Paediatr* 2008; 97:505–508.
71. Maldonado YA. Less common protozoan and helminth infections. In: *Infectious Diseases of the Fetus and Newborn Infant*, 7th edn (eds JS Remington, JO Klein, CB Wilson, V Nizet, Y Maldonado). Philadelphia: Elsevier, 2011. pp. 1042–1054.
72. Antibiotic Expert Group. *Therapeutic Guidelines: Antibiotic, Version 14.* Melbourne: Therapeutic Guidelines Limited, 2010.
73. Piola P, Nabasumba C, Turyakira E, et al. Efficacy and safety of artemether-lumefantrine compared with quinine in pregnant women with uncomplicated Plasmodium falciparum malaria: an open-label, randomised, non-inferiority trial. *Lancet Infect Dis* 2010; 10:762–769.
74. Manyando C, Kayentao K, D'Alessandro U, Okafor HU, Juma E, Hamed K. A systematic review of the safety and efficacy of artemether-lumefantrine against uncomplicated Plasmodium falciparum malaria during pregnancy. *Malar J* 2012; 11:141.
75. Garner P, Gülmezoglu AM. Drugs for preventing malaria in pregnant women. *Cochrane Database Syst Rev* 2006; Issue 4. Art. No.: CD000169. doi: 10.1002/14651858.CD000169.pub2
76. Orton LC, Omari AAA. Drugs for treating uncomplicated malaria in pregnant women. *Cochrane Database Syst Rev* 2008; Issue 4. Art. No.: CD004912. doi:10.1002/14651858.CD004912.pub
77. Gamble CL, Ekwaru JP, ter Kuile FO. Insecticide-treated nets for preventing malaria in pregnancy. *Cochrane Database Syst Rev* 2006; Issue 2. Art. No.: CD003755. doi: 10.1002/14651858.CD003755.pub2
78. Gilchrist M, Wong M, Mansour A, Isaacs D. An unusual cause of fever. *J Paediatr Child Health* 2012; 48:1039–1042.
79. Janka GE. Familial and acquired hemophagocytic lymphohistiocytosis. *Annu Rev Med* 2012; 63:233–246.

CHAPTER 19
Breast milk

Human breast milk has evolved as one of the most important defence mechanisms protecting the vulnerable newborn against infection.[1] Until the recent advent of neonatal intensive care, however, virtually all extremely pre-term infants died, so the breast milk produced by the mother of a pre-term infant has not necessarily evolved to have the same protective effect as for term infants. There is good evidence that a pre-term infant's mother's breast milk protects her infant against neonatal infections in industrialized countries[2] and in developing countries,[3] just as breast milk protects full-term babies against infections in industrialized[4] and developing countries[5] (Section 19.2 and Chapter 23). Breast milk also protects against necrotizing enterocolitis.[6, 7] One paediatrician put it succinctly, but in terms which may no longer be politically correct, "Breast milk is cheaper, cleaner and comes in cuter containers."

The limited knowledge about the possible mechanisms by which breast milk protects against infections will be considered in Section 19.1. Breast milk can also on occasion be a source of neonatal infection and the risks of acquiring infection from breast milk will also be considered (Section 19.4).

19.1 Mechanisms of defence against infection

Fresh human milk contains secretory IgA (sIgA) and soluble immunoglobulins, immune cells (T- and B-lymphocytes, macrophages and neutrophils), cytokines and cytokine receptors which modulate the immune response and many bioactive proteins, including ones such as lactoferrin with potent activity against microorganisms (Section 19.1.3). Breast milk also contains oligosaccharides (sometimes loosely called Bifidus factor) which actively promote the growth of bifidobacteria,[8] and there is growing evidence that bifidobacteria and other probiotics protect pre-term babies against NEC.[9, 10]

19.1.1 Immunoglobulins

sIgA, the major immunoglobulin class in human colostrum and milk, is a dimer of two IgA molecules linked by a polypeptide J-chain and associated with a secretory component. Specific sIgA antibodies against gastrointestinal and respiratory pathogens are probably a major factor in how human breast milk protects against gastroenteritis and respiratory infections.[11]

Other immunoglobulins, particularly IgM early in lactation but also IgG, IgD and IgE, are found in breast milk in lower concentrations than sIgA.[1]

19.1.2 Cells

Normal human breast milk contains large numbers of phagocytic cells, macrophages which are often IgA-associated, and neutrophils, as well as a small number of T-cells, even fewer B-cells and some epithelial cells. The precise function of these different cell types is still under investigation.

19.1.3 Bioactive proteins

Human breast milk contains many bioactive proteins, although their role in breastfed infants is unknown.[12] Some are involved in modulation of the immune system, including enhanced defence against pathogens; other important properties include enhanced nutrient absorption and growth promotion.[12] Antimicrobial activities include stimulation of beneficial (prebiotic) microorganisms, lysis or growth inhibition of pathogens and prevention of attachment or invasion of pathogenic bacteria. Bioactive proteins in breast milk with direct antimicrobial activity include the dominant

Evidence-Based Neonatal Infections, First Edition. David Isaacs.

whey protein, lactoferrin, lysozyme which lyses susceptible bacteria, α-lactalbumin which induces apoptosis and may be an important defence against tumours and fibronectin which aids macrophage function.[1, 12]

19.1.4 Cytokines

Many immunomodulatory cytokines are found in human breast milk, including interleukins IL-1β, IL-6, IL-8, IL-10 and IL-12, interferon-γ, TNF-α, and granulocyte and macrophage colony-stimulating factors (G-CSF and M-CSF). Their exact function is still uncertain.

19.2 Prevention of infection

There is good evidence (see Chapter 23) that human breast milk protects the following groups of babies:

- Pre-term neonates in industrialized countries against bacterial infections[4]
- Pre-term neonates in developing countries against bacterial infections[5]
- Full-term infants in industrialized countries against gastroenteritis and respiratory infections[11, 13]
- Full-term infants in developing countries against death from gastroenteritis and respiratory infections[7]

19.3 Prevention of necrotizing enterocolitis

There is strong evidence from a Cochrane Systematic Review that human breast milk compared with formula reduces the risk of necrotizing enterocolitis in pre-term or low birth-weight infants (see Chapter 11).[3]

19.4 Transmission of infection through human breast milk

19.4.1 Virus infections

A number of viruses can be detected in breast milk, particularly viruses that can persist, such as herpesviruses, hepatitis B virus, hepatitis C virus (HCV) and HIV. In general, mother-to-child transmission (MTCT) of virus causes the most severe disease when the virus is acquired transplacentally (e.g. VZV) or at the time of delivery (HSV, enteroviruses) and when the mother has not produced specific IgG antibodies to cross the placenta and protect the baby (see Chapter 17). In contrast, post-natal acquisition of viruses rarely results in severe neonatal infection. However, there are exceptions. The viruses transmitted by breast milk that are most critical in terms of causing significant chronic disease are the retroviruses, HIV and human T-lymphotropic virus type 1 (HTLV-1), while post-natally acquired cytomegalovirus (CMV) can cause severe, acute disease to extremely low birth-weight infants.

19.4.1.1 HIV

Question: Should HIV-positive mothers breastfeed in developing countries and in industrialized countries?

Breast milk transmission of HIV to an infant was first described in 1985, from a mother who acquired HIV from a post-natal blood transfusion.[14] Since then, risk factors for breast milk transmission of HIV have been shown to include the duration of breastfeeding, the mother's viral load and other maternal characteristics, characteristics of the breast milk and the type of breast-feeding.[15]

In an individual patient data meta-analysis of nine clinical trials in sub-Saharan Africa, the cumulative probability of transmission from HIV-infected women to their infants increased with increasing duration of breastfeeding (from 1.6% at age 3 months to 9.3% at age 18 months).[16] For children whose timing of infection was known, up to 44% of transmission could be attributed to breastfeeding.

Maternal factors associated with transmission of HIV by breastfeeding include younger maternal age and higher parity, recent HIV infection associated with high viral load and breast abnormalities, such as mastitis or breast abscess. More advanced maternal disease, with low CD4+ cell counts and higher maternal peripheral blood or human milk viral loads, is a risk factor for late post-natal transmission of HIV.[15]

Oral candidiasis (thrush) has been described as an infant risk factor associated with increased MTCT of HIV by breast milk, but this may be merely an epiphenomenon indicative of greater immune dysfunction.

The main breast milk-associated risk factor for HIV transmission is the breast milk viral load (both cell-free and cell-associated). Another characteristic of breast milk which may be associated with a higher risk of transmission is reduced concentrations of antiviral substances, such as lactoferrin, lysozyme and epidermal growth factor.[15]

Studies have shown that mixed feeding with breast milk and formula or solids is associated with a higher risk of transmission of HIV than exclusive breastfeeding.[16–20] It is thought that foods other than breast milk in early infancy may damage the gastrointestinal tract, causing increased permeability and allowing HIV in breast milk to penetrate.

Complete avoidance of breastfeeding may be a problem for women in some developing countries. Potential interventions to reduce or prevent transmission of HIV through maternal breast milk include decreasing the duration of breast milk exposure (either by complete avoidance of breastfeeding or by stopping breastfeeding early), reducing maternal infectivity (e.g. by using chemical or heat treatment of breast milk to lower breast milk HIV viral load or by giving the breastfeeding mother antiretroviral treatment), reducing factors which increase mother-to-child HIV transmission (e.g. mixed feeding, maternal breast problems, infant thrush).[15]

A Cochrane systematic review of the efficacy of interventions to decrease late post-natal MTCT of HIV identified six RCTs and one intervention cohort study.[15] Two trials examined eliminating or shortening the duration of exposure to breast milk from HIV-positive mothers.[21, 22] In a trial of breastfeeding versus formula feeding, the cumulative probability of the infant developing HIV infection was 36.7% at 24 months in the breastfeeding arm and 20.5% in the formula arm ($p = 0.001$), but at this age the rates of mortality and malnutrition were not significantly different in the two groups.[21] In a trial of early cessation of breastfeeding, HIV-free survival and mortality at 24 months was similar for children who ceased breastfeeding abruptly at around 4 months of age and children who continued breastfeeding for at least 6 months.[22]

A trial of maternal vitamin A supplementation surprisingly found more cases of HIV infection in children of mothers who were given vitamin A.[23] Maternal multivitamin supplements had no significant effect on HIV transmission.[23]

One intervention cohort study involving 1276 infants evaluated the effect of infant feeding modality on MTCT.[24] Breastfed children who also received solids during the first 6 months of life were significantly more likely than exclusively breastfed children to be infected with HIV (HR 10.9; 95% CI 1.5–78). The cumulative 3-month mortality in exclusively breastfed infants was 6.1% (4.7–7.9) compared with 15.1% (7.6–28.7) in infants given replacement feeds (HR 2.06; 1–4.27).[24]

Three trials evaluated antiretroviral prophylaxis to breastfeeding infants. In a trial in Botswana, breastfeeding plus zidovudine prophylaxis during the first 6 months of life (7-month HIV infection rate 9%) was less effective than formula feeding (7-month HIV infection rate 5.6%) in preventing post-natal HIV transmission.[25] The breastfeeding plus zidovudine infants had a lower mortality rate at 7 months, but mortality and HIV-free survival at 18 months were comparable.[25]

Two trials studied infant nevirapine prophylaxis for breastfed infants.[26, 27] In one study, which combined data from trials in Ethiopia, India, and Uganda, a 6-week course of nevirapine resulted in a significantly lower risk of HIV transmission at 6 weeks, but not at 6 months of age.[26] In a second study in Malawi of infants who were exclusively breastfed for 6 months, 14 weeks of either nevirapine alone (5.2%) or of nevirapine with zidovudine (6.4%) reduced MTCT at 9 months of age significantly compared to a control regimen of two-dose nevirapine prophylaxis (10.6%). HIV-free survival was significantly better at 9 months for both extended prophylaxis groups, and at 15 months in the extended nevirapine group.[27]

There are no randomized studies of heat-treating breast milk in developing countries. A small feasibility study of 20 mother–infant pairs in Zimbabwe showed that heat treatment of expressed breast milk is a possible option for feeding HIV-exposed, uninfected children after 6 months of age.[28]

Rarely, an HIV-positive mother in an industrialized country may want to breastfeed, and this can raise tricky child protection issues.[29, 30] In the past an HIV-positive woman who wanted to breastfeed triggered an immediate notification to child protection authorities. The risk of breastfeeding in a woman with undetectable virus load is low and needs to be weighed against the harms of trying to enforce no breastfeeding. Most authorities no longer feel an immediate notification is mandatory.

Recommendation: Complete avoidance of breastfeeding reduces mother-to-child HIV transmission, but is associated with significant morbidity (e.g. gastroenteritis) in many developing countries.[15] Two alternative strategies that reduce transmission for breastfed infants are, firstly, exclusive breastfeeding during the first few months of life as opposed to mixed feeding and secondly, extended use of antiretrovirals (nevirapine alone, or nevirapine with zidovudine).

In industrialized countries, where formula feeding is effectively as safe as breastfeeding, all HIV-positive mothers are counselled to use formula feeds and to avoid breastfeeding completely.

19.4.1.2 Human T-cell lymphotropic virus type 1

Human T-cell lymphotropic virus type I (HTLV-I) is a retrovirus, most prevalent in Japan, Africa, the Caribbean and South America, which can cause adult T-cell leukaemia, lymphoma and tropical spastic paraparesis.[31] Known modes of transmission include vertical transmission (predominantly through breastfeeding), transverse transmission (sexual intercourse), transfusion of infected blood products and sharing of needles and syringes.[31] Infected mothers and blood donors can be identified by screening.

The main route of MTCT is through breastfeeding. Although HTLV-1 proviral DNA can be detected in cord blood samples, HTLV-I proviruses in cord blood may be defective, and intrauterine transmission is rare. The placenta can be infected by HTLV-I, but infection does not reach the foetus. HTLV-I proviral DNA and antibodies against HTLV-I can also be detected in saliva, but there is no direct evidence to show that HTLV-I transmission via saliva occurs.[32]

Avoiding breastfeeding can prevent MTCT of HTLV-1 but, as with HIV, the risks of formula feeding in a resource-poor setting may outweigh the benefits.[33]

19.4.1.3 Cytomegalovirus

Like all herpesviruses, CMV persists after acquisition and can reactivate with or without causing symptoms. Using the sensitive technique of DNA amplification by polymerase chain reaction (PCR) it can be shown that CMV can be detected intermittently in breast milk from the majority of CMV-seropositive mothers.[34–38]

While post-natally acquired neonatal CMV infection is usually mild, the same is not true for extremely low birth-weight infants, who can develop severe, sometimes fatal disease.[34–39] A sepsis-like syndrome, thrombocytopenia, neutropenia, hepatitis and pneumonitis have all been described (see Chapter 17).

A literature search on breast milk transmission of CMV found three non-systematic reviews[34–36] and one non-Cochrane systematic review.[38] The non-Cochrane systematic review analysed studies from 1966 to 2008 on transmission of CMV via breast milk to pre-term infants and their outcome.[38] The reviewers included 26 studies. The proportion of CMV IgG seropositive mothers ranged from 52% to 100% (median 82%), and CMV IgG was detected in 67–97.2% (median 80%) of breast milk samples. The proportion of infants who became seropositive varied widely from 5.7% to 58.6%. Similarly, a wide range of infants from none to 34.5% (median 3.7%) developed symptomatic CMV disease and 0–13.8% (median 0.7%) developed severe sepsis-like syndrome. Pre-term infants with acquired symptomatic CMV infection had a low risk of mild neurologic and cognitive sequelae, without hearing impairment.[38] Finding an association between the presence of CMV in breast milk and the infant becoming infected with CMV does not prove that milk is the vehicle of infection, because CMV is also found in respiratory secretions and many other body fluids (see Section 17.1).

Question: Should pre-term babies be fed breast milk if their mothers are CMV seropositive?

Breast milk transmission of CMV can be prevented by using formula feeds instead of breast milk, but in extremely low birth-weight infants the benefits of breast milk in preventing NEC and bacterial infections far outweigh the benefits of preventing post-natal CMV acquisition. Possible interventions to reduce CMV transmission are to freeze the milk, which has been shown to reduce transmission and reduce the severity of CMV infection but not eliminate it totally, or to pasteurize the breast milk, which will destroy proteins and is likely to reduce many of the benefits of breast milk. The American Academy of Pediatrics suggests that short-term pasteurization may be less harmful to the beneficial constituents of human milk, but sits firmly on the fence by saying that decisions about breastfeeding of infants by CMV-seropositive mothers should "include consideration of the potential benefits of human milk and the risk of CMV transmission."[40]

Recommendation: The data do not support avoidance or pasteurization of breast milk for high-risk pre-term infants of CMV-positive mothers.

19.4.1.4 Varicella-zoster virus

Although VZV can be detected in the breast milk of mothers with chickenpox[41] and zoster,[42] the major risk to the infant comes from transplacentally acquired VZV in the absence of maternal IgG. Post-natally acquired VZV, even in the absence of IgG antibodies, is almost always benign, presumably because the viral load is far lower from post-natal than from transplacental exposure (see Chapter 17).

Babies whose mothers develop chickenpox around delivery are given varicella-zoster immunoglobulin and/or antivirals and the risk of severe neonatal chickenpox in a baby who has received suitable prophylaxis is negligible (see Chapter 17). There is no rational reason to separate a mother with chickenpox or zoster from her baby and no reason to stop her from breastfeeding.

VZV vaccine is a live attenuated vaccine. The vaccine strain has not been detected in breast milk, but it is possible that it could be transmitted in milk, although the risk to the infant is likely to be extremely low.[40, 43] If a VZV-seronegative woman is exposed to VZV post-natally, we recommend that she should be immunized with VZV vaccine and be counselled that it is probably safe to continue breastfeeding.

19.4.1.5 Herpes simplex virus

As with VZV, although HSV can sometimes be detected in breast milk, the infant is exposed to far greater loads of HSV by other routes, such as peri-partum exposure, and maternal HSV infection (oral or genital HSV) is not considered a contraindication to breastfeeding. However, it is recommended that a woman with a herpetic lesion on a breast or nipple should refrain from using the affected breast to breastfeed until the lesion or lesions resolve.[40]

19.4.1.6 Hepatitis B virus

Hepatitis B surface antigen (HBsAg) can be detected in breast milk from women who are chronically infected with hepatitis B virus (HBV). We found two non-Cochrane systematic reviews of breastfeeding and maternal chronic hepatitis B infection.[44, 45]

A systematic review of 32 studies of infants vaccinated against hepatitis B found that 4.3% of infants born to mothers with chronic hepatitis B were infected at 1 year of age, and it made no difference whether they were breastfed or formula fed, or whether or not the mothers were *e*-antigen positive.[44] A meta-analysis of 10 prospective randomized trials (1624 infants) found no significant difference in the rates of MTCT between breastfed and formula-fed infants at 6–12 months.[45]

Mothers should be screened for HBV infection in pregnancy. The infants of all HBV-seropositive mothers should be given immunoglobulin and vaccine at birth.[46] If immunoglobulin and vaccine have been given to the infant, there is no contraindication to an HBV-seropositive mother breastfeeding.[40] The incubation period of hepatitis B is long and there is no reason to delay initiation of breastfeeding until after the infant is immunized.[40]

19.4.1.7 Hepatitis C virus

Although HCV can be detected in breast milk, the major risk is transplacental transmission, which itself is primarily a function of maternal viral load (see Chapter 17). Transmission of HCV by breast milk has not been documented in HIV-negative women who are HCV positive.[47, 48] This does not mean that it is certain that HCV cannot be transmitted in breast milk, but that the risk is probably extremely low. It is generally considered to be so low that a woman who is HCV positive can be advised of the very low risk and told that it is fine to breastfeed, although it is generally advised that the baby should not feed from a breast with a cracked or bleeding nipple.[40, 47, 49]

19.4.2 Bacterial infections

19.4.2.1 Group B Streptococcus

GBS can be grown from breast milk in the absence of maternal symptoms such as mastitis. It has been reported in association with recurrent neonatal GBS infection on a number of occasions.[49, 50] However, it is known that infants treated for GBS infection remain colonized with GBS in the nasopharynx and gastrointestinal tract and that late-onset GBS infection can occur in formula-fed babies. For this reason, it is by no means certain that merely growing the same strain of GBS from the mother's milk of an infected baby means that the milk caused the infection. The literature of anecdotal reports is very unclear on this matter. A typical report is careful in the title to use the term 'in association with' but then, in the Abstract, reports "late-onset and recurrent GBS infection in newborn twins *resulting from* ingestion of maternal breast milk infected with GBS" (our italics).[50]

Thus the authors have jumped to the conclusion that the baby's infection was caused by the mother's milk with no supportive evidence.

GBS can rarely cause mastitis and, as discussed below (Section 19.4.2.2) a woman is advised not to breastfeed from a breast with active mastitis. In most cases, however, GBS is only ever grown from breast milk because a baby has developed late-onset GBS or, more frequently, recurrent GBS infection. Our preference is not to culture mother's milk in these situations, because even culturing the milk implies a possible causative link. The best action when GBS has been cultured from a mother's milk is not clear. One option is to counsel the mother to stop breastfeeding, but this seems overvigorous in the absence of strong evidence that breast milk *causes* late-onset or recurrent GBS infection. Furthermore, the inevitable guilt this will cause the mother means that neonatologists should want strong evidence before suggesting a mother's breast milk is a cause of her baby's recurrent infection. Another option is to counsel the mother of the association and let her decide. Whether the mother decides to breastfeed or not, she should be warned that if her infant develops fever, feeding difficulties, lethargy or other worrying signs or symptoms she should bring the infant for urgent review.

19.4.2.2 Mastitis and breast abscess

Mastitis and breast abscess are common, occurring in up to a third of all breastfeeding mothers.[51–53] *Staphylococcus aureus* is the commonest cause, including MRSA, although GBS, group A streptococci and Gram-negative bacilli can also cause mastitis and breast abscess. Some breast abscesses require surgical drainage. Both mastitis and breast abscess are extremely painful. While the advice to stop breastfeeding from the affected side[40] seems sensible, most women have already stopped feeding using the affected breast without being told to do so.

19.4.2.3 Mycobacterium tuberculosis

Mycobacterium tuberculosis can rarely cause mastitis or breast abscess in which case the mother should not breastfeed until she has been treated for 2 weeks.[40] *M. tuberculosis* may also be detected in breast milk in the absence of mastitis or breast abscess, usually in association with miliary tuberculosis. It is hardly ever necessary to separate a mother with tuberculosis from her infant (see Chapter 18). If a mother was found to have miliary tuberculosis around the time of delivery, the possibility of delaying breastfeeding until she had been treated for 2 weeks might be considered, but is probably unnecessary if the infant is being treated for congenital tuberculosis.

19.5 Breast milk expression

A Cochrane Systematic Review of methods of expressing breast milk found 23 studies, but only 10 (632 mothers) were suitable for analysis.[54] Electric pumps increased the volume of milk over 6 days compared to hand expression, but the standardized mean difference (MD) was only 1 mL. No difference in volume was found between simultaneous or sequential pumping, or between manual and electric pumps.[54]

Mothers provided with a relaxation tape produced more milk than mothers without such a tape (mean difference (MD) 34.7 mL per single expression, 95% CI 9.5–59.9, $p = 0.007$).[54]

No difference was found between methods of expressing milk regarding energy content, milk contamination or adverse effects. Maternal views on different methods varied. Economic aspects were not reported.[54]

A Cochrane Systematic Review of studies of medications to improve breast milk supply for mothers of pre-term babies found two studies of the anti-dopaminergic drug domperidone involving only 59 women. Domperidone was associated with a modest increase in expressed breast milk which did not reach statistical significance.[55] The authors did not look for studies of dark beer; Guinness has traditionally been used in the United Kingdom to increase mothers' milk supply but we could find only anecdotal evidence of its efficacy.

19.6 Human breast milk banks

Prior to 1981 and the description of the HIV epidemic, human breast milk banks were becoming increasingly popular as a way of providing human breast milk for pre-term babies whose mothers were unable or unwilling to provide milk themselves. The HIV epidemic raised fears of transmission of HIV by breast milk. However, it was subsequently shown that pasteurization, using heat treatment at 62.5°C for 30 minutes, completely destroys HIV. Heat treatment at 56°C for 30 minutes kills bacteria, inactivates HIV but may not completely destroy CMV and other viruses. Pasteurization at 62.5°C for 30 minutes inactivates HIV and CMV and decreases the titre of other viruses.[40]

Most human milk banks screen donors for blood-borne infections and discard milk from seropositive donors. Donor milk banks which belong to the Human Milk Banking Association of North America follow guidelines approved by the Food and Drug Administration (FDA) and Centers for Disease Control and Prevention (CDC) (https://www.hmbana.org/) and these include screening donors for HIV-1 and 2, HTLV-1 and 2, hepatitis C and syphilis.[40] The importance of such screening is shown by a retrospective review of the serological status of unpaid volunteers donating human milk to a regional milk bank in California over a 6-year period.[56] Of 1091 potential donors, 3.3% were positive on screening serology, including 6 for syphilis, 17 for hepatitis B, 3 for hepatitis C, 6 for HTLV and 4 for HIV.[56]

Similar best practice guidelines have been developed by National Institute for Health and Clinical Excellence (NICE) in the United Kingdom[57] and in Australia.[58, 59]

19.7 Accidental breast milk exposure

It is not uncommon in neonatal units that one mother's expressed breast milk is inadvertently fed to another mother's infant. Although the risk of transmitting an infection is extremely low, such an event usually causes huge anxiety. The recommended course of action is to treat the incident like any accidental exposure to body fluids.[40, 60] The donor mother should be told of the incident and asked if she would be willing to undergo an HIV test (or allow the result of a recent HIV test to be disclosed). The recipient's mother should be told of the incident and counselled that the risk is exceedingly low, almost certainly far lower than one in a million, which is generally considered a negligible risk. If the donor mother is HIV negative, no further action needs to be taken.[40, 60] This approach assumes that the risk of acquiring other infections from the donor mother's milk is negligible and that the donor has been screened for and is not chronically infected with hepatitis B.

19.8 Antimicrobials in breast milk

Lactating women may be prescribed antimicrobials and the paediatrician may be asked whether this is safe. In general only low levels of antimicrobials will appear in breast milk and it can be assumed that any antimicrobial that could safely be prescribed to a neonate is also safe for the mother of a breastfed baby. A review of the teratogenic potential of 11 commonly prescribed antibiotics found that all except chloramphenicol were compatible with lactation, although the strength of the data to make the safety recommendation varied.[61] The US National Library of Medicine publishes a Toxicology Data Network on http://toxnet.nlm.nih.gov/cgi-bin/sis/htmlgen?LACT, which can be searched for individual drugs.

Useful websites

- Human Milk Banking Association of North America for breast milk banks: https://www.hmbana.org/
- Toxicology Data Network for mother's drugs in breast milk: http://toxnet.nlm.nih.gov/cgi-bin/sis/htmlgen?LACT
- CDC link for accidental ingestion of another mother's milk: http://www.cdc.gov/breastfeeding/recommendations/other_mothers_milk.htm.

References

1. Wilson CB, Ogra PL. Human milk. In: *Infectious Diseases of the Fetus and Newborn Infant.* (eds JS Remington, JO Klein, CB Wilson, V Nizet, Y Maldonado). 7th edn. Philadelphia: Elsevier, 2011, 192–222.
2. Schanler RJ, Lau C, Hurst NM, Smith EO. Randomized trial of donor human milk versus preterm formula as substitutes for mothers' own milk in the feeding of extremely premature infants. *Pediatrics* 2005; 116:400–406.
3. Narayanan I, Prakash K, Gujral VV. The value of human milk in the prevention of infection in the high-risk low-birth-weight infant. *J Pediatr* 1981; 99:496–498.
4. Duijts L, Ramadhani MK, Moll HA. Breastfeeding protects against infectious diseases during infancy in industrialized countries. A systematic review. *Matern Child Nutr* 2009; 5:199–210.
5. WHO Collaborative Study Team on the Role of Breastfeeding on the Prevention of Infant Mortality. Effect of breastfeeding on infant and child mortality due to infectious diseases in less developed countries: a pooled analysis. *Lancet* 2000; 355:451–455.

6. Lucas A, Cole TJ. Breast milk and neonatal necrotising enterocolitis. *Lancet* 1990; 336:1519–1523.
7. Quigley M, Henderson G, Anthony MY, McGuire W. Formula milk versus donor breast milk for feeding preterm or low birth weight infants. *Cochrane Database Syst Rev* 2007, Issue 4. Art. No.: CD002971. doi: 10.1002/14651858.CD002971.pub2.
8. Kunz C. Historical aspects of human milk oligosaccharides. *Adv Nutr* 2012; 3:430S–439S.
9. AlFaleh K, Anabrees J, Bassler D, Al-Kharfi T. Probiotics for prevention of necrotizing enterocolitis in preterm infants. *Cochrane Database Syst Rev* 2011, Issue 3. Art. No.: CD005496. doi: 10.1002/14651858.CD005496.pub3.
10. Deshpande G, Rao S, Patole S, Bulsara M. Updated meta-analysis of probiotics for preventing necrotizing enterocolitis in preterm neonates. *Pediatrics* 2010; 125:921–930.
11. Quigley MA, Kelly YJ, Sacker A. Breastfeeding and hospitalization for diarrheal and respiratory infection in the United Kingdom Millennium Cohort Study. *Pediatrics* 2007; 119:e837–e842.
12. Lönnerdal B. Bioactive proteins in breast milk. *J Paediatr Child Health* 2013; 49(Supp 1):1–7
13. Kramer MS, Chalmers B, Hodnett ED, et al. PROBIT Study Group (Promotion of Breastfeeding Intervention Trial).Promotion of Breastfeeding Intervention Trial (PROBIT): a randomized trial in the Republic of Belarus. *J Am Med Assoc* 2001; 285:413–420.
14. Ziegler JB, Cooper DA, Johnson RO, Gold J. Postnatal transmission of AIDS-associated retrovirus from mother to infant. *Lancet* 1985; 1:896–898.
15. Horvath T, Madi BC, Iuppa IM, Kennedy GE, Rutherford GW, Read JS. Interventions for preventing late postnatal mother-to-child transmission of HIV. *Cochrane Database Syst Rev* 2009, Issue 1. Art. No.: CD006734. DOI: 10.1002/14651858.CD006734.pub2.
16. Breastfeeding and HIV International Transmission Study Group. Late postnatal transmission of HIV-1 in breast-fed children: An individual patient data meta-analysis. *J Infect Dis* 2004; 189:2154–2166.
17. Iliff PJ, Piwoz EG, Tavengwa NV, et al. Early exclusive breastfeeding reduces the risk of postnatal HIV-1 transmission and increases HIV-free survival. *AIDS* 2005; 19:699–708.
18. Nduati R, John G, Mbori-Ngacha D, et al. Effect of breastfeeding and formula feeding on transmission of HIV-1: a randomized clinical trial. *J Am Med Assoc* 2000; 283:1167–1174.
19. Mbori-Ngacha D, Nduati R, John G, et al. Morbidity and mortality in breastfed and formula-fed infants of HIV-1-infected women: A randomized clinical trial. *J Am Med Assoc* 2001; 286:2413–2420.
20. Coutsoudis A, Pillay K, Spooner E, Coovadia HM, Pembrey L, Newell ML. Morbidity in children born to women infected with human immunodeficiency virus in South Africa: does mode of feeding matter? *Acta Paediatr* 2003; 92:890–895.
21. Nduati R, John G, Mbori-Ngacha D, et al. Effect of breastfeeding and formula feeding on transmission of HIV-1: a randomized clinical trial. *J Am Med Assoc* 2000; 283:1167–1174.
22. Kuhn L, Aldrovandi GM, Sinkala M, et al. Effects of early, abrupt weaning on HIV-free survival of children in Zambia. *N Engl J Med* 2008; 359:130–141.
23. Fawzi WW, Msamanga GI, Hunter D, et al. Randomized trial of vitamin supplements in relation to transmission of HIV-1 through breastfeeding and early child mortality. *AIDS* 2002; 16:1935–1944.
24. Coovadia HM, Rollins NC, Bland RM, et al. Mother-to-child transmission of HIV-1 infection during exclusive breastfeeding in the first 6 months of life: an intervention cohort study. *Lancet* 2007; 369:1107–1116.
25. Thior I, Lockman S, Smeaton LM, et al. Breastfeeding plus infant zidovudine prophylaxis for 6 months vs formula feeding plus infant zidovudine for 1 month to reduce mother-to-child HIV transmission in Botswana: a randomized trial: the Mashi Study. *J Am Med Assoc* 2006; 296:794–805.
26. Bedri A, Gudetta B, Isehak A, et al. Extended-dose nevirapine to 6 weeks of age for infants to prevent HIV transmission via breastfeeding in Ethiopia, India, and Uganda: an analysis of three randomized controlled trials. *Lancet* 2008; 372:300–313.
27. Kumwenda NI, Hoover DR, Mofenson LM, et al. Extended antiretroviral prophylaxis to reduce breast-milk HIV-1 transmission. *N Engl J Med* 2008; 359:119–129.
28. Mbuya MN, Humphrey JH, Majo F, et al. Heat treatment of expressed breast milk is a feasible option for feeding HIV-exposed, uninfected children after 6 months of age in rural Zimbabwe. *J Nutr* 2010; 140:1481–1488.
29. Kuhn L, Aldrovandi G. Survival and health benefits of breastfeeding versus artificial feeding in infants of HIV-infected women: developing versus developed world. *Clin Perinatol* 2010; 37:843–862.
30. John-Stewart G, Nduati R. Should women with HIV-1 infection breastfeed their infants? It depends on the setting. *Adv Exp Med Biol* 2012; 743:289–297.
31. Verdonck K, Gonzalez E, Van Dooren S, Vandamme A-M, Vanham G, Gotuzzo E. Human T-lymphotropic virus 1: recent knowledge about an ancient infection. *Lancet Infect Dis* 2007; 7:266–281.
32. Fujino T, Nagata Y. HTLV-1 transmission from mother to child. *J Reprod Immunol* 2000; 47:197–206.
33. van Tienen C, Jakobsen M, Schim van der Loeff M. Stopping breastfeeding to prevent vertical transmission of HTLV-1 in resource-poor settings: beneficial or harmful? *Arch Gynecol Obstet* 2012; 286:255–256.
34. Jim WT, Shu CH, Chiu NC, et al. Role of breast milk in acquisition of cytomegalovirus infection: recent advances. *Pediatr Infect Dis J* 2004; 23:848–851.
35. Schliess MR. Role of breast milk in acquisition of cytomegalovirus infection: recent advances. *Curr Opin Pediatr* 2006; 18:48–52.
36. Stronati M, Lombardi G, Di Comite A, Fanos V. Breastfeeding and cytomegalovirus infections. *J Chemother* 2007; 19(Suppl 2):49–51.

37. Jim WT, Shu CH, Chiu NC, et al. High cytomegalovirus load and prolonged virus excretion in breast milk increase risk for viral acquisition by very low birth weight infants. *Pediatr Infect Dis J* 2009; 28:891–894.
38. Kurath S, Halwachs-Baumann G, Müller W, Resch B. Transmission of cytomegalovirus via breast milk to the prematurely born infant: a systematic review. *Clin Microbiol Infect* 2010; 16:1172–1178.
39. Nijman J, de Vries LS, Koopman-Esseboom C, Uiterwaal CS, van Loon AM, Verboon-Maciolek MA. Postnatally acquired cytomegalovirus infection in preterm infants: a prospective study on risk factors and cranial ultrasound findings. *Arch Dis Child Fetal Neonatal Ed* 2012; 97:F259–F263.
40. American Academy of Pediatrics. Human milk. In: *Red Rook: 2009 Report of the Committee on Infectious Diseases.* (eds LK Pickering, CJ Baker, DW Kimberlin, SS Long). 28th edn. Elk Grove Village, Il: American Academy of Pediatrics; 2009, 118–124.
41. Yoshida M, Yamagami N, Tezuka T, Hondo R. Case report: detection of varicella-zoster virus DNA in maternal breast milk. *J Med Virol* 1992; 38:108–110.
42. Yoshida M, Tezuka T, Hiruma M. Detection of varicella-zoster virus DNA in maternal breast milk from a mother with herpes zoster. *Clin Diagn Virol* 1995; 4:61–65.
43. Pinot de Moira A, Edmunds WJ, Breuer J. The cost-effectiveness of antenatal varicella screening with post-partum vaccination of susceptibles. *Vaccine* 2006; 27:1298–1307.
44. Zheng Y, Lu Y, Ye Q, et al. Should chronic hepatitis B mothers breastfeed? A meta-analysis. *BMC Public Health* 2011; 11:502.
45. Shi Z, Yang Y, Wang H. Breastfeeding of newborns by mothers carrying hepatitis B virus: a meta-analysis and systematic review. *Arch Pediatr Adolesc Med* 2011; 165:837–846.
46. Isaacs D, Kilham HA, Alexander S, Wood N, Buckmaster A, Royle J. Ethical issues in preventing mother-to-child transmission of hepatitis B by immunisation. *Vaccine* 2011; 29:6159–6162.
47. Indolfi G, Resti M. Perinatal transmission of hepatitis C virus infection. *J Med Virol* 2009; 81:836–843.
48. Valladares G, Chacaltana A, Sjogren MH. The management of HCV-infected pregnant women. *Ann Hepatol* 2010; 9(Suppl):92–97.
49. Cottrell EB, Chou R, Wasson N, Rahman B, Guise J-M. Reducing risk for mother-to-infant transmission of hepatitis C virus: a systematic review for the U.S. Preventive Services Task Force. *Ann Intern Med* 2013; 158:109–113.
50. Wang LY, Chen CT, Liu WH, Wang YH. Recurrent neonatal group B streptococcal disease associated with infected breast milk. *Clin Pediatr (Phila)* 2007; 46:547–549.
51. Gagneur A, Héry-Arnaud G, Croly-Labourdette S, et al. Infected breast milk associated with late-onset and recurrent group B streptococcal infection in neonatal twins: a genetic analysis. *Eur J Pediatr* 2009; 168:1155–1158.
52. Jahanfar S, Ng CJ, Teng CL. Antibiotics for mastitis in breastfeeding women. *Cochrane Database Syst Rev* 2009, Issue 1. Art. No.: CD005458. doi: 10.1002/14651858.CD005458.pub2.
53. Crepinsek MA, Crowe L, Michener K, Smart NA. Interventions for preventing mastitis after childbirth. *Cochrane Database Syst Rev* 2012, Issue 10. Art. No.: CD007239. doi: 10.1002/14651858.CD007239.pub3.
54. Becker GE, Cooney F, Smith HA. Methods of milk expression for lactating women. *Cochrane Database Syst Rev* 2011, Issue 12. Art. No.: CD006170. doi: 10.1002/14651858.CD006170.pub3.
55. Donovan TJ, Buchanan K. Medications for increasing milk supply in mothers expressing breastmilk for their preterm hospitalised infants. *Cochrane Database Syst Rev* 2012, Issue 3. Art. No.: CD005544. doi: 10.1002/14651858.CD005544.pub2.
56. Cohen RS, Xiong SC, Sakamoto P. Retrospective review of serological testing of potential human milk donors. *Arch Dis Child Fetal Neonatal Ed* 2010; 95:F118—F120.
57. NHS National Institute for Health and Clinical Excellence (NICE). Donor breast milk banks: the operation of donor milk bank services. London, NICE clinical guideline 93, Feb 2010. Available at: http://www.nice.org.uk/nicemedia/pdf/CG93FullGuideline.pdf
58. Hartmann BT, Pang WW, Keil AD, Hartmann PE, Simmer K; Australian Neonatal Clinical Care Unit. Best practice guidelines for the operation of a donor human milk bank in an Australian NICU. *Early Hum Dev* 2007; 83:667–673.
59. Simmer K, Hartmann B. The knowns and unknowns of human milk banking. *Early Hum Dev* 2009; 85:701–704.
60. Centers for Disease Control. Breastfeeding. Recommendation. Other mother's milk. What to do if an infant or child is mistakenly fed another woman's expressed breast milk. Available at: http://www.cdc.gov/breastfeeding/recommendations/other_mothers_milk.htm.
61. Nahum GG, Uhl K, Kennedy DL. Antibiotic use in pregnancy and lactation: what is and is not known about teratogenic and toxic risks. *Obstet Gynecol* 2006; 107:1120–1138.

CHAPTER 20
Surveillance

The word 'surveillance' is often used in neonatal infections (French: *surveiller* = to watch over).[1] Although the term surveillance has come to have a somewhat sinister meaning in terms of international spying, in neonatal infections it means watching, recording and monitoring in order to guide actions.

Surveillance can be used to mean surveillance of microorganisms within neonatal units (by taking admission and regular surveillance cultures, Section 20.1), of systemic infections on the neonatal unit (Section 20.2) or of antibiotic use (Section 20.3).

20.1 Surveillance cultures

Surveillance cultures are time consuming and costly, and it is appropriate to question their use and to assess whether they are effective and cost-beneficial.

20.1.1 Respiratory tract cultures

The original aim of surveillance cultures was to predict the organism causing sepsis. The rationale was that knowing the potential pathogens colonizing an infant could allow targeted empiric antibiotic therapy if that infant developed suspected sepsis.

Endotracheal tube suction results in transient bacteraemia, in 3 of 10 artificially ventilated infants in one study,[2] raising etiologic implications for sepsis. Reports in the 1970s suggested that the 'abnormal' organisms, primarily coliforms, colonizing the endotracheal tube or nasopharynx of infants on artificial ventilation correlated well with the organisms causing systemic sepsis.[3,4] One report suggested that only infants with pharyngeal colonization with abnormal organisms developed systemic sepsis, whereas infants whose pharyngeal cultures grew nothing or 'normal respiratory flora' (predominantly α-haemolytic streptococci) did not develop systemic sepsis.[2] These old reports led to a tendency to treat infants colonized with coliforms or other potential pathogens, still occasionally practised even though antibiotics do not eliminate colonization or prevent infection. There is no evidence that treating colonization is anything but harmful.

Subsequent studies found a poor correlation between the organisms colonizing the endotracheal tube and those causing sepsis, finding the same organism in only around 20% of cases.[5–8] This questioned the utility of endotracheal or nasopharyngeal surveillance cultures. Endotracheal colonization increases with increasing duration of intubation and infants with sepsis are no more likely to be colonized than matched control infants without sepsis.[5,6,9] In a longitudinal study, 354 ventilated infants had daily tracheal aspirate cultures, and 48 (14%) became septic.[9] Of these, 14 had early bacteraemia, six had intra-abdominal pathology and 28 had late-onset sepsis of unknown cause. The sensitivity of tracheal cultures in predicting blood culture organisms was 71% for early sepsis, 50% for late intra-abdominal sepsis and 93% (26 of 28) for other late-onset sepsis (overall 81%). However, most infants who never developed sepsis also had positive endotracheal cultures. The authors concluded that the only value of tracheal aspirate cultures is providing information about potential pathogens when sepsis occurs.[9] A once-weekly culture provides virtually the same information, reducing workload for NICU and laboratory staff considerably.

Neonatal intensive care is changing and the use of surfactant has meant that it is possible to remove endotracheal tubes and use continuous positive airways pressure (CPAP) much earlier. Nevertheless, the major risk factor for late-onset sepsis in NICUs is extreme prematurity and infants <1500 g on respiratory support, even CPAP, remain among the infants at highest risk for sepsis.

Evidence-Based Neonatal Infections, First Edition. David Isaacs.

We recommend sending **once-weekly cultures of respiratory secretions** (endotracheal tube aspirate or nasopharyngeal secretions) from infants receiving respiratory support (level III neonatal intensive care) for two reasons:

(1) **To direct antibiotic therapy**: if an infant receiving respiratory support develops suspected late-onset sepsis, the clinician wants to know about the antibiotic sensitivity of colonizing organisms.

(2) **Infection control**: finding an infant colonized with a highly pathogenic (e.g. *Pseudomonas aeruginosa*) or multi-resistant organism (e.g. MRSA) should trigger screening of other infants to assess if the organism is widespread and trigger extra infection control measures, for example isolation and/or cohorting, to prevent an outbreak (see Chapter 21).

In many centres multi-resistant organism surveillance is mandated.

20.1.2 Surface cultures

The role of routine surveillance surface cultures was called into question colourfully by Fulginiti and Ray,[10] who called them "an exercise in futility, wastefulness and inappropriate practice" after a study showed unacceptably low sensitivity, specificity and positive predictive values.[11] Colonization with potential pathogens did not increase the risk of developing sepsis. Some colonized babies developed sepsis with different organisms.[10, 11] Furthermore, clinician choice of empiric antibiotics ignored surface culture results.[10, 11] A UK study showed the number of surface cultures could be reduced substantially without jeopardizing patient safety.[12]

Regarding developing countries, in studies from India[13] and Bangladesh[14] skin and mucosal surface cultures did not predict the organisms causing late sepsis. An Estonian study found low predictive value for routine rectal and nasopharyngeal cultures, but did find that infants colonized with certain Gram-negative organisms (*Pseudomonas*, *Klebsiella*, *E. coli* and *Stenotrophomonas*) were more likely to develop Gram-negative sepsis; the authors suggested targeted screening might be useful.[15]

Routine surveillance cultures are not necessarily useless, but respiratory tract cultures (endotracheal or nasopharyngeal aspirate cultures) are more reliable than skin surface cultures (Section 20.1.1).

20.1.3 Admission cultures

It is generally recommended that an infant being transferred from another institution, especially one with multi-resistant organisms, should be isolated pending surveillance admission culture results. If isolation facilities are not available, strict infection control procedures are recommended, emphasizing hand washing, to prevent transmission of multi-resistant organisms. MRSA screening of new admissions to prevent outbreaks is particularly important for NICUs with no MRSA-colonized infants.[16, 17] On the other hand, when the prevalence of MRSA in referring units is known to be low, the cost of screening may outweigh the benefits.[18]

20.2 Sepsis surveillance

Reasons for surveillance and regular review of episodes of systemic sepsis include the following.

(1) Appropriateness of empiric antibiotic regimens: for both early-onset and late-onset sepsis it is important to know that the empiric antibiotic regimens employed by the NICU (or by different consultants if practices differ) cover the organisms being isolated.

(2) Early-onset sepsis: the incidence of early-onset GBS sepsis and the number and proportion of cases whose mothers did not receive recommended screening and/or intra-partum antibiotics gives important information about the need for and the effectiveness of GBS prevention measures (see Section 14.1.1).

(3) Surveillance of central-line-associated bacteraemias (CLABs) provides important benchmark information about whether current strategies to prevent CLABs are effective or additional measures are needed.

(4) Surveillance of the incidence of late-onset sepsis allows benchmarking against previous years and against other neonatal units.

(5) Episodes of sepsis with multi-resistant organisms (e.g. MRSA, ESBL-producing Gram-negative bacilli) and organisms of high virulence (e.g. *Pseudomonas*) have infection control implications.

(6) A high incidence of fungal infections should prompt review of policies on antibiotics and early enteral feeding, and duration of parenteral nutrition and endotracheal intubation (see Chapter 16).

(7) Changes in outcome of sepsis, particularly deaths, should prompt reflection on likely causes

(e.g. increased organism virulence, delayed clinical response).

20.2.1 Surveillance of central-line-associated bacteraemia

Surveillance of CLABs or central-line-associated bloodstream infections (CLABSIs) is mandated in some jurisdictions,[19] to allow benchmarking between neonatal units, to detect changes in incidence over time, and to assess the need for additional preventative measures.[20]

Essentially a CLAB or CLABSI is a bloodstream infection occurring in an infant with a central line in place where there is no other explanation for the infection. The current Centers for Disease Control and Prevention (CDC) National Nosocomial Infections Surveillance (NNIS) CLABSI definition is a significant bloodstream infection (fungaemia or bacteraemia) with no other apparent focus of infection where a central line has been *in situ* within 48 hours of the event.[20] An infant with a central line who develops necrotizing enterocolitis and whose blood cultures grow an enteric Gram-negative bacillus does not have a CLAB(SI), because an enteric origin of sepsis is probable.

Diagnostic difficulties include the complexity[19, 21] and multiplicity of definitions used in different studies, complicating comparisons.[22] Definitions vary according to the need for positive blood cultures to be collected peripherally or from the central line or catheter tip. There can be problems of interpretation when empiric antibiotics are given and a single blood culture grows a potential skin contaminant.

Interestingly, a German study found infants <1500 g had the same increased risk of bloodstream infection with peripheral venous cannulas as with central venous catheters compared with infants not needing IV access.[23] This suggests the neonate sick enough to need IV access is the problem not the central venous catheter.

In a non-Cochrane review, rates of CLAB ranged from 2.6 to 60 cases per 1000 central line days. CLABs were generally associated with increased mortality; odds ratios ranged from 2.8 to 9.5.[24] Six prospective before-and-after intervention studies showed that hand hygiene and educational programmes significantly reduced rates of CLAB. CLAB rates are higher in countries with limited resources and have a significant impact on mortality. It is important to use practical, low-cost, low-technology measures to prevent CLABs in low-income countries and to use surveillance to show that such interventions are effective.[23] There is strong evidence that many CLABs are preventable (see Chapter 23). Problems of definition do not negate the importance of CLAB surveillance.

20.2.2 Surveillance of nosocomial infections

Nosocomial infection surveillance aims to identify rising and/or unacceptably high nosocomial infection rates. Useful comparisons with other units depend on clear definitions of nosocomial infection.[25, 26] Definitions that include 'possible' or 'clinical' culture-negative sepsis will include infants without true sepsis, preventing valid comparison between different units or different countries. It is recommended strongly, therefore, to restrict surveillance to culture-proven episodes of nosocomial bacteraemia or meningitis. As discussed in Chapter 2, even comparison of rates of proven bacteraemia or meningitis can be complicated by differential exclusion or inclusion criteria for possible or likely contaminants.

In a 1999 US National Nosocomial Infections Surveillance System (NNISS) study of >13 000 nosocomial neonatal infections in 99 hospitals, the most frequent nosocomial infections in all birth-weight groups were bloodstream infections, followed by nosocomial pneumonia, then infections of the gastrointestinal tract, eye, ear, nose and throat.[25] CoNS were the most common pathogen, followed by *S. aureus*, enterococci, *Enterobacter* and *E. coli*. CoNS caused 58% of all nosocomial bloodstream infections and 88% of episodes of CoNS bacteraemia were associated with umbilical or central intravenous catheters.[25]

A Dutch single-centre study reported similar data.[27] The study used new definitions of neonatal nosocomial infections,[28] modified from CDC definitions for children <1 year of age and including the Clinical Risk Index for Babies (CRIB) severity score, which has been shown to have a reasonable correlation with risk of bacteraemia.[29] Bloodstream infection and pneumonia predominated; 59% of bloodstream infections were caused by CoNS. Enterobacteriaceae were identified as causing 25% of episodes of pneumonia. The main risk factors for nosocomial bloodstream infection were low birth weight and parenteral nutrition. The CRIB score did not predict nosocomial infections in a sub-group of infants <1500 g.[27]

In a study of nosocomial infections in six Italian neonatal units, the risk factors for nosocomial infection in neonates <1500 g were CPAP, a CRIB score of four or greater and gestation <28 weeks. For heavier neonates, the main risk factors were parenteral nutrition and congenital malformations.[30]

Surveillance of the incidence of nosocomial infections is time-consuming and its cost-effectiveness debatable.[1] An alternative to longitudinal surveillance is to use point-prevalence surveys to ascertain and compare rates of nosocomial infection in neonates on a single day.[31] One advantage of a point-prevalence survey that includes all in-patients is the ability to compare infected with non-infected patients to identify the risk factors for nosocomial infection. A point-prevalence survey in 29 US NICUs identified duration of stay, central intravascular catheters and parenteral nutrition as independent risk factors for nosocomial infection.[31]

20.2.3 Ventilator-associated pneumonia

Ventilator-associated pneumonia (VAP) is the second most frequently reported nosocomial infection in neonatal[25, 27] and paediatric[32, 33] intensive care units. Surveillance of VAP in neonatal units, however, is plagued by difficulties in its definition and diagnosis (see Chapter 8).[34] Recurrent, often transient, chest radiographic abnormalities are common with prolonged artificial ventilation and their interpretation (VAP or no VAP?) problematic.

A US prospective cohort study reported VAP rates of 6.5 per 1000 ventilator days for infants <28 weeks of gestation and 4 per 1000 ventilator days for infants ≥28 weeks. VAP was an independent predictor of mortality (OR 3.4; 95% CI 1.2–12.3) and the relative risk was 8 for neonates who stayed in the NICU >30 days. Patients with VAP stayed longer in the NICU than other infants (median: 138 vs 82 days).[35]

A retrospective Chinese cohort study of 259 NICU infants ventilated >48 hours reported 52 episodes of VAP (20.1%). The main pathogens identified were Gram-negative bacilli. Hospital stay was prolonged, but the mortality rate of the VAP group was no higher than controls (13.5% vs 12.1%). VAP was independently associated with re-intubation, duration of mechanical ventilation, endotracheal suctioning and treatment with opiates.[36]

In a Swiss NICU study, the rate of VAP in ventilated infants (12.5 of 1000 ventilator days) was significantly higher than the rate of pneumonia for infants on CPAP (1.8 of 1000 patient days).[37]

Prevention strategies have been proposed.[24] However, in many Western countries increased surfactant use has already virtually eradicated VAP,[37] rendering VAP surveillance unnecessary.

20.3 Antibiotic surveillance

Surveillance of antibiotic use is not widely advocated. Patterns of antibiotic use will depend on patient mix which will influence comparisons of antibiotic use between different hospitals. Nevertheless, antibiotic use surveillance in an institution can identify important changes over time and inter-hospital comparisons are possible.

In the adult literature, antibiotic use is usually expressed using the World Health Organization's defined daily doses (DDD).[38] DDD are based on a standard body weight and are not applicable to children because their body weight varies enormously, although one group used unmodified adult DDD to compare antibiotic use in different neonatal units.[39] An alternative is to use neonatal DDD based on a standard body weight of 2 kg.[40] However, the range of weights on most neonatal units varies from <500 g to >4 kg, calling this approach into question. Another alternative is to add up the total weight of an antibiotic prescribed to an NICU over a given period and divide it by the number of treatment days to give a drug use density.[41] In one study, the drug use density differed between units and was greater than the adult DDD per 100 days.[41] None of these methods takes into account adequately variations in the birth weights of neonates on different units. Since the best metric for assessing resistance-selection pressure is arguably a patient day on a given antibiotic, an important alternative is to express antibiotic use as the sum of days of antibiotics prescribed divided by the sum of the number of patient days over a given period. A figure of 25% means each baby spends an average of one in every 4 days on antibiotics. This method was used to show a 40% reduction in antibiotic use, attributed to the regular attendance on neonatal ward rounds of a paediatric infectious disease trainee who

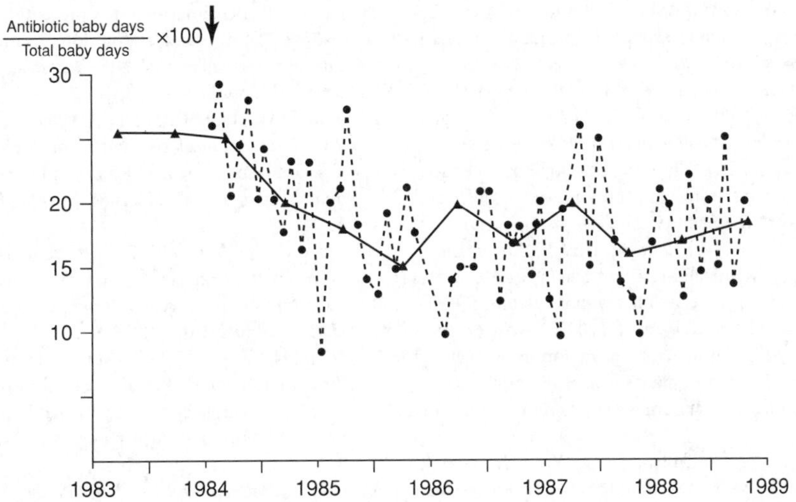

Figure 20.1 Antibiotic use over time expressed as the proportion of total infant days spent receiving antibiotics in Oxford NICU (adapted from Reference 42). The dotted line joins the monthly figure, while the continuous line joins the 6-monthly data. The arrow represents the date regular infectious disease ward rounds started.

continually questioned the need to continue prescribing antibiotics in the face of negative systemic cultures (Figure 20.1).[42]

Other measurements of antibiotic use that may be informative are the mean and median duration of antibiotic courses and the proportion of infants admitted to an NICU who ever received antibiotics. These measurements are probably most relevant for audit in an NICU where the case mix remains similar over time or for comparing different NICUs with similar patient case mix.

The above data only capture the extent and duration of antibiotic use. It may also be advisable to capture data on antibiotic days of broad spectrum antibiotic use, acknowledging that limited use of broad spectrum antibiotics may be necessary if there are concerns about antibiotic resistant organisms.

References

1. Gray JW. Surveillance of infection in neonatal intensive care units. *Early Hum Dev* 2007; 83:157–163.
2. Storm W. Transient bacteraemia following endotracheal suctioning in ventilated newborns. *Pediatrics* 1980; 65:487–490.
3. Harris H, Wirtschafter D, Cassady G. Endotracheal intubation and its relationship to bacterial colonization and systemic infection of newborn infants. *Pediatrics* 1976; 58:816–823.
4. Sprunt K, Leidy G, Redman W. Abnormal colonization of neonates in an intensive care unit: means of identifying neonates at risk of infection. *Pediatr Res* 1978; 12:998–1002.
5. Sherman MP, Chance KH, Goetzman BW. Gram's stains of tracheal secretions predict neonatal bacteraemia. *Am J Dis Child* 1984; 138:848–850.
6. Slagle TA, Bifano EM, Wolf JW, Gross SJ. Routine endotracheal cultures for the prediction of sepsis in ventilated babies. *Arch Dis Child* 1989; 64:34–38.
7. Webber S, Lindsell D, Wilkinson AR, Hope PL, Dobson SRM, Isaacs D. Neonatal pneumonia. *Arch Dis Child* 1990; 65:207–211.
8. Srinivasan HB, Vidyasagar D. Endotracheal aspirate cultures in predicting sepsis in ventilated neonates. *Indian J Pediatr* 1998; 65:79–84.
9. Bozaykut A, Ipek IO, Kilic BD. Predicting neonatal sepsis in ventilated neonates. *Indian J Pediatr* 2008; 75:39–42.
10. Fulginiti VA, Ray GG. Body surface cultures in the newborn infant. An exercise in futility, wastefulness and inappropriate practice. *Am J Dis Child* 1988; 142:19–20.
11. Evans ME, Schaffner W, Federspiel CF, Cotton RB, McKee Jr KT, Stratton CW. Sensitivity, specificity, and predictive value of body surface cultures in a neonatal intensive care unit. *J Am Med Assoc* 1988; 259:248–252.
12. Dobson S, Isaacs D, Wilkinson A, et al. Reduced use of surface cultures for suspected neonatal sepsis and surveillance is safe. *Arch Dis Child* 1992; 67:44–47.
13. Puri J, Revathi G, Faridi MM, Talwar V, Kumar A, Parkash B. Role of body surface cultures in prediction of sepsis in a neonatal intensive care unit. *Ann Trop Paediatr* 1995; 15:307–311.

14. Choi Y, Saha SK, Ahmed AS, et al. Routine skin cultures in predicting sepsis pathogens among hospitalized preterm neonates in Bangladesh. *Neonatology* 2008; 94:123–131.
15. Parm Ü, Metsvaht T, Sepp E, et al. Mucosal surveillance cultures in predicting Gram-negative late-onset sepsis in neonatal intensive care units. *J Hosp Infect* 2011; 78:327–332.
16. Dobson SR, Isaacs D, Wilkinson AR, Hope PL. Reduced use of surface cultures for suspected neonatal sepsis and surveillance. *Arch Dis Child* 1992; 67:44–47.
17. McDonald JR, Carriker CM, Pien BC, Trinh JV, Engemann JJ, Harrell LJ, et al. Methicillin-resistant *Staphylococcus aureus* outbreak in an intensive care nursery: potential for interinstitutional spread. *Pediatr Infect Dis J* 2007; 26:678–683.
18. Al Reyami E, Al Zoabi K, Rahmani A, Tamim M, Chedid F. Is isolation of outborn infants required at admission to the neonatal intensive care unit? *Am J Infect Control* 2009; 37:335–357.
19. Sarda V, Molloy A, Kadkol S, Janda WM, Hershow R, McGuinn M. Active surveillance for methicillin-resistant *Staphylococcus aureus* in the neonatal intensive care unit. *Infect Control Hosp Epidemiol* 2009; 30:854–860.
20. CDC. Device-associated module. Central Line-Associated Bloodstream Infection (CLABSI) Event. Centers for Disease Control, 2012. Available at: http://www.cdc.gov/nhsn/PDFs/pscManual/4PSC_CLABScurrent.pdf.
21. O'Grady NP, Alexander M, Burns LA, et al. Healthcare Infection Control Practices Advisory Committee (HICPAC). Guidelines for the prevention of intravascular catheter-related infections, 2011. CDC, 2011. Available at: http://www.cdc.gov/hicpac/pdf/guidelines/bsi-guidelines-2011.pdf.
22. Worth LJ, Brett J, Bull AL, McBryde ES, Russo PL, Richards MJ. Impact of revising the National Nosocomial Infection Surveillance System definition for catheter-related bloodstream infection in ICU: reproducibility of the National Healthcare Safety Network case definition in an Australian cohort of infection control professionals. *Am J Infect Control* 2009; 37:643–648.
23. Tomlinson D, Mermel LA, Ethier M-C, Anne Matlow A, Gillmeister B, Sung L. Defining bloodstream infections related to central venous catheters in patients with cancer: a systematic review. *Clin Infect Dis* 2011; 53:697–710.
24. Geffers C, Gastmeier A, Schwab F, Groneberg K, Rüden H, Gastmeier P. Use of central venous catheter and peripheral venous catheter as risk factors for nosocomial bloodstream infection in very-low-birth-weight infants. *Infect Control Hosp Epidemiol* 2010; 31:395–401.
25. Rosenthal VD. Central line-associated bloodstream infections in limited-resource countries: a review of the literature. *Clin Infect Dis* 2009; 49:1899–1907.
26. Richards MJ, Edwards JR, Culver DH, Gaynes RP. Nosocomial infections in pediatric intensive care units in the United States. National Nosocomial Infections Surveillance System. *Pediatrics* 1999; 103:e39.
27. van der Zwet WC, Kaiser AM, van Elburg RM, et al. Nosocomial infections in a Dutch neonatal intensive care unit: surveillance study with definitions for infection specifically adapted for neonates. *J Hosp Infect* 2005; 61:300–311.
28. Jarvis WR. Benchmarking for prevention: the Centers for Disease Control and Prevention's National Nosocomial Infections Surveillance (NNIS) system experience. *Infection* 2003; 31(Suppl 2):44–48.
29. Fowlie PW, Gould CR, Parry GJ, Phillips G, Tarnow-Mordi WO. CRIB (clinical risk index for babies) in relation to nosocomial bacteraemia in very low birthweight or preterm infants. *Arch Dis Child Fetal Neonatal Ed* 1996; 75:F49–F52.
30. Auriti C, Ronchetti MP, Pezzotti P, et al. Determinants of nosocomial infection in 6 neonatal intensive care units: an Italian multicenter prospective cohort study. *Infect Control Hosp Epidemiol* 2010; 31:926–933.
31. Sohn AH, Garrett DO, Sinkowitz-Cochran RL, et al. Pediatric Prevention Network. Prevalence of nosocomial infections in neonatal intensive care unit patients: Results from the first national point-prevalence survey. *J Pediatr* 2001; 139:821–827.
32. Foglia E, Meier MD, Elward A. Ventilator-associated pneumonia in neonatal and pediatric intensive care unit patients. *Clin Microbiol Rev* 2007; 20:409–425.
33. Garland JS. Strategies to prevent ventilator-associated pneumonia in neonates. *Clin Perinatol* 2010; 37:629–643.
34. CDC. Device-associated events. Ventilator-Associated Pneumonia Event. Centers for Disease Control, 2012. Available at: http://www.cdc.gov/nhsn/PDFs/pscManual/6pscVAPcurrent.pdf.
35. Apisarnthanarak A, Holzmann-Pazgal G, Hamvas A, Olsen MA, Fraser VJ. Ventilator-associated pneumonia in extremely preterm neonates in a neonatal intensive care unit: characteristics, risk factors, and outcomes. *Pediatrics* 2003; 112:1283–1289.
36. Yuan TM, Chen LH, Yu HM. Risk factors and outcomes for ventilator-associated pneumonia in neonatal intensive care unit patients. *J Perinat Med* 2007; 35:334–338.
37. Hentschel J, Brüngger B, Stüdi K, Mühlemann K. Prospective surveillance of nosocomial infections in a Swiss NICU: low risk of pneumonia on nasal continuous positive airway pressure? *Infection* 2005; 33:350–355.
38. WHO Collaborating Centre for Drug Statistics Methodology. Anatomical Therapeutic Chemical (ATC) Classification System: Guidelines for ATC Classification and DDD Assignment. http://www.whocc.no/atcddd/.
39. Liem TB, Krediet TG, Fleer A, Egberts TC, Rademaker CM. Variation in antibiotic use in neonatal intensive care units in the Netherlands. *J Antimicrob Chemother* 2010; 65:1270–1275.
40. Liem TB, Heerdink ER, Egberts AC, Rademaker CM. Quantifying antibiotic use in paediatrics: a proposal for neonatal DDDs. *Eur J Clin Microbiol Infect Dis* 2010; 29:1301–1313.
41. Valcourt K, Norozian F, Lee H, Raszynski A, Torbati D, Totapally BR. Drug use density in critically ill children and newborns: analysis of various methodologies. *Pediatr Crit Care Med* 2009; 10:495–499.
42. Isaacs D, Wilkinson AR, Moxon ER. Duration of antibiotic courses for neonates. *Arch Dis Child* 1987; 62:727–728.

CHAPTER 21
Infection control

21.1 Infection control programmes

All neonatal units know the importance of infection control measures, particularly hand washing, to reduce transmission of pathogens and need infection control programmes. However, there is considerable variation in the degree to which infection control is promoted, implemented, assessed, and reinforced. NICU outbreaks of neonatal infection are regularly attributed to breakdowns in good infection control practice. Ideally, hospitals have formal infection control programmes with regular education programmes covering hand washing and hygienic care of invasive devices such as intravascular catheters, with review of hand-washing compliance and rates of central-line associated bloodstream infections; and feedback combined with education to improve compliance.

Standard precautions protect any hospitalized patient against nosocomial infections. Transmission-based precautions are special precautions for patients colonized or infected with a pathogen deemed epidemiologically important in terms of transmissibility and/or virulence.

21.2 Standard precautions

Standard precautions apply to all hospital patients. They reduce transmission of organisms within hospitals using hygienic care of blood, body fluids, urine, faeces, and secretions (not sweat) and care when handling broken skin and mucous membranes.

21.2.1 Hand hygiene

The evidence that hand washing prevents nosocomial infections (see Section 23.2.1) and the value (or otherwise) of other infection control interventions such as gloves and gowns (see Section 23.2) is considered in Chapter 23. Neonatal units generally comply better with hand hygiene than paediatric intensive care units and general paediatric wards, but there is evidence that education, regular audits and feedback of compliance rates improve performance.[1]

Studies repeatedly show transmission of pathogens in neonatal units on the hands of staff.[2] Many outbreaks of neonatal infection have been attributed to poor staff hand hygiene, including Enterobacteriaceae (e.g. Klebsiella,[3,4] Serratia,[5,6] Enterobacter[7,8]), non-fermenters (e.g. Acinetobacter,[9,10] Pseudomonas,[11–13] Stenotrophomonas[14,15]) and MRSA.[16,17] Although Gram-negative bacilli can be carried on the hands of staff to infants, molecular evidence shows the Gram-negative bacilli causing invasive infections are often not detected on the hands of nursing staff or other infants.[18,19] Therefore, to reduce the incidence of Gram-negative bacillary neonatal infections, we may need to address the possibility of transmission from endogenous neonatal flora or environmental sources.

21.2.2 Intravenous catheter care

The Healthcare Infection Control Practices Advisory Committee (HICPAC) of the US Centers for Disease Control (CDC) publishes detailed, evidence-based guidelines on minimizing the risk of nosocomial infections covering the site of insertion, skin preparation and catheter care for peripheral and central catheters.[20]

Evidence-Based Neonatal Infections, First Edition. David Isaacs.

(Available free on www.cdc.gov/hicpac/pdf/guidelines/bsi-guidelines-2011.pdf).

21.3 Transmission-based precautions

21.3.1 Contact precautions

Contact precautions aim to prevent transmission of a potential pathogen from a colonized or infected infant to other infants. Potential pathogens include multi-resistant bacteria (e.g. MRSA, resistant Gram-negative bacilli), highly pathogenic bacteria (e.g. Pseudomonas) or viruses transmitted on hands (e.g. HSV, RSV). There is no good evidence that wearing gowns (see Section 23.2.2) or gloves (see Section 23.2.3) prevents nosocomial infections more than hand washing alone. Although some guidelines mandate wearing gloves and gowns for all contact precautions, they rarely quote rationale or evidence. Gloves and gowns are expensive, in terms of time and comfort as well as financially.

Wearing gloves, however, can be important to protect specific health-care workers from infection if the skin on their hands is broken due to eczema or cuts.

21.3.1.1 Cohorting

Patients needing contact precautions should only spread organisms to other patients on hands of staff, so hand washing alone should suffice. However, despite best intentions, no neonatal unit achieves 100% hand washing. Ideally, therefore, a patient requiring contact precautions should be placed in an isolation room, but these are often scarce. In their absence, infants infected or colonized with the same organism may need to be nursed in the same room or the same area of the nursery, a practice called 'cohorting'. Staffing permitting, nurses should also be cohorted: any one nurse only looks after infants colonized with the same organism or only looks after infants who are known not to be colonized. Newborn infants are cohorted with non-colonized infants.

21.3.2 Respiratory precautions

Respiratory precautions to prevent or reduce transmission of respiratory pathogens, are either droplet or airborne precautions, depending on particle size.[21]

21.3.2.1 Droplet precautions

Droplet precautions are for infections involving coughing or sneezing or where transmission can occur due to aerosols generated by respiratory care. Droplets are large and do not remain in the air long but can infect close contacts directly via the nasopharyngeal mucosa or conjunctiva. Droplet precautions comprise patient isolation, ideally in a single room with closed door, but otherwise by appropriate patient separation (at least 1 m bed separation with curtains closed). Droplet precautions are recommended for influenza and other respiratory viruses except RSV, for pertussis, and early in the course of meningococcal infection.[21] Staff should wear masks for personal protection unless immune.

21.3.2.2 Airborne precautions

Pathogens or spores carried on droplet nuclei or dust particles can remain airborne for long periods and travel long distances on natural air currents or currents generated by ventilation systems without filters. Airborne precautions ideally use special isolation rooms with negative air-pressure ventilation and high-efficiency particulate air (HEPA) filters or an external exhaust system. Staff should wear masks unless immune (e.g. to varicella). Airborne precautions are recommended for highly contagious airborne respiratory viruses such as measles and VZV and for TB (Section 21.4).

21.4 Environmental and workforce issues

21.4.1 Environmental

Recommendations and guidelines have been published about the ideal design and layout of NICUs.[22, 23] They specify the spacing between cots, the width of aisles, the proximity of sinks, and the cleaning properties of environmental surface (Figure 21.1). Guidelines may support clinicians negotiating with administrators, but evidence for the specifications is weak. Before and after studies support the argument that the physical environment is important, but the study design is not strong. For example, in a longitudinal US study the nosocomial infection rate fell from 5.6% on an old NICU with inadequate facilities to 0.9% when the unit moved to a new facility with isolation facilities, more

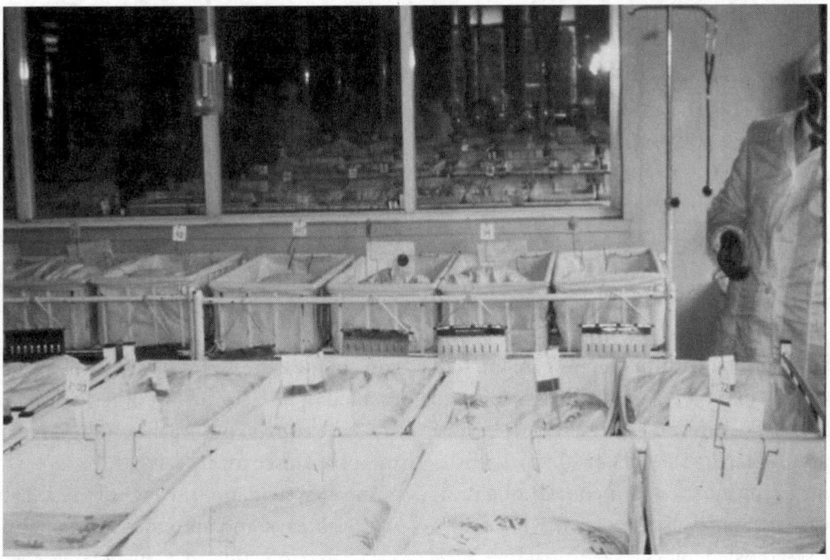

Figure 21.1 Crowding on a neonatal unit in a developing country which was experiencing an outbreak of *Staphylococcus aureus* infection. Note the cots in close proximity and no sinks visible.

sinks and more space between infants.[24] However, the unit also had 50% more nurses.[24]

21.4.2 Workload

The transmission of gentamicin-resistant Gram-negative bacilli on a UK NICU did not correlate with antibiotic use but correlated with two indicators of workload (Figure 21.2).[25] Transmission correlated with the number of unit baby days each week and even better with a score which also took into account the level of nursing care.[25]

One problem with assessing workload is that sicker infants require intensive nursing. NICUs with high-risk infants need more nursing staff and a higher

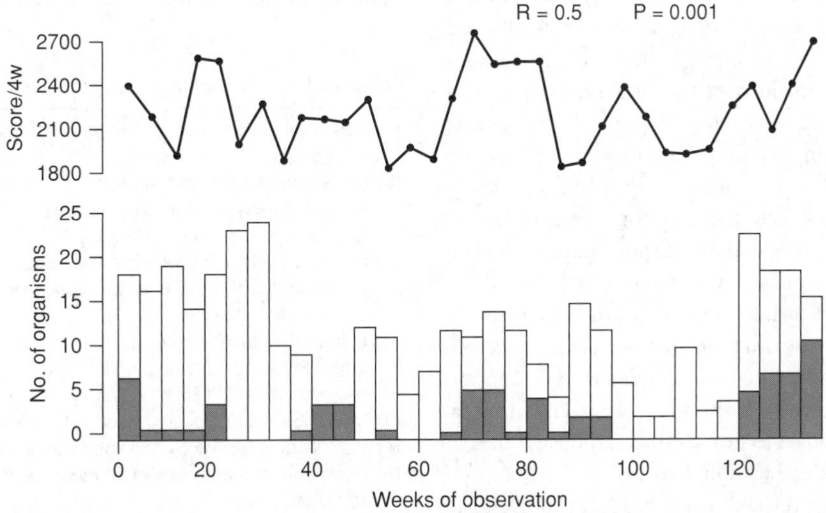

Figure 21.2 Significant association between workload score (top line) and transmission of antibiotic-resistant Gram-negative bacilli on a neonatal unit. Reprinted with permission from Reference 25.

nurse:patient ratio than NICUs looking after low-risk infants. However, less mature, high-risk infants are at increased risk of nosocomial infections. A large prospective UK study looked at outcomes in relation to patient volume, staffing and workload in 186 NICUs and attempted to adjust the outcomes for risk. The incidence of nosocomial bacteraemia increased with increasing patient volume.[26]

Two studies examined the effect of nursing workload on mortality but not specifically on nosocomial infections.[27, 28] An Australian single-centre study found improved infant survival with the highest infant/staff ratio.[27] A UK study of 54 NICUs found risk-adjusted mortality was inversely related to having specialist neonatal nurses (OR 0.67; 95% CI 0.42–0.97). Increasing the ratio to 1:1 of nurses with neonatal qualifications to high-risk infants was associated with a 48% decrease in risk-adjusted mortality (OR: 0.52, 95% CI 0.33, 0.83).[28] These studies emphasize the need for adequate staffing with specialist neonatal nurses. Hand washing by nurses[29] and physicians[30] deteriorates with increased workload. This largely explains the increased incidence of nosocomial infections with increasing workload, and shows adequate staffing of neonatal units is critical to prevent nosocomial infections.

21.5 Outbreak management

What constitutes an outbreak? Logically an outbreak should refer to more than one related case of infection on a neonatal unit. Clinically, however, an 'outbreak' might refer to a situation requiring an immediate enhanced infection control response. On occasion, a single infant developing sepsis (or even colonization) with a virulent organism, for example Pseudomonas (Section 21.5.1) or pertussis (Section 21.9), might suggest the need for action to prevent an outbreak. Similarly, diagnosing TB or varicella in a parent or staff member requires immediate action. In contrast, in some situations (e.g. a cluster of necrotizing enterocolitis in high-risk infants with no common organism identified and no known precipitating factors) a vigorous infection control response is likely to increase workload without benefit.

A systematic review[31] used the Outbreak Database, a free worldwide database for nosocomial outbreaks (available on www.outbreak-database.com), to compare neonatal nosocomial infection outbreaks with those occurring in other intensive care units. The authors reviewed 276 outbreaks from NICUs and 453 from other ICUs. Enterobacteriaceae were responsible for NICU outbreaks significantly more often than in other ICUs, where non-fermenters predominated. On average, 23.9 patients and 1.8 health-care workers were involved in NICU outbreaks. The average mortality in NICU outbreaks was 6.4% (1.5 newborns on average). In 48.6% of NICU outbreaks the authors were unable to identify the source. The most important infection control measures were significantly more often implemented in NICUs than in other ICUs. Currently there are 328 neonatal outbreaks on the database, which is a useful resource for research.[31]

In a systematic review of 125 articles regarding outbreaks and sporadic incidents of health-care-associated infections, Gram-positive cocci, viruses and fungi predominated in reports from Western units, while Gram-negative enteric bacilli, non-fermenters and fungi predominated in resource-poor settings.[32] Most outbreaks in either Western or developing countries were attributed to poor infection control practices.[32]

Table 21.1 outlines a suggested approach to outbreaks.[33, 34] A common question is whether or not to investigate for an environmental source. Outbreaks caused by water-loving organisms are more likely to have an environmental source and the possibility of a common environmental source should be considered

Table 21.1 Guidelines for management of an outbreak.

(1) Decide whether or not an outbreak or the potential for an outbreak exists

(2) If yes, convene meeting to decide:
- **a** is there likely to be a common source
- **b** where to nurse index case(s)
- **c** how to protect uninfected infants (and staff)
- **d** how to detect new cases, for example stool cultures for gram-negative bacilli
- **e** how often to meet to evaluate outcomes
- **f** how to record the outbreak: infected and uninfected persons, place and time

(3) Notify hospital and public health authorities if necessary

(4) Institute necessary infection control interventions

(5) Decide on frequency of regular meetings to assess the extent of outbreak

(6) Meet regularly and assess progress

(7) Decide when outbreak has ended

Table 21.2 Usual modes of spread of outbreaks, including environmental sources.

Organism	Usual mode of spread	Possible environmental sources
Acinetobacter	Hands of staff	Parenteral nutrition
Burkholderia	Hands of staff	Sinks, humidifiers, CVCs
Enterobacter cloacae	Hands of staff	Multiple dose medications
Enterobacter sakazakii	Powdered milk formula	
Klebsiella	Hands of staff	IV fluids, breast pump, disinfectant
MRSA	Hands of staff	Staff nasal carriage ('cloud adults')
Pseudomonas	Hands of staff	Sinks, taps/faucets, water bath, hand lotion
Salmonella	Hands of staff	Resuscitator, thermometer
Serratia	Hands of staff	Soap, shampoo, breast milk, breast pump, feeds, etc. (see Section 26.6.1)
Staphylococcus aureus	Hands of staff	Staff nasal carriage ('cloud adults')
Vancomycin-resistant enterococci	Hands of staff	

CVC, central venous catheter; IV, intravenous; MRSA, methicillin-resistant *S. aureus.*

earlier in outbreaks due to non-fermentative and other Gram-negative bacilli. Common modes of spread are outlined in Table 21.2.

21.6 Outbreaks due to non-fermentative Gram-negative bacilli

21.6.1 Pseudomonas

Most outbreaks of *P. aeruginosa* infections occur due to transmission on the hands of staff,[35] and unless there is a clear risk factor, intensive investigations for environmental sources are not recommended immediately. However, Pseudomonas are water-loving organisms and outbreaks of Pseudomonas outbreaks have been linked to water outlets including tap water which can be both the result and cause of hand colonization,[35, 36] faucets (taps)[37, 38] including electronic faucets,[38] and sinks.[39] Because organisms are transmitted from water outlets on the hands of staff, improved hand hygiene may suffice to terminate the outbreak. Other outbreaks of *P. aeruginosa* infection have been linked epidemiologically to a water bath used to thaw fresh frozen plasma,[40] contaminated hand lotion[41] and a contaminated blood gas analyser.[42]

Staff colonization may contribute to Pseudomonas outbreaks and should be considered. In an investigation of endemic *P. aeruginosa* on an NICU, staff with artificial fingernails and staff with nail wraps were more likely to have colonized hands and a healthcare worker with onychomycosis carried the epidemic strain.[43] Another outbreak was linked to a staff member with recurrent otitis externa with *P. aeruginosa.*[44]

Feeds may rarely cause Pseudomonas outbreaks. An outbreak of *P. aeruginosa* in a Spanish NICU was caused by contaminated feeding bottles prepared in the hospital feeding room.[45] In France an outbreak of 31 cases of *P. aeruginosa* infection including four deaths was caused by a contaminated milk bank pasteurizer and bottle warmer.[46]

Neonatal *P. aeruginosa* bacteraemia has a >50% mortality (see Section 14.2.7). Although most infants colonized with *P. aeruginosa* do not develop sepsis, it is an unwelcome colonizing organism on neonatal units. Identifying one colonized infant should raise consideration of precautions (isolating the infant and screening other infants for carriage) to prevent a possible outbreak.

Environmental pseudomonads are often contaminants and can sometimes cause pseudo-outbreaks or outbreaks of pseudo-bacteraemia. In one such pseudo-outbreak, multi-resistant pseudomonads were cultured from several infants using in-house culture media but not from commercial media. The in-house media, stored under the sink, was thought to have been contaminated by water splashed from the sink.[47] A pseudo-outbreak should be suspected when environmental pseudomonads are isolated in blood cultures from relatively well infants. However, environmental pseudomonads can cause central-line-associated infections occasionally. Reported outbreaks of infections with environmental pseudomonads may have been true or pseudo-outbreaks.[48]

21.6.2 Acinetobacter

Acinetobacter are non-motile, non-fermenting, aerobic Gram-negative coccobacilli found in soil and fresh water.[49] Outbreaks of infection on neonatal units are generally thought to be transmitted on the hands of staff.[50, 51] A systematic review of invasive Acinetobacter infections described 18 outbreaks, 16 of them in neonatal units, mostly causing bacteraemia and sometimes meningitis.[52] The outbreaks were caused by multiple different species, mainly *A. baumannii* (6 outbreaks) and *A. calcoaceticus* (5). Multi-drug resistant strains are increasingly reported.[50, 51] Many studies describe isolation of Acinetobacter from environmental sources including air conditioners, suction catheters and dressings and hands of health-care workers, but typing was not usually performed to confirm whether patient and environmental strains were identical.[52] In the only study which clearly showed that an environmental source caused an outbreak, an Acinetobacter strain was isolated from total parenteral nutrition solution.[53] An outbreak with a highly resistant Acinetobacter strain should trigger review of the empiric antibiotic regimen, which may need changing until the outbreak resolves.[51, 54]

21.6.3 *Burkholderia cepacia*

Neonatal outbreaks of *B. cepacia* have been linked with central venous catheters[55] and *B. cepacia* has been grown in environmental samples from the water in a delivery room oxygen humidifier; from ventilator water traps and a humidifier water trap in the neonatal unit;[54] and from sinks.[56] It is an environmental organism which can also cause pseudo-outbreaks of bacteraemia (or outbreaks of pseudo-bacteraemia),[57, 58] including one associated with a contaminated blood gas analyser.[57] Junior doctors collecting precious blood samples sometimes use the same syringe to inject blood into a blood gas analyser and then into blood culture bottles, causing pseudo-outbreaks.

21.7 Outbreaks due to Enterobacteriaceae

The Enterobacteriaceae are an important cause of nosocomial infections and of neonatal unit outbreaks. As their name suggests they are enteric organisms although can colonize the respiratory tract. They can all carry plasmid genes coding for extended spectrum β-lactamases (ESBLs).[59]

21.7.1 *Serratia marcescens*

S. marcescens is a hardy Gram-negative bacillus. The organism is usually transmitted via the hands of staff,[60, 61] but outbreaks have been linked with contaminated soap,[62–64] hand-washing brushes,[65] baby shampoo[66] and multi-dose bottles of liquid theophylline.[67] Outbreaks have been associated with feeds using contaminated milk bottles,[67] enteral feed additives[68] and breast pumps.[69, 70] Serratia produces a red pigment (which has been described to be a cause of the appearance of apparent blood-stained 'stigmata' on religious statues). *S. marcescens* may be grown from breast milk,[71] including one mother who reported her breast pump tubing had turned bright pink.[72] Contaminated delivery room tocogram transducers were the suspected source in one outbreak[67] and laryngoscopes[73] in another. Serratia was isolated from air conditioning ducts during one outbreak although the mode of spread was unclear.[74]

A systematic review of 34 outbreaks of *S. marcescens* in NICUs and PICUs, using genotyping to determine clonality, concluded that two or more temporally related cases of nosocomial infection should raise the suspicion of an outbreak.[59] The authors recommended enhanced infection control measures, including nursery screening of infants (with regular stool samples) and cohorting of colonized infants, as the initial outbreak response.[75] Environmental sampling from likely sources is only recommended if enhanced infection measures fail to contain the outbreak. An outbreak with a multi-resistant organism should trigger re-evaluation of empiric antibiotic treatment, in consultation with a paediatric infectious disease specialist or microbiologist.[59]

21.7.2 Enterobacter

E. cloacae is the major cause of reported Enterobacter outbreaks. A review of 26 outbreaks found that most were associated with over-crowding but found no common source, implying transmission on hands of staff. Two outbreaks were related to multiple-dose medications.[76]

E. sakazakii is an organism especially associated with contamination of powdered milk formula. It was recognized as a separate species in 1980 having previously been classified as a yellow-pigmented *E. cloacae*. It has recently been re-classified as *Cronobacter sakazakii*. It has been cultured from powdered milk formula in many different Western and developing countries.[77] It can cause isolated cases of sepsis, outbreaks of bacteraemia and meningitis[78, 79] and outbreaks of necrotizing enterocolitis.[80] A single case occurring in a bottle-fed infant should alert the clinician to the possibility of contaminated infant formula. Breastfeeding is protective and nosocomial Enterobacter infection is rarely described in exclusively breastfed infants.[81]

21.7.3 Klebsiella

Most outbreaks with Klebsiella species are linked to poor infection control and resolve with improved hand washing and other infection control measures,[82] suggesting spread on the hands of staff is the most common mode of transmission.[83]

Outbreaks have been described in association with contaminated dextrose-containing intravenous fluids.[84–86] One outbreak was associated with a contaminated breast milk pump[87] and one with contaminated disinfectant.[88]

21.7.4 *Escherichia coli*

E. coli can cause devastating outbreaks of neonatal diarrhoea in infant wards, although rarely described in neonatal units. *E. coli* are an important cause of early-onset and late-onset neonatal infections in developing countries[89] but outbreaks with infant-to-infant spread have not been reported.

21.7.5 Salmonella

Most neonatal Salmonella infections are transmitted from the mother at the time of delivery but the organism can be spread readily to other infants, presumably on the hands of staff. In developing countries devastating outbreaks of invasive neonatal Salmonella infection have been repeatedly traced to contaminated suction machines in the delivery room[90–92] or the neonatal unit.[92] Salmonella outbreaks have also been described in Western countries. One outbreak was traced to an asymptomatic infected mother with spread via a resuscitator in the labour ward operating theatre.[93] In another, Salmonella, spread from a mother and her child via inadequately disinfected thermometers in the labour suite and ward.[94]

21.8 Outbreaks due to *Staphylococcus aureus*

Infant-to-infant spread of *S. aureus* commonly occurs on the hands of staff.[95] Early recognition of bacteraemia is associated with improved outcome.[96]

Improved hand hygiene, screening infants for carriage, and cohorting colonized infants are the main approaches to controlling outbreaks.[95–103] Other more intensive infection control measures may need to be instituted.[95–103] Topical mupirocin is often recommended to eradicate carriage in staff and infants, but has not been studied formally in outbreaks and is not always successful.[100]

Investigation of staff is controversial. Outbreaks have been associated with infected eczema of the hands or ears (otitis externa) of staff. During an outbreak, any infected skin lesions should be cultured and referral for formal dermatologic assessment considered.

Airborne transmission has had a possible role in some outbreaks. The first report of 'cloud babies' in 1960 described increased airborne dissemination of *S. aureus* in babies with respiratory tract co-infection with viruses (adenovirus or enterovirus).[104] Some outbreaks of *S. aureus* were linked to staff with nasal carriage. The possibility of 'cloud adults' is supported by experiments in which nasal carriers of *S. aureus* given experimental rhinovirus infection developed increased staphylococcal shedding.[105, 106] However, the clinical significance and the need to screen staff for nasal carriage during *S. aureus* outbreaks remains uncertain. One recommendation is to assess and improve existing infection control measures first and only investigate staff nasal carriage if unsuccessful.

21.9 Outbreaks due to vancomycin-resistant enterococci

Neonatal outbreaks of vancomycin-resistant enterococci (VRE) infection are rare. Carriage is far more common than infection.[107–113] VRE carriage has been associated with prolonged use of vancomycin and prolonged hospital stay.[110] Published recommendations on prevention emphasize avoiding vancomycin use and good infection control practices, particularly screening for faecal carriage, cohorting colonized infants and rigorous infection control measures (Section 21.2.1).[114, 115]

21.10 *Bordetella pertussis*

Although high levels of maternal antibodies protect against neonatal pertussis infection,[116] most neonates are susceptible to infection with *B. pertussis*. The morbidity and mortality of pertussis is higher in neonates and infants <3 months old than at any other age.[117] The incubation period is 5–10 days. Infected neonates are usually afebrile and may present with apnoea without cough, although some develop increasingly severe paroxysmal cough. Whoop may or may not be present but colour change to red or purple during coughing paroxysms is classic and vomiting common.[117]

The source of infection is only identified in about half of all non-hospitalized infants with pertussis, usually a parent, more commonly the mother, or a sibling.[118–123] In hospitalized infants, however, members of staff are an important and often unrecognized source of infection. Infected infants do not have a strong cough so, although infected infants should be placed in strict respiratory isolation to protect other infants, diagnosing infected family and staff members arguably provides better protection.[124] Prevention is better than cure. Mathematical modelling suggests immunizing staff with a booster dose of pertussis vaccine would decrease the probability of secondary transmission from 49% without boosting to 2% if 95% of staff are boosted, and will decrease the final size of an outbreak.[125] It has been estimated that a programme to give staff a booster dose of acellular pertussis vaccine would be cost-effective at anything over 25% uptake.[126] Neonatal pertussis immunization is considered in Chapter 23.

A Cochrane systematic review of 13 trials of antibiotics in pertussis found short-term macrolide antibiotics (azithromycin for 3–5 days or clarithromycin or erythromycin for 7 days) were as effective as long-term (erythromycin for 10 days) at eradicating nasopharyngeal *B. pertussis* with fewer side effects.[127] Trimethoprim/sulfamethoxazole for 7 days was also effective.[127] All these antibiotics may cause problems in the neonatal period. Erythromycin has been associated with pyloric stenosis,[127, 128] while a report of pyloric stenosis in two of triplets given azithromycin[129] raises the possibility that this may be a class effect of all macrolides. Trimethoprim/sulfamethoxazole is generally avoided in infants because of safety concerns regarding displacement of bilirubin and haematologic adverse events.

21.11 *Mycobacterium tuberculosis*

There are many descriptions of neonatal exposure to an adult family or staff member with 'open TB' (cavitary respiratory TB, smear positive for *M. tuberculosis*) on neonatal units,[130–141] most resulting in extensive epidemiologic investigations.[142] It is generally recommended that exposed infants have a clinical examination, a chest radiograph and prophylactic isoniazid should be considered. A tuberculin skin test (TST) is usually delayed until the infant is 3–4 months old. If the TST is negative at 3–4 months and the infant is well, the infant is uninfected and any chemoprophylaxis can be stopped. In one outbreak, however, infants were not clinically evaluated or empirically treated for TB disease because the risk of transmission was felt to be negligible.[138] This illustrates that each outbreak needs to be considered on its merits to assess the degree of risk (see Section 18.1.7).

Neonatal BCG vaccine is not routinely recommended in outbreaks because of unknown efficacy and because BCG interferes with interpretation of a later TST. However, neonatal BCG vaccine is usually recommended when the index case is infected with a multi-resistant strain of *M. tuberculosis*.

The risk of nosocomial neonatal TB from nursery exposure to an infected health-care worker is low,[130–141] but neonatal TB is potentially devastating. One report described two neonates who developed miliary TB following nursery exposure to a nurse's aide with cavitatory TB[131] and another report documented five neonates with pulmonary TB from a common nursery exposure.[133] Because TB is spread almost exclusively from adults by respiratory droplets, important factors for neonatal unit transmission include ventilation, room size, proximity to the index case, infectiousness of the index case and duration of contact. The duration of time spent sharing a room with the index case is the key determinant influencing transmission.[143]

Investigations of TB outbreaks are extremely time-consuming and costly and generate great anxiety. Prevention is ideal and screening all staff for TB is critical.

Children with primary TB are not considered infectious, but infants with congenital TB often have extensive pulmonary involvement with large numbers of acid-fast bacilli (AFB).[144] Transmission from infants with congenital TB to health-care workers has been described rarely, but never to other infants.[145–150] An infant diagnosed with congenital TB should be isolated until it is known whether or not they are AFB positive and therefore infectious. Infection control precautions and screening of exposed infants and staff should be reviewed in the light of whether or not either the infant with congenital TB or the infant's mother was infectious.

The diagnosis of TB should be based on clinical grounds and confirmed by **accredited** laboratory tests, including radiology, tuberculin skin testing, histopathology and microbiology testing. These do not include antibody tests. Serologic antibody testing for *M. tuberculosis* is widely practiced in the private sector in India, costing an estimated US$15 million annually, despite strong evidence that serologic tests are unreliable for diagnosis[151] and strong recommendations against their use.[152]

21.12 Herpes simplex virus infection

Most neonatal HSV is acquired at the time of delivery (90–95%) but 5–10% is acquired post-natally.[153, 154] Both HSV-1 and HSV-2 can cause devastating neonatal HSV infection (see Chapter 17). This brief section covers prevention of transmission of HSV from staff to neonates.

About half of all staff will have previously been infected with HSV and will shed HSV intermittently in saliva despite being completely asymptomatic.[153, 154] Reassuringly, nosocomial HSV infection is comparatively rare. However, staff members with active cold sores (oral herpes) may be more infectious and pose a higher risk of nosocomial infection. There is no formal evidence on how to manage staff members with cold sores but guidelines quite reasonably suggest they should be excluded from the neonatal unit until the cold sores have crusted over.[153, 154] Most authorities recommend topical acyclovir to speed recovery and decrease infectivity.

21.13 Varicella zoster virus infection

The greatest risk to neonates is if they acquire VZV infection perinatally, when they may be exposed to a high titre of virus transplacentally in the absence of specific maternal antibody (see Chapter 17).

However, post-natal acquisition of VZV through respiratory exposure can occasionally result in severe neonatal varicella infection.[155] VZV spreads efficiently by airborne spread: a person with chickenpox infects about 85% of susceptible household contacts, although zoster is less infectious.[156] The greatest risk is to infants with no maternal antibody, either because their mothers are seronegative and/or because they are born preterm before maternal IgG has crossed the placenta. Varicella zoster immunoglobulin (ZIG or VZIG), a preparation with high titre antibodies purified from donors, does not prevent varicella infection in exposed neonates but reduces the severity of the disease.[157]

When a neonate is potentially exposed to VZV from a staff member, parent, sibling or visitor with chickenpox or zoster, the first critical decision is what constitutes a 'true and substantial exposure'. Transient exposure is not considered to represent a significant risk of infection. For newborns, substantial exposure is defined as sharing the same hospital room with an infectious patient or direct face-to-face contact with an infectious person.[156] Brief contact, for example with X-ray technicians or housekeeping personnel, is less likely to result in VZV transmission.[156] Direct contact exposure is defined as face-to-face contact with an infectious person while indoors. Some experts have recommended 5 minutes or more of direct contact and some 60 minutes or more as constituting significant exposure, with no data to support either assumption.[156, 158] No action is required if the potential exposure is not considered significant.[156, 158] The next consideration is who is infectious. A member of staff, parent or visitor who develops chickenpox or zoster at an exposed surface is deemed infectious from 48 hours before the rash appears until the rash is completely crusted over.

It is generally recommended that all exposed infants born <28 weeks of gestation will have insufficient maternal antibody to be protected and should be given ZIG (the US guideline is for infants of birth weight <1000 g or <28 weeks,[156] the Australian guideline is for ≤ 28 weeks[158]). For more mature infants, only those lacking VZV antibody are at risk: this can be determined by performing urgent maternal serology.[158] The US guideline does not recommend ZIG for healthy term infants even with no history of maternal varicella,[156] whereas the Australian recommendation is to give ZIG to any seronegative neonate born >28 weeks with significant VZV exposure,[158] which is what about half of all US clinicians say they would do in practice.[159] Previously it was recommended to give ZIG up to 4 days after exposure, but a more recent recommendation is that ZIG can be given up to 10 days after exposure, although evidence of efficacy between 4 and 10 days post-exposure is weak.[160] It is recommended to place all infants exposed to VZV who remain in hospital in protective isolation from 7 to 21 days after exposure (7–28 days if given ZIG which can prolong the incubation period).[158]

References

1. Erasmus V, Daha TJ, Brug H, et al. Systematic review of studies on compliance with hand hygiene guidelines in hospital care. *Infect Control Hosp Epidemiol* 2010; 31:283e94.
2. Gastmeier P, Loui A, Stamm-Balderjahn S, Hansen S, Zuschneid I, Sohr D, et al. Outbreaks in neonatal intensive care units - they are not like others. *Am J Infect Control* 2007; 35:172–176.
3. Gupta A. Hospital-acquired infections in the neonatal intensive care unit–Klebsiella pneumoniae. *Semin Perinatol* 2002; 26:340–345.
4. Cassettari VC, da Silveira IR, Dropa M, et al. Risk factors for colonisation of newborn infants during an outbreak of extended-spectrum beta-lactamase-producing *Klebsiella pneumoniae* in an intermediate-risk neonatal unit. *J Hosp Infect* 2009; 71:340–347.
5. Dessì A, Puddu M, Testa M, Marcialis MA, Pintus MC, Fanos V. *Serratia marcescens* infections and outbreaks in neonatal intensive care units. *J Chemother* 2009; 21:493–499.
6. Voelz A, Müller A, Gillen J, et al. Outbreaks of *Serratia marcescens* in neonatal and pediatric intensive care units: clinical aspects, risk factors and management. *Int J Hyg Environ Health* 2010; 213:79–87.
7. Hervas JA, Ballesteros F, Alomar A, Gil J, Benedi VJ, Alberti S. Increase of Enterobacter in neonatal sepsis: a twenty-two-year study. *Pediatr Infect Dis J* 2001; 20:134–140.
8. Dalben M, Varkulja G, Basso M, et al. Investigation of an outbreak of *Enterobacter cloacae* in a neonatal unit and review of the literature. *J Hosp Infect* 2008; 70:7–14.
9. Hu J, Robinson JL. Systematic review of invasive Acinetobacter infections in children. *Can J Infect Dis Med Microbiol* 2010; 21:83–88.
10. McGrath EJ, Chopra T, Abdel-Haq N, et al. An outbreak of carbapenem-resistant *Acinetobacter baumannii* infection in a neonatal intensive care unit: investigation and control. *Infect Control Hosp Epidemiol* 2011; 32:34–41.
11. Foca M, Jakob K, Whittier S, et al. Endemic Pseudomonas aeruginosa infection in a neonatal intensive care unit. *N Engl J Med* 2000; 343:695–700.
12. Foca MD. Pseudomonas aeruginosa infections in the neonatal intensive care unit. *Semin Perinatol* 2002; 26:332–339.
13. Crivaro V, Di Popolo A, Caprio A, et al. Pseudomonas aeruginosa in a neonatal intensive care unit: molecular epidemiology and infection control measures. *BMC Infect Dis* 2009; 9:70.
14. Gulcan H, Kuzucu C, Durmaz R. Nosocomial Stenotrophomonas maltophilia cross-infection: three cases in newborns. *Am J Infect Control* 2004; 32:365–368.
15. Looney WJ. Role of Stenotrophomonas maltophilia in hospital-acquired infection. *Br J Biomed Sci* 2005; 62:145–154.
16. Geva A, Wright SB, Baldini LM, Smallcomb JA, Safran C, Gray JE. Spread of methicillin-resistant *Staphylococcus aureus* in a large tertiary NICU: network analysis. *Pediatrics* 2011; 128:e1173–e1180.
17. Huang YC, Lien RI, Su LH, Chou YH, Lin TY. Successful control of methicillin-resistant *Staphylococcus aureus* in endemic neonatal intensive care units–a 7-year campaign. *PLoS One* 2011; 6:e23001.
18. Waters V, Larson E, Wu F, et al. Molecular epidemiology of gram-negative bacilli from infected neonates and health care workers' hands in neonatal intensive care units. *Clin Infect Dis* 2004; 38:1682–1687.
19. Larson EL, Cimiotti JP, Haas J, et al. Gram-negative bacilli associated with catheter-associated and non-catheter-associated bloodstream infections and hand carriage by healthcare workers in neonatal intensive care units. *Pediatr Crit Care Med* 2005; 6:457–461.
20. O'Grady NP, Alexander M, Burns LA, the Healthcare Infection Control Practices Advisory Committee. Guidelines for the prevention of intravenous catheter-related infections, 2011. CDC 2011. Available at: http://www.cdc.gov/hicpac/pdf/guidelines/bsi-guidelines-2011.pdf
21. Siegel JD, Rhinehart E, Jackson M, Chiarello L, the Healthcare Infection Control Practices Advisory Committee. 2007 Guideline for isolation precautions: preventing transmission of infectious agents in healthcare settings. CDC 2007. Available at: http://www.cdc.gov/hicpac/pdf/isolation/Isolation2007.pdf
22. British Association of Perinatal Medicine. Standards for hospitals providing neonatal intensive and high dependency care. 2nd edition. *BEPM* 2001. Available at: http://www.bapm.org/publications/documents/guidelines/hosp_standards.pdf

23. White RD, Consensus Committee on Recommended Standards for Newborn intensive care unit (NICU) design. Recommended standards for newborn ICU design. *J Perinatal* 2006; 26: S2–S18.
24. Goldmann DA, Durbin Jr WA, Freeman J. Nosocomial infections in a neonatal intensive care unit. *J Infect Dis* 1981; 144:449–459.
25. Isaacs D, Catterson J, Hope PL, Wilkinson AR, Moxon ER. Factors influencing colonisation with gentamicin-resistant Gram negative organisms in the neonatal unit. *Arch Dis Child* 1988; 63:533–535.
26. Tucker J; UK Neonatal Staffing Study Group. Patient volume, staffing, and workload in relation to risk-adjusted outcomes in a random stratified sample of UK neonatal intensive care units: a prospective evaluation. *Lancet* 2002; 359:99–107.
27. Callaghan LA, Cartwright DW, O'Rourke P, Davies MW. Infant to staff ratios and risk of mortality in very low birthweight infants. *Arch Dis Child Fetal Neonatal Ed* 2003; 88:F94–F97.
28. Hamilton KE, Redshaw ME, Tarnow-Mordi W. Nurse staffing in relation to risk-adjusted mortality in neonatal care. *Arch Dis Child Fetal Neonatal Ed* 2007; 92:F99–F103.
29. Knoll M, Lautenschlaeger C, Borneff-Lipp M. The impact of workload on hygiene compliance in nursing. *Br J Nurs* 2010; 19:S18–S22.
30. Pittet D, Simon A, Hugonnet S, Pessoa-Silva CL, Sauvan V, Perneger TV. Hand hygiene among physicians: performance, beliefs, and perceptions. *Ann Intern Med* 2004; 141:1–8.
31. Outbreak Database. Worldwide Database for Nosocomial Outbreaks. [Neonatal]: http://www.outbreak-database.com/QueryResults/QueryPage.aspx
32. Srivastava S, Shetty N. Healthcare-associated infections in neonatal units: lessons from contrasting worlds. *J Hosp Infect* 2007; 65:292–306.
33. Curtis C, Shetty N. Recent trends and prevention of infection in the neonatal intensive care unit. *Curr Opin Infect Dis* 2008; 21:350–356.
34. Haas JP, Trezza LA. Outbreak investigation in a neonatal intensive care unit. *Semin Perinatol* 2002; 26:367–378.
35. Trautmann M, Lepper PM, Haller M. Ecology of Pseudomonas aeruginosa in the intensive care unit and the evolving role of water outlets as a reservoir of the organism. *Am J Infect Control* 2005; 33(5 Suppl 1):S41–S49.
36. Rogues AM, Boulestreau H, Lashéras A, et al. Contribution of tap water to patient colonisation withPseudomonas aeruginosa in a medical intensive care unit. *J Hosp Infect* 2007; 67:72–78.
37. Reuter S, Sigge A, Wiedeck H, Trautmann M. Analysis of transmission pathways of Pseudomonas aeruginosa between patients and tap water outlets. *Crit Care Med* 2002; 30:2222–2228.
38. Yapicioglu H, Gokmen TG, Yildizdas D, et al. *Pseudomonas aeruginosa* infections dueto electronic faucets in a neonatal intensive care unit. *J Paediatr Child Health* 2012;48:430–434.
39. Crivaro V, Di Popolo A, Caprio A, et al. *Pseudomonas aeruginosa* in a neonatal intensive care unit: molecular epidemiology and infection control measures. *BMC Infect Dis* 2009; 9:70.
40. Muyldermans G, de Smet F, Pierard D, et al. Neonatal infections with *Pseudomonas aeruginosa* associated with a waterbath used to thaw fresh frozen plasma. *J Hosp Infect* 1998; 39:309–314.
41. Becks VE, Lorenzoni NM. *Pseudomonas aeruginosa* outbreak in a neonatal intensive care unit: a possible link to contaminated hand lotion. *Am J Infect Control* 1995; 23:396–398.
42. Garland SM, Mackay S, Tabrizi S, Jacobs S. *Pseudomonas aeruginosa* outbreak associated with a contaminated bloodgas analyser in a neonatal intensive care unit. *J Hosp Infect* 1996; 33:145–151.
43. Foca M, Jakob K, Whittier S, et al. Endemic *Pseudomonas aeruginosa* infection in a neonatal intensive care unit. *N Engl J Med* 2000; 343:695–700.
44. Zawacki A, O'Rourke E, Potter-Bynoe G, Macone A, Harbarth S, Goldmann D. An outbreak of *Pseudomonas aeruginosa* pneumonia and bloodstream infection associated with intermittent otitis externa in a healthcare worker. *Infect Control Hosp Epidemiol* 2004; 25:1083–1089.
45. Sánchez-Carrillo C, Padilla B, Marín M, et al. Contaminated feeding bottles: the source of an outbreak of *Pseudomonas aeruginosa* infections in a neonatal intensive care unit. *Am J Infect Control* 2009; 37:150–154.
46. Gras-Le Guen C, Lepelletier D, Debillon T, Gournay V, Espaze E, Roze JC. Contamination of a milk bank pasteuriser causing a *Pseudomonas aeruginosa* outbreak in a neonatal intensive care unit. *Arch Dis Child Fetal Neonatal Ed* 2003; 88:F434–F435.
47. Heard S, Lawrence S, Holmes B, Costas M. A pseudo-outbreak of Pseudomonas on a special care baby unit. *J Hosp Infect* 1990; 16:59–65.
48. Bouallègue O, Mzoughi R, Weill FX, et al. Outbreak of *Pseudomonas putida* bacteraemia in a neonatal intensive care unit. *J Hosp Infect* 2004; 57:88–91.
49. Bergogne-Berezin E, Towner K. *Acinetobacter* spp. as nosocomial pathogens: Microbiological, clinical, and epidemiologic features. *Clin Microbiol Rev* 1996; 9:148–165.
50. Chan PC, Huang LM, Lin HC, et al. Control of an outbreak of pandrug-resistant *Acinetobacter baumannii* colonization and infection in a neonatal intensive care unit. *Infect Control Hosp Epidemiol* 2007; 28:423–429.
51. McGrath EJ, Chopra T, Abdel-Haq N, et al. An outbreak of carbapenem-resistant *Acinetobacter baumannii* infection in a neonatal intensive care unit: investigation and control. *Infect Control Hosp Epidemiol* 2011; 32:34–41.
52. Hu J, Robinson JL. Systematic review of invasive Acinetobacter infections in children. *Can J Infect Dis Med Microbiol* 2010; 21:83–88.
53. De Vegas E, Nieves B, Araque M, Velasco E, Ruiz J, Vila J. Outbreak of infection with *Acinetobacter* strain RUH 1139 in an intensive care unit. *Infection Control Hosp Epidemiol* 2006; 27:397–403.

54. Zingg W, Posfay-Barbe KM, Pittet D. Healthcare-associated infections in neonates. *Curr Opin Infect Dis* 2008; 21:228–234.
55. Lee JK. Two outbreaks of Burkholderia cepacia nosocomial infection in a neonatal intensive care unit. *J Paediatr Child Health* 2008; 44:62–66.
56. Lucero CA, Cohen AL, Trevino I, et al. Outbreak of *Burkholderia cepacia* complex among ventilated pediatric patients linked to hospital sinks. *Am J Infect Control* 2011; 39:775–778.
57. Gravel-Tropper D, Sample ML, Oxley C, Toye B, Woods DE, Garber GE. Three-year outbreak of pseudobacteremia with *Burkholderia cepacia* traced to a contaminated blood gas analyzer. *Infect Control Hosp Epidemiol* 1996; 17:737–740.
58. Manzar S, Nair AK, Pai MG, Al-Khusaiby SM. Pseudo-outbreak of *Burkholderia cepacia* in a neonatal intensive care unit. *J Hosp Infect* 2004; 58:159.
59. Paterson DL. Resistance in gram-negative bacteria: enterobacteriaceae. *Am J Med* 2006; 119(6 Suppl 1):S20–S28.
60. Dessì A, Puddu M, Testa M, Marcialis MA, Pintus MC, Fanos V. *Serratia marcescens* infections and outbreaks in neonatal intensive care units. *J Chemother* 2009; 21:493–499.
61. Voelz A, Müller A, Gillen J, et al. Outbreaks of *Serratia marcescens* in neonatal and pediatric intensive care units: clinical aspects, risk factors and management. *Int J Hyg Environ Health* 2010; 213:79–87.
62. Archibald LK, Corl A, Shah B, et al. *Serratia marcescens* outbreak associated with extrinsic contamination of 1% chlorxylenol soap. *Infect Control Hosp Epidemiol* 1997; 18:704–709.
63. Sartor C, Jacomo V, Duvivier C, Tissot-Dupont H, Sambuc R, Drancourt M. Nosocomial *Serratia marcescens* infections associated with extrinsic contamination of a liquid nonmedicated soap. *Infect Control Hosp Epidemiol* 2000; 21: 196–199.
64. Rabier V, Bataillon S, Jolivet-Gougeon A, Chapplain JM, Beuchée A, Bétrémieux P. Hand washing soap as a source of neonatal *Serratia marcescens* outbreak. *Acta Paediatr* 2008;97:1381–1385.
65. Anagnostakis D, Fitsialos J, Koutsia C, Messaritakis J, Matsaniotis N. A nursery outbreak of *Serratia marcescens* infection. Evidence of a single source of contamination. *Am J Dis Child* 1981; 135:413–414.
66. Madani TA, Alsaedi S, James L, et al. *Serratia marcescens*-contaminated baby shampoo causing an outbreak among newborns at King Abdulaziz University Hospital, Jeddah, Saudi Arabia. *J Hosp Infect* 2011; 78:16–19.
67. Fleisch F, Zimmermann-Baer U, Zbinden R, et al. Three consecutive outbreaks of *Serratia marcescens* in a neonatal intensive care unit. *Clin Infect Dis* 2002; 34:767–773.
68. Berthelot P, Grattard F, Amerger C, et al. Investigation of a nosocomial outbreak due to *Serratia marcescens* in a maternity hospital. *Infect Control Hosp Epidemiol* 1999; 20:233–236.
69. Bayramoglu G, Buruk K, Dinc U, Mutlu M, Yilmaz G, Aslan Y. Investigation of an outbreak of *Serratia marcescens* in a neonatal intensive care unit. *J Microbiol Immunol Infect* 2011; 44:111–115.
70. Moloney AC, Quoraishi AH, Parry P, Hall V. A bacteriological examination of breast pumps. *J Hosp Infect* 1987; 9:169–174.
71. Gransden WR, Webster M, French GL, Phillips I. An outbreak of *Serratia marcescens* transmitted by contaminated breast pumps in a special care baby unit. *J Hosp Infect* 1986; 7:149–154.
72. Faro J, Katz A, Berens P, Ross PJ. Premature termination of nursing secondary to *Serratia marcescens* breast pump contamination. *Obstet Gynecol* 2011;117:485–486.
73. Cullen MM, Trail A, Robinson M, Keaney M, Chadwick PR. *Serratia marcescens* outbreak in a neonatal intensive care unit prompting review of decontamination of laryngoscopes. *J Hosp Infect* 2005; 59:68–70.
74. Uduman SA, Farrukh AS, Nath KN, et al. An outbreak of *Serratia marcescens* infection in a special-care baby unit of a community hospital in United Arab Emirates: the importance of the air conditioner duct as a nosocomial reservoir. *J Hosp Infect* 2002; 52:175–180.
75. Giles M, Harwood HM, Gosling DA, Hennessy D, Pearce CT, Daley AJ. What is the best screening method to detect *Serratia marcescens* colonization during an outbreak in a neonatal intensive care nursery? *J Hosp Infect* 2006; 62:349–352.
76. Dalben M, Varkulja G, Basso M, et al. Investigation of an outbreak of *Enterobacter cloacae* in a neonatal unit and review of the literature. *J Hosp Infect* 2008; 70:7–14.
77. Muytjens HL, Roelofs-Willemse H, Jaspar GH. Quality of powdered substitutes for breast milk with regard to members of the family *Enterobacteriaceae*. *J Clin Microbiol* 1988; 26:743–746.
78. Centers for Disease Control and Prevention (CDC). *Enterobacter sakazakii* infections associated with the use of powdered infant formula–Tennessee, 2001. *MMWR Morb Mortal Wkly Rep* 2002; 51:297–300.
79. Drudy D, Mullane NR, Quinn T, Wall PG, Fanning S. *Enterobacter sakazakii*: an emerging pathogen in powdered infant formula. *Clin Infect Dis* 2006;42:996–1002.
80. van Acker J, de Smet F, Muyldermans G, Bougatef A, Naessens A, Lauwers S. Outbreak of necrotizing enterocolitis associated with *Enterobacter sakazakii* in powdered milk formula. *J Clin Microbiol* 2001; 39:293–297.
81. Ray P, Das A, Gautam V, Jain N, Narang A, Sharma M. *Enterobacter sakazakii* in infants: novel phenomenon in India. *Indian J Med Microbiol* 2007; 25:408–410.
82. Gupta A. Hospital-acquired infections in the neonatal intensive care unit–*Klebsiella pneumoniae*. *Semin Perinatol* 2002; 26:340–345.
83. Dashti AA, Jadaon MM, Gomaa HH, Noronha B, Udo EE. Transmission of a *Klebsiella pneumoniae* clone harbouring genes for CTX-M-15-like and SHV-112 enzymes in a neonatal intensive care unit of a Kuwaiti hospital. *J Med Microbiol* 2010; 59:687–692.
84. Ross BS, Peter G, Dempsey JM, Oh W. Klebsiella pneumoniae nosocomial epidemic in an intensive care nursery due

to contaminated intravenous fluid. *Am J Dis Child* 1977; 131:712.
85. Lalitha MK, Kenneth J, Jana AK, et al. Identification of an IV-dextrose solution as the source of an outbreak of Klebsiella pneumoniae sepsis in a newborn nursery. *J Hosp Infect* 1999; 43:70–73.
86. Moore KL, Kainer MA, Badrawi N, et al. Neonatal sepsis in Egypt associated with bacterial contamination of glucose-containing intravenous fluids. *Pediatr Infect Dis J* 2005; 24:590–594.
87. Donowitz LG, Marsik FJ, Fisher KA, Wenzel RP. Contaminated breast milk: A source of Klebsiella bacteremia in a newborn intensive care unit. *Rev Infect Dis* 1981; 3:716–720.
88. Reiss I, Borkhardt A, Füssle R, Sziegoleit A, Gortner L. Disinfectant contaminated with Klebsiella oxytoca as a source of sepsis in babies. *Lancet* 2000; 356:310.
89. Zaidi AKM, Thaver D, Ali AS, Khan TA. Pathogens associated with sepsis in newborns and young infants in developing countries. *Pediatr Infect Dis J* 2009; 28:S10–S18.
90. Ip HM, Sin WK, Chau PY, Tse D, Teoh-Chan CH. Neonatal infection due to *Salmonella worthington* transmitted by a delivery-room suction apparatus. *J Hyg (Lond)* 1976; 77:307–314.
91. Khan MA, Abdur-Rab M, Israr N, et al. Transmission of *Salmonella worthington* by oropharyngeal suction in hospital neonatal unit. *Pediatr Infect Dis J* 1991; 10:668–672.
92. Mahajan R, Mathur M, Kumar A, Gupta P, Faridi MM, Talwar V. Nosocomial outbreak of *Salmonella typhimurium* infection in a nursery intensive care unit (NICU) and paediatric ward. *J Commun Dis* 1995; 27:10–14.
93. Umasankar S, Mridha EU, Hannan MM, Fry CM, Azadian BS. An outbreak of *Salmonella enteritidis* in a maternity and neonatal intensive care unit. *J Hosp Infect* 1996; 34:117–122.
94. McAllister TA, Roud JA, Marshall A, Holland BM, Turner TL. Outbreak of*Salmonella eimsbuettel* in newborn infants spread by rectal thermometers. *Lancet* 1986;1:1262–1264.
95. Carey AJ, Long SS. *Staphylococcus aureus*: a continuously evolving and formidable pathogen in the neonatal intensive care unit. *Clin Perinatol* 2010; 37:535–546.
96. Isaacs D, Fraser S, Hogg G, Li HY. *Staphylococcus aureus* infections in Australasian neonatal nurseries. *Arch Dis Child Fetal Neonatal Ed* 2004; 89:F331–F335.
97. Vergnano S, Menson E, Smith Z, et al. Characteristics of invasive *Staphylococcus aureus* in United Kingdom neonatal units. *Pediatr Infect Dis J* 2011; 30:850–854.
98. El Helali N, Carbonne A, Naas T, et al. Nosocomial outbreak of staphylococcal scalded skin syndrome in neonates: epidemiological investigation and control. *J Hosp Infect* 2005; 61:130–138.
99. Bertini G, Nicoletti P, Scopetti F, Manoocher P, Dani C, Orefici G. *Staphylococcus aureus* epidemic in a neonatal nursery: a strategy of infection control. *Eur J Pediatr* 2006; 165:530–535.
100. Lepelletier D, Corvec S, Caillon J, Reynaud A, Rozé JC, Gras-Leguen C. Eradication of methicillin-resistant *Staphylococcus aureus* in a neonatal intensive care unit: which measures for which success? *Am J Infect Control* 2009; 37:195–200.
101. Song X, Cheung S, Klontz K, Short B, Campos J, Singh N. A stepwise approach to control an outbreak and ongoing transmission of methicillin-resistant *Staphylococcus aureus* in a neonatal intensive care unit. *Am J Infect Control* 2010; 38:607–611.
102. Neylon O, O'Connell NH, Slevin B, et al. Neonatal staphylococcal scalded skin syndrome: clinical and outbreak containment review. *Eur J Pediatr* 2010; 169:1503–1509.
103. Vergnano S, Menson E, Smith Z, et al. Characteristics of invasive *Staphylococcus aureus* in United Kingdom neonatal units. *Pediatr Infect Dis J* 2011; 30:850–854.
104. Eichenwald HF, Kotsevalov O, Fasso LA. The "cloud baby": an example of bacterial-viral interaction. *Am J Dis Child* 1960; 100:161–173.
105. Sherertz RJ, Reagan DR, Hampton KD, et al. A cloud adult: the *Staphylococcus aureus*-virus interaction revisited. *Ann Intern Med* 1996; 124:539–547.
106. Bassetti S, Bischoff WE, Walter M, et al. Dispersal of*Staphylococcus aureus* into the air associated with a rhinovirus infection. *InfectControl Hosp Epidemiol* 2005; 26:196–203.
107. Malik RK, Montecalvo MA, Reale MR, et al. Epidemiology and control of vancomycin-resistant enterococci in a regional neonatal intensive care unit. *Pediatr Infect Dis J* 1999; 18:352–356.
108. Lee HK, Lee WG, Cho SR. Clinical and molecular biological analysis of a nosocomial outbreak of vancomycin-resistant enterococci in a neonatal intensive care unit. *Acta Paediatr* 1999; 88:651–654.
109. Yüce A, Karaman M, Gülay Z, Yulug N. Vancomycin-resistant enterococci in neonates. *Scand J Infect Dis* 2001; 33:803–805.
110. Khan E, Sarwari A, Hasan R, et al. Emergence of vancomycin-resistant Enterococcus faecium at a tertiary care hospital in Karachi, Pakistan. *J Hosp Infect* 2002; 52:292–296.
111. Singh N, Léger MM, Campbell J, Short B, Campos JM. Control of vancomycin-resistant enterococci in the neonatal intensive care unit. *InfectControl Hosp Epidemiol* 2005; 26:646–649.
112. Ergaz Z, Arad I, Bar-Oz B, et al. Elimination of vancomycin-resistant enterococci from a neonatal intensive care unit following an outbreak. *J Hosp Infect* 2010; 74:370–376.
113. Lee WG, Ahn SH, Jung MK, Jin HY, Park IJ. Characterization of avancomycin-resistant *Enterococcus faecium* outbreak caused by 2 genetically different clones at a neonatal intensive care unit. *Ann Lab Med* 2012; 32:82–86.
114. Recommendations for preventing the spread of vancomycin resistance. Recommendations of the Hospital Infection Control Practices Advisory Committee (HICPAC). *MMWR Recomm Rep* 1995; 44(RR-12):1–13.
115. Siegel JD, Rhinehart E, Jackson M, et al. The Healthcare Infection Control Practices Advisory Committee (HICPAC). Management of multidrug-resistant organisms in healthcare settings, 2006. CDC, 2006. Available at: http://www.cdc.gov/hicpac/pdf/MDRO/MDROGuideline2006.pdf

116. Van Rie A, Wendelboe AM, Englund JA. Role of maternal pertussis antibodies in infants. *Pediatr Infect Dis J* 2005; 24(5 Suppl):S62–S65.
117. Hoppe JE. Neonatal pertussis. *Pediatr Infect Dis J* 2000; 19:244–247.
118. Crowcroft NS, Booy R, Harrison T, et al. Severe and unrecognised: pertussis in UK infants. *Arch Dis Child* 2003; 88:802–806.
119. Elliott E, McIntyre P, Ridley G, et al. National study of infants hospitalized with pertussis in the acellular vaccine era. *Pediatr Infect Dis J* 2004;23:246–252.
120. Wendelboe AM, Van Rie AM, Salmaso SP, Englund JA. Duration of immunity against pertussis after natural infection or vaccination. *Pediatr Infect Dis J* 2005; 24(5 Supp):S58–S61.
121. Chuk LM, Lambert SB, May ML, et al. Pertussis in infants: how to protect the vulnerable? *Commun Dis Intell* 2008; 32:449–456.
122. de Greeff SC, Mooi F, Westerhof A, et al. Pertussis disease burden in the household: how to protect young infants. *Clin Infect Dis* 2010; 50:1339–1345.
123. Jardine A, Conaty S, Lowbridge C, et al. Who gives pertussis to infants? Source of infection for laboratory confirmed cases less than 12 months of age during an epidemic, Sydney, 2009. *Comm Dis Intell* 2010; 34:116.
124. Bryant KA, Humbaugh K, Brothers K, et al. Measures to control an outbreak of pertussis in a neonatal intermediate care nursery after exposure to a healthcare worker. *Infect Control Hosp Epidemiol* 2006; 27:541–545.
125. Greer AL, Fisman DN. Keeping vulnerable children safe from pertussis:preventing nosocomial pertussis transmission in the neonatal intensive care unit. *Infect Control Hosp Epidemiol* 2009; 30:1084–1089.
126. Greer AL, Fisman DN. Use of models to identify cost-effective interventions: pertussis vaccination for pediatric health care workers. *Pediatrics* 2011; 128:e591–e599.
127. Altunaiji SM, Kukuruzovic RH, Curtis NC, Massie J. Antibiotics for whooping cough (pertussis). Cochrane Database of Systematic Reviews 2007, Issue 3. Art. No.: CD004404. DOI: 10.1002/14651858.CD004404.pub3.
128. Maheshwai N. Are young infants treated with erythromycin at risk for developing hypertrophic pyloric stenosis? *Arch Dis Child* 2007; 92:271–273.
129. Morrison W. Infantile hypertrophic pyloric stenosis in infants treated with azithromycin. *Pediatr Infect Dis J* 2007; 26:186–188.
130. Light IJ, Saidleman M, Sutherland JM. Management of newborns after nursery exposure to tuberculosis. *Am Rev Resp Med* 1974; 109:415–419.
131. Steiner P, Rao M, Victoria MS, Rudolph N, Buynoski G. Miliary tuberculosis in two infants after nursery exposure: epidemiologic, clinical and laboratory findings. *Am Rev Respir Dis* 1976; 113:267–271.
132. Burk JR, Bahar D, Wolf FS, Greene J, Bailey WC. Nursery exposure of 528 newborns to a nurse with pulmonary tuberculosis. *South Med J* 1978; 71:7–10.
133. Kim KI, Lee JW, Park JH, et al. Pulmonary tuberculosis in five young infants with nursery exposure: clinical, radiographic and CT findings. *Pediatr Radiol* 1998; 28:836–840.
134. Lee LH, Le Vea, CM, Graman PS. Congenital tuberculosis in a neonatal intensive care unit: case report, epidemiological investigation, and management of exposures. *Clin Infect Dis* 1998; 27:474–477.
135. Nivin B, Nicholas P, Gayer M, Frieden TR, Fujiwara PI. A continuing outbreak of multidrug-resistant tuberculosis with transmission in a hospital nursery. *Clin Infect Dis* 1998; 26:303–307.
136. Sen M, Gregson D, Lewis J. Neonatal exposure to active pulmonary tuberculosis in a health care professional. *CMAJ* 2005; 172:1453–1455.
137. Isaacs D, Jones CA, Dalton D, et al. Exposure to open tuberculosis on a neonatal unit. *J Paed Child Health* 2006; 42:557–559.
138. Nania JJ, Skinner J, Wilkerson K, et al. Exposure to pulmonary tuberculosis in a neonatal intensive care unit: unique aspects of contact investigation and management of hospitalized neonates. *Infect Control Hosp Epidemiol* 2007; 28:661–665.
139. Ohno H, Ikegami Y, Kishida K, et al. A contact investigation of the transmission of *Mycobacterium tuberculosis* from a nurse working in a newborn nursery and maternity ward. *J Infect Chemother* 2008; 14:66–71.
140. Millership SE, Anderson C, Cummins AJ, Bracebridge S, Abubakar I. The risk to infants from nosocomial exposure to tuberculosis. *Paediatr Infect Dis J* 2009; 28:915–916.
141. Borgia P, Cambieri A, Chini F, et al. Suspected transmission of tuberculosis in a maternity ward from a smear-positive nurse: preliminary results of clinical evaluations and testing of neonates potentially exposed, Rome, Italy, 1 January to 28 July 2011. *Euro Surveill* 2011; 16(40) pii: 19984.
142. Jensen PA, Lambert LA, Iademarco MF, Ridzon R; CDC. Guidelines for preventing the transmission of *Mycobacterium tuberculosis* in health-care settings, 2005. *MMWR Recomm Rep* 2005;54(RR-17):1–141.
143. Richeldi L, Ewer K, Losi M, et al. T cell-based tracking of multidrug resistant tuberculosis infection after brief exposure. *Am J Respir Crit Care Med* 2004; 170:288–295.
144. Peng W, Yang J, Liu E. Analysis of 170 cases of congenital TB reported in the literature between 1946 and 2009. *Pediatr Pulmonol* 2011; 46:1215–1224.
145. Rabalais G, Adams G, Stover B. PPD skin test conversion in health-care workers after exposure to *Mycobacterium tuberculosis* infection in infants. *Lancet* 1991; 338:826.
146. Machin GA, Honoré LH, Fanning EA, Molesky M. Perinatally acquired neonatal tuberculosis: report of two cases. *Pediatr Pathol* 1992; 12:707–716.
147. Lee LH, LeVea CM, Graman PS. Congenital tuberculosis in a neonatal intensive care unit: case report, epidemiological investigation, and management of exposures. *Clin Infect Dis* 1998; 27:474–477.
148. Pillay T, Adhikari M. Congenital tuberculosis in a neonatal intensive care. *Clin Infect Dis* 1999; 29:467–468.

149. Saitoh M, Ichiba H, Fujioka H, Shintaku H, Yamano T. Connatal tuberculosis in an extremely low birth weight infant: case report and management of exposure to tuberculosis in a neonatal intensive care unit. *Eur J Pediatr* 2001; 160: 88–90.
150. Laartz BW, Narvarte HJ, Holt D, Larkin JA, Pomputius 3rd WF. Congenital tuberculosis and management of exposures in a neonatal intensive care unit. *Infect Control Hosp Epidemiol* 2002; 23:573–579.
151. Steingart KR, Henry M, Laal S, et al. A systematic review of commercial serological antibody tests for the diagnosis of pulmonary tuberculosis. *Thorax* 2007; 62:911–918.
152. Tuberculosis Coalition for Technical Assistance. *International Standards for TuberculosisCare (ISTC)*, 2nd edition. Tuberculosis Coalition for Technical Assistance, The Hague, 2009. Available on: http://www.istcweb.org/documents/ISTC_Report_2ndEd_Nov2009.pdf.
153. Sauerbrei A, Wutzler P. Herpes simplex and varicella-zoster virus infections during pregnancy: current concepts of prevention, diagnosis and therapy. Part 1: herpes simplex virus infections. *Med Microbiol Immunol* 2007; 196:89–94.
154. Anzivino E, Fioriti D, Mischitelli M, Bellizzi A, Barucca V, Chiarini F, et al. Herpes simplex virus infection in pregnancy and in neonate: status of art of epidemiology, diagnosis, therapy and prevention. *Virol J* 2009; 6:40.
155. Rubin L, Leggiadro R, Elie MT, Lipsitz P. Disseminated varicella in a neonate: implications for immunoprophylaxis of neonates postnatally exposed to varicella. *Pediatr Infect Dis* 1986; 5:100–102.
156. Miller E, Cradock-Watson JE, Ridehalgh MK. Outcome in newborn babies given anti-varicella-zoster immunoglobin after perinatal maternal infection with varicella-zoster virus. *Lancet* 1989; 2:371–373.
157. CDC. Prevention of varicella: recommendations of the Advisory Committee on Immunization Practices (ACIP). *MMWR* 2007;56(No. RR-4). Available at: http://www.cdc.gov/mmwr/preview/mmwrhtml/rr5604a1.htm.
158. Palasanthiran P, Starr M, Jones C. *Management of perinatal infections.* Australasian Society for Infectious Diseases (ASID). Sydney, 2002. Available at: http://www.asid.net.au/images/Documents/Guidelines/Management%20of%20Perinatal%20Infections%20ASID%202002%20rev%202007.pdf
159. Wurzel CL, Rubin LG, Krilov LR. Varicella zoster immunoglobulin after postnatal exposure to varicella: survey of experts. *Pediatr Infect Dis J* 1987; 6:466–470.
160. Centers for Disease Control and Prevention (CDC). FDA approval of an extended period for administering VariZIG for postexposure prophylaxis of varicella. *MMWR Morb Mortal Wkly Rep* 2012; 61:212.

CHAPTER 22

Developing countries

This book is intended to be relevant both to clinicians in Western countries and to clinicians in developing countries. This chapter covers issues that are primarily relevant to developing countries.

22.1 Antenatal care

Intuitively, improved antenatal care, particularly on a community basis, should prevent congenital infections such as congenital syphilis, should reduce the incidence of neonatal tetanus by immunizing mothers (see Chapter 23, Section 23.5.1.4) and should reduce the incidence of pre-term birth and, therefore, of neonatal infections. However, supportive evidence is scarce.[1, 2] Antenatal interventions are cheap compared to perinatal interventions but save fewer lives.[3] A review of within-country variation in maternal newborn and child health interventions in 54 low-income countries found that antenatal visit attendance varied more than any other intervention except skilled birth attendants.[4] Improved antenatal care is important for many reasons,[2] but scientific proof that it reduces congenital and neonatal infections would be invaluable.

22.2 Birth

22.2.1 Trained birth attendants

The majority of deliveries in developing countries take place in the home, not at a health-care facility. The presence of a skilled birth attendant is one of the most important factors in a good neonatal outcome. A Cochrane systematic review of studies which compared untrained with trained traditional birth attendants[5] found one cluster randomized trial which showed that trained traditional birth attendants were associated with significant reductions in stillbirths, perinatal and all-cause neonatal deaths and with an 83% reduction in puerperal sepsis (95% CI 77–87).[6]

22.2.2 Clean birth practices

A non-Cochrane systematic review found low-quality evidence that birth attendant hand washing was associated with a 19% reduction in all-cause neonatal mortality (95% CI 1–34), 30% reduction in cord infection (95% CI 35–62) and 49% reduction in neonatal tetanus (95% CI 35–62).[7]

Subsequently, the use of **sterile delivery packs** was studied in three cluster randomized trials in nearly 20 000 home births in South Asia (Bangladesh, India and Nepal).[8] The delivery packs consisted of a boiled blade and thread, soap, gloves and plastic sheet. The kits were only used for 18.4% of deliveries in Bangladesh and India and 5.7% in Nepal. However, when the packs were used, neonatal mortality was reduced by about half and death from sepsis was reduced by 72% (OR 0.28, 95% CI 0.39–0.68).[8] Use of a clean delivery kit was not always accompanied by clean delivery practices, but use of a plastic sheet during delivery, a boiled blade to cut the cord, a boiled thread to tie the cord, and antiseptic to clean the umbilicus were each significantly associated with relative reductions in mortality. Each additional one of these clean delivery practices used was associated with a 16% relative reduction in neonatal mortality (OR 0.84, 95% CI 0.77–0.92).[8] Delivery packs are cheap and apparently extremely effective but under-used and their use should be promoted vigorously.

22.2.3 Cord care

A non-Cochrane systematic review found moderate-quality evidence that chlorhexidine cord applications in the first 24 hours of life are associated with a 34%

Evidence-Based Neonatal Infections, First Edition. David Isaacs.

reduction in all-cause neonatal mortality (95% CI 5–54) and low-quality evidence that antimicrobial cord applications are associated with a 63% reduction in all-cause neonatal mortality (95% CI 41–86).[7] Since this review and an earlier Cochrane systematic review of umbilical cord care,[9] community-based cluster RCTs in Bangladesh[10] and in Pakistan[11] showed that cord care using topical chlorhexidine reduced omphalitis and all-cause mortality from home deliveries and was more effective than attempts to promote hand washing (see Section 23.3.1, Table 23.3).

22.2.4 Whole body skin cleaning

A non-Cochrane systematic review found seven RCTs and two before-and-after studies that evaluated single cleansing of the whole body with chlorhexidine.[12] Pooled analysis showed no significant effect on neonatal mortality rate and reported sepsis rates had substantial heterogeneity. The authors found no conclusive evidence for any beneficial effect after single skin cleansing with chlorhexidine. Umbilical cord care is effective (Section 22.2.3) and should take precedence.

22.3 Community-based interventions

22.3.1 Case management

In developing countries where the majority of infants are born at home with limited access to antenatal and perinatal care, case management (early identification and treatment of infants with infections) in primary care settings has been a major policy initiative promoted by the World Health Organization.

A non-Cochrane systematic review and meta-analysis of 13 controlled trials of neonatal care by community health workers in India involving 192 000 births reported a 27% reduction in all-cause neonatal mortality in resource-poor settings (95% CI 17–35).[13] The interventions were a mix of preventative and therapeutic. They were most effective when the baseline neonatal mortality rate was high (>50 per 1000 live births) although still statistically significant at lower mortality rates.[13]

It is important to be able to use simple clinical criteria to identify neonates in the community with systemic sepsis and/or pneumonia.[14, 15] Two systematic reviews of clinical signs that predict severe infection in infants <60 days old brought to a developing country health-care facility concluded the most valuable signs and symptoms were feeding difficulty, convulsions, fever or hypothermia, reduced activity, tachypnoea, severe chest in-drawing, grunting and cyanosis. Other signs associated with sepsis were pallor and poor capillary return.[16, 17]

A non-Cochrane meta-analysis of seven controlled studies of pneumonia case management reported a 27% reduction in all-cause mortality and a 42% reduction in mortality due to neonatal pneumonia.[18] A non-Cochrane systematic review identified four non-randomized concurrently controlled studies of oral antibiotics for neonatal pneumonia which showed a 25% reduction in all-cause mortality (95% CI 11–36) and a 42% reduction (95% CI 18–59) in mortality of neonatal pneumonia (Figure 22.1).[19] Injectable antibiotics are likely to be more effective than oral in neonatal pneumonia, but are not always available in developing countries (see Section 8.1.8).

A large cluster randomized trial from Bangladesh illustrates the value of case management for neonatal

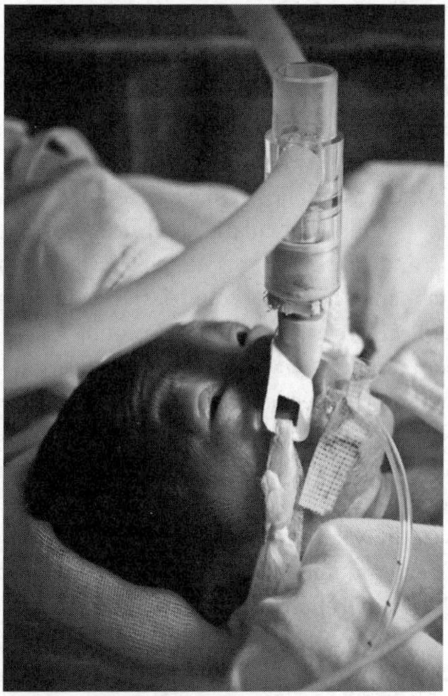

Figure 22.1 Neonatal pneumonia requiring nasal continuous positive airways pressure. Photograph by Philip Cruz.

sepsis and some of the problems.[20, 21] Clusters of pregnant women were randomly allocated to home care, community care or comparison arms. In the home-care arm, female community health workers made antenatal home visits, post-natal home visits and they treated or referred sick neonates. In the community-care arm, qualified providers promoted birth and newborn-care preparedness and care seeking solely through group sessions. In the last 6 months of the 30-month intervention, neonatal mortality was reduced in the home-care arm by 34% (95% CI 7–53) compared with the comparison arm but mortality was not reduced in the community-care arm.[20] The case fatality rate for infected neonates was 4.4% if treated by community health workers, 14.2% by qualified medical providers and 28.5% by other unqualified providers or untreated. Compared with neonates who were untreated or treated by unqualified providers, neonates treated by community health workers had a 78% reduction in mortality (95% CI 29–93) and those treated by qualified providers had a 39% reduction (95% CI 1–63). However, referral compliance even for very severe diseases was only 34% and home-treatment acceptance was 43%,[21] showing that one problem will be putting effective interventions into practice.[22]

22.4 Pathogens

The predominant pathogens causing early-onset infections in many developing countries in Africa, Asia, Latin America and the Middle East are Gram-negative enteric bacilli, particularly Klebsiella species and *E. coli*, and *Staphylococcus aureus*.[23] GBS is uncommon in many developing countries[23] but an important cause of early sepsis in some Asian countries.[24]

There are limited data on home deliveries. The 4 commonest pathogens reported with almost equal frequency from 7–28 days of age are *S. aureus*, GBS, *Streptococcus pneumoniae* and non-typhoidal Salmonella species.[14]

There are very limited data on antibiotic susceptibility of community-acquired pathogens in Africa and Asia.[25–27] Available data suggest common pathogens such as *S. aureus* and Klebsiella have reduced susceptibility to almost all commonly used antibiotics.[25] *S. pneumoniae* are usually susceptible to penicillin but not co-trimoxazole.[25] One review of 10 studies found that 72% of *E. coli* were resistant to ampicillin, 78% to cotrimoxazole (trimethoprim–sulfamethoxazole) and 19% resistant to third generation cephalosporins.[26] Klebsiella species were almost 100% resistant to ampicillin, 45% to cotrimoxazole and 66% to third generation cephalosporins.[26] Methicillin resistance of *S. aureus* was rare but 46% were resistant to cotrimoxazole.[26] A subsequent study from Kolkata, India reported that over 80% of Gram-negative bacilli causing early-onset sepsis exhibited multi-drug resistance to ampicillin, third generation cephalosporins and gentamicin indicating that these multi-resistant organisms circulate widely in the community. The mortality from Gram-negative sepsis was high.[27] A more recent non-Cochrane systematic review and meta-analysis of 19 studies from 13 countries found up to 40% of cases were resistant or had reduced susceptibility to ampicillin/penicillin, gentamicin and third generation cephalosporins.[28]

22.5 Antibiotics

The appropriate choice of empiric antibiotics depends on the antibiotic susceptibility of local organisms causing neonatal sepsis. This makes it unwise to be prescriptive about empiric antibiotic regimens, which may anyway be dictated in part by cost. As discussed in Chapter 5 (see Section 5.1.3) the WHO currently recommends the use of ampicillin or penicillin G plus gentamicin to treat suspected community-acquired late-onset sepsis in developing countries but up to 40% of infections are caused by organisms resistant or with reduced susceptibility to ampicillin/penicillin and gentamicin and to third generation cephalosporins.[28] An editorial on combating antibiotic resistance sub-titled 'The war against error' advised against one size fits all recommendations and recommended that antibiotic regimens be tailored to local epidemiology. The editorial also stressed that bacteria have evolved resistance genes over millions of years, so escalation to use increasingly broad-spectrum antibiotics to chase resistance is doomed to failure.[29]

Oral antibiotics are effective in the case management of pneumonia.[30] Parenteral antibiotics are needed for serious infections. A review suggested that procaine penicillin G plus gentamicin or ceftriaxone alone were the preferred regimens for serious neonatal infections in the community and primary care because they could be given once daily and were safe and effective.[31]

There are very few RCTs of antibiotics in neonatal infection.[32] An RCT compared failure rates of three clinic-based antibiotic regimens in 0–59 day-old infants with possible serious bacterial infection whose families refused hospitalization in Karachi communities with high neonatal mortality rates >45/1000 live births.[33] Eligible infants were randomly assigned to 7 days of: (i) procaine penicillin plus gentamicin or (ii) ceftriaxone alone, or (iii) oral cotrimoxazole (trimethoprim–sulfamethoxazole) plus gentamicin. The primary outcome was treatment failure (defined as death or either, deterioration or no improvement after 2 days on antibiotics). There were 13 of 145 failures (9%) with penicillin–gentamicin, 22 of 145 with ceftriaxone (15.1%) and 26 of 143 with cotrimoxazole–gentamicin (18.2%). Treatment failure was significantly higher with cotrimoxazole–gentamicin compared to penicillin–gentamicin (RR 2.0, 95% CI 1.1–3.8). The difference between the ceftriaxone and penicillin–gentamicin groups approached statistical significance (RR 1.7, 95% CI 0.9–3.2). By 14 days, there were 2 deaths in the penicillin–gentamicin group, 3 in the ceftriaxone group, and 11 in the cotrimoxazole–gentamicin group. The authors concluded that outpatient therapy with injectable antibiotics is an effective option when hospitalization of sick infants is not possible, that procaine penicillin–gentamicin was superior to cotrimoxazole–gentamicin and that ceftriaxone may be less effective.[33]

In developing countries antibiotics are often continued despite negative cultures and increasingly broad-spectrum antibiotics are often added without evidence of infection.[34, 35] The wonderful name '**spiraling empiricism**' was used to describe this unjustifiable escalation of antibiotic treatment of suspected but undocumented infections.[36] The main danger is selection of highly resistant organisms,[35] a phenomenon that appears to be getting worse.[27] Cost is another major problem of using expensive broad-spectrum antibiotics in many developing countries, for individual families and for the country.

Good neonatal practice needs access to a reliable microbiology laboratory performing culture and antimicrobial susceptibility. Clinicians need to trust the culture results and stop unnecessary antibiotic therapy when systemic cultures are negative. If cultures are positive, clinicians should 'step down,' that is stop broad-spectrum antibiotics and change to the narrowest-spectrum antibiotic regimen possible.

22.6 Cost-effectiveness

Even if interventions are effective in reducing neonatal morbidity and mortality in developing countries it is also important to show that they are cost-effective in comparison to other competing health-care interventions. For example, if an immunization programme was cheaper, easier to implement and saved more lives, it would be foolish to spend scarce resources on another community-based programme.

A cost-effectiveness analysis of 21 interventions for maternal and newborn health found the most cost-effective mix of interventions in both sub-Saharan Africa and South East Asia was a community-based newborn care package, followed by maternal antenatal care (tetanus toxoid, screening for pre-eclampsia, screening and treatment of asymptomatic bacteriuria and syphilis); skilled birth attendants; and emergency obstetric and neonatal care around and after birth. Screening and treatment of maternal syphilis, community-based management of neonatal pneumonia, and antenatal steroids were relatively less cost-effective in South East Asia.[37] The authors estimated that achieving 95% coverage of all the included interventions would halve neonatal and maternal deaths. They concluded that community preventive interventions for newborn babies and primary care interventions for mothers and newborn babies are extremely cost-effective, but universal access to clinical services is also needed to achieve the 2015 millennium goal of the United Nations to reduce child mortality by two-thirds and maternal mortality by three-quarters by 2015 (goals 4 and 5, respectively).[37, 38]

22.7 Feasibility

Experts consulted about research priorities to reduce global neonatal infection-related mortality by 2015 identified barriers affecting the delivery of existing cost-effective health-care interventions as the main priority.[39] The main areas identified were promotion of preventative home-care practices and strategies to increase the coverage and quality of management of neonatal infections in health-care facilities and in the community. Research into health systems and policy was seen as critical to improve neonatal outcomes from infection.[39]

References

1. Bhutta ZA, Darmstadt GL, Hasan BS, Haws RA. Community-based interventions for improving perinatal and neonatal health outcomes in developing countries: a review of the evidence. *Pediatrics* 2005; 115(2 Suppl):519–617.
2. Saugstad OD. Reducing global neonatal mortality is possible. *Neonatology* 2011; 99:250–257.
3. Darmstadt GL, Walker N, Lawn JE, Bhutta ZA, Haws RA, Cousens S. Saving newborn lives in Asia and Africa: cost and impact of phased scale-up of interventions within the continuum of care. *Health Policy Plan* 2008; 23:101–117.
4. Barros AJ, Ronsmans C, Axelson H, et al. Equity in maternal, newborn, and child health interventions in Countdown to 2015: a retrospective review of survey data from 54 countries. *Lancet* 2012; 379:1225–1233.
5. Sibley LM, Sipe TA, Brown CM, Diallo MM, McNatt K, Habarta N. Traditional birth attendant training for improving health behaviours and pregnancy outcomes. Cochrane Database of Systematic Reviews 2007, Issue 3. Art. No.: CD005460. doi: 10.1002/14651858.CD005460.pub2.
6. Jokhio AH, Winter HR, Cheng KK. An intervention involving traditional birth attendants and perinatal and maternal mortality in Pakistan. *N Engl J Med* 2005; 352:2091–2098.
7. Blencowe H, Cousens S, Mullany LC, et al. Clean birth and postnatal care practices to reduce neonatal deaths from sepsis and tetanus: a systematic review and Delphi estimation of mortality effect. *BMC Public Health* 2011; 11(Suppl 3):S11.
8. Seward N, Osrin D, Li L, et al. Association between clean delivery kit use, clean delivery practices, and neonatal survival: pooled analysis of data from three sites in South Asia. *PLoS Med* 2012; 9:e1001180. doi: 10.1371/journal.pmed.1001180
9. Zupan J, Garner P, Omari AAA. Topical umbilical cord care at birth. Cochrane Database of Systematic Reviews 2004, Issue 3. Art. No.: CD001057. doi: 10.1002/14651858.CD001057.pub2.
10. Arifeen SE, Mullany LC, Shah R, et al. The effect of cord cleansing with chlorhexidine on neonatal mortality in rural Bangladesh: a community-based, cluster-randomised trial. *Lancet* 2012; 379:1022–1028.
11. Soofi S, Cousens S, Imdad A, Bhutto N, Ali N, Bhutta ZA. Topical application of chlorhexidine to neonatal umbilical cords for prevention of omphalitis and neonatal mortality in a rural district of Pakistan: a community-based, cluster-randomised trial. *Lancet* 2012; 379:1029–1036.
12. Sankar MJ, Paul VK. Efficacy and safety of whole body skin cleansing with chlorhexidine in neonates - A systemic review. *Pediatr Infect Dis J* 2013; 32(6):e227–e234.
13. Gogia S, Ramji S, Gupta P, Gera T, Shah D, et al. Communtiy based newborn care: a systematic review and metaanalysis of evidence: UNICEF-PHI series on newborn and child health, India. *Indian Pediatr* 2011; 48:537–546.
14. Bang AT, Bang RA, Reddy MH, et al. Simple clinical criteria to identify sepsis or pneumonia in neonates in the community needing treatment or referral. *Pediatr Infect Dis J* 2005; 24:335–341.
15. Darmstadt GL, Baqui AH, Choi Y; Bangladesh Projahnmo-2 (Mirzapur) Study. Validation of a clinical algorithm to identify neonates with severe illness during routine household visits in rural Bangladesh. *Arch Dis Child* 2011; 96:1140–1146.
16. Opiyo N, English M. What clinical signs best identify severe illness in young infants aged 0-59 days in developing countries? A systematic review. *Arch Dis Child* 2011; 96:1052–1059.
17. Coghill JE, Simkiss DE. Which clinical signs predict severe illness in children less than 2 months of age in resource poor countries? *J Trop Pediatr* 2011; 57:3–8.
18. Sazawal S, Black RE. Pneumonia Case Management Trials Group. Effect of pneumonia case management on mortality in neonates, infants, and preschool children: a meta-analysis of community-based trials. *Lancet Infect Dis* 2003; 3:547–556.
19. Zaidi AK, Ganatra HA, Syed S, et al. Effect of case management on neonatal mortality due to sepsis and pneumonia. *BMC Public Health* 2011; 11(Suppl 3):S13.
20. Baqui AH, El-Arifeen S, Darmstadt GL, Ahmed S, Mannan I, Rahman SM, et al. Effect of community-based newborn-care intervention package implemented through two service-delivery strategies in Sylhet district, Bangladesh: a cluster-randomised controlled trial. *Lancet* 2008; 371:1936–1944.
21. Baqui AH, Arifeen SE, Williams EK, Ahmed S, Mannan I, Rahman SM, et al. Effectiveness of home-based management of newborn infections by community health workers in rural Bangladesh. *Pediatr Infect Dis J* 2009; 28:304–310.
22. Bhutta Z, Zaidi AK, Thaver D, Humayun Q, Ali S, Darmstadt GL. Management of newborn infections in primary care settings: a review of the evidence and implications for policy? *Pediatr Infect Dis J* 2009; 28(1 Suppl):S22–S30.
23. Zaidi AKM, Thaver D, Ali AS, Khan TA. Pathogens associated with sepsis in newborns and young infants in developing countries. *Pediatr Infect Dis J* 2009; 28:S10–S18.
24. Tiskumara R, Fakharee SH, Liu CQ, et al. Neonatal infections in Africa. *Arch Dis Fetal Neonatal Ed* 2009; 94:F144–F148.
25. Thaver D, Ali SA, Zaidi AKM. Antimicrobial resistance among neonatal pathogens in developing countries. *Pediatr Infect Dis J* 2009; 28(1 Suppl):S19–S21.
26. Lubell Y, Ashley EA, Turner C, Turner P, White NJ. Susceptibility of community-acquired pathogens to antibiotics in Africa and Asia in neonates -an alarmingly short review. *Trop Med Int Health* 2011; 16:145–151.
27. Viswanathan R, Singh AK, Basu S, Chatterjee S, Sardar S, Isaacs D. Multi-drug resistant gram negative bacilli causing early neonatal sepsis in India. *Arch Dis Child Fetal Neonatal Ed* 2012; 97: F182–F187.
28. Downie L, Armiento R, Subhi R, et al. Community acquired infant and neonatal sepsis in developing countries: efficacy

of WHO's currently recommended antibiotics: a systematic review and meta-analysis. *Arch Dis Child* 2013; 98:146–154.

29. Isaacs D, Andresen D. Combating antibiotic resistance: the war on error. *Arch Dis Child* 2013; 98:90–91.
30. Darmstadt GL, Batra M, Zaidi AKM. Oral antibiotics in the management of serious neonatal bacterial infections in developing country communities. *Pediatr Infect Dis J* 2009; 28(1 Suppl):S31–S36.
31. Darmstadt GL, Batra M, Zaidi AKM. Parenteral antibiotics for the treatment of serious neonatal bacterial infections in developing country settings. *Pediatr Infect Dis J* 2009; 28(1 Suppl):S37–S42.
32. Gordon A, Jeffery HE. Antibiotic regimens for suspected late onset sepsis in newborn infants. Cochrane Database of Systematic Reviews 2005, Issue 3. Art. No.: CD004501. doi: 10.1002/14651858.CD004501.pub2.
33. Zaidi AK, Tikmani SS, Warraich HJ, et al. Community-based treatment of serious bacterial infections in newborns and young infants: a randomized controlled trial assessing three antibiotic regimens. *Pediatr Infect Dis J* 2012; 31:667–672.
34. Isaacs D. Neonatal sepsis: the antibiotic crisis. *Indian Pediatrics* 2005; 42:1–6.
35. Isaacs D. Unnatural selection: reducing antibiotic resistance in neonatal units. *Arch Dis Child Fetal Neonatal Ed* 2006; 91:F72–F74.
36. Kim JH, Gallis HA. Observations on spiralling empiricism: its causes, allure and perils, with particular reference to antibiotic therapy. *Am J Med* 1989; 87:201–206.
37. Adam T, Lim SS, Mehta S, et al. Cost effectiveness analysis of strategies for maternal and neonatal health in developing countries. *BMJ* 2005; 331:1107.
38. Evans DB, Adam T, Tan-Torres Edejer T, et al. Achieving the millennium development goals for health: Time to reassess strategies for improving health in developing countries? *BMJ* 2005; 331:1133.
39. Bahl R, Martines J, Ali N, et al. Research priorities to reduce global mortality from newborn infections by 2015. *Pediatr Infect Dis J* 2009; 28(1 Suppl):S43–S48.

CHAPTER 23

Prevention of neonatal infections

A review of the literature on adjunctive treatments to prevent neonatal infection identified three non-Cochrane systematic reviews which included different modalities for prevention of neonatal infections.[1–3] This chapter will consider four different categories of intervention: feed-related, infection control, physical environment and immunomodulatory agents.

23.1 Feeding-related interventions

23.1.1 Breast milk

Although few paediatricians doubt the value of breast milk, the evidence of its efficacy in preventing neonatal infections is not particularly strong. It is hard to imagine anyone ever performing a large trial in which babies are randomized to receive human breast milk or formula.

There are a number of reasons for expecting breast milk to be protective against infection. Breast milk contains secretory IgA, lactoferrin and oligosaccharides called prebiotics with antibacterial activity (see Chapter 19).) Lack of breast milk could be described as the commonest immune deficiency of infancy.[4]

A Cochrane systematic review and meta-analysis of five trials which compared donor breast milk with pre-term formula on growth and development in pre-term infants demonstrated a statistically significantly higher incidence of necrotizing enterocolitis (NEC) in the formula-fed group: typical relative risk 2.5 (95% CI 1.2, 5.1); number needed to harm: 33 (95% CI 17, 100).[5] In the only study which reported rates of infection, extremely pre-term infants <30 weeks of gestation whose mothers intended to breastfeed were randomized to receive either pasteurized donor milk or pre-term formula if their own mother's milk supply became insufficient.[6] The rate of clinical and proven late-onset infection between infants who received donor milk (29%) was the same as infants who received pre-term formula (30%), but significantly lower (23%) for infants who received exclusively mother's milk ($p = 0.02$). Furthermore, infants who received mother's milk had a significantly lower incidence of proven gram-negative bloodstream infection (6%) than donor milk (14%) or pre-term formula (22%), ($p < 0.01$).[6]

In a non-randomized study from India gave expressed human milk to 4 of 31 infants <1500 g given breast milk but 17 of 31 given standard nursery formula developed nosocomial infections ($p < 0.001$).[7]

An observational study from Ghana found that delayed initiation of breastfeeding increased neonatal mortality.[8] The adverse effects of delaying breast feeds started within an hour of birth and there was a marked dose response: neonatal mortality increased progressively with delay up to day 7. Initiation of breastfeeding after day 1 was associated with a 2.4-fold increase in neonatal mortality.[8] A possible explanation is that total protein and immunoglobulin levels in breast milk are highest on day 1, halve by day 2 and slowly decrease thereafter.[8]

There are stronger data regarding infant breastfeeding and infections. A systematic review of breastfeeding and mortality in developing countries with a high prevalence of HIV infection found that breastfeeding in the first 6 months protected against death from diarrhoeal diseases and respiratory infections.[9] In another study of infants in Ghana, India and Peru, non-breastfed infants were more than 10 times as likely to die.[10]

Studies from Western countries confirm that breastfeeding prevents infections. In a cluster-randomized

Evidence-Based Neonatal Infections, First Edition. David Isaacs.

trial of breast-feeding promotion in Belarus maternity hospitals, breastfeeding was associated with a reduction in diarrhoeal but not respiratory infections.[11] In a UK study, exclusive breastfeeding compared with no breastfeeding was associated with a reduction in hospitalization in infancy for both diarrhoeal and respiratory infections.[12] In a non-Cochrane systematic review of breastfeeding in industrialized countries, breastfeeding protected against diarrhoeal infections in 6 of 8 studies and against respiratory infections in 13 of 16 studies.[13]

Mother's breast milk is strongly recommended for pre-term infants in developing and Western countries and preferred for term infants in both developing and Western countries, unless the mother is HIV positive (Table 23.1 and Chapter 17).

Breast milk transmission of infections (e.g. CMV, GBS, HIV) is considered in Chapter 19.

23.1.2 Early enteral feeding

Early enteral feeding could reduce late-onset neonatal infections by reducing the need for central venous access and parenteral nutrition, both known risk factors for late-onset sepsis (see Section 2.2.4).

Theoretical suggestions that early enteral feeds might predispose to NEC have been refuted by trial-based evidence (see Chapter 11).[17–19] A Cochrane systematic review of nine trials (754 infants) comparing early trophic feeding versus fasting for infants <1500 g found no difference in the incidence of NEC.[17] Only two trials reported rates of sepsis. One RCT compared minimal enteral nutrition from days 2 to 7 with fasting, but feeds were increased at the same rate from day 8 and not surprisingly there was no difference in incidence of sepsis.[20] Another RCT randomized infants <1750 g to trophic feeds or (0.5–1 mL/hour plus parenteral nutrition from day 3 until ventilator support finished) or parenteral nutrition alone.[14] Trophic feeding infants had significantly fewer infections (mean 0.5 vs. 1.2 episodes of culture-proven sepsis), received less parenteral nutrition (mean difference 11.5 days), grew better and were discharged home earlier.[14] The additional infections in the parenteral nutrition group were mainly due to catheter-associated organisms (CoNS and to a lesser extent *S. aureus*).[14]

In a retrospective study from Israel of infants <1500 g, 42% developed nosocomial infection and 9% NEC.[21] Enteral feeding was introduced at the same age (3–4 days) in infants who did and did not develop NEC. However, enteral feeding was introduced significantly later (4.8 vs. 2.8 days) in infants who developed late-onset infection. The mean age at start of feeding fell consistently over the 6-year study period, correlating with a concomitant fall in late-onset infections. This study is susceptible to confounding: the fall in infections with time could be due to many other factors.[21]

Although more RCTs would be welcome, the evidence from one well-conducted RCT[14] and one observational study[21] supports early trophic feeds for very low birth-weight infants as being beneficial and not harmful (Table 23.1).

23.1.3 Probiotics

Probiotics, naturally occurring gut bacteria such as Lactobacillus and Bifidobacterium found in the stools of full-term breastfed infants, can be given as live microbial supplements to colonize the gastrointestinal tract.

A Cochrane systematic review found 16 randomized or quasi-randomized trials of probiotics in 2842 pre-term infants.[15] Probiotics were associated with significant reductions in severe NEC (typical relative risk (RR) 0.35, 95% CI 0.24–0.52) and in mortality (typical RR 0.40, 95% CI 0.27–0.60). There was no reduction in nosocomial infections (typical RR 0.90, 95% CI 0.76–1.07).[15] A non-Cochrane systematic review found similar reductions in NEC and mortality with no difference in rates of blood culture-proven late-onset infection.[16] Neither review reported sepsis caused by probiotic organisms, one theoretical concern that has been raised.

These findings have provoked controversy (see Chapter 11). The largest studies were in Italy, Taiwan and Turkey and some critics have questioned their applicability to other settings. Different probiotic formulations were used and in some countries probiotics are not licensed for neonatal use. At the time of writing, results are awaited from large RCTs in Western countries which will provide more evidence (Table 23.1).

Probiotics do not reduce mortality by reducing sepsis or NEC. Interestingly, however, prolonged antibiotics are associated with increased all-cause mortality and NEC in very low birth-weight infants.[22, 23] It is tempting to postulate that probiotics act by replacing protective gut micro-organisms eradicated by broad-spectrum antibiotics.

Table 23.1 Feeding-related interventions to prevent neonatal infection.

Intervention	Level of evidence	No. of infants	Outcomes	Conclusions
Breast milk	RCT of donor milk or pre-term formula in infants <30 weeks started on mother's milk in the United States[6]	243	Mother's milk reduced clinical and proven late-onset sepsis and reduced proven gram-negative bloodstream infection in pre-term US infants	Breast milk recommended to reduce late-onset infections in pre-term infants in developing countries and Western countries
	Controlled trial of expressed breast milk versus formula in infants <1500 g in India[7]	62	Breast milk reduced infections in low birth-weight infants in India	Breast milk strongly recommended for pre-term infants in developing countries
	Systematic review comparing donor milk with formula in pre-term infants[5]	816	Breast milk is associated with lower risk of necrotizing enterocolitis (NEC)	Breast milk protects against NEC and is strongly recommended for all infants at risk of NEC
	Cohort study in Ghana[9]	10 947	Initiation of breastfeeding within 1 hour of birth reduces neonatal mortality	In developing countries, breastfeeding should be initiated within 1 hour of birth
	Individual patient data meta-analysis of six cohort studies in developing countries[8]	17 982	Breast milk is associated with lower risk of death from gastroenteritis and infectious respiratory disease	Breast milk recommended in developing countries to reduce mortality from diarrhoeal and respiratory infections
	Prophylactic cluster RCT of breastfeeding promotion in Belarus infants[10]	17 046	Breastfeeding reduced gastroenteritis (and atopic eczema) in first 12 months after birth	Breast milk recommended in Western countries to reduce incidence of diarrhoeal and respiratory infections
	Cohort study in UK infants[11]	15 890	Breastfeeding reduced hospitalizations from diarrheal and respiratory infections.	Breast milk recommended in Western countries to reduce hospitalizations for infections
	Cohort study in Dutch infants[12]	4164	Breastfeeding reduced incidence of diarrhoeal and respiratory infections	Breast milk recommended in Western countries to reduce diarrhoeal and respiratory infections
Early enteral feeding	RCT in UK infants[14]	100	Early trophic feeds reduced late-onset infections compared with delayed feeds	Early enteral feeding strongly recommended
Probiotics	Cochrane systematic review[15]	2842	Significant reduction in mortality and in NEC in very low birth-weight infants, but not in neonatal infections. Some concerns about general applicability of trial results	Not currently recommended for all very low birth-weight infants pending the results of further trials
	Non-Cochrane systematic review[16]	2176		
Prebiotics	Non-Cochrane systematic review in pre-term infants	126	No reduction in neonatal infection	Not recommended
	Non-Cochrane systematic review in full-term infants	1459	No reduction in neonatal infection	Not routinely recommended

Source: Adapted from Reference 2 with permission.

23.1.4 Prebiotics

Prebiotics are non-digestible oligosaccharide food components that selectively stimulate the growth or activity of non-pathogenic bacteria in the colon.[24] In a systematic review and meta-analysis of four RCTs in 126 pre-term infants prebiotic supplemented formula increased stool colony counts of probiotic organisms (bifidobacteria and lactobacilli), but there was no effect on the rates of infection.[25] A systematic review of six RCTs in 1459 full-term infants found that prebiotics did not affect neonatal infections.[26] (Table 23.1).

23.2 Infection control measures

23.2.1 Hand washing

Hand hygiene (hand washing) is compulsory in the computer microchip industry, because microchips can be permanently damaged if handled with unwashed hands, and non-compliant workers can be disciplined or even dismissed.[27] Hospitals are busy and stressful and hand washing lapses when health-care workers' workload increases.[28] Nevertheless, it is not easy to explain to parents that health-care workers forget to wash their hands when they are busy. It is shameful that microchips are valued higher than babies.[29]

Does hand hygiene reduce nosocomial infections? Studies of improved hand hygiene and nosocomial neonatal infections are generally before-and-after intervention studies which often do not measure compliance (Table 23.2). A systematic review of hand hygiene and nosocomial infections found only 35 studies that met the inclusion criteria and concluded 'the varied nature of the interventions used and the diverse factors affecting the acquisition of health-care associated infections make it difficult to show the specific effect of hand hygiene alone'.[41] In Western countries most of the reduction is in CoNS infections,[30–32] although before-and-after studies suggest improved hand hygiene also reduces spread of virulent or multi-resistant colonizing pathogens[33, 34] and respiratory virus infections.[35]

In developing countries, there are few well-conducted studies. Introduction of an infection control programme in Bangladesh emphasizing improved hand washing was followed by a 61% decrease in

Table 23.2 Infection control interventions to prevent neonatal infection.

Intervention	Level of evidence	No. of infants	Outcomes	Conclusions
Hand hygiene	Before and after studies of variable quality[30–35, 36]	Unknown	Reduction in nosocomial infections and, in Bangladesh, reduction in deaths from infection[35]	Good hand hygiene strongly recommended despite relatively low-level evidence
Gowns	Cochrane review[37] including two good quality randomized studies	3811	No reduction in infections	Gowns not routinely recommended
Gloves	A neonatal study compared gloves plus alcohol rub with hand washing[37]	337	Reduction in nosocomial infection but could have been due to improved compliance with hand hygiene	Gloves not routinely recommended. Gloves only recommended for high-risk invasive or dirty procedures
	Cluster-randomized adult ICU study[38]	9139	No reduction in MRSA or VRE transmission	
Clusters of infection control measures	Interventional studies. Six intervention NICUs compared with 66 control hospitals[39]	24 872	Reduction in CoNS infections greater in intervention hospitals than in control hospitals. Intervention cost-saving	Cluster interventions recommended if feasible for Western or developing countries with high rates of nosocomial infections
	18 NICUs before and after bundle and checklist introduced[40]		67% reduction in central-line-associated infections	

culture-proven sepsis and in deaths from clinical (82%) or culture-proven sepsis (50%).[42]

How well do we wash our hands?

A non-Cochrane systematic review found 96 empiric studies on compliance with hand hygiene, 65 in intensive care units.[43] The overall median compliance rate was an embarrassing 40% and rates were lower in intensive care units (30–40%) than elsewhere, presumably due to workload. Doctors (32%) were worse than nurses (48%).[43]

Does it matter what we use for hand hygiene?

Alcohol rubs remove more bacteria from hands than soap and water,[44] but there is little evidence that this equates with fewer nosocomial infections. A cross-over study in two US neonatal units compared a traditional antiseptic hand-wash with an alcohol hand sanitizer. Infection rates and microbial counts on nurses' hands were no different, although nurses' skin improved when using alcohol.[45] In an Italian study, nosocomial infections were reduced when a standardized hand hygiene programme was introduced using chlorhexidine antimicrobial soap and alcohol-based hand rubs compared with plain detergent (triclosan) but the study did not examine compliance.[46] Soap and water were more effective than alcohol rubs in reducing office workers' infections in a cluster-randomized study in Finland,[47] but were no different when compared in US elementary schoolchildren.[48] A large cluster-randomized surgical study in Kenya found no difference in surgical site infections irrespective of whether alcohol-based rub or plain soap and water was used for surgical hand preparation.[36] Alcohol-based hand rubs are cheap and a good alternative when continuous clean water is unavailable.[36]

How can we improve hand hygiene compliance?

Medical and nursing staff and other health-care workers are well aware that hand washing is important, but compliance is a major issue. A Cochrane systematic review found only four studies of hand hygiene compliance describing different interventions with inconclusive results.[37] In a non-Cochrane systematic review, low compliance was associated with high activity levels and with physician involvement.[43] Compliance was higher in association with dirty tasks, availability of alcohol-based hand rub or gel, improved accessibility of hand hygiene materials and with performance feedback.[43]

An Australian children's hospital reported a sustained increase in hand hygiene compliance from 23% in 2006 to 87% in 2011 following a 'Clean hands save lives' campaign involving education, improving alcohol-based hand rub accessibility at points of patient care, monitoring staff practices and feeding back performance data.[37] This was associated with a decline in nosocomial bacteraemia and in transmission of multi-resistant organisms.[49]

23.2.2 Gowns

A Cochrane systematic review of gowning by attendants and visitors in neonatal units found that only two of eight studies were of good quality. *Not* wearing gowns was associated with a trend to lower death rate (typical RR 0.84, 95% CI 0.70–1.02). Gowning had no effect on nosocomial infections (typical RR 1.24, 95% CI 0.90–1.71).[50] Routine gowning is not recommended (Table 23.2).

23.2.3 Gloves

There is no evidence that gloves have any advantage over hand hygiene. A Hong Kong sequential study compared 36 months of conventional hand washing with 36 months of alcohol hand rub used by workers wearing non-sterile gloves.[51] Nosocomial infections fell but compliance was not assessed. Universal gloving did not reduce transmission of MRSA or VRE compared with standard infection control practices in a large cluster-randomized trial in US adult intensive care units.[38]

Routine use of gloves is expensive and unpopular with staff. Gloving is obviously important for high-risk invasive procedures such as central venous catheter insertion and to protect staff with broken skin on their hands, for example, eczema, against infections (Table 23.2).

23.2.4 Clusters of infection control interventions

Clusters of different infection control interventions introduced simultaneously have become popular in adult and paediatric intensive care units. Sequential studies or preferably cluster-randomized trials can be used to evaluate efficacy of the whole cluster. This does not generate evidence on individual components which may not matter if the cluster is effective and cost-effective. The Vermont Oxford Network leads the way in this field in neonatal infection prevention, initially in Western countries and subsequently in resource-poor settings.[39, 52]

In a sequential before-and-after study late-onset CoNS infections fell from 22% to 16.6% of infants <1500 g in US neonatal units assigned to a 3-year collaborative quality improvement intervention.[39] Nosocomial infections with other organisms did not fall.[39] The intervention reduced the costs of neonatal care while the costs rose in control hospitals and the intervention was assessed as cost-effective.[52]

An innovative study compared 15 differences in infection control practices in US NICUs with high and low rates of nosocomial infections, shared them with all the hospitals and let individual NICUs decide which practice differences to implement.[53] The network nosocomial infection rate fell from 3.8 to 2.9 episodes per 1000 patient-days.[53]

A statewide intervention in New York State aimed to reduce central-line-associated bacteraemias (CLABs). All 18 NICUs adopted central-line insertion and maintenance bundles and checklists to monitor their use. The before and after study found a 67% reduction in rates of CLAB (95% CI 59–73).[40]

A Canadian cluster-randomized study assigned six NICUs to a cluster of evidence-based interventions to reduce nosocomial infections (strategic placement of hand cleaner dispensers, measures to reduce skin breaks and measures to reduce duration of antibiotics) and six NICUs to interventions to reduce bronchopulmonary dysplasia (BPD).[54, 55] There was a significant reduction in BPD but a non-significant reduction in nosocomial infections. Cost-effectiveness was not assessed.[55]

23.3 Physical interventions

23.3.1 Umbilical cord care

Historically, improved umbilical cord care was associated with dramatic reductions in omphalitis and in skin (impetigo) and systemic infections (osteomyelitis, disseminated sepsis) with *Staphylococcus aureus*.[56, 57] A Cochrane systematic review of umbilical cord care found 21 studies (8959 participants) mainly from high-income countries.[58] Antiseptics reduced colonization with *S. aureus* significantly by about half. Umbilical infection was rare (about 1%) and not reported in most studies. Antiseptic cord care compared with dry cord care was associated with a non-significant but almost 50% reduction in umbilical infection (9 of 1431 vs. 18 of 1400, RR 0.53, 95% CI 0.25, 1.13).[58]

Evidence of the importance of cord care is much stronger in developing countries, particularly three recent cluster-randomized trials. A community-based study in Nepal randomized over 15 000 infants to cord care with 4% chlorhexidine, soap and water or dry cord care.[59] Topical chlorhexidine reduced severe omphalitis by 75% (95% CI 47–88) compared to dry cord care and reduced mortality by 34% (95% CI 5–54) for infants enrolled within 24 hours of birth.[59] In Bangladesh, 29 760 babies were randomized to single cleansing with chlorhexidine as soon as possible after birth, multiple cleansing daily chlorhexidine for 7 days or dry cord care.[60] Neonatal mortality was 20% lower in the single-cleansing group than dry cord care. Severe omphalitis was reduced in the multiple-cleansing but not the single-cleansing group compared to dry cord care. A Pakistan study randomized 9741 babies to combinations of chlorhexidine or promotion of hand washing in the family. Hand-washing promotion was ineffective, but chlorhexidine was associated with a 42% reduction in omphalitis (95% CI 18–59) and a 38% reduction in mortality (95% CI 15–55).[61]

There were no safety concerns with the use of chlorhexidine which is strongly recommended in developing countries (Table 23.3).

23.3.2 Skin barrier therapy

Skin barrier therapy using emollient ointments may reduce heat loss and skin breakdown in very pre-term babies and possibly nosocomial infections. A Cochrane systematic review[62] of four RCTs (1304 infants) reported borderline increased incidence of any nosocomial infection in babies who received skin barrier therapy (RR 1.20, 95% CI 1–1.43), almost entirely due to CoNS infections in babies 501–750 g (RR 1.31, 95% CI 1.02–1.70). However, 92% of the babies in the Cochrane review came from a single US study performed by the Cochrane authors, using a proprietary product, Aquaphor, comprising petrolatum, mineral oil, mineral wax and lanolin alcohol.

Studies in developing countries led by Gary Darmstadt and colleagues from Johns Hopkins University, Baltimore show sunflower seed oil is cheap and highly effective at reducing infections and deaths in pre-term

Table 23.3 Physical interventions to prevent neonatal infection.

Intervention	Level of evidence	No. of infants	Outcomes	Conclusions
Umbilical cord care	Cochrane systematic review[58]	8959	No difference in infections but not always studied	Routine umbilical cord care with a topical antiseptic such as chlorhexidine is strongly recommended in Western and developing countries
	Subgroup of Cochrane review[58]	2831	Topical antiseptics reduced umbilical infection by 47% (non-significant) compared to dry cord care	
	Cluster-randomized study in Nepal[59]	15 136	Topical chlorhexidine reduced omphalitis by 75% and deaths by 34%	
	Cluster-randomized study in Bangladesh[60]	29 760	Chlorhexidine reduced omphalitis and mortality but results varied between single and multiple applications	
	Cluster-randomized study in Nepal[61]	9741	Chlorhexidine reduced omphalitis by 42% and mortality by 38%	
Skin barrier therapy	Cochrane systematic review of infants <1500 g[62]	1304	Skin emollients (mainly Aquaphor) increased infections due to CoNS (mainly in US infants <750 g)	Sunflower oil strongly recommended for very pre-term babies in developing countries
	RCT in infants <34 weeks in Egypt[63]	103	Sunflower oil reduced infections by 54%	More studies needed in Western countries
	RCT in infants <33 weeks in Bangladesh[64, 65]	497	Sunflower oil reduced infections by 41% and deaths by 26%; Aquaphor reduced deaths by 32%	
Kangaroo care	Cochrane systematic review[66]	2518	Kangaroo care reduced nosocomial infections by 58% and mortality by 40%	Kangaroo care strongly recommended in resource-poor developing countries
Delayed cord clamping	Two small RCTs in pre-term infants[66]	107	One study showed reduced late-onset infections with delayed cord clamping, the other not	Results awaited from large RCT currently underway

babies.[63–65] An Egyptian study of infants <34 weeks of gestation found that 8 hourly topical sunflower oil was associated with a 46% reduction (95% CI 19–74) in nosocomial infections.[64] The cost was about US $0.20 a course. An RCT of infants <33 weeks in Bangladesh compared sunflower oil or Aquaphor with untreated controls.[65, 67] Either sunflower oil or Aquaphor reduced nosocomial infections by 40%, although only the former result reached significance.[64] When the study was continued, they both reduced mortality significantly: sunflower oil by 26% (95% CI 1–45) and Aquaphor by 34% (95% CI 8–49).[65, 67]

The number needed to treat (NNT) is three or four babies. The total cost is less than US $1 to save a life. This is arguably the most cost-effective intervention in neonatal infection prevention.

23.3.3 Kangaroo care

Kangaroo care or kangaroo mother care was developed by Edgar Rey in 1978 in Bogota, Colombia, as an alternative to conventional methods of caring for low birth-weight infants, because of a local lack of incubators and a high rate of nosocomial infections.[68] The name refers to using skin-to-skin contact between a mother and her

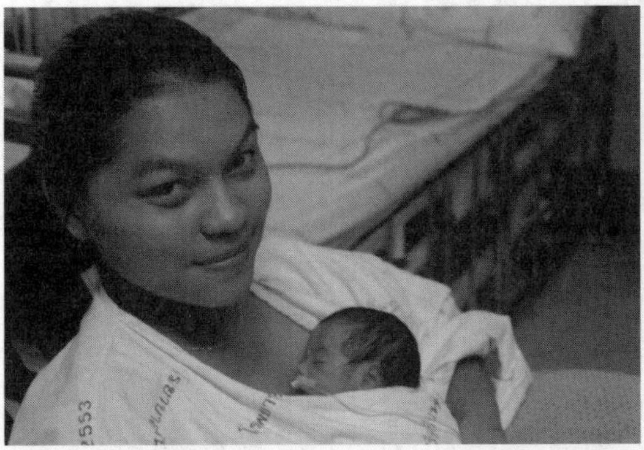

Figure 23.1 Kangaroo care (photograph courtesy of Prof Heather Jeffery).

newborn to provide warmth and comfort: babies are placed between the mother's breasts and held in place with a wrap (Figure 23.1). Rey likened this to a baby kangaroo in its mother's pouch. A mother can share the role with others, especially the baby's father.

In a Cochrane systematic review of 16 RCTs (2518 babies) kangaroo care reduced mortality at 40–41 weeks (typical RR, 0.60, 95% CI 0.39–0.93), reduced nosocomial infections (typical RR 0.42, 95% CI 0.24–0.73), reduced hypothermia by 79% and reduced length of hospital stay by a mean of 2.4 days.[66]

Kangaroo care is a cheap and highly effective intervention in resource-poor countries where neonatal special and intensive care is unavailable and/or unaffordable (Table 23.3). Its use has not been studied adequately in Western countries.

23.3.4 Delayed cord clamping

Delayed umbilical cord clamping for pre-term deliveries improves haematocrit and circulation and reduces intraventricular haemorrhage (IVH). In an RCT of babies delivered <32 weeks of gestation, delayed cord clamping (at 30–45 seconds) reduced blood culture-proven infection compared to immediate (5–10 seconds) clamping (1 of 36 delayed vs. 8 of 36 immediate clamping, $p = 0.03$). Infants with sepsis had significantly lower haematocrits at birth.[69] An underpowered Israeli study of 35 pre-term infants (29 <1500 g) found no effect on the incidence neonatal infections.[70]

A Cochrane systematic review of timing of cord clamping on maternal and neonatal outcomes did not examine NEC or neonatal infection.[71] Another Cochrane systematic review looked at the effect of delayed cord clamping on NEC but not on neonatal infection.[72] At least one large RCT is underway which will compare neonatal infections in pre-term babies following immediate or delayed cord clamping.

23.4 Immunomodulatory interventions

23.4.1 Polyclonal intravenous immunoglobulin

A Cochrane systematic review of polyclonal IVIG to prevent neonatal infections identified 19 RCTs in 4986 pre-term or very low birth-weight infants.[73] There was a significant reduction in one or more episodes of any bloodstream infection (RR 0.85, 95% CI 0.74, 0.98). The absolute risk difference was small: 3% for any proven bloodstream infection and 4% for any 'serious infection'. There was no reduction in mortality, NEC, IVH or length of hospital stay.[73] The reduction in serious infection, without reduction in other adverse outcomes, was judged by the Cochrane review authors as being of marginal clinical significance. The NNT was 33 to prevent one bloodstream infection and 25 to prevent one 'serious infection'. The authors concluded, unusually for a Cochrane review, that further studies were not warranted and advised basing decisions on use on the costs and values assigned to the clinical outcomes.[73] There are no published cost-effectiveness analyses of prophylactic IVIG, which is almost certainly not cost-effective compared to other effective health-care interventions and cannot be recommended (Table 23.4).

23.4.2 Anti-staphylococcal immunoglobulins

Staphylococci are of major importance in neonatal infection. CoNS cause over half of all late-onset infections in Western countries. MSSA and MRSA infections are important late-onset pathogens in all countries and important early-onset pathogens in many developing countries. Researchers have developed various type-specific antibodies targeted at different antigenic markers of the Staphylococcus.[81–83]

A Cochrane systematic review[81] of three RCTs of anti-staphylococcal IVIG compared to placebo showed

Table 23.4 Immunomodulatory interventions to prevent neonatal infection.

Intervention	Level of evidence	Number of infants	Outcomes	Conclusions
IVIG (polyclonal)	Cochrane systematic review of RCTs in pre-term infants[69]	4986	Infection reduced by 3%, but no effect on mortality. Cost-effectiveness unknown	Not recommended. No further similar RCTs needed. Unlikely to be cost-effective
IVIG (monoclonal)	Cochrane systematic review[70]	2694	No difference in mortality, sepsis or other adverse outcomes	Not recommended
G-CSF or GM-CSF	Cochrane systematic review of four prophylactic RCTs[70]	639	No difference in mortality or sepsis	Not recommended. More RCTs needed
Lactoferrin	Cochrane systematic review[74] but only one RCT[75, 76]	472	Lactoferrin reduced incidence of late-onset bacterial and fungal infection sepsis in infants <1500 g	More RCTs needed to confirm protection and evaluate effects on disability-free survival
Heparin	Two RCTs[77, 78]	411	One showed no effect, one showed heparin infusion significantly reduced culture-proven sepsis	More RCTs needed
Selenium	Cochrane systematic review of three RCTs[79]	583	Selenium reduces sepsis, but two of the three studies were in areas with low soil selenium	More RCTs needed
Glutamine	Cochrane systematic review[80]	2365	No difference in mortality or sepsis	Not recommended

Source: Adapted from Reference 2 with permission.

no difference in sepsis, mortality or other adverse outcomes in two RCTs ($n = 2488$) of INH-A21 (Veronate), an antibody to 'microbial surface components recognizing adhesive matrix molecules' (RR 1.07; 95% CI 0.94–1.22), and in an RCT ($n = 206$) of Altastaph, which targets capsular polysaccharide antigens (RR 0.86; 95% CI 0.32–2.28). Further RCTs are in progress (Table 23.4).

23.4.3 Colony-stimulating factors

A Cochrane systematic review of G-CSF or GM-CSF in neonates found three prophylaxis studies (359 neonates) which did not show a significant reduction in mortality (RR 0.59, 95% CI 0.24–1.44).[84] The primary outcome of sepsis was not evaluable because of unsatisfactory definitions of infection. In one study the incidence of systemic infection in a subgroup of infants <32 weeks of gestation who were neutropoenic or at high risk of developing post-natal neutropoenia was reduced from 53% to 31%, but the numbers were small ($n = 31$) and the difference not statistically significant (RR 0.59, 95% CI 0.25–1.39).[85]

A subsequent multi-centre trial randomized 280 neonates <31 weeks of gestation with low birth weight (<10th percentile) within 72 hours of birth to receive GM-CSF for 5 days or standard care.[86] Although neutrophil counts rose more rapidly in the GM-CSF babies, there was no significant difference in sepsis-free survival for all infants. A meta-analysis of this and previous published trials showed no evidence of survival benefit.[86]

Colony-stimulating factors are not indicated for prophylaxis to prevent systemic infection in high-risk neonates (Table 23.4).

23.4.4 Lactoferrin

Lactoferrin is a naturally occurring glycoprotein with antimicrobial activity (see Chapter 6).[74,87,88]

A Cochrane systematic review[74] found one eligible RCT of bovine lactoferrin.[75] This Italian trial randomized 472 infants <1500 g to oral lactoferrin alone, lactoferrin plus the probiotic *Lactobacillus rhamnosus* GG or placebo from birth until 30 days. Late-onset sepsis was significantly lower in the groups that received lactoferrin alone (RR 0.34, 95% CI 0.17–0.70) or lactoferrin in combination with *L. rhamnosus* GG (RR 0.27, 95% CI 0.12–0.60).[75] The incidence of NEC was significantly reduced with lactoferrin and *L. rhamnosus* GG (RR 0.05, 95% CI 0.00–0.90), but not oral lactoferrin alone (RR 0.33, 95% CI 0.09–1.17). No adverse effects due to lactoferrin were observed. A subsequent secondary analysis of the data found that invasive fungal infection was significantly lower with bovine lactoferrin alone (0.7%) or plus *L. rhamnosus* GG (2%) than with placebo (7.7%).[76]

One double-blind RCT found that formula-fed infants whose formula was supplemented with bovine lactoferrin in the first 12 months of life had significantly fewer respiratory infections than unsupplemented formula-fed infants (0.15 vs. 0.5 episodes/year).[89]

More studies of lactoferrin are in progress (Table 23.4).

23.4.5 Heparin

Heparin can prolong the duration of central venous catheters. An RCT found that infants who had heparin infusion had a slightly higher though not statistically different rate of suspected or proven sepsis than controls (10 of 100 vs. 6 of 101).[77] In a subsequent RCT, heparin in total parenteral nutrition significantly reduced culture-proven catheter-related sepsis (RR 0.57, 95% CI 0.32– 0.98; NNT 9, 95% CI 4.6–212.4).[78] More data are needed (see Table 23.4).

23.4.6 Selenium

Selenium is an essential trace element and a component of many proteins including glutathione peroxidase, which helps protect against oxidative damage. Selenium deficiency is associated with impairment of T-cell-mediated immunity and B-cell function.[79] Selenium deficiency is associated with increased susceptibility to oxidative lung injury in animal models. Low blood selenium concentrations in pre-term infants have been suggested as a potential risk factor for sepsis, chronic neonatal lung disease and retinopathy of prematurity.

A Cochrane systematic review identified three RCTs of parenteral or enteral selenium supplementation for pre-term or very low birth-weight infants.[79] Two trials were from geographical areas with low population selenium concentrations. Meta-analysis ($n = 583$) showed that selenium supplementation was associated with a significant reduction in the number of infants with sepsis (summary RR 0.73, 95% CI 0.57–0.93; NNT 10, 95% CI 5.9, 50). Supplementation with selenium was not associated with improved survival or reduced neonatal chronic lung disease or retinopathy of prematurity. Selenium supplementation should be studied more and considered for pre-term infants in areas with very low soil selenium levels (Table 23.4).

23.4.7 Glutamine

Glutamine is an amino acid that is synthesized endogenously, although endogenous biosynthesis may be insufficient when there is severe metabolic stress. Glutamine supplementation improves clinical outcomes in critically ill adults and it has been postulated that it might benefit pre-term infants, particularly <1500 g. A Cochrane systematic review found seven good quality trials of glutamine supplementation, three enteral and four parenteral, involving 2365 very low birth-weight neonates.[80] Glutamine supplementation had no statistically significant effect on neonatal infections, NEC, mortality or neurodevelopment at 18 months.[80]

23.5 Immunization

23.5.1 Maternal immunization

Maternal immunization can protect the mother and potentially the foetus and/or infant.

Population use of **rubella** immunization in infancy, as measles, mumps, rubella (MMR) vaccine, has virtually eliminated congenital rubella syndrome in Western countries.[90, 91] Similarly universal immunization of a population against **hepatitis B** protects women from developing chronic hepatitis B virus infection and therefore prevents mother-to-child transmission.[91] Other examples of childhood immunization which include girls and so protect the unborn foetus or newborn infant when the girl becomes a mother include vaccines against **varicella-zoster virus**, **pertussis** and **tetanus**. One can also argue that other childhood vaccines give indirect protection by keeping the mother healthy.

In general vaccines are rarely advised for pregnant women because of theoretical safety concerns. The devastating effect of pandemic H1N1 influenza on pregnant women and their foetuses, however, resulted in large numbers of pregnant women being immunized safely against influenza and increased provider confidence in intrapartum immunization. Vaccines that might be given intrapartum to pregnant women specifically to protect the newborn infant are considered below.

23.5.1.1 Influenza vaccine

Influenza vaccine is recommended by US and Australian advisory committees for women who will be in the second or third trimester of pregnancy in the influenza season, because of the increased morbidity of influenza for pregnant women.[92, 93] The maternal and foetal morbidity was particularly severe with pandemic influenza A/H1N1 (pandemic 'swine flu') when at least 75 pregnant women in the United States died from influenza and survivors were more likely to deliver pre-term and low birth-weight infants.[94]

In an RCT from Bangladesh, maternal influenza immunization at about 32 weeks of gestation reduced laboratory-proven influenza in infants in the first 6 months of life by 63% (95% CI 5–85).[95, 96]

Antepartum and intrapartum influenza immunization is recommended for women who will be or are pregnant to protect the mother, the foetus and the newborn baby (Table 23.5).

23.5.1.2 Pertussis vaccine

Pertussis continues to circulate and reported incidence is increasing in many Western countries despite high population coverage. Possible reasons include waning immunity from acellular vaccines or increased diagnosis due to increased awareness or more sensitive laboratory tests, for example, polymerase chain reaction (PCR). Infants in the first 3 months of life are most at risk of fatal infection (see Chapter 14), yet will have received no or only one dose of vaccine when exposed to pertussis. Strategies to protect very young infants indirectly include intrapartum maternal immunization and 'cocooning'. The policy of cocooning is based on the fact that about 50% of infants with pertussis can be shown to have acquired pertussis from a parent, usually the mother, and 25% from siblings or grandparents. Cocooning involves immunizing parents (the mother post-natally) and possibly other relatives to reduce the risk of neonatal exposure. There is at best weak evidence that cocooning actually prevents infection and cost-effectiveness analyses suggest it is not cost-effective compared with other health-care interventions.[104]

Intrapartum maternal immunization with pertussis or a pertussis-containing vaccine is another possible approach.[104] Such an approach has not been scientifically proven to prevent neonatal or infant infections, but an expert analysis of the costs and likely efficacy compared to cocooning suggests intrapartum maternal immunization is likely to prevent more infections and save more lives at a lower cost than cocooning. However, protection was based on serologic criteria and there are no proven serologic correlates for pertussis protection. Surprisingly, in view of the lack of formal evidence of efficacy, the US Advisory Committee on Immunization Practices (ACIP) recommended giving a booster dose of tetanus toxoid, reduced diphtheria and acellular pertussis vaccine (tdap) intrapartum to any pregnant woman who had not received a booster previously (or post-natally if not given intrapartum).[105] (Table 23.5).

23.5.1.3 Pneumococcal immunization

The highest incidence of invasive pneumococcal disease is in the first few months of life. Maternal intrapartum pneumococcal immunization is one possible strategy to protect the neonate and young infant. There is indirect evidence that this would protect infants: studies in the Philippines and Finland showed that infants of mothers immunized intrapartum with the polysaccharide vaccine had high antibody levels until 4 months old.[106, 107] There is a good correlation for pneumococcal infection between antibody levels and protection. However, there are no studies that have yet shown neonatal or infant protection and further studies are awaited.

23.5.1.4 Tetanus immunization

Pregnant women in developing countries who never received tetanus vaccine can be immunized safely in pregnancy to prevent neonatal tetanus.[97, 108] A Cochrane systematic review found two RCTs.[97] One study of 1919 infants assessed the effectiveness of tetanus toxoid in preventing neonatal tetanus deaths.[109] After a single dose, the RR was 0.57 (95%

Table 23.5 Maternal and neonatal immunizations to prevent neonatal infection and protect the foetus and newborn infant.

Intervention	Level of evidence	No. of infants	Outcomes	Conclusions
Intrapartum maternal inactivated influenza vaccine	One RCT.[94] Large number of observational studies	340	Infants protected against influenza for first 6 months	We recommend antepartum and intrapartum influenza immunization of women who will be or are pregnant to protect the foetus and newborn baby
Intrapartum maternal pertussis vaccine	No RCTs	0	No evidence of efficacy from any studies	Recommended in the United States, but we do not recommend its use until safety and efficacy data are available
Intrapartum pneumococcal vaccine	No RCTs	0	Serological evidence but no evidence of protective efficacy in neonatal or infants	Not recommended. Neonatal and infant data needed
Maternal intrapartum tetanus vaccine	Cochrane systematic review of RCT s in pregnant women or women of childbearing age[97]	10 560	Vaccine safe and highly effective in reducing deaths from neonatal tetanus	Strongly recommended
BCG vaccine	Non-Cochrane meta-analysis[98, 99]	361 443	Vaccine safe and immunogenic (except in severe T-cell deficiency, including HIV), no tolerance	Strongly recommended where tuberculosis endemic
Neonatal polio vaccine	No RCTs		Vaccine safe and immunogenic, no tolerance	Strongly recommended where polio endemic
Neonatal pneumococcal vaccine	Two RCTs[100, 101]	619	Vaccine safe and immunogenic, no tolerance, but not superior to standard schedule	Not recommended yet
Neonatal pertussis vaccine	Two RCTs[102, 103]	197	Vaccine safe and immunogenic early, no tolerance, but some reduction in antibody titres to other antigens	Not recommended yet. Large RCTs needed

CI 0.26–1.24) and vaccine effectiveness was 43%. After two or three doses the RR was 0.02 (95% CI 0.00–0.30) and vaccine effectiveness 98%. The RR of cases of neonatal tetanus after at least one dose of tetanus toxoid was 0.20 (95% CI 0.10–0.40) and vaccine effectiveness 80%. Another study of 8641 children showed that one or two doses of maternal tetanus–diphtheria toxoid vaccine reduced all-cause neonatal deaths by 32% (95% CI 18–44) and deaths at 4–14 days by 62% (95% CI 45–73).[110] Neither study reported any maternal ill effects of immunization. A non-Cochrane systematic review estimated that immunization of pregnant women or women of childbearing age with at least two doses of tetanus toxoid reduces mortality from neonatal tetanus by 94% (95% CI 80–98).[111]

23.5.2 Neonatal immunization

There are theoretical concerns that neonatal immunization might result in immunologic tolerance. A paper in 1965 suggested that neonates immunized at birth with pertussis vaccines not only failed to respond well to the vaccine but responded less well than controls to subsequent doses of pertussis vaccine.[112] They interpreted this as meaning that the infant's immune system interpreted the pertussis antigens as being 'self-antigens' and so did not recognize them as foreign, becoming 'tolerant' to them. Subsequent studies suggest the neonate can respond to a number of vaccines, perhaps because of newer adjuvants, without developing tolerance.[113]

A non-Cochrane review reported that studies demonstrate that the neonatal immune system is specifically adapted for early post-natal life rather than being 'immature'.[113] Memory B cells, not antibody-secreting plasma cells, are induced preferentially and neonatal T-cell responses are polarized away from potentially deleterious T-helper type 1 cytokines. The authors commented that in small trials birth doses of acellular pertussis and pneumococcal conjugate vaccines are immunogenic and do not appear to lead to tolerance, although vaccine interference is a potential problem.[113]

23.5.3 Neonatal BCG vaccine

BCG vaccine is effective when given at birth or in infancy. A non-Cochrane meta-analysis of 5 RCTs and 11 case-control studies of BCG vaccine in neonates and infants showed an overall protective efficacy against tuberculosis (TB) disease of 74% (95% CI 62–83) estimated from 4 RCTs and of 52% (95% CI 38–64) from 9 case-control studies.[98] BCG had 65% protective efficacy against death from TB (95% CI 12–86), 64% against TB meningitis (95% CI 30–82) and 78% against disseminated TB (95% CI 58–88). Better studies reported greater efficacy.[98]

A further analysis of the above meta-analysis selected 26 of the original 70 studies involving 361 443 infants and estimated the efficacy of BCG against TB as an average of 50% across all ages of vaccination.[99] BCG vaccine protected against both pulmonary and extra-pulmonary TB.[99]

Observational studies have suggested BCG may also have non-specific beneficial effects on survival. A randomized trial compared BCG at birth (early BCG) with delayed BCG in infants <2500 g in Guinea-Bissau.[114] The pre-trial infant mortality was 250 per 1000. Infant mortality was only 101 per 1000 during the trial. In the primary analysis, infant mortality was reduced by 17%, mainly due to fewer cases of neonatal sepsis, respiratory infection and fever. The impact of early BCG on infant mortality was most marked for children weighing <1.5 kg (MRR = 0.43, 95% CI 0.21–0.85). This study[114] and another from India showing that tuberculin skin conversion rates for full-term and 34–35 week gestation infants given BCG was 80%[115] show that pre-term infants of 34 weeks of gestation and above can be immunized with BCG vaccine at birth.

A large South African study showed that percutaneous BCG vaccine was as safe and effective as intradermal BCG vaccine.[116]

23.5.4 Neonatal polio vaccine

Birth doses of polio vaccine are immunogenic and do not induce tolerance.[117, 118] Birth doses of polio vaccine are an important component of the strategy for the global elimination of poliomyelitis.

23.5.5 Neonatal hepatitis B vaccine

Mothers with chronic hepatitis B infection, particularly if *e* antigen positive, are at risk of passing hepatitis B infection to their newborn infant at the time of delivery, unless the infant is protected by immunization and antibody. The infected newborn becomes chronically infected but never develops antibodies, presumably because of tolerance. If the carrier mother is *e* antigen positive (highly infective), the calculated risk to the infant without intervention is 75.2%, but this risk can be reduced to 6% by giving vaccine and immunoglobulin at birth. If the mother is surface antigen positive but *e* antigen negative, the risk to the infant without intervention is 10.3%, reduced to 1% by giving vaccine and immunoglobulin.[119, 120] The vaccine is composed of purified hepatitis B surface antigen. Presumably the infant mounts an immunologic response to vaccine but not wild-type virus because adjuvant in the vaccine stimulates the immune response.

23.5.6 Neonatal pneumococcal conjugate vaccine

The incidence of pneumococcal invasive disease is higher in the first year of life than at any other age. In developing countries, invasive pneumococcal infection can infect infants <3 months old and cause major morbidity and mortality.[112] A birth dose of pneumococcal conjugate vaccine is safe, is immunogenic, primes for memory, and does not cause B-cell or T-cell tolerance.[100, 101] However, two small RCTs in developing countries suggest that a birth dose of pneumococcal vaccine does not give significantly higher levels of antibodies than the standard schedule.[100, 101] Studies are needed on the efficacy of birth dose pneumococcal conjugate vaccine.

23.5.7 Neonatal pertussis vaccine

Pertussis continues to circulate in Western countries despite high levels of infant immunization (Section 23.5.1.2 and Chapter 14). A RCT comparing a birth dose of acellular pertussis vaccine plus routine 2-, 4- and 6-month immunizations with birth dose hepatitis B vaccine plus routine immunizations found the birth dose of pertussis induced higher pertussis antibodies at 3 months of age[102] but not 7 months, primed well without tolerance,[121] but elicited some 'bystander' reduction in hepatitis B, Hib and diphtheria antibody titres, of dubious clinical significance.[102, 121] An RCT compared acellular pertussis vaccine (Pa) at birth and 1 month with Pa at birth and with controls. All infants also received standard 2-, 4- and 6-month immunizations. The birth plus 1-month infants had higher pertussis antibody levels at 2 months without tolerance.[103] These studies show that a birth dose of acellular vaccine can induce early pertussis antibody responses without tolerance, but large RCTs are needed to show whether this translates into clinical effectiveness and the effect on responses to other vaccine antigens.

23.6 Prophylactic antibiotics

A Cochrane systematic review[122] found three small randomized controlled studies of prophylactic antibiotics in neonates with central venous catheters from the 1990s.[123–125] Prophylactic antibiotics decreased the rate of proven bacterial sepsis (typical RR 0.38, 95% CI 0.18, 0.82), but had no effect on overall mortality (typical RR 0.68, 95% CI 0.31, 1.51).[122] The authors of the review queried the clinical importance in view of the lack of effect on mortality or neurodevelopmental outcome and the lack of data on resistant organisms and concluded that routine use of prophylactic antibiotics for infants with central venous catheters could not be recommended.[122] The available data do not support the use of prophylactic antibiotics for infants with umbilical venous catheters,[126] umbilical arterial catheters[127] or intercostal drains.[128]

One RCT found that infants whose central venous catheters were locked with heparin that contained vancomycin had a lower incidence of CLAB with CoNS than infants who had heparin locks.[129] However, asymptomatic hypoglycaemia developed in infants in both groups, which is an enormous safety concern. No vancomycin-resistant enterococci or staphylococci were detected, but detecting vancomycin-resistant *S. aureus* is difficult. Long-term prophylactic vancomycin is not recommended because of the danger of antibiotic resistance.

23.7 Maternal antibiotics for pre-term rupture of membranes

In a Cochrane review of 22 trials (6800 women and babies) prophylactic maternal antibiotics for pre-term rupture of membranes (PROM) were associated with statistically significant reductions in chorioamnionitis (average RR 0.66, 95% CI 0.46–0.96) and in neonatal infection (RR 0.67, 95% CI 0.52–0.85) compared with no antibiotics or placebo.[130] Prophylactic antibiotics reduced the number of babies born within 48 hours by 29% and within 7 days by 21%. However, amoxicillin–clavulanate was associated with a significant increase in neonatal NEC (RR 4.72, 95% CI 1.57–14.23).[130] The authors of the Cochrane review pointed out the lack of evidence of reduced mortality or long-term benefit and concluded that the decision to prescribe antibiotics for PROM is not clear-cut.[130] They also said the antibiotic regimen of choice was uncertain and is likely to depend on local epidemiology.

References

1. Borghesi A, Tzialla C, Decembrino L, Manzoni P, Stronati M. New possibilities of prevention of infection in the newborn. *J Matern Fetal Neonatal Med* 2011; 24(Suppl 2):28–30.
2. Tarnow-Mordi W, Isaacs D, Dutta S. Adjunctive immunologic interventions in neonatal sepsis. *Clin Perinatol* 2010; 37:481–499.
3. Cohen-Wolkowiez M, Benjamin Jr DK, Capparelli E. Immunotherapy in neonatal sepsis: advances in treatment and prophylaxis. *Curr Opin Pediatr* 2009; 21:177–181.
4. Hanson LA. Session 1: feeding and infant development breast-feeding and immune function. *Proc Nutr Soc* 2007; 66:384–396.
5. Quigley M, Henderson G, Anthony MY, McGuire W. Formula milk versus donor breast milk for feeding preterm or low birth weight infants. *Cochrane Database Syst Rev*

2007; Issue 4. Art. No.: CD002971. doi: 10.1002/14651858.CD002971.pub2
6. Schanler RJ, Lau C, Hurst NM, Smith EO. Randomized trial of donor human milk versus preterm formula as substitutes for mothers' own milk in the feeding of extremely premature infants. *Pediatrics* 2005; 116:400–406.
7. Narayanan I, Prakash K, Gujral VV. The value of human milk in the prevention of infection in the high-risk low-birth-weight infant. *J Pediatr* 1981; 99:496–498.
8. Edmond KM, Zandoh C, Quigley MA, Amenga-Etego S, Owusu-Agyei S, Kirkwood BR. Delayed breastfeeding initiation increases risk of neonatal mortality. *Pediatrics* 2006; 117:e380–e386.
9. WHO Collaborative Study Team on the Role of Breastfeeding on the Prevention of Infant Mortality. Effect of breastfeeding on infant and child mortality due to infectious diseases in less developed countries: a pooled analysis. *Lancet* 2000; 355:451–455.
10. Bahl R, Frost C, Kirkwood BR, et al. Infant feeding patterns and risks of death and hospitalization in the first half of infancy: multicentre cohort study. *Bull World Health Org* 2005; 83:418–426.
11. Kramer MS, Chalmers B, Hodnett ED, et al.; PROBIT Study Group (Promotion of Breastfeeding Intervention Trial). Promotion of Breastfeeding Intervention Trial (PROBIT): a randomized trial in the Republic of Belarus. *J Am Med Assoc* 2001; 285:413–420.
12. Quigley MA, Kelly YJ, Sacker A. Breastfeeding and hospitalization for diarrheal and respiratory infection in the United Kingdom Millennium Cohort Study. *Pediatrics* 2007; 119:e837–e842.
13. Duijts L, Ramadhani MK, Moll HA. Breastfeeding protects against infectious diseases during infancy in industrialized countries. A systematic review. *Matern Child Nutr* 2009; 5:199–210.
14. McClure RJ, Newell SJ. Randomised controlled trial of clinical outcome following trophic feeding. *Arch Dis Child Fetal Neonatal Ed* 2000; 82:F29–F33.
15. AlFaleh K, Anabrees J, Bassler D, Al-Kharfi T. Probiotics for prevention of necrotizing enterocolitis in preterm infants. *Cochrane Database Syst Rev* 2011; Issue 3. Art. No.: CD005496. doi: 10.1002/14651858.CD005496.pub3
16. Deshpande G, Rao S, Patole S, Bulsara M. Updated meta-analysis of probiotics for preventing necrotizing enterocolitis in preterm neonates. *Pediatrics* 2010; 125:921–930.
17. Bombell S, McGuire W. Early trophic feeding for very low birth weight infants. *Cochrane Database Syst Rev* 2009; Issue 3. Art. No.: CD000504. doi: 10.1002/14651858.CD000504.pub3
18. Morgan J, Young L, McGuire W. Slow advancement of enteral feed volumes to prevent necrotising enterocolitis in very low birth weight infants. *Cochrane Database Syst Rev* 2011; Issue 3. Art. No.: CD001241. doi: 10.1002/14651858.CD001241.pub3
19. Morgan J, Young L, McGuire W. Delayed introduction of progressive enteral feeds to prevent necrotising enterocolitis in very low birth weight infants. *Cochrane Database Syst Rev* 2011; Issue 3. Art. No.: CD001970. doi: 10.1002/14651858.CD001970.pub3
20. Mosqueda E, Sapiegiene L, Glynn L, Wilson-Costello D, Weiss M. The early use of minimal enteral nutrition in extremely low birth weight newborns. *J Perinatol* 2008; 28:264–269.
21. Flidel-Rimon O, Friedman S, Lev E, Juster-Reicher A, Amitay M, Shinwell ES. Early enteral feeding and nosocomial sepsis in very low birthweight infants. *Arch Dis Child Fetal Neonatal Ed* 2004; 89:F289–F292.
22. Cotten CM, Taylor S, Stoll B, et al. Prolonged duration of initial empirical antibiotic treatment is associated with increased rates of necrotizing enterocolitis and death for extremely low birth weight infants. *Pediatrics* 2009; 123:58–66.
23. Alexander VN, Northrup V, Bizzarro MJ. Antibiotic exposure in the newborn intensive care unit and the risk of necrotizing enterocolitis. *J Pediatr* 2011; 159:392–397.
24. Roberfroid M, Gibson GR, Hoyles L, et al. Prebiotic effects: metabolic and health benefits. *Br J Nutr* 2010; 104(Suppl 2):S1–S63.
25. Srinivasjois R, Rao S, Patole S. Prebiotic supplementation of formula in preterm neonates: a systematic review and meta-analysis of randomised controlled trials. *Clin Nutr* 2009; 28:237–242.
26. Rao S, Srinivasjois R, Patole S. Prebiotic supplementation in full-term neonates: a systematic review of randomized controlled trials. *Arch Pediatr Adolesc Med* 2009; 163:55–64.
27. Goldmann D. System failure versus personal accountability—the case for clean hands. *N Engl J Med* 2006; 355:121–123.
28. Pittet D, Simon A, Hugonnet S, Pessoa-Silva CL, Sauvan V, Perneger TV. Hand hygiene among physicians: performance, beliefs, and perceptions. *Ann Intern Med* 2004; 141:1–8.
29. Isaacs D. Hand washing. *J Paediatr Child Health* 2012; 48:457.
30. Kilbride HW, Wirtschafter DD, Powers RJ, Sheehan MB. Implementation of evidence-based potentially better practices to decrease nosocomial infections. *Pediatrics* 2003; 111:e519–e533.
31. Sharek PJ, Benitz WE, Abel NJ, Freeburn MJ, Mayer ML, Bergman DA. Effect of an evidence-based hand washing policy on hand washing rates and false-positive coagulase negative staphylococcus blood and cerebrospinal fluid culture rates in a level III NICU. *J Perinatol* 2002; 22:137–143.
32. Lam BC, Lee J, Lau YL. Hand hygiene practices in a neonatal intensive care unit: a multimodal intervention and impact on nosocomial infection. *Pediatrics* 2004; 114:e565–e571.
33. Royle J, Halasz S, Eagles G, Gilbert G, Dalton D, Jelfs P, Isaacs D. Outbreak of extended spectrum beta-lactamase producing *Klebsiella pneumoniae* in a neonatal unit. *Arch Dis Child Fetal Neonatal Ed* 1999; 80:F64–F68.
34. Brown SM, Lubimova AV, Khrustalyeva NM, et al. Use of an alcohol-based hand rub and quality improvement interventions to improve hand hygiene in a Russian

neonatal intensive care unit. *Infect Control Hosp Epidemiol* 2003; 24:172–179.
35. Jefferson T, Del Mar CB, Dooley L, et al. Physical interventions to interrupt or reduce the spread of respiratory viruses. *Cochrane Database Syst Rev* 2011; Issue 7. Art. No.: CD006207. doi: 10.1002/14651858.CD006207.pub4
36. Nthumba PM, Stepita-Poenaru E, Poenaru D, et al. Cluster-randomized, crossover trial of the efficacy of plain soap and water versus alcohol-based rub for surgical hand preparation in a rural hospital in Kenya. *Br J Surg* 2010; 97:1621–1628.
37. Gould DJ, Moralejo D, Drey N, Chudleigh JH. Interventions to improve hand hygiene compliance in patient care. *Cochrane Database Syst Rev* 2010; Issue 9. Art. No.: CD005186. doi: 10.1002/14651858.CD005186.pub3
38. Huskins WC, Huckabee CM, O'Grady NP, et al.; STAR*ICU Trial Investigators. Intervention to reduce transmission of resistant bacteria in intensive care. *N Engl J Med* 2011; 364:1407–1418.
39. Horbar JD, Rogowski J, Plsek PE, et al. Collaborative quality improvement for neonatal intensive care. NIC/Q Project Investigators of the Vermont Oxford Network. *Pediatrics* 2001; 107:14–22.
40. Schulman J, Stricof R, Stevens TP, et al; New York State Regional Perinatal Care Centers. Statewide NICU central-line-associated bloodstream infection rates decline after bundles and checklists. *Pediatrics* 2011; 127:436–444.
41. Backman C, Zoutman DE, Marck PB. An integrative review of the current evidence on the relationship between hand hygiene interventions and the incidence of health care-associated infections. *Am J Infect Control* 2008; 36:333–348.
42. Darmstadt GL, Ahmed NU, Saha SK, et al. Infection control practices reduce nosocomial infections and mortality in preterm infants in Bangladesh. *J Perinatol* 2005; 25:331–335.
43. Erasmus V, Daha TJ, Brug H, et al. Systematic review of studies on compliance with hand hygiene guidelines in hospital care. *Infect Control Hosp Epidemiol* 2010; 31:283e94.
44. Girou E, Loyeau S, Legrand P, Oppein F, Brun-Buisson C. Efficacy of handrubbing with alcohol based solution versus standard handwashing with antiseptic soap: randomised clinical trial. *BMJ* 2002; 325:362.
45. Savolainen-Kopra C, Haapakoski J, Peltola PA, et al. Hand washing with soap and water together with behavioural recommendations prevents infections in common work environment: an open cluster-randomized trial. *Trials* 2012; 13:10.
46. Capretti MG, Sandri F, Tridapalli E, Galletti S, Petracci E, Faldella G. Impact of a standardized hand hygiene program on the incidence of nosocomial infection in very low birth weight infants. *Am J Infect Control* 2008; 36:430–435.
47. Vessey JA, Sherwood JJ, Warner D, Clark D. Comparing hand washing to hand sanitizers in reducing elementary school students' absenteeism. *Pediatr Nurs* 2007; 33:368–372.
48. Larson EL, Cimiotti J, Haas J, et al. Effect of antiseptic handwashing vs alcohol sanitizer on health care-associated infections in neonatal intensive care units. *Arch Pediatr Adolesc Med* 2005; 159:377–383.
49. Jamal A, O'Grady G, Harnett E, Dalton D, Andresen D. Improving hand hygiene in a paediatric hospital: a multimodal quality improvement approach. *BMJ Qual Saf* 2012; 21:171–176.
50. Webster J, Pritchard MA. Gowning by attendants and visitors in newborn nurseries for prevention of neonatal morbidity and mortality. *Cochrane Database Syst Rev* 2003; Issue 2. Art. No.: CD003670. doi: 10.1002/14651858.CD003670
51. Ng PC, Wong HL, Lyon DJ, et al. Combined use of alcohol hand rub and gloves reduces the incidence of late onset infection in very low birthweight infants. *Arch Dis Child Fetal Neonatal Ed* 2004; 89:F336–F340.
52. Rogowski JA, Horbar JD, Plsek PE, et al. Economic implications of neonatal intensive care unit collaborative quality improvement. *Pediatrics* 2001; 107:23–29.
53. Bloom BT, Craddock A, Delmore PM, et al. Reducing acquired infections in the NICU: observing and implementing meaningful differences in process between high and low acquired infection rate centers. *J Perinatol* 2003; 23:489–492.
54. Lee SK, Aziz K, Singhal N, et al. Improving the quality of care for infants: a cluster randomized controlled trial. *Can Med Assoc J* 2009; 181:469–476.
55. McGuire W, Fowlie PW. Bridging the gaps: getting evidence into practice. *Can Med Assoc J* 2009; 181:457–458.
56. Forshall I. Septic umbilical arteritis. *Arch Dis Child* 1957; 32:25–30.
57. Cushing AH. Omphalitis: a review. *Pediatr Infect Dis* 1985; 4:282–285.
58. Zupan J, Garner P, Omari AAA. Topical umbilical cord care at birth. *Cochrane Database Syst Rev* 2004; Issue 3. Art. No.: CD001057. doi: 10.1002/14651858.CD001057.pub2
59. Mullany LC, Darmstadt GL, Khatry SK, et al. Topical applications of chlorhexidine to the umbilical cord for prevention of omphalitis and neonatal mortality in southern Nepal: a community-based, cluster-randomised trial. *Lancet* 2006; 367:910–918.
60. Arifeen SE, Mullany LC, Shah R, et al. The effect of cord cleansing with chlorhexidine on neonatal mortality in rural Bangladesh: a community-based, cluster-randomised trial. *Lancet* 2012; 379:1022–1028.
61. Soofi S, Cousens S, Imdad A, Bhutto N, Ali N, Bhutta ZA. Topical application of chlorhexidine to neonatal umbilical cords for prevention of omphalitis and neonatal mortality in a rural district of Pakistan: a community-based, cluster-randomised trial. *Lancet* 2012; 379:1029–1036.
62. Conner JM, Soll R, Edwards WH. Topical ointment for preventing infection in preterm infants. *Cochrane Database Syst Rev* 2003; Issue 4. Art. No.: CD001150. doi: 10.1002/14651858.CD001150.pub2
63. Edwards WH, Conner JM, Soll RF; Vermont Oxford Network Neonatal Skin Care Study Group. The effect of prophylactic ointment therapy on nosocomial sepsis rates and skin integrity in infants with birth weights of 501 to 1000g. *Pediatrics* 2004; 113:1195–1203.

64. Darmstadt GL, Badrawi N, Law PA, et al. Topically applied sunflower seed oil prevents invasive bacterial infections in preterm infants in Egypt: a randomized, controlled clinical trial. *Pediatr Infect Dis J* 2004; 23:719–725.
65. Darmstadt GL, Saha SK, Ahmed AS, et al. Effect of topical treatment with skin barrier-enhancing emollients on nosocomial infections in preterm infants in Bangladesh: a randomized controlled trial. *Lancet* 2005; 365:1039–1045.
66. Conde-Agudelo A, Belizán JM, Diaz-Rossello J. Kangaroo mother care to reduce morbidity and mortality in low birthweight infants. *Cochrane Database Syst Rev* 2011; Issue 3. Art. No.: CD002771. doi: 10.1002/14651858.CD002771.pub2
67. Darmstadt GL, Saha SK, Ahmed AS, et al. Effect of skin barrier therapy on neonatal mortality rates in preterm infants in Bangladesh: a randomized, controlled, clinical trial. *Pediatrics* 2008; 121:522–529.
68. Rey E, Martinez H. Rational management of the premature infant [Manejo racional del niño prematuro]. *I Curso de Medicina Fetal y Neonatal.* Bogota, Colombia: Universidad Nacional, 1983: 137–151.
69. Mercer JS, Vohr BR, McGrath MM, Padbury JF, Wallach M, Oh W. Delayed cord clamping in very preterm infants reduces the incidence of intraventricular hemorrhage and late-onset sepsis: a randomized, controlled trial. *Pediatrics* 2006; 117:1235–1242.
70. McDonald SJ, Middleton P. Effect of timing of umbilical cord clamping of term infants on maternal and neonatal outcomes. *Cochrane Database Syst Rev* 2008; Issue 2. Art. No.: CD004074. doi: 10.1002/14651858.CD004074.pub2
71. Rabe H, Reynolds GJ, Diaz-Rosello JL. Early versus delayed umbilical cord clamping in preterm infants. *Cochrane Database Syst Rev* 2004; Issue 4. Art. No.: CD003248. doi: 10.1002/14651858.CD003248.pub2
72. Kugelman A, Borenstein-Levin L, Kessel A, Riskin A, Toubi E, Bader D. Immunologic and infectious consequences of immediate versus delayed umbilical cord clamping in premature infants: a prospective, randomized, controlled study. *J Perinat Med* 2009; 37:281–287.
73. Ohlsson A, Lacy J. Intravenous immunoglobulin for preventing infection in preterm and/or low birth weight infants. *Cochrane Database Syst Rev* 2004; Issue 1. Art. No.: CD000361. doi: 10.1002/14651858
74. Pammi M, Abrams SA. Oral lactoferrin for the prevention of sepsis and necrotizing enterocolitis in preterm infants. *Cochrane Database Syst Rev* 2011; Issue 10. Art. No.: CD007137. doi: 10.1002/14651858.CD007137.pub3
75. Manzoni P, Rinaldi M, Cattani S, et al. Bovine lactoferrin supplementation for prevention of late-onset sepsis in very low-birth-weight neonates: a randomized trial. *J Am Med Assoc* 2009; 302:1421–1428.
76. Manzoni P, Stolfi I, Messner H, et al. Bovine lactoferrin prevents invasive fungal infections in very low birth weight infants: a randomized controlled trial. *Pediatrics* 2012; 129:116–123.
77. Shah PS, Kalyn A, Satodia P, et al. A randomized, controlled trial of heparin versus placebo infusion to prolong the usability of peripherally placed percutaneous central venous catheters (PCVCs) in neonates: the HIP (Heparin Infusion for PCVC) study. *Pediatrics* 2007; 119:e284–e291.
78. Birch P, Ogden S, Hewson M. A randomised, controlled trial of heparin in total parenteral nutrition to prevent sepsis associated with neonatal long lines: the Heparin in Long Line Total Parenteral Nutrition (HILLTOP) trial. *Arch Dis Child Fetal Neonatal Ed* 2010; 95:F252–F257.
79. Darlow BA, Austin N. Selenium supplementation to prevent short-term morbidity in preterm neonates. *Cochrane Database Syst Rev* 2003; Issue 4. Art. No.: CD003312. doi: 10.1002/14651858.CD003312
80. Tubman RTRJ, Thompson S, McGuire W. Glutamine supplementation to prevent morbidity and mortality in preterm infants. *Cochrane Database Syst Rev* 2008; Issue 1. Art. No.: CD001457. doi: 10.1002/14651858.CD001457.pub3
81. Shah PS, Kaufman DA. Antistaphylococcal immunoglobulins to prevent staphylococcal infection in very low birth weight infants. *Cochrane Database Syst Rev* 2009; Issue 2. Art. No.: CD006449. doi:10.1002/14651858
82. Patti JM. Vaccines and immunotherapy for staphylococcal infections. *Int J Artif Organs* 2005; 28:1157–1162.
83. Kaufman D. Veronate (Inhibitex). *Curr Opin Investig Drugs* 2006; 7:172–179.
84. Carr R, Modi N, Doré CJ. G-CSF and GM-CSF for treating or preventing neonatal infections. *Cochrane Database Syst Rev* 2003; Issue 3. Art. No.: CD003066. doi: 10.1002/14651858
85. Carr R, Modi N, Doré CJ, El-Rifai R, Lindo D. A randomised controlled trial of prophylactic GM-CSF in human newborns less than 32 weeks gestation. *Pediatrics* 1999; 103:796–802.
86. Carr R, Brocklehurst P, Doré CJ, Modi N. Granulocyte-macrophage colony stimulating factor administered as prophylaxis for reduction of sepsis in extremely preterm, small for gestational age neonates (the PROGRAMS trial): a single-blind, multicentre, randomised controlled trial. *Lancet* 2009; 373:226–233.
87. Valenti P, Antonini G. Lactoferrin: an important host defence against microbial and viral attack. *Cell Mol Life Sci* 2005; 62:2576–2587.
88. Gifford JL, Hunter HN, Vogel HJ. Lactoferricin: a lactoferrin-derived peptide with antimicrobial, antiviral, antitumor and immunological properties. *Cell Mol Life Sci* 2005; 62:2588–2598.
89. King Jr JC, Cummings GE, Guo N, et al. A double-blind, placebo-controlled, pilot study of bovine lactoferrin supplementation in bottle-fed infants. *J Pediatr Gastroenterol Nutr* 2007; 44:245–251.
90. Marin M, Broder KR, Temte JL, Snider DE, Seward JF; Centers for Disease Control and Prevention (CDC). Use of combination measles, mumps, rubella, and varicella vaccine: recommendations of the Advisory Committee on Immunization Practices (ACIP). *MMWR Recomm Rep* 2010; 59(RR-3):1–12.

91. Australian Government Department of Health and Ageing. *Australian Immunisation Handbook*, 10th edn. Canberra: Government Publishing, 2012. Available at: http://www.health.gov.au/internet/immunise/publishing.nsf/Content/Handbook-rubella (accessed 14 August 2013)
92. CDC. Prevention and control of influenza with vaccines. Recommendations of the Advisory Committee on Immunization Practices (ACIP), 2010. MMWR 2010; 59(No. RR-8).
93. MMWR. Prevention and control of influenza with vaccines: recommendations of the Advisory Committee on Immunization Practices, 2011. MMWR Weekly Reports 2011; 60: 1128-32.Available at: http://www.cdc.gov/mmwr/preview/mmwrhtml/mm6033a3.htm (accessed 14 August 2013)
94. Centers for Disease Control and Prevention (CDC). Maternal and infant outcomes among severely ill pregnant and postpartum women with 2009 pandemic influenza A (H1N1)–United States, April 2009–August 2010. *Morb Mortal Wkly Rep* 2011; 60: 1193–1196.
95. Zaman K, Roy E, Arifeen SE, et al. Effectiveness of maternal influenza immunization in mothers and infants. *N Engl J Med* 2008; 359:1555–1564.
96. Steinhoff MC, Omer SB, Roy E, et al. Neonatal outcomes after influenza immunization during pregnancy: a randomized controlled trial. *Can Med Assoc J* 2012; 184(6):645–653.
97. Lassi ZS, Haider BA, Bhutta ZA. Community-based intervention packages for reducing maternal and neonatal morbidity and mortality and improving neonatal outcomes. *Cochrane Database Syst Rev* 2010; Issue 11. Art. No.: CD007754. doi: 10.1002/14651858.CD007754.pub2
98. Colditz GA, Berkey CS, Mosteller F, et al. The efficacy of bacillus Calmette-Guérin vaccination of newborns and infants in the prevention of tuberculosis: meta-analyses of the published literature. *Pediatrics* 1995; 96:29–35.
99. Brewer TF. Preventing tuberculosis with bacillus Calmette-Guerin vaccine: a meta-analysis of the literature. *Clin Infect Dis* 2000; 31(Supp3):S64–S67.
100. Scott JA, Ojal J, Ashton L, Muhoro A, Burbidge P, Goldblatt D. Pneumococcal conjugate vaccine given shortly after birth stimulates effective antibody concentrations and primes immunological memory for sustained infant protection. *Clin Infect Dis* 2011; 53:663–670.
101. van den Biggelaar AH, Pomat W, Bosco A, et al. Pneumococcal conjugate vaccination at birth in a high-risk setting: no evidence for neonatal T-cell tolerance. *Vaccine* 2011; 29:5414–5420.
102. Knuf M, Schmitt HJ, Wolter J, et al. Neonatal vaccination with an acellular pertussis vaccine accelerates the acquisition of pertussis antibodies in infants. *J Pediatr* 2008; 152:655–660.
103. Wood N, McIntyre P, Marshall H, Roberton D. Acellular pertussis vaccine at birth and one month induces antibody responses by two months of age. *Pediatr Infect Dis J* 2010; 29:209–215.
104. Mooi FR, de Greeff SC. The case for maternal vaccination against pertussis. *Lancet Infect Dis* 2007; 7:614–624.
105. CDC. Updated recommendations for use of tetanus toxoid, reduced diphtheria and acellular pertussis vaccine (Tdap) in pregnant women and persons who have or anticipate having close contact with an infant aged <12 months. Advisory Committee on Immunization Practices (ACIP), 2011. *Morb Mortal Wkly Rep* 2011; 60: 1424–1426.
106. Quiambao BP, Nohynek HM, Käyhty H, et al. Immunogenicity and reactogenicity of 23-valent pneumococcal polysaccharide vaccine among pregnant Filipino women and placental transfer of antibodies. *Vaccine* 2007; 25:4470–4477.
107. Holmlund E, Nohynek H, Quiambao B, Ollgren J, Käyhty H. Mother-infant vaccination with pneumococcal polysaccharide vaccine: persistence of maternal antibodies and responses of infants to vaccination. *Vaccine* 2011; 29:4565–4575.
108. Demicheli V, Barale A, Rivetti A. Vaccines for women to prevent neonatal tetanus. *Cochrane Database Syst Rev* 2005; Issue 4. Art. No.: CD002959. doi: 10.1002/14651858.CD002959.pub2
109. Newell KW, Duenas Lehmann A, LeBlanc DR, Garces Osorio N. The use of toxoid for the prevention of tetanus neonatorum. Final report of a double-blind controlled field trial. *Bull World Health Org* 1966; 35:863–871.
110. Black RE, Huber DH, Curlin GT. Reduction of neonatal tetanus by mass immunization of non-pregnant women: duration of protection provided by one or two doses of aluminium-adsorbed tetanus toxoid. *Bull World Health Org* 1980; 58: 927–930.
111. Blencowe H, Lawn J, Vandelaer J, Roper M, Cousens S. Tetanus toxoid immunization to reduce mortality from neonatal tetanus. *Int J Epidemiol* 2010; 39(Suppl 1):i102–i109.
112. Provenzano RW, Wetterlow LH, Sullivan CL. Immunization and antibody response in the newborn infant. I. Pertussis inoculation within twenty-four hours of birth. *N Engl J Med* 1965; 273:959–965.
113. Wood N, Siegrist CA. Neonatal immunization: where do we stand? *Curr Opin Infect Dis* 2011; 24:190–195.
114. Aaby P, Roth A, Ravn H, et al. Randomized trial of BCG vaccination at birth to low-birth-weight children: beneficial nonspecific effects in the neonatal period? *J Infect Dis* 2011; 204:245–252.
115. Thayyil-Sudhan S, Kumar A, Singh M, Paul VK, Deorari AK. Safety and effectiveness of BCG vaccination in preterm babies. *Arch Dis Child Fetal Neonatal Ed* 1999; 81:F64–F66.
116. Hawkridge A, Hatherill M, Little F, et al; South African BCG trial team. Efficacy of percutaneous versus intradermal BCG in the prevention of tuberculosis in South African infants: randomised trial. *BMJ* 2008; 337:a2052.
117. el-Sayed N, el-Gamal Y, Abbassy AA, et al. Monovalent type 1 oral poliovirus vaccine in newborns. *N Engl J Med* 2008; 359:1655–1665.
118. Waggie Z, Geldenhuys H, Sutter RW, et al. Randomized trial of type 1 and type 3 oral monovalent poliovirus vaccines in newborns in Africa. *J Infect Dis* 2012; 205:228–236.

119. Lee C, Gong Y, Brok J, Boxall EH, Gluud C. Hepatitis B immunisation for newborn infants of hepatitis B surface antigen-positive mothers. *Cochrane Database Syst Rev* 2006; Issue 2. Art. No.: CD004790. doi: 10.1002/14651858.CD004790.pub2
120. Isaacs D, Kilham HA, Alexander S, Wood N, Buckmaster A, Royle J. Ethical issues in preventing mother-to-child transmission of hepatitis B by immunisation. *Vaccine* 2011; 29:6159–6162.
121. Knuf M, Schmitt HJ, Jacquet JM, et al. Booster vaccination after neonatal priming with acellular pertussis vaccine. *J Pediatr* 2010; 156:675–678.
122. Jardine LA, Inglis GDT, Davies MW. Prophylactic systemic antibiotics to reduce morbidity and mortality in neonates with central venous catheters. *Cochrane Database Syst Rev* 2008; Issue 1. Art. No.: CD006179. doi: 10.1002/14651858.CD006179.pub2
123. Spafford PS, Sinkin RA, Cox C, Reubens L, Powell KR. Prevention of central venous catheter-related coagulase-negative staphylococcal sepsis in neonates. *J Pediatr* 1994; 125:259–263.
124. Harms K, Herting E, Kron M, Schiffmann H, Schulz-Ehlbeck H. Randomized, controlled trial of amoxicillin prophylaxis for prevention of catheter-related infections in newborn infants with central venous silicone elastomer catheters. *J Pediatr* 1995; 127:615–619.
125. Cooke RWI, Nycyk A, Okuonghuae H, Shah V, Damjanovic V, Hart CA. Low-dose vancomycin prophylaxis reduces coagulase-negative staphylococcal bacteraemia in very low birth weight infants. *J Hosp Infect* 1997; 37:297–303.
126. Inglis GDT, Davies MW. Prophylactic antibiotics to reduce morbidity and mortality in neonates with umbilical venous catheters. *Cochrane Database Syst Rev* 2005; Issue 4. Art. No.: CD005251. doi: 10.1002/14651858.CD005251.pub2
127. Inglis GDT, Jardine LA, Davies MW. Prophylactic antibiotics to reduce morbidity and mortality in neonates with umbilical artery catheters. *Cochrane Database Syst Rev* 2007; Issue 4. Art. No.: CD004697. doi: 10.1002/14651858.CD004697.pub3
128. Stewart A, Inglis GDT, Jardine LA, Koorts P, Davies MW. Prophylactic antibiotics to reduce morbidity and mortality in newborn infants with intercostal catheters. *Cochrane Database Syst Rev* 2012; Issue 4. Art. No.: CD008173. doi: 10.1002/14651858.CD008173.pub2
129. Garland JS, Alex CP, Henrickson KJ, McAuliffe TL, Maki DG. A vancomycin-heparin lock solution for prevention of nosocomial bloodstream infection in critically ill neonates with peripherally inserted central venous catheters: a prospective, randomized trial. *Pediatrics* 2005; 116:e198–e205.
130. Kenyon S, Boulvain M, Neilson JP. Antibiotics for preterm rupture of membranes. *Cochrane Database Syst Rev* 2010; Issue 8. Art. No.: CD001058. doi: 10.1002/14651858.CD001058.pub2

CHAPTER 24

Neonatal antimicrobials

Neonates present particular problems in prescribing compared with older children and adults. Oral absorption is variable making oral therapy unreliable in general, although there are exceptions. There are differences in hepatic and renal function which can affect drug metabolism. The extracellular fluid volume is proportionally higher in newborns, so antibiotics like aminoglycosides which are distributed in the extracellular space achieve lower peak levels than older children for a comparable per kilogram dose and persist longer. Pharmacokinetic studies on which recommended doses and dose intervals are based show variation by gestational age, birth weight, growth retardation and post-natal age, so dosing recommendations are often complex.

Drug toxicity is a greater problem in neonates. The grey baby syndrome, a syndrome of cardiovascular collapse, shock and death with chloramphenicol, affected neonates but not older children and is probably due to immature hepatic enzymes.[1] Sulfonamides can displace bilirubin bound to albumin and cause kernicterus.[2,3] Cefoperazone, ceftriaxone and dicloxacillin can also displace bilirubin[4] and although they have not yet been shown to cause kernicterus, they should not be used in jaundiced infants.

The intravenous (IV) route is always preferred to the intramuscular (IM) route for parenteral use in newborns whenever possible because of pain and the risk of causing skin abscesses.

Whenever possible antibiotic levels should be measured to ensure drug levels are not sub-therapeutic and to minimize toxicity.

24.1 Penicillins

Penicillin is an antibacterial produced naturally by the mould *Penicillium notatum*, discovered by Fleming in 1929 but not purified until 1940 by Florey, Chain and colleagues in Oxford. Most penicillins in therapeutic use are semi-synthetic derivatives prepared by adding acyl side chains to the β-lactam penicillin ring.

There are *in vitro* and animal model data, although relatively few human *in vivo* data, that the time that serum concentrations of penicillin remain above the minimum inhibitory concentration (MIC) of an organism is the main determinant of successful eradication of the organism. The same is true for other β-lactam antibiotics.

24.1.1 Penicillin

Penicillin is a β-lactam antibiotic (it has a central β-lactam ring) and acts by interfering with bacterial wall synthesis by binding to penicillin-binding proteins. It is cheap and extremely safe and penicillin (or ampicillin) remains the antibiotic of choice for susceptible organisms, including group B streptococcus, *Listeria monocytogenes*, penicillin-sensitive *Staphylococcus aureus*, penicillin-sensitive *Streptococcus pneumoniae* and *Treponema pallidum*. It is excreted renally.

Mechanisms of resistance to penicillin include the production of β-lactamase enzymes (primarily by enteric gram-negative bacilli although penicillinases produced by *S. aureus* are also examples of β-lactamases), alteration in penicillin-binding proteins (e.g. *S. pneumoniae* strains with reduced penicillin susceptibility) and decreased outer membrane permeability of Gram-negative bacilli.[5]

There are three main parenteral formulations of penicillin:

- **Penicillin G** (aqueous penicillin G): can be given IV or IM and has a half-life of 1.5–10 hours depending on age and birth weight.

Evidence-Based Neonatal Infections, First Edition. David Isaacs.

- **Procaine penicillin** (procaine penicillin G): can only be given IM and can be used to give a daily dose in developing country settings.
- **Benzathine penicillin** (benzathine penicillin G): a single IM dose gives low levels of penicillin for 12 days or more and has been used to treat neonatal syphilis if central nervous system involvement has been excluded.

Although CSF penetration of penicillins is relatively poor, the CSF levels achieved exceed the MIC of susceptible organisms by 50- to 100-fold. Penicillin G is the antibiotic of choice to treat group B streptococcal and meningococcal meningitis and also pneumococcal meningitis caused by fully sensitive strains.

Oral penicillin is administered as penicillin V (phenoxymethyl penicillin). Neonatal absorption is generally considered too unreliable to guarantee effective levels, although there are anecdotal reports of the successful use of penicillin V to complete treatment of osteomyelitis due to susceptible organisms.[6, 7]

Dosing of penicillin is complicated by the use either of units of penicillin or of milligrams of penicillin. The conversion factor is 1666 units per milligram of penicillin so 1 million units is 600 mg of penicillin.

24.1.2 Ampicillin

There is relatively little to choose between ampicillin and penicillin G, the two β-lactam antibiotics most commonly used to provide gram-positive cover in the empiric treatment of early-onset sepsis. Ampicillin has a slightly broader spectrum than penicillin G: it is more active *in vitro* against enterococci (faecal streptococci) and has activity against some gram-negative bacilli including *Escherichia coli*, Proteus, Salmonella and *Haemophilus influenzae*. Ampicillin is also more active *in vitro* against *L. monocytogenes* although there is no evidence that ampicillin produces better outcomes than penicillin G in treating listeriosis.

Because of its broader spectrum, ampicillin predisposes to Candida infection more than penicillin G. Other adverse events seen in older children such as rash and diarrhoea are rare in neonates treated with ampicillin.

Parenteral ampicillin gives CSF levels sufficient to treat meningitis with susceptible organisms. Amoxicillin is better absorbed than ampicillin and is preferred for oral therapy.

24.1.3 Extended-spectrum penicillins

24.1.3.1 Piperacillin

Piperacillin is a semi-synthetic acylureidopenicillin derived from piperazine and ampicillin which belongs to the acylampicillins and has a broader spectrum than ampicillin. It has the highest *in vitro* activity of the extended-spectrum antibiotics against *Pseudomonas aeruginosa*. It is active against ampicillin-sensitive streptococci including enterococci, against many other gram-negative enteric bacilli but not against most *S. aureus*. Piperacillin-resistant strains of *Bacteroides fragilis* are common. Piperacillin has to be given parenterally.

Piperacillin is not active against β-lactamase-producing organisms, including extended-spectrum β-lactamase (ESBL) producers. It is often used in combination with the β-lactamase inhibitor tazobactam to improve coverage of β-lactamase-producing gram-negative bacilli and *S. aureus*. Because Pseudomonas do not usually produce ESBL, piperacillin alone is preferable to piperacillin–tazobactam for treating Pseudomonas infection. However, in many places piperacillin is hard to obtain and has been almost replaced by piperacillin–tazobactam.

Pseudomonas can develop resistance to piperacillin during therapy due to the induction of chromosomal β-lactamase production, active efflux and/or altered permeability.

There is evidence that over-use of piperacillin–tazobactam selects for multi-resistant gram-negative bacteria and for vancomycin-resistant enterococci.[8, 9]

24.1.3.2 Ticarcillin

Ticarcillin is a semi-synthetic carboxypenicillin with activity against *P. aeruginosa*. Like piperacillin it is often used in combination with a β-lactamase inhibitor, in this case clavulanic acid, to improve coverage of β-lactamase-producing gram-negative bacilli and *S. aureus*. Ticarcillin–clavulanate is active against most anaerobes including *B. fragilis*. There is a trend to use ticarcillin–clavulanate rather than ticarcillin alone, although ticarcillin is preferable for sensitive Pseudomonas. Ticarcillin is inactive against enterococci and most *S. aureus*.

There is evidence that over-use of ticarcillin–clavulanate can select for multi-resistant gram-negative bacteria and for vancomycin-resistant enterococci.[9, 10]

24.1.3.3 Azlocillin

Azlocillin is a semi-synthetic acylureidopenicillin with activity against *P. aeruginosa* and with a similar spectrum of activity to piperacillin, although with less activity against Klebsiella species and other Enterobacteriaceae than mezlocillin and piperacillin.

24.1.3.4 Mezlocillin

Mezlocillin is a semi-synthetic acylureidopenicillin which is less active against *P. aeruginosa* than piperacillin and azlocillin.

24.1.4 Anti-staphylococcal penicillins

Several semi-synthetic penicillins have been developed which are resistant to the simple β-lactamases (penicillinases) produced by *S. aureus.* These include methicillin (sometimes called meticillin), nafcillin, oxacillin, cloxacillin, flucloxacillin and dicloxacillin. Dicloxacillin can displace bilirubin bound to albumin and is particularly prone to cause phlebitis and is not recommended in neonates. There is relatively little to choose between the different anti-staphylococcal penicillins and the preferred anti-staphylococcal penicillin varies across the Atlantic more due to fashion than any evidence of superior efficacy. Oxacillin is rather less stable to hydrolysis by staphylococcal β-lactamases than the others, and methicillin and nafcillin are the most stable, but the clinical significance of these differences is unclear.

An anti-staphylococcal antibiotic is the treatment of choice for penicillin-resistant *S. aureus* but penicillin is preferred for the 10% or so of strains of penicillin-sensitive *S. aureus.* Most CoNS strains are resistant to the anti-staphylococcal penicillins. The anti-staphylococcal penicillins have only modest activity against penicillin-sensitive streptococci, meningococci and gonococci, so penicillin is preferred for confirmed infections with these organisms. The anti-staphylococcal penicillins are inactive against enterococci, enteric gram-negative bacilli and *H. influenzae.*

24.2 Cephalosporins

The cephalosporins are antibiotics based on cephalosporin C, produced by the mould *Cephalosporium acremonium,* first cultivated from sewage in Sardinia in 1948 and later purified by Abraham and colleagues in Oxford. All the cephalosporins have a β-lactam ring and are stable to staphylococcal β-lactamases.

The cephalosporins have been classified into generations as further modifications are made, a classification with uses and limitations.[11] With increasing generation there is improved stability to β-lactamases. In general, the following apply:

- First-generation cephalosporins (including cefazolin, cephalothin, cephalexin) are active against most gram-positive organisms except enterococci, MRSA and Listeria, but have only limited activity against gram-negative organisms.
- Second-generation cephalosporins (including cefuroxime, cefoxitin, cefaclor) have improved activity against Gram-negative bacilli compared with first-generation cephalosporins.
- Third-generation cephalosporins (including cefotaxime, ceftriaxone, ceftazidime, cefoperazone) are active against many gram-negative enteric bacilli, although only ceftazidime and cefoperazone are active against Pseudomonas. Enterococci and Listeria are resistant to all cephalosporins.
- Fourth-generation cephalosporins (cefepime, cefpirome) are active against many gram-negative enteric bacilli including Pseudomonas. There are few studies in neonates and they should be reserved for infections with multi-resistant organisms not susceptible to other antibiotics.

Use of third-generation cephalosporins is associated with Darwinian selection of multi-resistant gram-negative bacteria, may cause the emergence of vancomycin-resistant enterococci and is associated with an increased incidence of invasive candidiasis.[12–14]

24.2.1 Cefazolin

The first-generation cephalosporin cefazolin is active against β-lactamase-producing *S. aureus* but not MRSA and is active against streptococci including modest activity against penicillin-sensitive pneumococci but not against enterococci. It is inactive against

Enterobacteriaceae and *B. fragilis*. It does not penetrate the CSF.

24.2.2 Cephalothin

The first-generation cephalosporin cephalothin (or cefolatin) is still useful as an antibiotic with anti-staphylococcal activity. It is active against streptococci including penicillin-sensitive pneumococci but not against enterococci or Listeria. It is active against some wild-type gram-negative bacilli such as *E. coli*, *Proteus mirabilis* and Klebsiella spp. It is susceptible to many β-lactamases produced by gram-negative bacteria and lacks activity against Salmonella, Citrobacter, Enterobacter and Pseudomonas. It does not penetrate the CSF.

24.2.3 Cephalexin (cefalexin)

Cephalexin is an oral antibiotic relatively resistant to staphylococcal β-lactamases, thus useful to treat staphylococcal infections and very well absorbed if oral therapy is required. It is somewhat less active than other first-generation cephalosporins against other gram-positive cocci. It is active against many gram-negative bacilli, but is degraded by enterobacterial β-lactamases, while Citrobacter, Enterobacter and Serratia species are all inherently resistant to cephalexin.

24.2.4 Cefuroxime

Cefuroxime can be used parenterally or orally. It is resistant to most gram-negative β-lactamases and so is active against many Enterobacteriaceae, although Acinetobacter, *Serratia marcescens* and *P. aeruginosa* are inherently resistant. Some strains of *Burkholderia cepacia* are susceptible. *B. fragilis* are resistant. CSF penetration is good if the meninges are inflamed. Cefuroxime axetil can be used orally in children >3 months but is rarely used in neonates.

24.2.5 Cefotaxime

Cefotaxime is active against many gram-positive cocci including *S. aureus* and streptococci and against most gram-negative enteric bacilli. Organisms inherently resistant to cefotaxime include the pseudomonads, *P. aeruginosa* and *Stenotrophomonas maltophilia*, enterococci, Listeria and *B. fragilis*. *Enterobacter cloacae* and related organisms may appear susceptible on initial isolation but treatment-emergent resistance is common due to the induction of chromosomal cephalosporinases. CSF penetration is good, particularly if the meninges are inflamed.

24.2.6 Ceftriaxone

The spectrum of activity of ceftriaxone is virtually identical to cefotaxime. The advantage of ceftriaxone is that it can be given less frequently. The main disadvantage is that it can displace bilirubin from albumin so should not be used when there is a risk of causing kernicterus. In addition there has been concern that co-administration of ceftriaxone with calcium-containing solutions may lead to precipitation in lines and to vascular occlusion. Five post-marketing reports of fatal cases caused the US Food and Drug Administration (FDA) to issue a warning in 2007 about co-administration of ceftriaxone with calcium-containing solutions. A review of seven cases (six fatal) found that the incidence was unknown, but questioned the role of using higher than FDA-approved doses, of giving an intravenous 'push' and of giving the total daily dose as a single infusion.[15] Ceftriaxone can precipitate in the neonatal gall bladder causing biliary sludge and obstruction.[16] It seems prudent to avoid ceftriaxone in the neonatal period,[17] particularly as cefotaxime covers the same spectrum of organisms and appears safer.

24.2.7 Ceftazidime

Ceftazidime is active against *P. aeruginosa* and *B. cepacia*, and otherwise has similar antimicrobial activity to cefotaxime, although less active against *S. aureus*. The clearance and the volume of distribution of ceftazidime increases with gestational age and ceftazidime clearance increases significantly with rising glomerular filtration rate.[18]

24.2.8 Cefoperazone

Cefoperazone has moderate anti-pseudomonal activity,[19] but its use has been superseded by other cephalosporins with better activity against *P. aeruginosa* and Burkholderia.

24.2.9 Cefepime

Cefepime is a fourth-generation cephalosporin active against *P. aeruginosa* and also, because of low affinity for cephalosporinases, against most Citrobacter, Enterobacter and Serratia. Listeria is inherently resistant. Cefepime is not active against most anaerobes. Cefepime has been studied in neonates[20, 21] and penetrates CSF well.[22] Because it has an extremely broad spectrum, there is a high risk that its widespread use will drive multi-drug resistance, so it should be reserved for treatment of neonates proven to be infected with highly resistant organisms for which there is no better choice of antibiotics.

24.3 Aztreonam

Aztreonam is a monobactam with a β-lactam ring not attached to another ring, unlike the penicillins and cephalosporins. Monobactams are produced by bacteria whereas penicillins and cephalosporins are produced by moulds. Although other monobactams were developed and studied, aztreonam is the only one in active use. Aztreonam is a synthetic construct of an antibiotic produced by the potentially pathogenic gram-negative bacterium *Chromobacter violaceum.* It is active against many gram-negative bacilli, but relatively resistant to *P. aeruginosa* and *B. fragilis.* It is inactive against most gram-positive organisms including *S. aureus*, pneumococci and enterococci. It can be given IM but is not absorbed enterally. Its pharmacokinetics has been studied in the neonate,[23] but aztreonam is not widely used in the neonatal period. Its use should be reserved for infections with highly resistant organisms. For example, aztreonam is not destroyed by metallo-β-lactamases[24] which destroy carbapenems such as meropenem.

24.4 Carbapenems

The carbapenems are antibiotics produced by streptomycetes. They have broad spectrum activity against most gram-positive cocci, except MRSA, and many gram-negative bacilli. The carbapenems are potent drivers of the selection of multi-resistant organisms. The carbapenems contain a β-lactam ring and although they are resistant to hydrolysis by most β-lactamases produced by gram-negative bacilli, they can be destroyed by metallo-β-lactamases (also called carbapenemases).[24, 25] Empiric use of the carbapenems should be avoided if at all possible, because of the considerable risk of selecting for MRSA, VRE, *Clostridium difficile*, Candida and highly resistant organisms including metallo-β-lactamase-producing organisms that are resistant to almost all available antibiotics (see Chapter 5).[24–26]

24.4.1 Meropenem

Meropenem is a semi-synthetic carbapenem slightly less active than imipenem against gram-positive organisms but with better anti-anaerobic activity.[27, 28] It is not active against MRSA.

It has good CSF penetration. It is not absorbed enterally. It is less likely than imipenem–cilastatin to cause convulsions.[27] It should not be used as empiric therapy and should only be used as directed therapy for proven infection with organisms resistant to suitable alternatives because of the high risk of selecting for highly resistant organisms.[26–29]

24.4.2 Imipenem–cilastatin

Imipenem is active against many gram-positive and gram-negative organisms. It is active against MSSA but has reduced activity against MRSA, although more active than meropenem against MRSA. Imipenem is active against *P. aeruginosa* and most other pseudomonads, but not *S. maltophilia.* It is active against Listeria and most anaerobes.

Imipenem is degraded by renal dehydropeptidase enzymes, so is used in combination with the dehydropeptidase inhibitor cilastatin.

A case series which reported an unexpectedly high rate of seizures (7 of 21) in children with bacterial meningitis treated with imipenem–cilastatin[30] raised concerns about neurotoxicity in neonates.[31] A non-Cochrane review reported rates of seizures of 3–33% associated with imipenem–cilastatin use at different ages, but <1% for the other carbapenems meropenem, doripenem and ertapenem.[32] Imipenem–cilastatin is thought to cause seizures by binding to γ-aminobutyric acid (GABA) receptors.[32] Although there are few reports of seizures with imipenem in neonates, many neonates have other risk factors for seizures and meropenem is the preferred carbapenem.

24.5 Glycopeptides

The glycopeptides are produced by soil actinomycetes and have a central heptapeptide core with sugars attached. There is strong epidemiologic evidence that the use of the glycopeptides avoparcin and actaplanin as additives in animal feeds selects for vancomycin-resistant enterococci (VRE) in animals and birds and their transfer to humans.[33, 34] Avoparcin, which is related to vancomycin and teicoplanin, is now banned in most countries. The use of antibiotics in animal husbandry is arguably an example of human greed exceeding common sense.

24.5.1 Vancomycin

Vancomycin was discovered and developed in the 1950s to treat staphylococcal infections, but because of toxicity (mainly red man syndrome due to histamine release caused by rapid administration) its use was superseded by newer anti-staphylococcal agents. However, vancomycin was resurrected to cope with the emergence of MRSA and has proved an effective and safe antibiotic with activity against most gram-positive organisms, including MRSA, other staphylococci and streptococci including enterococci, Listeria and gram-positive anaerobes including Clostridia. Vancomycin is inactive against gram-negative bacteria.

Resistance to vancomycin can occur in enterococci (VRE) and vancomycin-insensitive *S. aureus* (VISA) strains and vancomycin-resistant *S. aureus* (VRSA) strains have been described. Fortunately symptomatic neonatal infections with VRE, VISA or VRSA are rare.[35] This may be due in part to the 1995 Centers for Disease Control recommendation to introduce measures to reduce vancomycin use in hospitals.[36] Introduction of antimicrobial stewardship guidelines to reduce vancomycin use is highly effective.[37, 38]

Early reports of vancomycin use in the 1950s reported nephrotoxicity and ototoxicity, now thought to have been substantially due to impurities. Subsequent studies have reported that vancomycin is generally well tolerated in the neonatal period, although relatively few infants have been studied systematically for ototoxicity.[39–42] Rapid infusion can cause 'red man syndrome' with erythroderma, tachycardia and an appearance sometimes termed shock or anaphylaxis but which rapidly resolves when the infusion is stopped. It is due to histamine release caused by too rapid administration, is not IgE mediated, is not a true allergic reaction and is not a contraindication to continuing the drug at a slower rate.[42, 43]

A New Zealand study of infants from NICU routinely investigated for hearing loss by measuring oto-acoustic emissions found a background rate of failed tests of 7% (85 of 1233) for infants who did not receive gentamicin or vancomycin, no increased risk with gentamicin alone (42 of 949 or 4%), but a significantly increased risk with vancomycin alone (9 of 41 or 22%) and with both gentamicin and vancomycin (17 of 124 or 14%).[44] This study was not randomized and is likely to be confounded by the fact that sicker infants will tend to receive antibiotics. There are multiple reasons for neonates to develop ototoxicity. Furthermore oto-acoustic emissions are a screening test for deafness and do not confirm the diagnosis. However, the difference between vancomycin and gentamicin is at least intriguing and warrants further study. It is a further reason to reduce vancomycin use and to monitor therapeutic drug levels.

Vancomycin levels in CSF are far higher in neonates treated with intravenous vancomycin than in older children.[40, 45] CSF penetration is good in neonates and the use of intrathecal vancomycin is discouraged (see Section 7.10).

Therapeutic drug monitoring (TDM) for vancomycin is recommended strongly, although monitoring regimens vary.[46] A number of studies show that the pharmacokinetics of vancomycin in neonates and infants can be described best by a one-compartment model,[47–49] whereas in adults a two-compartment model fits the data better.[49] While vancomycin has often been given in intermittent doses, recent data suggest a continuous infusion achieves more stable serum levels without nephrotoxicity.[50–53] A loading dose of 20 mg/kg followed by a continuous infusion of 30 mg/kg/day usually achieves a target serum vancomycin level of 25 mg/L without renal toxicity.[53] If intermittent dosing is used, vancomycin should be infused over 30–60 minutes to avoid causing red man syndrome. The aim of therapeutic drug monitoring is to ensure adequate therapeutic levels and to avoid accumulation. Trough levels are measured before an intermittent dose is given and should be 10–20 mg/L to ensure vancomycin is being cleared adequately and is not accumulating. Peak levels are no longer recommended in older children and adults. When measured in intermittent neonatal dosing they were usually measured 15–30 minutes after the third dose (once a steady state has been achieved) aiming at levels of 20–30 mg/L (20–30 μg/mL) for sepsis and 30–40 mg/L for meningitis. With vancomycin infusion it is recommended to aim for vancomycin levels of 10–30 mg/L after achieving a steady state.[50–53]

24.5.2 Teicoplanin

Teicoplanin is a glycopeptide with a similar spectrum of activity to vancomycin, sometimes been used in Europe but rarely in North America.[54–57] It is more active than vancomycin against susceptible strains of *S. aureus*, pneumococcus, group A streptococci and enterococci, but less active against some CoNS, particularly *S. haemolyticus*.[54] It causes less nephrotoxicity than vancomycin and does not cause red man syndrome. Vancomycin-resistant enterococci of the VanA type are also resistant to teicoplanin but VanB VRE strains are usually sensitive. There are insufficient pharmacokinetic data to recommend its routine use. A review of teicoplanin in newborns recommended a loading dose of 10–20 mg/kg followed by a dose of 8–10 mg/kg 24 hourly.[56]

24.6 Linezolid

Linezolid is a member of a novel class of synthetic antimicrobial agents called oxazolidinones. It is active against many gram-positive organisms including MSSA and MRSA, CoNS, enterococci including vancomycin-resistant enterococci, pneumococci (including penicillin-resistant pneumococci), Listeria, Bacillus and Corynebacterium species.[58] It has no useful activity against gram-negative organisms.

The main toxic adverse effects of linezolid described in adults and older children are more likely with prolonged use and are neurologic (permanent peripheral neuropathy) and haematologic (anaemia, thrombocytopenia).[59] A systematic review of five studies and eight case reports of linezolid use in neonates found that courses of 10–28 days were safe and effective.[60] However, the ability of these studies to detect significant peripheral neuropathy remains in question.[61]

Systematic reviews show linezolid is superior to glycopeptides (vancomycin or teicoplanin) in treating nosocomial or MRSA pneumonia in adults.[62, 63] Linezolid is expensive and concerns about peripheral neuropathy and the need to preserve novel antimicrobial agents mean it should be reserved for infections with resistant gram-positive organisms which have not responded to conventional antibiotics, for example, persistent MRSA bacteraemia on adequate doses of vancomycin. Linezolid has been used successfully in the treatment of multi-resistant tuberculosis.[64, 65]

24.7 Daptomycin

Daptomycin is a semi-synthetic lipopeptide derived from the streptomycete *Streptomyces roseosporus*. Its structure resembles the polymyxins. It is active against gram-positive organisms including MRSA and VRE. There are anecdotal reports of successful treatment of neonatal MRSA infections unresponsive to other antibiotics[66–68] and of neonatal VRE infection.[69] It can cause irreversible muscle toxicity in adults so routine creatine kinase monitoring is recommended. Concerns about toxicity dictate its use only as a last resort to treat gram-positive infections unresponsive to other antibiotics or organisms resistant to all other alternative antibiotics.

24.8 Macrolides and lincosamides

The macrolides are a large group of antibiotics produced by Streptomyces or its relatives active against many gram-positive organisms, intracellular organisms such as atypical mycobacteria and Chlamydia, *Bordetella pertussis* and gram-positive anaerobes. Macrolides used in neonates include erythromycin, azithromycin and spiramycin (for toxoplasmosis). The lincosamides, clindamycin and lincomycin, share a target with the macrolides and have a similar activity spectrum but a novel structure. Lincomycin is produced naturally by *Streptomyces lincolnensis* and clindamycin is a semi-synthetic derivative of lincomycin. They are active against most community strains of MRSA. There are no data on lincomycin use in neonates, which is not recommended.

24.8.1 Erythromycin

Erythromycin binds to bacterial ribosomes and interferes with protein synthesis. It can be used orally in its base form but enteric-coated to prevent gastric acid degradation or in the form of stearate salt or propionate, ethylsuccinate, estolate or acistrate esters which are less bitter and have improved pharmacokinetic properties. In neonates the estolate achieves slightly higher serum levels than the ethylsuccinate form.[70] Erythromycin is not usually used parenterally in neonates because it tends to damage blood vessels and extravasation can cause tissue necrosis. Erythromycin has been associated with the development of pyloric stenosis[71, 72] which has also been described with azithromycin and may be a class effect.[73] Because of selective reporting it is not possible to give the exact risk of pyloric stenosis, but the increased risk appears to occur with all oral preparations.[72] Erythromycin causes more adverse effects, particularly diarrhoea and other gastro-intestinal symptoms, than the other macrolides.[74]

24.8.2 Clindamycin

Clindamycin is a lincosamide active against gram-positive organisms such as *S. aureus*, including most community strains of MRSA (for which it is most useful in neonatology), and also streptococci including many resistant pneumococci. It is active against many anaerobes and for this reason has been used in the management of necrotizing enterocolitis (see Chapter 11). It can cause pseudo-membranous colitis in adults but this is exceedingly rare in neonates. Excretion is mainly hepatic and is prolonged in very pre-term infants.[75, 76]

24.9 Aminoglycosides

Aminoglycosides are naturally occurring or semi-synthetic antibiotics active against a wide range of gram-negative bacilli. Streptomycin, produced by a soil organism *Streptomyces griseus,* was identified in 1944 and gentamicin, produced by *Micromonospora purpurea,* in 1963. Streptomycin and kanamycin are now used rarely, because of ototoxicity and resistance respectively, but other aminoglycosides are still used extensively. They have limited CSF penetration of uninflamed meninges but were used successfully in gram-negative meningitis historically. The outcome of gram-negative meningitis in neonates and infants treated with ampicillin and gentamicin was surprisingly good, even in the face of widespread ampicillin resistance.[77, 78]

Aminoglycosides bind to the bacterial ribosome and interfere with protein synthesis and they also damage the bacterial cell membrane. Aminoglycosides have a dose-dependent bactericidal effect. They also exhibit a post-antibiotic effect, whereby bacterial growth continues to be inhibited after aminoglycoside levels fall, due to persistence of intracellular aminoglycoside bound to ribosomes. These properties caused clinicians to investigate the use of once-daily aminoglycosides. Systematic reviews of studies in all age groups,[79] children[80] and patients with febrile neutropoenia[81] or cystic fibrosis[82] show once-daily or extended-interval dosing is as effective as multiple daily dosing and reduces nephrotoxicity and possibly ototoxicity. A Cochrane review of 11 neonatal studies comparing once-daily with multiple daily doses of gentamicin found equal efficacy, minimal toxicity with either regimen but better serum levels with once-daily dosing.[83]

Traditionally, aminoglycosides were given by the intramuscular rather than the intravenous route to avoid high serum levels, but studies showed levels are similar with either route and that antibacterial efficacy is predicted best by a high peak level or area under the concentration–time curve. The intravenous route is, therefore, now preferred.

The aminoglycosides can cause ototoxicity and sometimes permanent hearing impairment by accumulation in the perilymph of the inner ear leading to damage to the sensory cells of the inner ear and to the vestibular and cochlear branches of the VIII nerve. Such ototoxicity is associated primarily with long duration of use, because aminoglycosides accumulate in otolymph and renal tissue, even if serum levels are maintained at recommended levels.[84, 85] Hence it is recommended not to continue aminoglycosides for longer than 7 days in neonates unless essential. Ototoxicity is also associated with prolonged high levels, particularly in association with other ototoxic and nephrotoxic drugs or with impaired renal function. Despite long-standing concern about ototoxicity there is little evidence that therapeutic use of gentamicin and other aminoglycosides in neonatal intensive care units causes neonatal deafness. Neonates requiring intensive care are subject to multiple potentially ototoxic insults and deafness may be multifactorial. There are no randomized controlled studies that have examined hearing in infants randomized to receive aminoglycosides or non-aminoglycoside antibiotics. One cohort study found that infants who received gentamicin were no more likely to fail hearing screening tests than infants who did not whereas vancomycin, in contrast, was associated with a significant increase in test failure (Section 24.5.1).[44] Another study of 'critically ill' infants <1500 g found those who received gentamicin in the first week of life were no more likely than who did not to fail oto-acoustic emission screening.[86] However, critically ill infants >1500 g who had serum gentamicin concentrations >10 μg/mL (>10 mg/L) were twice as likely to fail hearing screening as infants with gentamicin levels <10 μg/mL and there was a dose effect with rising serum gentamicin levels.[86]

24.9.1 Gentamicin

Gentamicin has been used and studied more than any other aminoglycoside in the neonatal period. It has activity against a wide range of gram-negative bacilli including *P. aeruginosa* and Enterobacteriaceae and also has activity which may be clinically useful against *S. aureus*, coagulase-negative staphylococci and Listeria, although it would never be recommended as monotherapy for these indications. Streptococci are intrinsically aminoglycoside resistant although there is *in vitro* synergy when gentamicin is given with penicillin to a sensitive streptococcus such as GBS.

Acquired resistance is usually due to gentamicin-modifying enzymes which degrade gentamicin but do not always confer resistance to other aminoglycosides, so that an outbreak with a gentamicin-resistant organism may resolve by switching to another empiric aminoglycoside such as netilmicin if the organism is sensitive.[87] However, when gentamicin resistance is due to a non-specific decrease in aminoglycoside uptake it is usually associated with resistance to all aminoglycosides.

Extended-interval dosing of gentamicin appears to be as effective as intermittent dosing and while neonatal studies have not shown reduced nephro- or ototoxicity with extended dosing,[83] studies in other groups have shown that extended dosing is less toxic than intermittent dosing.[79–82] One question when using extended dosing is how to monitor serum levels. Peak levels are not useful and while trough levels can be and often are used to show whether or not there is accumulation, it may be more useful to take blood say 12–21 hours after a dose and use a nomogram to determine the optimum timing of the next dose. Nomograms that predicted steady-state gentamicin concentrations of <0.5 or <1 mg/L based on pharmacokinetic data from 341 neonates performed well in practice (Figures 24.1a and 24.1b).[88] The nomogram for <0.5 mg/L could be used to minimize the risk of toxicity whereas the nomogram for <1 mg/L might be preferred for more critical infections. These nomograms used data mainly from infants <7 days old and might not be appropriate for more mature infants.[88]

In developing countries a simplified dosing schedule for gentamicin based on extended intervals saves time. Studies in Bangladesh and India established a suitable regimen of a fixed dose of 10 mg 48 hourly for infants <2000 g, 10 mg 24 hourly for 2000–2500 g and 13.5 mg 24 hourly for infants >2500 g (Table 24.1),[89, 90] which has been evaluated and found to be safe.[91]

The initial doses for intermittent dosing of gentamicin are given in Table 24.1 for clinicians who prefer to stay with intermittent dosing until further data are available. If intermittent dosing is used, it is unnecessary to measure serum gentamicin levels (except possibly for medicolegal purposes) if gentamicin is stopped after 48 hours. However, if gentamicin is continued >48 hours, therapeutic drug monitoring is essential to minimize toxicity and ensure adequate therapeutic levels. The peak level taken 30–60 minutes after a dose should be 6–8 μg/mL (6–8 mg/L), while the trough level taken just before a dose should be <2 μg/mL (>2 mg/L).

24.9.2 Amikacin

Amikacin is a semi-synthetic derivative of kanamycin A (which comes from *Streptomyces kanamyceticus*). Amikacin is relatively resistant to degradation by plasmid-mediated enzymes that mediate resistance to gentamicin and tobramycin. Some North American neonatal units wisely refrain from using amikacin, to ensure amikacin can be reserved for empiric treatment if widespread resistance to other aminoglycosides becomes a problem. In many developing countries widespread aminoglycoside resistance is indeed a major problem and amikacin is used commonly.[92, 93] However, resistance can emerge during treatment with *P. aeruginosa* and Serratia so amikacin should be used responsibly. In particular, it should be stopped if systemic cultures are negative and not continued because of concerns about resistance and about cumulative toxicity.

Amikacin can cause oto- and nephrotoxicity. Amikacin clearance depends on gestational age and post-natal age and is reduced in intrauterine growth retardation.[94, 95] Small studies did not show any toxicity with once-daily compared with intermittent dosing of amikacin,[96–98] but too few infants were studied to guarantee its safety. Different dosing regimens have been proposed[99] but the largest pharmacokinetic

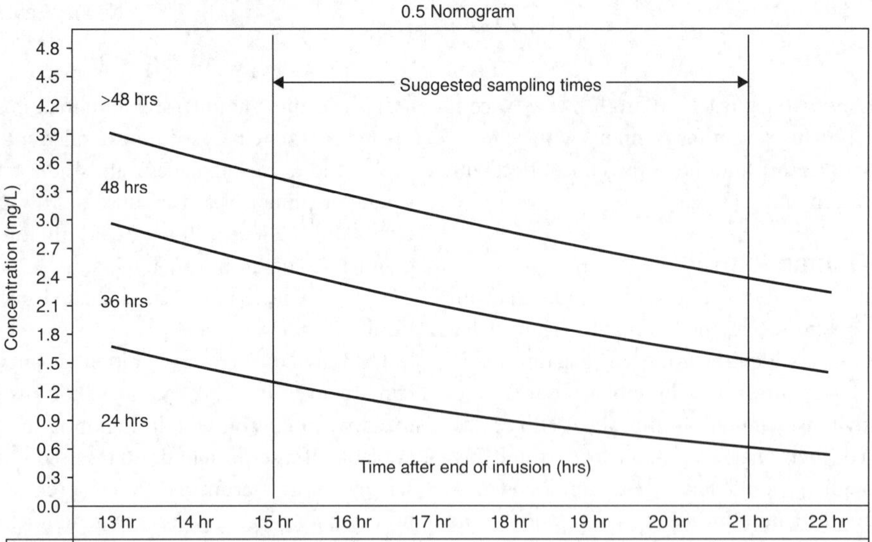

	13 hr	14 hr	15 hr	16 hr	17 hr	18 hr	19 hr	20 hr	21 hr	22 hr
24 hrs	1.7	1.5	1.3	1.1	1.0	0.9	0.6	0.7	0.6	0.5
36 hrs	3.0	2.7	2.5	2.3	2.1	2.0	1.8	1.7	1.5	1.4
48 hrs	3.9	3.7	3.5	3.2	3.1	2.9	2.7	2.5	2.4	2.2

Cut-off concentrations (mg/L)

(a)

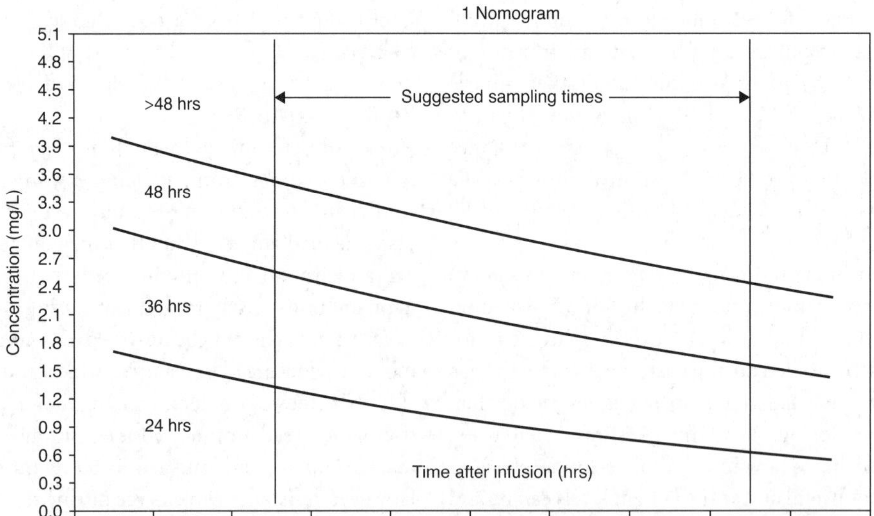

	13 hr	14 hr	15 hr	16 hr	17 hr	18 hr	19 hr	20 hr	21 hr	22 hr
24 hrs	2.4	2.2	2.0	1.8	1.6	1.5	1.3	1.2	1.1	1.0
36 hrs	3.8	3.5	3.3	3.1	2.9	2.7	2.6	2.4	2.2	2.1
48 hrs	4.7	4.5	4.2	4.0	3.9	3.7	3.5	3.3	3.2	3.0

Cut-off concentrations (mg/L)

(b)

Figure 24.1 (a) Once-daily gentamicin 0.5 mg/L nomogram for neonates. Plot measured concentration–time point. If concentration falls within 24-hour area, give 4 mg/kg every 24 hours. If time point in another zone, use that interval (e.g. if concentration 2.9 mg/L 16 hours after first-dose infusion give doses every 48 hours). If concentration in >48-hour zone, measure a second concentration at 48 hours: if concentration is indeed above desired trough value withhold dose for an additional period of time, depending on how high the concentration was, and give further doses cautiously. Reprinted with permission from Reference 88 (R1213). Copyright 2008 American Society of Health-System Pharmacists, Inc. All rights reserved. (b) Once-daily gentamicin 1 mg/L nomogram for neonates. Use as for (a). Reprinted with permission from Reference 88 (R1213). Copyright 2008 American Society of Health-System Pharmacists, Inc. All rights reserved.

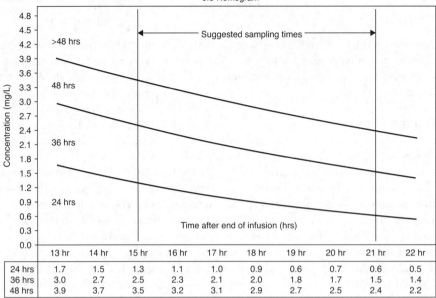

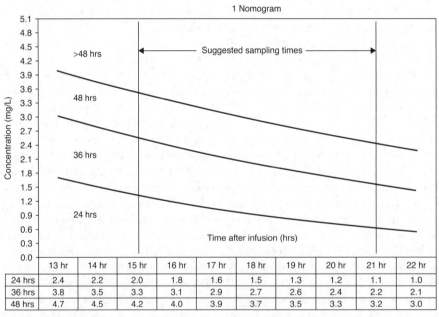

Table 24.1 Recommended antibiotic doses and intervals.

Antibiotic	Route	Dose and frequency	Notes
Acyclovir	IV	20 mg/kg/dose 8 hourly for 2 weeks for HSV (3 weeks for HSV encephalitis) 20 mg/kg/dose 8 hourly for VZV	See Chapter 17
Amikacin	IV, IM	<800 g: 16 mg/kg/dose 48 hourly if <14 days old <800 g: 20 mg/kg/dose 42 hourly if ≥14 days old 800–1200 g: 16 mg/kg/dose 42 hourly if <14 days old 800–1200 g: 20 mg/kg/dose 36 hourly if ≥14 days old 1200–2000 g: 15 mg/kg/dose 36 hourly if <14 days old 1200–2000 g: 19 mg/kg/dose 30 hourly if ≥14 days old 2000–2800 g: 13 mg/kg/dose 30 hourly if <14 days old 2000–2800 g: 18 mg/kg/dose 24 hourly if ≥14 days old >2800 g: 12 mg/kg/dose 24 hourly if <14 days old >2800 g: 17 mg/kg/dose 20 hourly if ≥14 days old	Data on extended daily dosing based on Reference 95 IV preferred to IM Poorly absorbed orally
Amoxicillin	IV, IM, (oral)	Sepsis: 50 mg/kg/dose Meningitis: 100 mg/kg/dose <7 days old 12 hourly 1–3 weeks 8 hourly 4 weeks or more 6 hourly	IV preferred to IM Oral not used to treat systemic sepsis or meningitis
Amphotericin B	IV	0.5-1 mg/kg/day IV once daily	Liposomal amphotericin not recommended (see Chapter 16)
Ampicillin	IV or IM	Sepsis: 50 mg/kg/dose Meningitis: 100 mg/kg/dose <7 days old 12 hourly 1–3 weeks 8 hourly 4 weeks or more 6 hourly	IV preferred to IM
Aztreonam	IV, IM	30 mg/kg/dose	Not absorbed orally
Cefazolin	IV, IM	20 mg/kg/dose 12 hourly >1 week 8 hourly if term	
Cefepime	IV, IM	50 mg/kg/dose 12 hourly <7 days old 12 hourly >1 week 8 hourly	Reserve use for proven infection with highly resistant organism
Cefotaxime	IV, IM	50 mg/kg/dose <7 days old 12 hourly (8 hourly if term) >1 week 8 hourly	Not active against Pseudomonas
Ceftazidime	IV, IM	50 mg/kg/dose 12 hourly if pre-term (BWt <1200 g) BWt >1200 g 8 hourly	
Ceftriaxone	IV, IM	50 mg/kg/dose once daily	Use cefotaxime in preference because of safety concerns (Section 24.2.6). Do not use if jaundiced. Do not use with calcium infusions
Cefuroxime	IV, IM	25 mg/kg/dose <7 days old 12 hourly 1–3 weeks 8 hourly 4 weeks or more 6 hourly	Cefuroxime axetil oral preparation rarely used in neonates
Cephalexin (cefalexin)	Oral	25 mg/kg/dose <7 days old 12 hourly 1–3 weeks 8 hourly 4 weeks or more 6 hourly	No parenteral preparation
Cephalothin (cefalotin)	IV	20 mg/kg/dose <7 days old 12 hourly >1 week 8 hourly	

(*continued*)

Table 24.1 (*Continued*)

Antibiotic	Route	Dose and frequency	Notes
Ciprofloxacin	IV, oral	10 mg/kg/dose 12 hourly	
Clindamycin	IV, IM, oral	5 mg/kg/dose <1200 g 12 hourly 1200–2000 g 8 hourly >2000 g 8 hourly (6 hourly >1 week old)	Higher doses of 10 mg/kg/dose 8 hourly can be used for term infants with community MRSA infection
Cloxacillin	IV, IM, (oral)	Sepsis: 50 mg/kg/dose Meningitis: 100 mg/kg/dose <7 days old 12 hourly >1 week 6 to 8 hourly	IV preferred to IM Can be given orally at 25 mg/kg/dose 6–8 hourly for less severe infections
Daptomycin	IV	6 mg/kg/dose 12 hourly	Poor oral absorption
Erythromycin	Oral	10 mg/kg/dose <7 days old 12 hourly >1 week 8 hourly	IV causes tissue necrosis
Flucloxacillin	IV, IM, oral	Sepsis: 50 mg/kg/dose Meningitis: 100 mg/kg/dose <7 days old 12 hourly >1 week 6 to 8 hourly	IV preferred to IM Can be given orally at 25 mg/kg/dose 6–8 hourly for less severe infections
Fluconazole	IV, oral	Loading dose: 25 mg/kg Treatment dose 12 mg/kg/24 hourly Prophylaxis dose: 6 mg/kg twice weekly (or 72 hourly)	See Chapter 16 Adjust dose for renal failure
Flucytosine (5-fluorocytosine)	IV, oral	Dose: 25–100 mg/kg/dose 24 hourly	Do not use as monotherapy as resistance develops rapidly. Monitor drug levels
Gentamicin	IV, IM	Extended dosing: <1200 g 5 mg/kg/dose 48 hourly >1200 g 4 mg/kg/dose 24 hourly Extended dosing in developing countries: <2000 g 10 mg *dose* 48 hourly 2000–2500 g 10 mg *dose* 24 hourly >2500 g 13.5 mg *dose* 24 hourly Intermittent dosing: 2.5 mg/kg/dose: <1200 g 18 hourly 1200–2000 g 12 hourly >2000 g 8 hourly	Suggest using nomogram (Figures 24.1a and 24.1b) to determine dosing interval if using extended interval dosing Monitor drug levels if intermittent dosing used for more than 48 hours. Aim for peak level of 6–8 μg/mL (mg/L) and trough <2 μg/mL
Imipenem–cilastatin	IV, IM	20 mg/kg/dose 12 hourly >1 week 8 hourly >2000 g	Meropenem preferred because of risk of seizures
Linezolid	IV, oral	10 mg/kg/dose < 7 days 12 hourly >1 week 8 hourly	
Meropenem	IV, IM	20 mg/kg/dose 12 hourly >1 week 8 hourly >2000 g	Do not use for empiric therapy unless no alternatives are available
Methicilin (or meticillin)	IV, IM	Sepsis: 50 mg/kg/dose Meningitis: 100 mg/kg/dose <7 days old 12 hourly >1 week 6 to 8 hourly	IV preferred to IM Rarely used now
Metronidazole	IV, oral	Loading dose 15 mg/kg for all infants Then 7.5 mg/kg/dose: <34 weeks 12 hourly 34–40 weeks 8 hourly >40 weeks 6 hourly	Based on Reference 121

115. Aggarwal P, Dutta S, Garg SK, Narang A. Multiple dose pharmacokinetics of ciprofloxacin in preterm babies. *Indian Pediatr* 2004; 41:1001–1007.
116. van den Oever HL, Versteegh FG, Thewessen EA, van den Anker JN, Mouton JW, Neijens HJ. Ciprofloxacin in preterm neonates: case report and review of the literature. *Eur J Pediatr* 1998; 157:843–845.
117. Krcméry Jr V, Filka J, Uher J, et al. Ciprofloxacin in treatment of nosocomial meningitis in neonates and in infants: report of 12 cases and review. *Diagn Microbiol Infect Dis* 1999; 35:75–80.
118. Isaacs D, Slack MPE, Wilkinson AR, Westwood AW. Successful treatment of Pseudomonas ventriculitis with ciprofloxacin. *J Antimicrob Chemother* 1986; 17:535–538.
119. Hata A, Honda Y, Asada K, Sasaki Y, Kenri T, Hata D. Mycoplasma hominis meningitis in a neonate: case report and review. *J Infect* 2008; 57:338–343.
120. Watt KM, Massaro MM, Smith B, Cohen-Wolkowiez M, Benjamin Jr DK, Laughon MM. Pharmacokinetics of moxifloxacin in an infant with Mycoplasma hominis meningitis. *Pediatr Infect Dis J* 2012; 31:197–199.
121. Suyagh M, Collier PS, Millership JS, et al. Metronidazole population pharmacokinetics in preterm neonates using dried blood-spot sampling. *Pediatrics* 2011; 127:e367–e374.
122. Cohen-Wolkowiez M, Ouellet D, Smith PB, et al. Population pharmacokinetics of metronidazole evaluated using scavenged samples from preterm infants. *Antimicrob Agents Chemother* 2012; 56:1828–1837.
123. Webber SA, Tuohy P. Bacteroides fragilis meningitis in a premature infant successfully treated with metronidazole. *Pediatr Infect Dis J* 1988; 7:886–887.
124. Ziebold C. Delayed etiologic diagnosis of meningitis in an extremely low birth weight newborn. *Pediatr Infect Dis J* 2010; 29:383, 388–389.
125. Patel S, DeSantis ER. Treatment of congenital tuberculosis. *Am J Health Syst Pharm* 2008; 65:2027–2031.
126. Skevaki CL, Kafetzis DA. Tuberculosis in neonates and infants: epidemiology, pathogenesis, clinical manifestations, diagnosis, and management issues. *Paediatr Drugs* 2005; 7:219–234.
127. Baley JE, Meyers C, Kliegman RM, et al. Pharmacokinetics, outcome of treatment, and toxic effects of amphotericin B and 5-fluorocytosine in neonates. *J Pediatr* 1990; 116:791–797.
128. Holler B, Omar SA, Farid MD, et al. Effects of fluid and electrolyte management on amphotericin B-induced nephrotoxicity among extremely low birth weight infants. *Pediatrics* 2004; 113:e608–e616.
129. Turkova A, Roilides E, Sharland M. Amphotericin B in neonates: deoxycholate or lipid formulation as first-line therapy - is there a 'right' choice? *Curr Opin Infect Dis* 2011; 24:163–171.
130. Blyth CC, Hale K, Palasanthiran P, O'Brien T, Bennett MH. Antifungal therapy in infants and children with proven, probable or suspected invasive fungal infections. *Cochrane Database Syst Rev* 2010; Issue 2. Art. No.: CD006343. doi: 10.1002/14651858.CD006343.pub2
131. Ascher SB, Smith PB, Watt K, et al. Antifungal therapy and outcomes in infants with invasive Candida infections. *Pediatr Infect Dis J* 2012; 31:439–443.
132. Wade KC, Wu D, Kaufman DA,et al; National Institute of Child Health and Development Pediatric Pharmacology Research Unit Network. Population pharmacokinetics of fluconazole in young infants. *Antimicrob Agents Chemother* 2008; 52:4043–4049.
133. Wade KC, Benjamin Jr DK, Kaufman DA, et al. Fluconazole dosing for the prevention or treatment of invasive candidiasis in young infants. *Pediatr Infect Dis J* 2009; 28:717–723.
134. Piper L, Smith PB, Hornik CP, et al. Fluconazole loading dose pharmacokinetics and safety in infants. *Pediatr Infect Dis J* 2011; 30:375–378.
135. Manzoni P, Rizzollo S, Franco C, et al. Role of echinocandins in the management of fungal infections in neonates. *J Matern Fetal Neonatal Med* 2010; 23(Suppl 3): 49–52.
136. Somer A, Törün SH, Salman N. Caspofungin therapy in immunocompromised children and neonates. *Expert Rev Anti Infect Ther* 2011; 9:347–355.
137. Kaufman DA. Challenging issues in neonatal candidiasis. *Curr Med Res Opin* 2010; 26:1769–1778.
138. Caudle KE, Inger AG, Butler DR, Rogers PD. Echinocandin use in the neonatal intensive care unit. *Ann Pharmacother* 2012; 46:108–116.
139. Manzoni P, Benjamin DK, Hope W, et al. The management of Candida infections in preterm neonates and the role of micafungin. *J Matern Fetal Neonatal Med* 2011; 24(Suppl 2):24–27.
140. Cohen-Wolkowiez M, Benjamin Jr DK, Piper L, et al. Safety and pharmacokinetics of multiple-dose anidulafungin in infants and neonates. *Clin Pharmacol Ther* 2011; 89:702–707.
141. Somer A, Törün SH, Salman N. Caspofungin therapy in immunocompromised children and neonates. *Expert Rev Anti Infect Ther* 2011; 9:347–355.
142. Mohamed WA, Ismail M. A randomized, double-blind, prospective study of caspofungin vs. amphotericin B for the treatment of invasive candidiasis in newborn infants. *J Trop Pediatr* 2012; 58:25–30.
143. Baley JE, Meyers C, Kliegman RM, et al. Pharmacokinetics, outcome of treatment, and toxic effects of amphotericin B and 5-fluorocytosine in neonates. *J Pediatr* 1990; 116:791–797.
144. Gill CJ, Sabin LL, Tham J, Hamer DH. Reconsidering empirical cotrimoxazole prophylaxis for infants exposed to HIV infection. *Bull World Health Organ* 2004; 82:290–297.
145. Aizire J, Fowler MG, Wang J, et al. Extended prophylaxis with nevirapine and cotrimoxazole among HIV-exposed uninfected infants is well tolerated. *AIDS* 2012; 26:325–333.
146. Springer C, Eyal F, Michel J. Pharmacology of trimethoprim-sulfamethoxazole in newborn infants. *J Pediatr* 1982; 100:647–650.

147. Mulhall A, de Louvois J, Hurley R. Efficacy of chloramphenicol in the treatment of neonatal and infantile meningitis: a study of 70 cases. *Lancet* 1983; 1:284–287.
148. Feder Jr HM, Osier C, Maderazo EG. Chloramphenicol: A review of its use in clinical practice. *Rev Infect Dis* 1981; 3:479–491.
149. Mulhall A, de Louvois J, Hurley R. Chloramphenicol toxicity in neonates: its incidence and prevention. *Br Med J (Clin Res Ed)* 1983; 287:1424–1427.
150. West BC, DeVault Jr GA, Clement JC, Williams DM. Aplastic anemia associated with parenteral chloramphenicol: review of 10 cases, including the second case of possible increased risk with cimetidine. *Rev Infect Dis* 1988; 10:1048–1051.
151. Fraunfelder FT, Bagby Jr GC, Kelly DJ. Fatal aplastic anemia following topical administration of ophthalmic chloramphenicol. *Am J Ophthalmol* 1982; 93:356–360.
152. Hartmann C, Peter C, Hermann E, et al. Successful treatment of vancomycin-resistant *Enterococcus faecium* ventriculitis with combined intravenous and intraventricular chloramphenicol in a newborn. *J Med Microbiol* 2010; 59:1371–1374.

Index

Evidence-Based Neonatal Infections, First Edition. David Isaacs.